W9-DIW-252

HORMONES

Anthony W. Norman

*Department of Biochemistry and
Division of Biomedical Sciences
University of California
Riverside, California*

Gerald Litwack

*Fels Research Institute
Temple University School of Medicine
Philadelphia, Pennsylvania*

1987

ACADEMIC PRESS, INC.

Harcourt Brace Jovanovich, Publishers

Orlando   San Diego   New York   Austin
Boston   London   Sydney   Tokyo   Toronto

ACADEMIC PRESS, INC.
Orlando, Florida 32887

United Kingdom Edition published by
ACADEMIC PRESS INC. (LONDON) LTD.
24–28 Oval Road, London NW1 7DX

Library of Congress Cataloging in Publication Data

Norman, A. W. (Anthony W.), Date
    Hormones.

    Includes bibliographies and index.
    1. Hormones. I. Litwack, Gerald. II. Title.
[DNLM: 1. Hormones. 2. Molecular Biology.
WK 102 N842h]
QP571.N66   1986   612.4   85-20044
ISBN 0–12–521440–5 (alk. paper)

PRINTED IN THE UNITED STATES OF AMERICA

87 88 89 90   9 8 7 6 5 4 3 2 1

Contents

Preface

The last decades have brought startling advances in our understanding of endocrinology. Of paramount importance is the large increase in the number of legitimate hormones, which now number more than 100, as well as the application of the modern concepts and methodologies of biochemistry and molecular biology to endocrinological research. It is now feasible to approach virtually all classical topics in endocrinology at the cellular and molecular levels.

This book provides a comprehensive treatment of human hormones viewed in the light of modern theories of hormone action and in the context of our current understanding of subcellular and cellular architecture and classical organ physiology. The book is intended for use by first-year medical students, graduate students, and advanced undergraduates in the biological sciences. Also, physicians-in-training should be cognizant of new insights into the etiology of endocrine-related diseases and appreciative of the contribution of basic science to the development of new treatments which are possible through the application of molecular biology and biochemistry to the classic domain of endocrinology. For example, who could have predicted a decade ago that hormonal receptors, or components of hormonal receptors, as well as key cell growth factors could be associated with oncogenes and the cellular expression of certain forms of cancer? Increasingly, medical school curricula are being revised to include a significant coverage of molecular endocrinology. The curriculum for advanced undergraduate biology majors is also being expanded to include molecular endocrinology. Graduate students in medical or biological sciences, including immunology, entomology, genetics, anatomy, physiology, and biochemistry, will inevitably encounter, either in the classroom or in excursions into the modern scientific literature, the contributions and impact of modern endocrinology. It is hoped that this book will fill the void that currently exists for resource materials for teaching cellular and molecular endocrinology and that it will be employed as an equal partner with most standard biochemistry textbooks to provide a comprehensive and balanced coverage of this realm of biology.

Our book presumes that the reader will have been exposed in detail to the fundamental areas of biochemistry, including enzymology, structure and function of macromolecules and the other bioorganic substances of intermediary metabolism, as well as to selected topics in molecular biology. In addition, an understanding of cell biology, cellular and subcellular organization, and mammalian physiology will be useful. It is the tetrad of biochemistry, molecular biology, and cell and organ physiology that provides the principles and biological "facts of life" that are critical to our modern understanding of hormones.

The book provides two introductory chapters followed by seventeen chapters on selected endocrinological topics pertinent to man. The first chapter presents the first principles of hormone action. These include a discussion of the structural and functional classification of hormones and a detailed presentation of current general theories of mechanisms of hormone action at both the cellular and subcellular levels. Chapter 2 provides a detailed presentation of the seven classes of steroid hormones and their chemistry, biosynthesis, and metabolism. These introductory chapters are followed by sixteen chapters that address either a classical endocrine system, e.g., hypothalamic hormones (Chapter 3), posterior pituitary hormones (Chapter 4), anterior pituitary hormones (Chapter 5), thyroid hormones (Chapter 6), pancreatic hormones (Chapter 7), gastrointestinal hormones (Chapter 8), calcium regulating hormones (Chapter 9), adrenal corticoids (Chapter 10), hormones of the adrenal medulla (Chapter 11), androgens (Chapter 12), estrogens and progestins (Chapter 13), hormones of pregnancy and lactation (Chapter 14), or newer domains of hormone action which are now essential to a comprehensive understanding of hormone action, including prostaglandins (Chapter 16), thymus hormones (Chapter 17), and pineal hormones (Chapter 18). The book concludes (Chapter 19) with a presentation of hormones of the future, i.e., cell growth factors. Chapter 15, Hormones of the Kidney, of necessity is not devoted exclusively to a single hormone system; it focuses on the hormones, excluding 1,25-dihydroxyvitamin D (Chapter 9), which are made (erythropoietin, kallikreins) or which act (aldosterone, vasopressin) in the kidney.

Each of the last seventeen chapters is organized in parallel fashion. Thus, each chapter has the following sections: (a) introduction; (b) human anatomical–morphological relationships; (c) chemistry; (d) biochemistry; (e) biological and molecular action of the hormone(s); (f) clinical aspects; and (g) reference citations. The clinical aspects section is not intended to be comprehensive, but rather to provide for the medical student an introduction/resume of key disease states and contemporary medical problems related to the hormone(s) deficiency or excess. In addition, Appendices C and D will provide insight into the definition and incidence rate of prominent endocrine-related disease states. Each chapter is highly illustrated with respect both to human physiology and anatomy and to the details and models of hormone action. Each chapter culminates with a listing of key reference citations, including books and review articles as well as recent research papers.

The book also contains eight appendices: (A) a table listing over 100 hormones; (B) a table of the blood concentrations of major hormones; (C) a list of prominent endocrine disorders; (D) a table of the rate of incidence of principal endocrine disease diagnoses; (E) a tabulation of Nobel prizes awarded in endocrinology and related areas; (F) a table of the genetic code; (G) a table of the three-letter and single-letter abbreviations for amino acids; and (H) a tabulation of the units of scientific measurement.

A major challenge to modern publication techniques as well as to authors is the ability of scientists to obtain the primary amino acid sequence of large proteins/hormones as well as the complementary DNA sequence (cDNA) of nucleotides and genomic sequence of nucleotides for proteins of interest. Thus, modern triumphs of molecular endocrinology include the primary amino acid sequence of prolactin (199 amino acid residues), the cDNA sequence of the steroid receptors for glucocorticoids (4800 nucleotides) and estradiol (3600 nucleotides), as well as the genomic organization of several hormones, e.g., insulin (1720 nucleotides). The dilemma to the authors was whether to include such extensive and detailed information in a volume that is intended for use as a textbook. Clearly, most students will not study protein amino acid sequences or cDNA sequence at the individual amino acid or nucleotide level. Yet we feel it instructive for the student to realize and appreciate the intrinsic complexity and detail of information pertaining to hormones which molecular endocrinologists can now almost routinely achieve. Accordingly, the authors have included many sequences of large peptide hormones as well as cDNA sequences. We have chosen in some instances to limit their format to a single-page "miniprint" rather than to extend their presentation over two or three pages. Interested readers should utilize a magnifying or "reading" glass to facilitate their study (e.g., see Figs. 5-4, 5-7, 7-13, 10-16A, 10-20B, and 13-15).

The text is related to biochemical endocrinology courses we have taught to first-year medical students and graduate students at the University of California–Riverside and Temple University. The authors hope that the uniform organization of the chapters and the subdivision of topics within each chapter will allow instructors to select the level of coverage they require from a comprehensive one to one focusing on only the subcellular mode of action of the hormones. We would like to acknowledge the students at UC–Riverside in Biochemistry 120 who used a draft of this textbook. From their comments and from our co-instructors, Professors H. L. Henry and R. A. Luben, we received much useful feedback.

In addition we would like to thank our professional colleagues who have individually read and critiqued the various chapters. These include: Julius Axelrod (18), Om P. Bahl (5), John D. Baxter (6, 10), Esther Breslow (4), Josiah Brown (6), Ralph A. Bradshaw (19), P. Michael Conn (3), Michael P. Czech (19), Leonard J. Deftos (9), Isidore Edelman (15), John H. Exton (11), H. Hugh Fudenberg (17), W. F. Ganong (3), Jack Geller (12), Allan L. Goldstein (17), Jack Gorski (1), Oscar Hechter (4), Bernard L. Horecker (17), Benita S. Katzenellenbogen (1), Leonard D. Kohn (5), William E. M. Lands (16), Joseph Larner (7), J. B. Lee (16), Robert J. Lefkowitz (11), Choh Hao Li (5), Marc E. Lippman (13), Walter Lovenberg (18), Joseph Meites (3), R. Curtis Morris (9), Allan Munck (10), William D. Odell (14), Jack H. Oppenheimer (6), Peter W. Ramwell (16), Russel J. Reiter (18), Herbert H. Samuels (1, 6), David A. Sirbasku (19), Melvin S. Soloff (4), Donald F. Steiner (97), E. Brad Thompson (10), Sidney Udenfriend (11), Larry Vickery (2), John H. Walsh (8), Owen N. Witte (15), and Richard J. Wurtman (18). We would like to thank Dr. A. Geoffrey Norman, Dr. Valerie Leathers, and Dr. Helen L. Henry, who all read major portions of the manuscript and provided essential feedback. If our book has merit it is due largely to the contributions of our scientific mentors and colleagues as well as those individuals who read various sections of the manuscript. Shortcomings still remaining are, of course, completely the responsibility of the authors.

We are also indebted to numerous authors and publishers for permission to reproduce figures and tables that were originally published elsewhere. In particular we recognize the masterful skill of Dr. Thomas Lentz and thank the publisher W. B. Saunders for allowing us to utilize numerous of his outstanding line drawings (based on electron micrographs) taken from his book *Cell Fine Structure*. Thanks are also due to Dr. Laurie Paavola of the Department of Anatomy, Temple University School of Medicine, who allowed us to reproduce several of her own drawings of various cells and their morphological components in relation to hormone function.

The authors have been privileged to utilize the skills of Ms. Patti Mote, a scientific illustrator, who prepared original line drawings or anatomical ink washes for approximately 120 of the 442 figures published in the book. Throughout the entire publication process, Ms. Mote was always a positive force striving for simplicity, accuracy, and clarity in our illustrations.

Also, the authors have been fortunate to have the services of a series of dedicated, loyal, and patient secretaries over the 6 years in which the typescript was being written or revised. In the early phases this included Ms. Sherry Bataglia, Ms. Cassie Wooten, Ms. Marcia Johnson, Ms. Pam Moore, and Ms. Jerri Flagg, and in the latter phases Mrs. Sharon Herbert, Mrs. Ann Hall, Mrs. Grace Jones, and Mrs. Lean Gill (who retyped several cDNA sequences); we thank you all! The authors are also indebted to the production staff of Academic Press–Orlando for their professional assistance during this project.

Finally we wish to express appreciation to our families in Philadelphia (Ellie, Geoffrey, Kate, Claudia, David, and Debbie) and in Riverside (Helen, Thea, Jacqueline, and Derek) who were most understanding of the long hours and absence from home that were required to produce the final manuscript.

Anthony W. Norman
Riverside, California

Gerald Litwack
Philadelphia, Pennsylvania

Chapter 1

General Considerations of Hormones

1

I. CLASSIFICATION OF HORMONES

A. Introduction

The classic categories of hormones, based upon their chemical structures, are steroids, polypeptides, and amino acid and fatty acid-derived compounds. Each of these classes excepting the last has been considered for many years to be the exclusive products of endocrine glands. These substances are synthesized and stored in endocrine gland cells awaiting the appropriate signal for their release, usually by a process of exocytosis into the bloodstream. When the hormones are polypeptides, creating a problem of permeability from the extracellular space to the interior of small blood vessels, the local capillaries are usually fenestrated (i.e., thinning or opening of the walls to allow permeation of polypeptides) to accommodate this need. Once in the bloodstream, the endocrine hormone can travel to a distant cellular target which it recognizes through high-affinity receptors located on the surface of its cellular membrane (polypeptide and certain amino acid-derived hormones; see Fig. 1-1) or within its cytoplasm or cellular nucleus (steroid hormones). The receptor for the amino acid-derived hormone, thyroxine or triiodothyronine, is located within the nuclear genome of the target cell. Increasing evidence suggests that steroid hormone receptors (especially for estrogens and vitamin D_3) reside within the nucleus and do not have cytoplasmic locations except by artifact after the cell is broken. The situation for the glucocorticoid receptor is less clear.

As time progresses, our understanding of what a hormone is must be redefined. A growing realization is that classical endocrine hormones and neurotransmitters may be more similar than different. Thus, we treat epinephrine as a hormone of the adrenal medulla and norepinephrine as a major neurotransmitter, but their structures (Fig. 1-2) are obviously similar and their activities, for example, on vascular cells, may clearly overlap. The hormones with nervous activity which operate across synapses may be defined as paracrine hormones, those substances which are secreted like traditional endocrine hormones, but which operate over a shorter, defined distance, as shown in Fig. 1-3. The opioid peptides, like β-endorphin and the enkephalins, may be a recent example of paracrines, in some cases, and of endocrines as well, in other cases. Finally, we must recognize a newer class of hormones which can be gathered under the heading of autocrine hormones. These are hormones that are synthesized and released by the same cell upon which the hormones act. They may also act on neighboring cells. Examples of autocrine hormones would be the prostaglandins and some of their

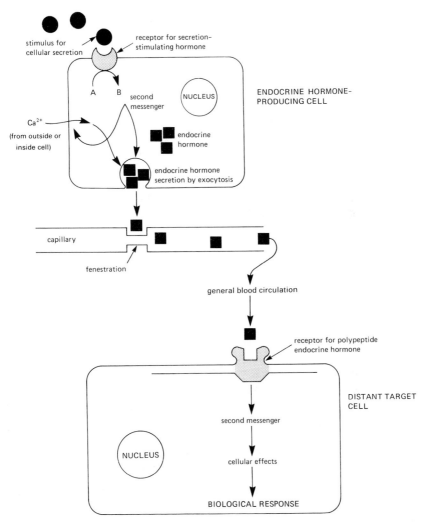

Figure 1-1. Overview of traditional endocrine hormone glandular cell; release and action.

relatives, such as thromboxanes, leukotrienes, and prostacyclin, the last of which also may have somewhat traditional endocrine hormone-like activity (Fig. 1-4). Consequently, we conceive of three major groups of hormones based not on their structures or on the nature of their receptors as much as on the extent of their radius of action: endocrine, paracrine, and autocrine in the order of decreasing effective distances (see Table 1-1).

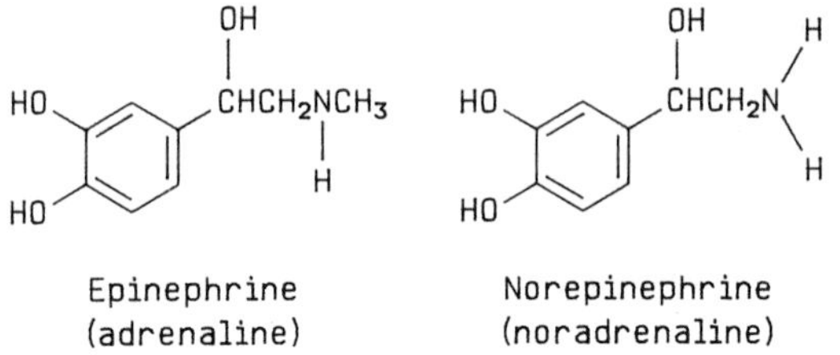

4

OH   OH   H
| | /
HO   CHCH₂NCH₃   HO   CHCH₂N
| \
HO   H   HO   H

Epinephrine   Norepinephrine
(adrenaline)   (noradrenaline)

Figure 1-2. Structures of the hormone, epinephrine, and the neurotransmitter, norepinephrine.

We also need to recognize that nature occasionally constructs a mechanism, in addition to the use of receptors, as a means to ensure that hormones, often produced in minute amounts, will be sequestered at the target site and not diluted out in the general blood circulation. Obviously, paracrine and autocrine hormones have this inherent advan-

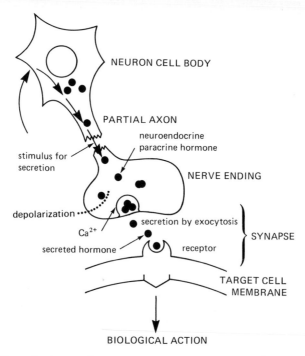

Figure 1-3. Example of a neurohormone operating in a synapse. In the case of some amine hormones or neurotransmitters, their synthesis may be confined to the nerve ending, whereas other substances are synthesized in the cell body and transported to the nerve ending as shown here.

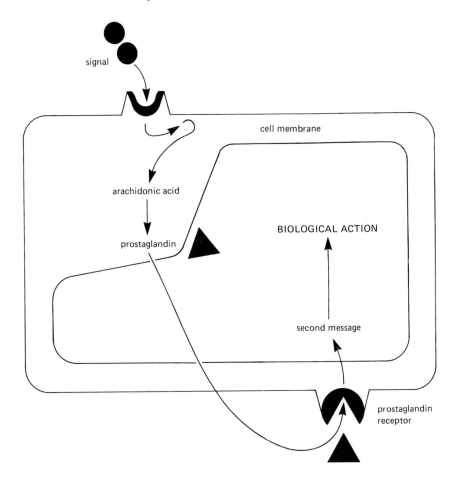

Figure 1-4. Example of an autocrine hormone operating on the same cell which released it. The active hormone may reach its receptor from the cell interior without having been secreted first, as shown in this example.

tage, but another means to this end is through a closed circulation. An example of this is the secretion of the hypothalamic releasing hormones into a closed portal system ensuring that most of these hormones will be delivered to the anterior pituitary, which contains the target cells for these releasing hormones (Fig. 1-5).

Another way to classify hormones is on the basis of their source. Thus, we can construct a list of hypothalamic hormones, anterior pituitary hormones (those of the adenohypophysis and the *pars intermedia*),

6

Table 1–1. Classes of Hormones Based on Distance of Action[a]

Class	Endocrine	Paracrine	Autocrine
Polypeptide	++++	(+)	
Steroid	++++		
Amino acid-derived	++++	++++	
Fatty acid-derived	+		++++

[a] + signs indicate the extent of secretory type. "Endocrine" means that the class of hormones is secreted, usually by exocytosis, and travels through the bloodstream to distant target cells; "paracrine" indicates that the cell secretes this class of hormones and they travel only a short distance to neighboring cellular targets; "autocrine" means that a class of hormones is secreted by a cell which may act on that cell's own receptors.

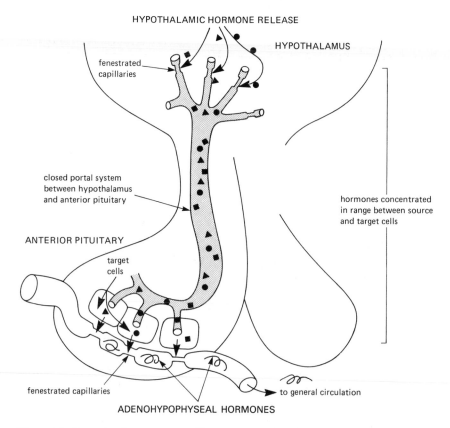

Figure 1-5. Example of conservation of hormone concentration between source and target by a closed portal delivery system.

posterior pituitary hormones, thyroid hormones, gastrointestinal hormones, brain hormones, kidney hormones, adrenal medulla hormones, ovarian hormones, testicular hormones, luteal hormones, and so on.

We now realize that the domain of endocrinology has become a science of signaling or communication mechanisms involving substances in a much broader category than previously connoted by "endocrine hormones." Logically, any substance that operates at the cellular level, generated either externally or internally, which conveys to that cell a message to stop, start, or modulate a cellular process will come under the pervue of modern endocrinology. In recognition of this fact, we have preferred to entitle this book "Hormones" rather than "Endocrinology," since the latter term refers to the limited category of substances operating over long distances.

B. The Hormones

A list of most of the known hormones in terms of our broader definition of signals in a communication system appears in a table as Appendix A.

II. RECEPTORS FOR HORMONES

As this is a subject of intensive research, the final classification of hormone receptors must await future developments. However, considerable information is available, enough to make some generalizations.

Virtually all of the receptors of polypeptide hormones reside in the surface of the cell membrane. These receptors, when bound with ligand, may have some mobility in the membrane, or receptor subunits or other components of the signaling system may move about. Structurally, the receptors for insulin and IGF_1 resemble the subunit structure of gamma globulin (Fig. 1-6).

On the other hand, the activated steroid receptors studied thus far appear to be represented by a single polypeptide chain (glucocorticoid receptor, progesterone receptor). In the activated form, some steroid receptors may be more complex and dissociate (glucocorticoid receptor) or polymerize (estrogen receptor) during activation, although dissociation as a true event in activation could be an *in vitro* artifact and much more research is needed on this topic (see Section II,D and III,I,3 for a brief explanation of the activation process). In the case of the estrogen receptor, activation may include the dimerization of two identical subunits. One idea, discussed by J. Baxter in 1983, is that steroid hormone receptors evolved from genes encoding steroid dehydrogenase enzymes

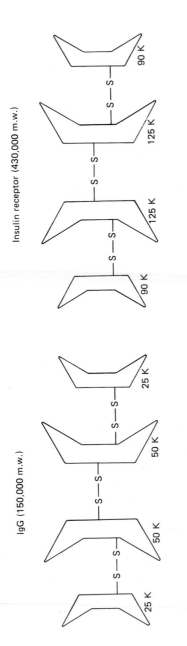

IgG (150,000 m.w.)

25 K 50 K 50 K 25 K

Insulin receptor (430,000 m.w.)

90 K 125 K 125 K 90 K

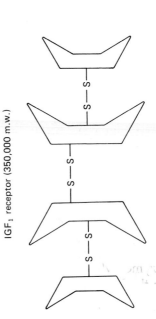

IGF₁ receptor (350,000 m.w.)

Figure 1-6. Subunit structures of IgG, insulin, and IGF receptors.

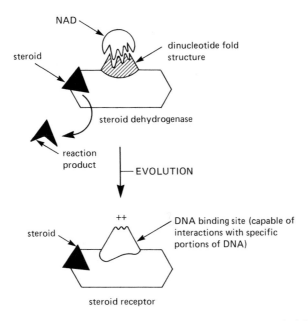

Figure 1-7. Speculation that steroid receptors evolve from steroid dehydrogenase enzymes.

(recently, one scientist has expressed reservations about the uniqueness of the glucocorticoid receptor and suggested that it may actually be a metabolizing enzyme itself which exhibits receptor actions). These are NAD enzymes which contain a dinucleotide fold. The dinucleotide fold to which the NAD coenzyme binds could have evolved into a specific DNA binding site. There is also evidence of direct binding of the progesterone receptor complex with upstream sequences of the ovalbumin gene (which is controlled by progesterone). Significantly higher affinities of the receptor complex for the gene sequence are involved than would be expected of nonspecific interactions with DNA. The idea of evolution of the steroid receptors from their respective dehydrogenases is pictured in Fig. 1-7. This theory should be testable in the near future, since monoclonal antibodies to steroid receptors are becoming available. If the speculation in Fig. 1-7 is correct, considerable homology should be evident between the enzyme and the receptor. Such homologies should extend to antigenic groupings (epitopes) yielding cross-reactions of receptor and dehydrogenase using panels of monoclonal antibodies directed against receptor. It should be possible ultimately to compare primary amino acid sequences of these two proteins or of the sequences of genes encoding these entities. Recently, the gene sequences of glucocorticoid and estradiol receptors have become known and there is considerable homology between their DNA binding domains and the *erb*-a oncogene, a DNA binding protein.

III. MECHANISMS OF HORMONE ACTION

A. Cell Membrane Constituents

Although the precise content of substances which comprise the cell membrane differs in different cell types, many components are common to all membranes. These are lipids (including phospholipids and glycolipids), proteins, and glycoproteins. The cell membrane that encloses the cell resembles the internal membranes, such as those associated with the nucleus, mitochondria, and microsomes. The approximate lipid compositions of different cell membranes are presented in Table 1-2.

The lipids consist in two portions: a head group and a tail. The head groups are charged (hydrophilic), while the tails are uncharged (hydrophobic). They form bilayers spontaneously oriented so that the heads form on the water sides and the tails are internal. This resembles the basic structure of the cell membrane and provides for a negative charge on the head side of the membrane. This arrangement is pictured in Fig. 1-8. Included in the membrane are various proteins, some of which are receptors, ion and other small molecule transporters, and enzymes. The specific proteins vary from cell type to cell type depending on the special membrane functions required by a given cell. Some of the proteinaceous

Table 1–2. Lipid Compositions of Different Cell Membranes (% of Lipid Weight)[a]

Lipid	Liver plasma membranes	Erythrocyte membranes	Mitochondria	ER
Cholesterol	17	23	3	6
Phosphatidylethanolamine	7	18	35	17
Phosphatidylserine	4	7	2	5
Phosphatidylcholine	24	17	39	40
Sphingomyelin	19	18	0	5
Glycolipids	7	3	Trace	Trace
Others	22	13	21	27

[a] This table was adapted with permission from B. Alberts, D. Bray, J. Lewis, M. Raff, K. Roberts, and J. D. Watson, "Molecular Biology of the Cell." Garland Publishing Co., New York, 1983.

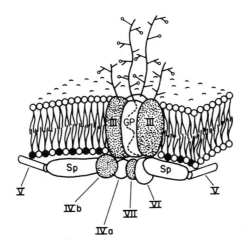

Figure 1-8. Speculative model based on the human erythrocyte major glycoprotein oligomeric complex. Phosphatidylserine and phosphatidylglycerol (dark circles) are distributed asymmetrically. GP, Glycophorin; III, component 3; IVa, component 4.1; IVb, component 4.2; V, component 5 or actin; VI, component 6 or GP-3-D; VII, component 7; Sp, spectrin. Reproduced from G. L. Nicolson, *in* "Biological Regulation and Development" (R. F. Goldberger and K. R. Yamamoto, eds.), Vol. 3A, p. 222. Plenum, New York, 1982.

constituents span the membrane so as to make contact with both the extracellular space and the cytoplasm while others do not, but can translocate to either side. Proteins that span the membrane are called intrinsic or integral proteins. Extrinsic proteins are those associated with the periphery of the membrane, but which may not be associated directly with the phospholipid layer. The cell membrane interacts with the fibrillar and tubular structures in the cytoplasm, facilitating dynamic movements of portions of the membrane into the cell (e.g., during internalization of ligand–receptor complexes). Thus, membrane components may connect with proteins called spectrin, actin, and others, visualized partly in Fig. 1-8.

Fluid Cell Membrane Model

In the context of the model described above, it is believed that various conditions, such as changes in the metabolism of phospholipids and responses to various signals via receptor interactions, can lead to changes in fluidity of the membrane which allow proteins to move within the membrane. This movement can generate productive interactions that can result in stimulation of enzymatic activities on the cytoplasmic side of the cell membrane, or other events. A model showing this type of motion is presented in Fig. 1-9.

12

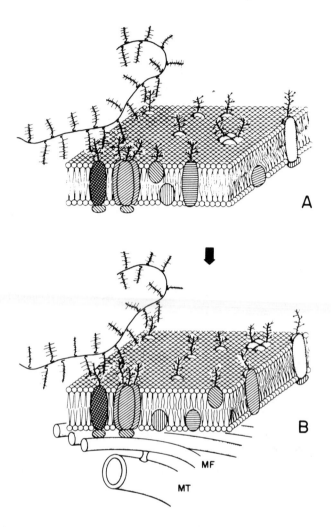

Figure 1-9. Model of a fluid mosaic membrane showing distribution and mobility of cell membrane receptors. (A) Integral transmembrane glycoproteins occur in a domain of the membrane of different lipid composition; a glycosaminoglycan molecule is shown associated with the carbohydrate side chains of the glycoproteins. (B) Aggregation of some of the glycoproteins stimulates attachment of cytoskeletal components: microfilaments (MF) and microtubules (MT) to peripheral membrane components on cytoplasmic surface. Other unattached integral membrane proteins are capable of lateral motion. Reproduced from G. L. Nicolson, *in* "Biological Regulation and Development" (R. F. Goldberger and K. R. Yamamoto, eds.), Vol. 3A, p. 225. Plenum, New York, 1982.

B. Polypeptide Hormones

As stated before, polypeptide hormones have receptors located on the membranes of target cells. The activities of the hormone–receptor complexes may be divided into two classes. Class I receptors produce changes in cell metabolism and behavior, usually rapidly, after binding hormonal ligand. Here the effects are more or less developed at the cell membrane. In contrast, Class II receptors are characterized by internalization of the ligand–receptor complex. It is unclear exactly what the purposes of Class II receptor internalization might be. Among the possibilities are the following: a means to degrade the ligand after it has promoted some action (or not) at the cell membrane; a means to degrade the receptor; a means to degrade the ligand to a product that is active in the cell's interior or to liberate an unaltered ligand inside the cell to bind to interior receptors (e.g., on the nuclear membrane) to produce a mitogenic effect; a means to degrade the receptor to an active fragment that would operate within the cell; and, finally, and perhaps most importantly, it may be the off-signal for activity at the cell membrane level. Hormones have immediate effects at the cell membrane and in some

Table 1–3. Characteristics of Some Well-Known Polypeptide Hormones

Hormone	Action at cell membrane	Internalized ligand–receptor complex	Known intracellular receptors[a]
Insulin	Glucose transporter of adipocyte; insulin second messenger in liver and other cells; may enhance activity of IGF receptor; receptor autophosphorylates	Yes	Perinuclear membrane
Glucagon	Stimulates adenylate cyclase	Not known	Not known
EGF	Phosphorylation of tyrosyl peptides	Yes	(Mitogenic effect)
TSH	Increases adenylate cyclase activity and iodide transport in thyroid follicular cell membrane	Yes	(Mitogenic effect)
IGF$_1$	Increases glucose transport in some cells	Yes	(Mitogenic effect)
IGF$_2$		Yes	(Mitogenic effect)
NGF		Yes	(Mitogenic effect)

[a] Although there are known intracellular binding sites resembling receptors, physiological actions cannot yet be ascribed to them.

cases have long-term effects through processes generated at the membrane or after internalization. Some of these activities are summarized in Table 1-3.

In terms of a polypeptide hormone that produces a mitogenic effect on a cell, a possibility is to view the internalization process as a means to generate a mitogenically active fragment of the hormone or its undegraded structure inside the cell so that it can interact in some way (receptor) with the nucleus to increase the rate of DNA replication. Perhaps some of these intracellular products can lead to activators of DNA polymerase α, the replicative enzyme. As a pure speculation, an internal fragment of growth hormone may have somatomedin-like activity (see Chapter 5). Internalization of GH and its subsequent degradation to release such a fragment might enable the activation of IGF receptors after the fragment passes to the exterior of the cell. A mitogenic effect could then be produced through this process. Alternatively the putative fragment could stimulate the nucleus in some way (receptors?) to amplify the rate of DNA replication in growing cells. Finally, it seems possible that some specific protein may be phosphorylated through a receptor-associated protein kinase and carry the message of the hormone to the interior of the cell.

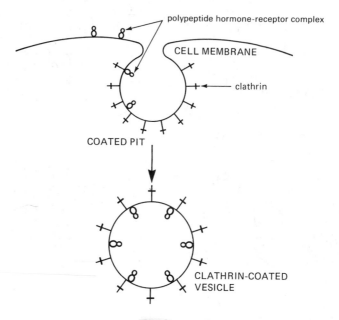

Figure 1-10. Diagrams of coated pit and vesicle.

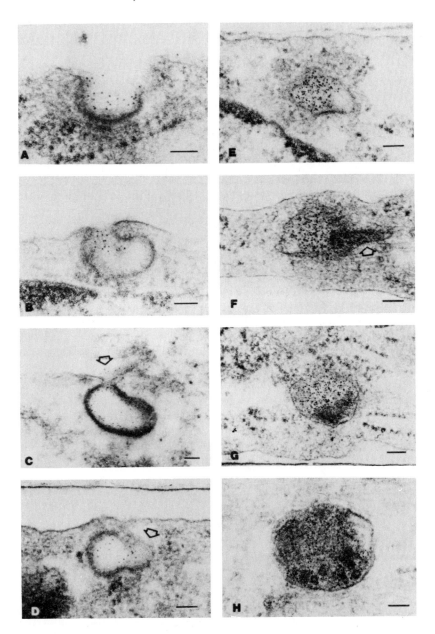

Figure 1-11. Stages in endocytosis of LDL-ferritin and its subsequent appearance in the lysosome. Fibroblasts were incubated with 47.5 μg/ml LDL-ferritin for 2 hr, 4°C, washed, and warmed at 37°C for various times (bar: 1000 Å). (A) Typical coated pit. (B) Transformation of coated pit into endocytotic vesicle. (C) Formation of a coated vesicle; arrow indi-

C. Mechanism of Internalization of Polypeptide Hormone–Receptor Complexes

Internalization has been shown to apply to insulin–receptor complexes, to EGF–receptor complexes, and to others. This process is referred to as *adsorptive* endocytosis. Polypeptides bind to receptors in coated pits which are indented sites on the plasma membrane. The coated pit invaginates into the cytoplasm, forming a coated vesicle containing hormone–receptor complexes. The vesicles then shed their coats, fuse with each other, and either receptors are returned to the cell surface after subsequent fusion with the Golgi apparatus or they fuse with lysosomes and the contents may be degraded. Formation of a coated vesicle is shown in Fig. 1-10.

Photographs of a coated pit and endocytotic vesicle are shown in Fig. 1-11. Recent evidence suggests that the forming coated vesicle is a molecular filter accounting for the selectivity of the contents. Diameters of coated vesicles are in the range of 50–150 nm. Coated vesicles from adrenal medulla are shown in Fig. 1-12. The major protein component of the coated vesicle is clathrin, a nonglycosylated protein of 180,000 molecular weight. Its primary sequence appears to be highly conserved. Clathrin makes up 70% of the total protein of coated vesicles; 5% is made up of polypeptides of about 35,000 molecular weight, while various other polypeptides, 50,000–100,000 molecular weight, are present. Coated vesicles have a remarkable surface structure resembling a lattice comprised of hexagons or pentagons. Three clathrins probably contribute to each polyhedral vertex and two clathrins contribute to each edge. Thus, the smallest structures would contain 12 pentagons plus 4 to 8 hexagons with 84 or 108 clathrin molecules. A 200-nm-diameter coated vesicle would have about 1000 clathrin molecules. Clathrin can form flexible lattices to act as scaffolds to form vesicles during budding. Actual electron micrographs of the budding vesicle are shown in Fig. 1-13. By

---

cates that some of the LDL-ferritin is left on the surface of the cell as the plasma membrane begins to fuse to form vesicle. (D) Fully formed coated vesicle; arrow shows loss of cytoplasmic coat on one side. (E) Endocytotic vesicle that has completely lost cytoplasmic coat. (F) Irregularly shaped endocytotic vesicle; arrow shows region of increased electron density with lumen. (G) Similar to (F) with more electron-dense material in lumen. (H) Secondary lysosome containing LDL-ferritin. Reproduced with permission from R. G. W. Anderson, M. S. Brown, and J. L. Goldstein, Role of the coated endocytotic vesicle in the uptake of receptor-bound low-density lipoprotein in human fibroblasts. *Cell* **10**, 351–364 (1977). © 1977 by MIT.

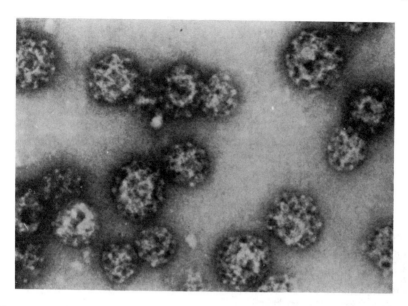

Figure 1-12. Electron micrograph of isolated coated vesicles magnified 125,000 times from adrenal medulla. Reproduced from B. M. F. Pearse and M. S. Bretscher, Membrane recycling by coated vesicles. *Annu. Rev. Biochem.* **50,** 85–101 (1981). © 1981 by Annual Reviews Inc.

this mechanism the ligands in the vesicle are delivered to the lysosome and degraded. Some specially active degradation product(s) or the intact hormone itself may emerge to promote the long-term effects of the original polypeptide hormone. Alternatively, long-term effects may occur through activities of second messenger molecules generated by action at the cell membrane.

D. Mechanism of Certain "Immediate" Effects of Polypeptide Hormones at the Cell Membrane; Stimulation of Adenylate Cyclase

Many polypeptide hormones (e.g., glucagon, PTH, VIP, calcitonin, ACTH, TSH, FSH, LH, vasopressin, and angiotensin) stimulate intracellular levels of cyclic AMP by causing the activation of target cell membrane adenylate cyclase. Polypeptide hormone receptors form oligomeric complexes with GTP regulatory proteins and inhibit the GTP regulatory proteins from reacting with GTP. Hormones bind to receptors on the cell membrane and release the inhibitory constraints im-

18

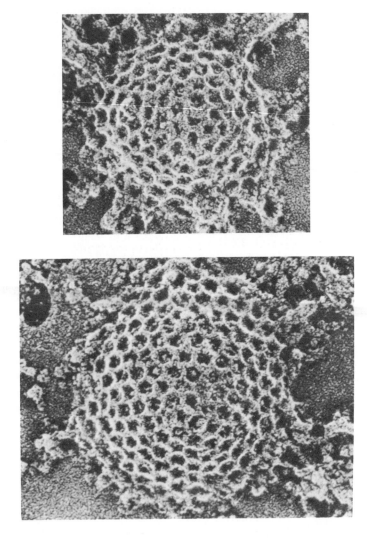

Figure 1-13. Regions of fibroblast-coated membranes at intermediate stages of the budding process demonstrated by deep etching and rotary replication using a method of J. E. Heuser. Reproduced from B. M. F. Pearse and M. S. Bretscher, Membrane recycling by coated vesicles. *Annu. Rev. Biochem.* **50,** 85–101 (1981). © 1981 by Annual Reviews Inc.

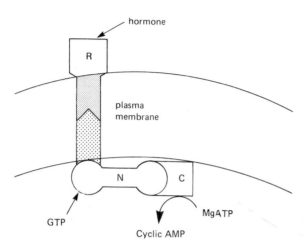

Figure 1-14. Schematic model of the components and organization of the glucagon-stimulated adenylate cyclase. The receptor, R, is visualized as spanning the plasma membrane and having different segments (indicated by shading and cross-hatched areas) which have functions for binding the hormone, attachment to the membrane, and linkage with the nucleotide regulation subunit that binds GTP. The N unit is postulated to form a bridge between R and the catalytic component, C, of the membrane at the internal face of the membrane. Reproduced with permission from M. Rodbell, The role of hormone receptors and GTP regulatory proteins in membrane transduction. *Nature (London)* **284**, 17–22 (1980). © 1980 Macmillan Journals Limited.

posed by the receptors, permitting the GTP regulatory proteins to interact with adenylate cyclase. This interaction leads to a functional adenylate cyclase and ATP is converted to cyclic AMP. M. Rodbell has proposed a theoretical model for hormones that activate adenylate cyclase, as shown in Fig. 1-14. The model envisions at least three classes of components: (1) the receptor or R component, which is located at the outer surface of the membrane and contains the high-affinity binding site for the hormone; (2) a nucleotide regulatory component, N, at the inner surface of the membrane; and (3) also on the inner face of the membrane is the catalytic subunit, C, of adenylate cyclase. A key feature of this model is the nucleotide regulatory subunit, N. Two types of N units have been distinguished functionally: One, N_S, mediates stimulation and the other, N_I, inhibition of the adenylate cyclase. Normally, the N and R components exist in the membrane separately from C as R:N aggregates or oligomers. The precise topological relationship between the R:N oligomers and C in the plasma membrane and the role of membrane lipids in this relationship are unknown.

When the hormone binding site of R is unoccupied, R inhibits interac-

uncoupling-aggregation
"turn-off" cycle

disaggregation-coupling
"turn-on" cycle

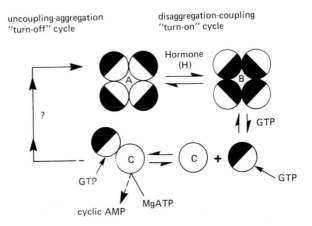

Figure 1-15. A model for coupling of the receptor–nucleotide regulatory subunits (R:N) to the catalytic subunit (C) of adenylate cyclase. Dark halves of circles represent hormone (H) binding sites of receptor; light halves of circles represent GTP binding subunits. Note that binding of hormone causes a change in conformation, rendering subunits able to bind to GTP and disaggregate. Also, the role of hormone (glucagon) and GTP in this process is indicated. Reproduced with permission from M. Rodbell, The role of hormone receptors and GTP regulatory proteins in membrane transduction. *Nature (London)* **284**, 17–22 (1980). © 1980 Macmillan Journals Limited.

tion of N with GTP. However, binding of hormone to R triggers release of the contraints imposed on N so that there is an enhanced regulatory activity when N binds GTP, which then leads to breakdown of the R:N oligomers to a monomeric R:N complex. This monomeric R:N next reacts with C to form the holoenzyme form of adenylate cyclase, as shown in Fig. 1-14. Then, depending on the type of R and N units interacting with C, the holoenzyme induces either an increased or decreased production of cyclic AMP. Figure 1-15 presents further details of this model. An essential aspect is the regulatory actions of GTP. Depending on whether N is stimulating, N_S, or inhibitory, N_I, either positive or negative cooperativity may result in the activation of the adenylate cyclase.

Association of N_S or N_I with C is reversible and is driven by the binding of guanine nucleotides. The relationship between hormone binding (K_d) and action (K_{act}) on glucagon-mediated activation of adenylate cyclase is complicated by the fact that two ligands, glucagon and GTP, are required for action. Direct binding studies with radioactive ^{125}I-labeled glucagon revealed that GTP at concentrations required for activation of adenylate cyclase in the presence of hormone converted 90% of the receptors to a state with a higher K_d and K_{act}.

Thus, association of the macromolecular components R:N and C enhances the binding affinity of the small ligands (hormone and GTP). In this "uncoupled" equilibrium model, the final concentration of the activated holoenzyme is a function of the relative concentrations of both macromolecular components and small ligands. In the overall equilibrium, all R:N complexes have equal potential to form complexes with C, but the amount of R:N:C formed is limited by the concentration of C. In the case of liver membranes and glucagon, the concentration of C may be only 10% of R and N. It should be appreciated that not all polypeptide hormones operate by this mechanism. Some will directly or indirectly stimulate the uptake of calcium ions perhaps by an effect on the calcium ion channel or by an effect through a second messenger which would be something other than cyclic AMP. Actions of this sort are characterized by oxytocin on the mammary gland myoepithelial cell or the myometrial cell (see Fig. 4-15), epinephrine on the liver membrane α receptor (Chapter 11), and others. Mechanisms occur with hormones such as insulin which may have an entirely unique second messenger, as will be discussed later.

E. Role of Phospholipid Metabolism at the Cell Membrane

Obviously there are important alterations in cell membrane constituents when a hormone is liganded to its receptor on the cell membrane surface. Based on recent work, it is apparent that association of hormones with receptors in the cell membrane may stimulate phospholipid metabolism. Concomitantly, receptor unmasking may occur enhancing the sensitivity of the target cell. Such changes may be involved in the movements of ions, such as calcium, into the cell. These changes could play a role in the regulation of arachidonic acid metabolism. Arachidonic acid is the major precursor of prostaglandins. Some of the important points of this process are illustrated in Fig. 1-16. The hormone binds to receptor, causing some alterations in the membrane which lead to the metabolism of triphosphoinositide to inositol triphosphate and diacylglycerol. Diacylglycerol is an activator of protein kinase C which may phosphorylate specific proteins in the cell membrane and cytoplasm. These phosphorylated products undoubtedly exert specific cellular actions. Inositol triphosphate releases calcium ions from stores in the endoplasmic reticulum. Calcium ions appear to be a second messenger for a number of reactions, and they can stimulate protein kinase, exocytosis, and others.

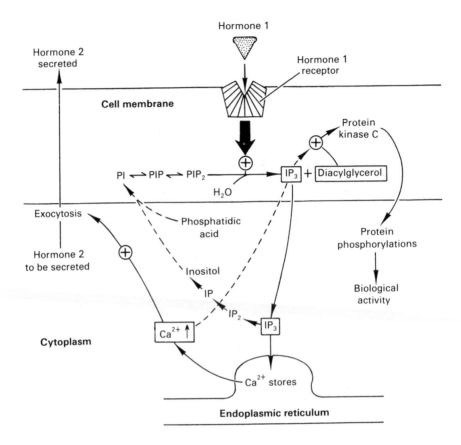

Figure 1-16. Hormone action on phospholipid metabolism in cell membrane of responsive cell. In this example, hormone 1 may act to cause the secretion of hormone 2. Hormone 1 binds to a receptor in the cell membrane, causing a stimulation, direct or indirect, of the hydrolysis of phosphatidylinositol-4,5-bisphosphate (PIP_2) to form inositol-1,4,5-triphosphate (IP_3) and diacylglycerol, which are second messengers. Diacylglycerol stimulates the activity of protein kinase C that phosphorylates proteins and produces biological actions. IP_3 enters the cytoplasm and stimulates the release of Ca^{2+} from endoplasmic reticulum stores into the cytoplasm. Increased cytoplasmic Ca^{2+} produces exocytosis (secretion) of hormone 2 from the cell. IP_3 is subsequently degraded by dephosphorylation to inositol diphosphate (IP_2), inositol monophosphate (IP), and to inositol which subsequently is combined with phosphatidic acid to produce phosphatidylinositol (PI) and with subsequent phosphorylations is converted to phosphatidylinositolphosphate (PIP) and finally to phosphatidylinositol bisphosphate (PIP_2) and readied for another round of the cycle. Increased cytoplasmic Ca^{2+} levels also stimulate protein kinase C activity.

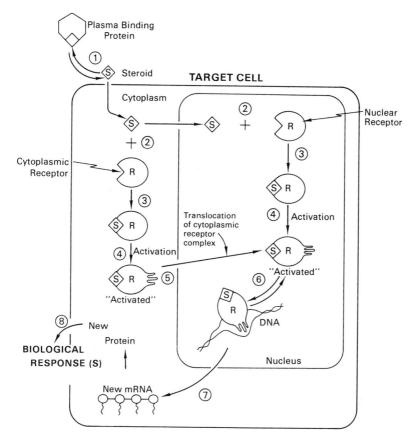

Figure 1-17. Overview of steroid hormone action on a target cell. A steroid hormone(s) is carried by a plasma binding protein which protects the ligand and serves as the circulatory transporter. The equilibrium between bound and free hormone (1) in blood favors the bound form with an affinity, K_{a_1}, of about 10^8 moles-liter. The unbound steroid enters the target cell probably by free diffusion. Inside the cell, it binds to the unoccupied receptor (2) to form the unactivated complex (3). This reaction occurs either in the cytoplasm or in the nucleus as indicated by the two pathways. After activation (4), the cytoplasmic receptor complex is either translocated to the nucleus (5) and/or exhibits an increased affinity for DNA (6) and binds to presumptive high-affinity binding sites upstream from the genes (6) regulated by the hormones. Transcription increases and mRNAs are translocated (7) to the cytoplasm for translation, leading to enhanced levels of phenotypes which alter metabolism (8).

24

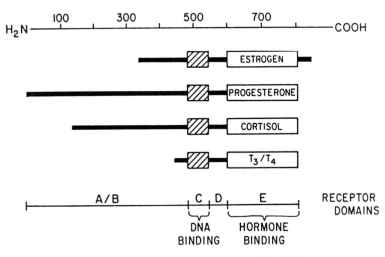

Figure 1-18. Schematic comparison of steroid and thyroid (T_3/T_4) hormone receptors predicted amino acid sequences as deduced from cloning and sequence analysis of appropriate complementary DNA. The steroid receptor can be divided into six regions. Region E, the hormone-binding domain (which lies in the carboxyl portion of the receptor), and particularly region C, the DNA-binding domain (approximately 66 amino acid residues with two pairs of cysteines) have a significant (17% and 45–55%, respectively) structural homology while Regions A/B (the immunogenic domain) and the hydrophilic Region D have little or no significant homology. Sequence comparisons have revealed similarities between the protein product of the v-erb-A oncogenes and all of these receptors. Thus, the steroid receptors, probably also including the 1,25-dihydroxyvitamin D_3 receptor, and the thyroid receptor, all may have evolved from a common ancestor gene. Modified with permission from S. Green and P. Chambon, A superfamily of potentially oncogenic hormone receptors. *Nature (London)* **324,** 615–617 (1986).

F. Mechanisms of Action of Steroid and Thyroid Hormones

Steroid and thyroid hormones have mechanisms that are quite different from the polypeptide hormones. Steroid hormones (such as cortisol, progesterone, estradiol, or 1,25-dihydroxyvitamin D_3) have their receptors located largely in the cell nucleus and to some extent also in the cytoplasm but not the cell membrane. The thyroid hormone receptor is known to be localized in the nucleus (see Chapter 6). The free steroid enters the target cell, probably by free diffusion (although that is not certain) as outlined Fig. 1-17; the steroid or thyroid hormone, once inside the cell, binds to the unoccupied receptor and becomes activated (or transformed) to the DNA binding form, where it interacts directly with the genes whose transcription it stimulates (or represses). Next, transcription of target genes is enhanced, mRNAs are produced in higher than basal levels, and these are translocated to the cytoplasm and translated into proteins/enzymes whose effects on cellular metabolism constitute the cellular responses attributable to the steroid hormone in question.

Recent evidence (see Fig. 1-18) suggests that steroid hormone receptors belong to a family of regulatory proteins whose ability to control gene expression is dependent on the binding of their hormone ligand. The control of gene expression by these receptor proteins appears to be achieved through the interaction of trans-acting proteins with the cis-acting DNA-promoter elements (the steroid receptor). A structural similarity is apparent among selected regions of many steroid receptors and the thyroid hormone receptor with the *v*-erb-A oncogene. This suggests that all of these proteins have evolved from a primordial receptor gene. These proteins may have arisen over evolutionary time to match the increasing developmental and physiological demands of more complex eukaryotes.

G. Impact of Molecular Biology on Understanding Hormone Action

1. General Considerations

In recent years, the field of molecular biology has unveiled many of the intricate steps in the process of gene transcription and maturation of messenger RNA. Some of the steps in this process are outlined in Fig. 1-19. Thus, steroid–receptor complexes, which act at the level of transcription, could theoretically operate at any one of the numerous steps in the process: unwinding of DNA, facilitating the binding of RNA polymerase; constitution of active polymerase with associated proteins; any of the reactions associated with the maturation of hnRNA to fully matured mRNA; or the transport of the mRNA ribonucleoprotein particles (informasomes) from the nucleus to the cytoplasm for translation in the polysome. The receptor could also play a role in the stabilization of mRNA. A straightforward view is that the receptor complex binds to high-affinity binding sites on or near the genes whose transcription is stimulated by the hormone. Recently, this possibility has been tested with encouraging results. Steroid–receptor complexes have been bound directly to flanking sequences of genes which are stimulated by the specific hormone. In one case the purified glucocorticoid–receptor com-

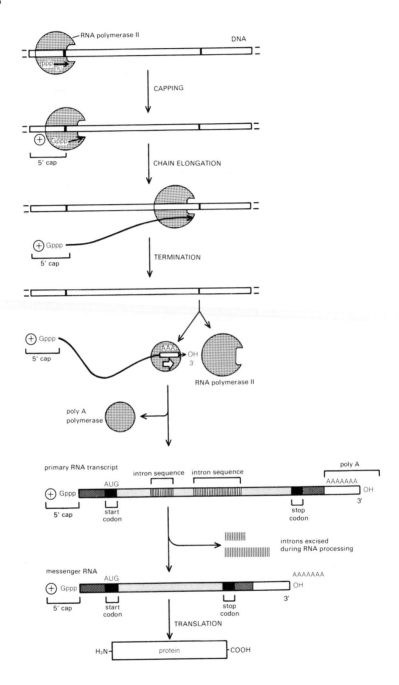

plex has been bound directly to the mammary tumor virus gene at an upstream flanking sequence; in another case, the progesterone–receptor complex has been bound with high affinity to a site upstream from the ovalbumin gene. These sequences which contain the receptor binding site can be determined in two ways: (1) If a series of known sequences containing the gene and various extents of upstream (left-handed) sequences are available, it is possible to deduce the steroid–receptor binding site by difference. A polynucleotide known to contain the receptor binding site can be fused with a heterologous gene, and that gene can then be shown to be stimulated by the steroid (receptor) complex. (2) With known sequences available, as in (1), protection experiments can be done, testing the action of DNase in the presence or absence of bound receptor complex. The receptor complex should protect its binding site from the action of the nuclease, thus availing the receptor binding site sequence. Specific sequences have been proposed for the acceptors of the progesterone receptor upstream from the chicken ovalbumin gene and for the glucocorticoid receptor upstream of the integrated mouse mammary tumor virus gene and upstream of the PEPCK (phosphoenolpyruvate carboxykinase) gene. A picture of the PEPCK gene with flanking sequences and a table showing the sequences of specific regulatory sites are given in Fig. 1-20. One idea is that steroid receptors may bind to enhancer regions of DNA which may be similar from gene to gene under the control of a specific steroid. The relatively large number (thousands) of steroid–receptor complexes that enter the nucleus in order to generate a transcriptional response may be explained by the thermodynamics of the binding process. Thus, an excess of such complexes would be required for binding to low-affinity sites and subsequent searching of the DNA strands until a high-affinity site is encountered to generate an increased rate of binding of RNA polymerase to the start (of transcription) site.

2. Gene Cloning

The ability to clone genes or portions of genes with varying amounts of information flanking the gene sequence aids in the understanding of the regulation of transcription, including the operation of steroid hor-

Figure 1-19. Overview of processes of transcription (top) and translation (bottom). The transcriptional process consists of synthesis of RNA by RNA polymerase II, capping at the 5' end, and addition of poly A at the 3' end. The positive charge at the cap is the result of methylation of the nitrogen at the 7 position of guanine. The mRNA is further processed by excision of intron information, leading to the mature mRNA which is translated in the cytoplasm. Reproduced from B. Alberts, D. Bray, J. Lewis, M. Raft, K. Roberts, and J. D. Watson, "Molecular Biology of the Cell." Garland Publishing Co., New York, 1983.

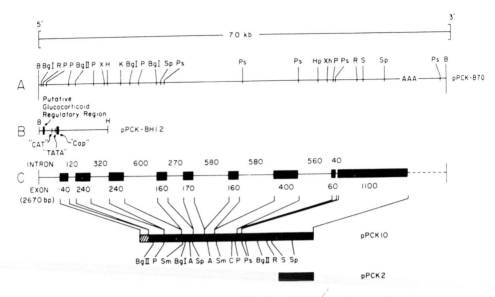

Putative regulatory sequences in the control region of the P-enolpyruvate carboxykinase gene

Base number	Specific area	Nucleotide sequence
+1 to +12	Cap site	5' A-C-T-G-T-G-C-T-A-G-G-T 3'
−39 to −32	"TATA box"	T-A-A-T-A-A-T -A
−84 to −77	"CAT box"	G-A-C-T-C-A-A-C-T
−230 to −207	Putative glucocorticoid regulatory region	A-A-A-T-G-T-G-C-A-G-C-C A-G-C-A-G-C-A-T-A-T-G-A

The specific sequences are numbered relative to the most 5' base in the cap site, which is arbitrarily assigned position +1. This data is drawn from an 800-bp sequence of a single strand at the 5' end of pPCK-BH1.2.

Figure 1-20. Structure of the gene for rat cytosolic phosphoenolpyruvate carboxykinase. (A) Detailed restriction map of the gene with flanking sequences at both ends. (B) Hypothetical regulatory sequences which are defined in the table beneath the figure. (C) Gene structure with exons (heavy black boxes) and introns (connecting lines). Numbers represent the average number of nucleotides in each exon or intron. Reproduced from H. Yoo-Warren, J. E. Monahan, J. Short, H. Short, A. Bruzel, A. Wynshaw-Boris, H. M. Meisner, D. Samols, and R. W. Hanson, Isolation and characterization of the gene coding for cytosolic phosphoenolpyruvate carboxykinase (GTP) from the rat. *Proc. Natl. Acad 'Sci. U.S.A.* **80,** 3656–3660 (1983).

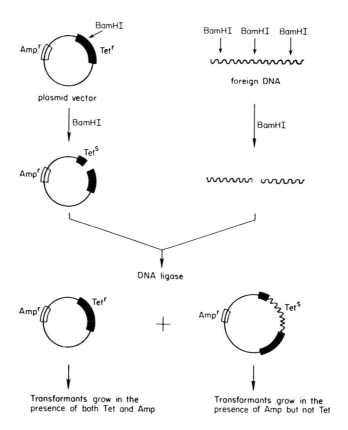

Figure 1-21. Cloning DNA in a plasmid vector involving inactivation of the plasmid gene for tetracycline resistance (Tet^r), while the gene for ampicillin resistance (Amp^r) remains intact. Reproduced from T. Maniatis, E. F. Fritsch, and J. Sambrook, "Molecular Cloning: A Laboratory Manual." Cold Spring Harbor Lab., Cold Spring Harbor, New York, 1982.

mone receptors cited above. Genes can be separated from the cellular DNA by cutting with various restriction nucleases which have different nucleotide base sequence specificities. The cleaved products can be separated by gel electrophoresis. DNAs can be incorporated into a bacterial plasmid that grows and replicates the specific DNA which can be recognized subsequently by hybridization with a labeled cDNA probe. The gene can also be integrated into the genome of a host cell and subsequently expressed. For cloning in plasmids, the plasmid DNA is split with a specific restriction endonuclease and the gene to be inserted is joined *in vitro* to the split ends of the plasmid DNA. The new recombinant plasmid is subsequently used to transform bacteria. In general, the plasmids selected carry two antibiotic resistance markers, as shown in Fig. 1-21. In this example, ampicillin-sensitive *Escherichia coli* can be transformed by the recombinant plasmid to ampicillin resistance. Since the restriction enzyme of choice, in this case, cuts the tetracycline resistance gene, colonies growing, after transformation, in the presence of tetracycline have a low probability of carrying the cloned gene, whereas the gene for ampicillin resistance remains intact (Fig. 1-21) and colonies will be selected on the basis of tetracycline sensitivity and ampicillin resistance.

H. Cellular Location of Steroid Hormone Action

Two lines of evidence lead to consideration of alternatives to the generalized mechanism of action of steroid hormones shown in Fig. 1-17. C. Szego's laboratory observes specific binding of estrogen to target cell membranes. As an extension of this finding, she concludes that the mechanism of estrogen action will follow from the membrane possibly reaching the nucleus after the steroid–receptor complex has fused with the lysosome which would be the transporting vehicle in the translocation step. This view would not explain the ability of cytosolic steroid–receptor complexes to bind to isolated nuclei, in the presumed absence of lysosomes, unless some remain attached to the partially purified nuclei. Alternatively, the *in vitro* binding to isolated nuclei may occur by a process different from the physiological one.

Unoccupied 1,25-dihydroxyvitamin D_3 receptors have been reported to be located in target cell nuclei, providing isotonic salt solutions with buffer near neutrality are used in the absence of sucrose. This finding fortifies the view that all steroid receptors, except glucocorticoid receptor, resemble the thyroid hormone receptor and that cytoplasmic concentrations may be the result of artifactual extractions from the nucleus after cell breakage. This conception aligns with P. Sheridan's for the estradiol receptor. Recent work from the laboratories of J. Gorski and G. Greene provides strong evidence for the nuclear location of the unoccupied estrogen receptor.

I. Receptor Polymorphism

1. Multiple Forms

The tendency in the past has been to regard receptors as unique or monolithic entities. This idea stems from the attractive hypothesis that cellular differentiation is directed exclusively by the arrangement of proteins on the genome. Thus, steroid hormone receptors which operate on the genome directly could be guided to high-affinity sites depending on whether those sites were "open" or "closed" by proteins. Differentiation would dictate the availability of gene binding sites by having differing protein decoration of the genome in specific cell types. This would ensure that cell type specific proteins could be transcribed in response to a specific hormone, explaining distinct responses to the same hormone in different cell types. However, recent investigations have provided evidence of multiplicity of steroid hormone receptors and of peptide hormone receptors, in some cases. The difficulty with these proposals lies in the possibility that so-called second forms of receptors may be proteolytic products of the monolithic forms which could be generated after the breakage of the cell. Because of this, multiplicity or polymorphism has not been well accepted.

2. Antagonist Receptors

A very recent development has been information suggesting that steroid hormone antagonists, previously conceived only to compete with the native ligand at its binding site, may, in addition to competing with agonist hormone for receptor binding, bind to and operate through a protein distinct from the hormone receptor.

3. Multiple Forms and the Process of Activation

Again, the steroid receptors have been more easily studied with respect to the process of activation, sometimes referred to as transformation, than the peptide hormone receptors. By activation, in this context, is meant the conversion of a form of the steroid–receptor complex, which cannot bind to DNA or to nuclei, to a form that can perform these functions. This process has been proposed to be of physiological importance rather than merely being a test-tube phenomenon. Because activation can usually be achieved in crude systems simply by heating, many considered, since the cell is at 37°, that activation is immediate upon binding the receptor by the hormonal ligand. This view is still popular. From *in vitro* studies, the activation step appears to involve a change in size of the unactivated precursor and availability of groups on the activated receptor which were formerly not measurable. It is uncertain whether disaggregation, or aggregation, as the case may be, actually occurs in the physiological process or is an *in vitro* artifact. It is also unclear whether the unactivated glucocorticoid receptor, large aggregate is a homopolymer, consisting only of steroid binding receptor entities, or whether it is a heteropolymer, consisting of the steroid binding protein plus some other nonreceptor proteins and perhaps other components.

The activation reaction became approachable when the unactivated precursor and activated form(s) were first physically separated. This was accomplished by rapid ion-exchange chromatography. Thus, the minimal multiplicity of steroid binding forms was shown to be the unactivated precursor and the activated form(s) which proved to be clearly resolvable. Although several theories exist for the activation reaction mechanism, this subject is in its infancy.

J. Second Messengers

A second messenger is a substance whose actual or relative concentration increases inside the cell in response to the primary hormone. Its function is to convey the primary hormonal signal and to translate it into metabolic changes within the target cell. Examples of second messengers are as follows: cyclic AMP, cyclic GMP, calcium ions (with or

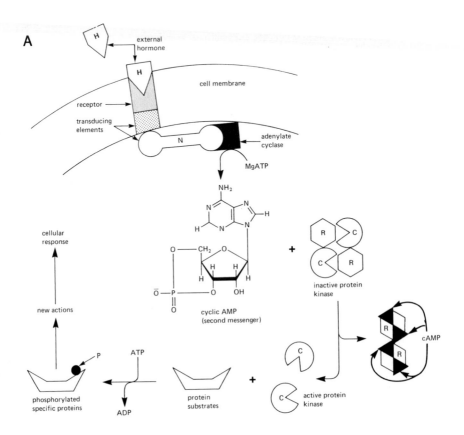

B

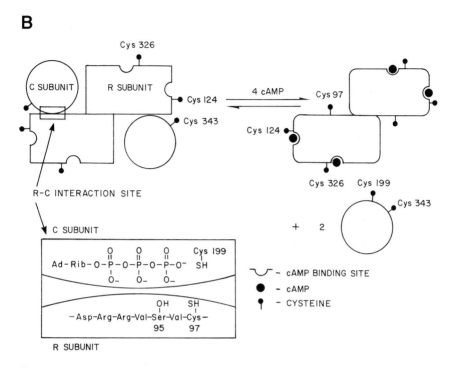

Figure 1-22. (A) Overview of the mechanism of activation of a protein kinase by elevated cytosolic levels of cyclic AMP. H, Hormone; N, guanine nucleotide binding protein; P, phosphate; R, regulatory subunit; C, catalytic subunit; cAMP, cyclic AMP. (B) Biochemical details of the activation of protein kinase II from porcine heart. The inactive protein kinase is diagrammed on the left and shows the accessible sulfhydryl groups and the biochemical nature of the sites of interaction between the regulatory (R) and catalytic (C) subunits (boxed inset). The portion of the R subunit shown in the inset includes the autophosphorylation site (Ser-95) followed by Cys-97. On the right side is drawn the activated catalytic subunits with the R cyclic AMP complexes above. Reproduced from N. C. Nelson and S. S. Taylor, Selective protection of sulfhydryl groups in cAMP-dependent protein kinase. II. *J. Biol. Chem.* **258,** 10981–10987 (1983).

without calmodulin), arachidonic acid, inositol triphosphate, diacylglycerol, and messengers that apparently regulate phosphoprotein phosphatases. Examples of hormones which stimulate cyclic AMP levels are typified in the general mechanism shown in Fig. 1-22A. Figure 1-22B shows a more detailed model of protein kinase, including the interaction sites between the R (regulatory) and C (catalytic) subunits. The elevated levels of cyclic AMP in the cell cytoplasm lead to the activation of protein kinase(s) (Fig. 1-15) and the phosphorylation of specific proteins. The

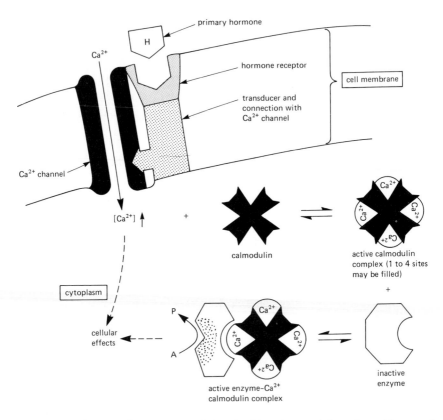

Figure 1-23. The second messenger activity of calcium ions and the action of increased cytoplasmic calcium together with calmodulin. In this model a specific hormone (H) usually a polypeptide, interacts with receptor in the outer cell membrane. This leads to conformational changes which directly stimulate the opening of or constitution of the calcium ion channel so that the flux of Ca^{2+} favors an increase in the cytoplasmic pool. Calcium ions can affect cellular processes directly or they may bind to calmodulin. The Ca^{2+}–calmodulin complex can then bind to certain enzymes which are activated. Either free Ca^{2+} or the calmodulin liganded form produce changes in cellular metabolism. As this is a speculative scheme, there are other alternatives. Among these would be the production of a second messenger, as yet unknown, which could, in turn, influence the uptake of Ca^{2+}. Also we must consider that Ca^{2+} could be bound to the inner membrane in some way and simply released into the cytoplasm by the product of the hormone–receptor complex. Finally, it is possible that cytoplasmic Ca^{2+} may derive in part from other cellular compartments, such as the endoplasmic reticulum or the mitochondria. Where the cellular response is to secrete another substance, possibly a second hormone, Ca^{2+} is usually required in the exocytosis mechanism.

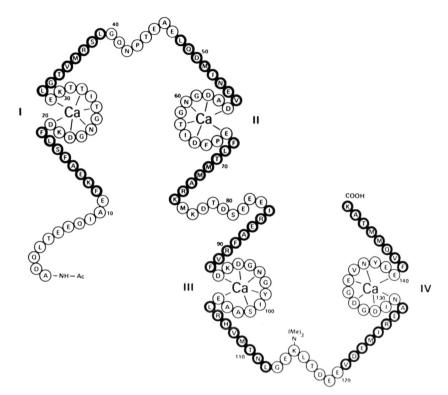

Figure 1-24. Sequence of bovine brain calmodulin using the standard one-letter code for amino acid residues. A, Ala; D, Asp; E, Glu; F, Phe; G, Gly; H, His; I, Ile; K, Lys; L, Leu; M, Met; N, Asn; P, Pro; Q, Gln; R, Arg; S, Ser; T, Thr; V, Val; Y, Tyr. The four proposed Ca^{2+} binding domains with the stretches of α helix (darker circles) are indicated. Domains III and IV contain the two tyrosyl residues; the single trimethyllysyl residue lies between domains III and IV. Domain III also contains the single histidyl residue. Note the homology especially between domains I and III and between domains II and IV. Reproduced from C. B. Klee, T. H. Crouch, and P. G. Richman, Calmodulin. *Annu. Rev. Biochem.* **49,** 489–515 (1980).

net reaction for activation of protein kinase by cyclic AMP can be written as

$$R_2C_2 + 4 \text{ cyclic AMP} = 2C + 2R \cdot 4 \text{ cyclic AMP}$$

The mechanisms involving increases in cytoplasmic calcium ions are quite obscure. There is the suggestion that the hormone receptor in the membrane can somehow interact with the elements of the calcium channel directly (Fig. 1-23). In this scheme, calcium either can act by itself or as a ligand of calmodulin (Fig. 1-24).

Very recently, suggestions of a new kind of second messenger have come forth. These refer especially to insulin action so far, but may

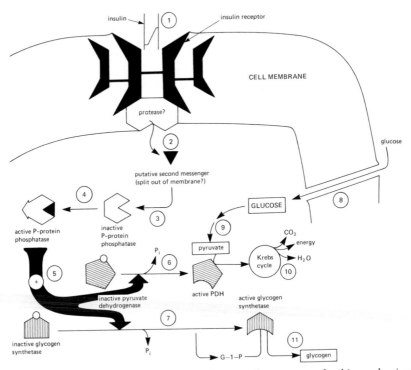

Figure 1-25. Speculative mechanism of insulin second messenger. In this mechanism, insulin binds to its cell membrane receptor (1) and through this interaction stimulates a protease in the cell membrane (which could be part of the insulin receptor). Through the action of the stimulated protease, the second messenger, presumably a polypeptide, is split out of the membrane (2). This second messenger stimulates phosphoprotein phosphatases, (3) and (4), in cytosol and in internal membranes to activate glycogen synthetase, (5)–(7), and pyruvate dehydrogenase, (5) and (6). Elevated blood levels of glucose, which evoked the insulin secretion, enter the liver cell (8). The glucose is metabolized to pyruvate (9), acetyl-CoA, and then is oxidized in the Krebs cycle (10). Glucose is also utilized through the glycogen synthetase pathway (11) to form glycogen. This mechanism, mediated by a second messenger, would explain the glucose utilizing effect of insulin and, consequently, its glucose lowering activity in blood.

eventually develop into a family of similar substances, perhaps small polypeptides, which regulate the activities of phosphoprotein phosphatases, and their actions may produce cascade-like effects. An overall mechanism is summarized in Fig. 1-25.

Thus, by stimulating the activity of phosphoprotein phosphatase through the action of this putative second messenger, the subsequent activation of pyruvate dehydrogenase and glycogen synthetase occurs because these enzymes are active in the dephosphorylated forms but not in the phosphorylated forms. Alternatively, a phosphorylated protein of high molecular weight may appear in the cytoplasm as a result of insulin–receptor interaction. Clearly, the insulin second messenger remains to be identified. Other second messenger actions will be encountered in appropriate sections of the book, but those presented here should acquaint the reader with the second messenger concept.

K. Cascade Mechanisms

A cascade mechanism is an amplification system whereby an initial reaction sets off multiple second reactions, each of which sets off multi-

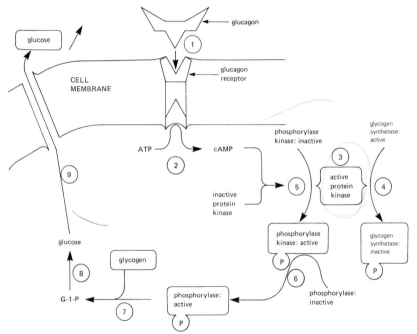

Figure 1-26. A cascade mechanism from cell surface hormonal signal to cellular metabolic response: glucagon and glycogenolysis. Glucagon combines with its cell membrane receptor (1), which stimulates the activity of adenylate cyclase, possibly mediated by a transducing element, on the cytoplasmic side of the membrane (2). Resulting increased level of cyclic AMP activates protein kinase (3) by a mechanism shown in Fig. 1-22A. Protein kinase subunits catalyze the phosphorylation of inactive phosphorylase kinase (5) and of active glycogen synthetase (4) to produce the phosphorylated inactive form (6) which produces glycogenolysis (7) to form glucose-1-P (G-1-P), which is further metabolized to glucose (8). Glucose is transported to the extracellular space and to the circulation. This represents a cascade system because each stimulated step after hormone binding is accomplished by an enzyme that can turn over multiple substrate molecules.

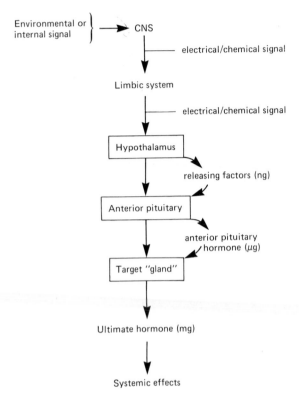

Figure 1-27. Hormonal cascade of signals from CNS to ultimate hormone. The target "gland" refers to the last hormone-producing tissue in the cascade which is stimulated by an appropriate anterior pituitary hormone. Examples would be thyroid gland, adrenal cortex, and liver.

ple third reactions, and so on. A classical biochemical cascade mechanism is generated by the action of a hormone, such as glucagon, at the cell membrane to produce an increase in cyclic AMP, as shown in Fig. 1-22A. The cascade may be visualized in terms of the alterations of cellular metabolism which generate the cellular response; glycogenolysis to avail glucose to the extracellular space is an example. This is shown in Fig. 1-26.

Another important concept involving a true cascade mechanism is the series of signals from the central nervous system through the hypothalamus to the terminal hormone, as shown in Fig. 1-27. The cascade effect may be produced by a single event or signal in the external or internal environment. Either by electrical or chemical transmission, a

signal is sent to the limbic system and then to the hypothalamus, resulting in secretion of a releasing hormone into the closed portal system
connecting the hypothalamus and anterior pituitary. Releasing hormones may be secreted in nanogram amounts and have half-lives of
about 3–7 min. In turn they signal the release of the appropriate anterior
pituitary hormones which may be secreted in microgram amounts with
half-lives on the order of 20 min or longer. The anterior pituitary hormone elicits the secretion of the ultimate hormone which may be secreted in milligram amounts and may be fairly stable. Thus, in terms of
increasing stability of hormones as one proceeds down this cascade
together with increasing amounts of hormones elaborated down the
cascade, an amplification of a single event at the outset could involve a
factor of thousands to a millionfold. The ultimate hormone will operate
on its receptors in many cell types, and these hormone–receptor complexes may stimulate the appearance of many phenotypes, augmenting
the amplification built into the cascade system even further. Although
not all signaling mechanisms involve this entire system, a good many
do, as will be exemplified in later chapters.

IV. EVOLUTION OF HORMONES

This problem deals with the question of how a given chemical structure comes to represent a specific signal to a cell to change its metabolism in accordance with specific changes in the extracellular environment. G. Tomkins referred to this problem as the "metabolic code." One
approach is from the vantage point of prebiotic biochemistry. After the
primordial cells were formed, their nutrition could have been based on
the most plentiful organic materials in the environment. Some of these
could have been polypeptides. As a major nutrient became used up by
all the similar primordial cells, that limiting nutrient may have become a
signal for the next major nutrient source in the environment, and so on
through a large series of shifts from one nutrient to another and the
utilization of the previous limiting substance as a signal for the next
available abundant nutrient. Thus, a primary nutrient might have resembled insulin or glucagon at one stage, and as it became limiting and
its structure "remembered" by the cell, the next major nutrient might
have been carbohydrate, like glucose; this is all imaginary, but perhaps
it is a line worth investigating as our knowledge of prebiotic biochemistry expands.

Some of the polypeptide hormones are very ancient and even when
branches have occurred, it is apparent that divergent forms, for exam-

ple, GH and PRL, were derived from a common ancestral gene. It is important that many hormones, such as cyclic AMP and now even steroid hormones as well as polypeptides such as insulin, are being found in cells across the species from man to bacteria.

G. Tomkins viewed cyclic AMP as a model system because of its ubiquity in biological regulation. He acknowledged that cyclic AMP acts as a symbol for carbon source starvation in most microorganisms, and ppGpp (guanosine 5'-diphosphate 3'-diphosphate) acts as a symbol for nitrogen or amino acid deficiency. He emphasized that metabolic signals need bear no structural relationship to the molecules which promote their accumulation in a nutritional or metabolic crisis (i.e., cyclic AMP is not a chemical analog of glucose). The ability of these second messengers to fluctuate rapidly in a cell ensured responsiveness to environmental conditions. Thus, the metabolic code is the expression of a particular signal which represents a unique state in the environment. Cyclic AMP may have become associated with carbon source starvation as a result of "idling" of a primordial kinase which normally catalyzed glucose phosphorylation with ATP. In the absence of glucose, cyclic AMP might have been derived from the unused ATP. In the same sense, ppGpp may have been derived from GTP during the idling of protein synthesis as a result of amino acid deprivation. Under this condition, the GTP, which would have been utilized in protein synthesis, could have been converted to ppGpp and come to symbolize amino acid starvation. G. Tomkin's speculations were made in an attempt to understand how specific structures have come to be symbols for specific environmental conditions.

V. PHYSICAL PARAMETERS OF HORMONE–RECEPTOR INTERACTIONS

Ligand–receptor interactions can be viewed as simple monomolecular reactions conforming to

$$\{H\} \ + \ \{R\} \underset{k_{-1}}{\overset{k_{+1}}{\rightleftharpoons}} \{RH\}$$

where H is the hormone, R is the unoccupied receptor, and RH is the hormone–receptor complex. This analysis focuses on the ligand interaction at low temperature and limits the reaction by precluding activation or subsequent activities of the receptor complex. Normally, these in-

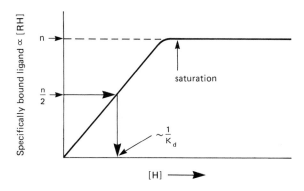

Figure 1-28. Determination of saturating amount of ligand.

teractions would be carried out at low temperature to limit the approach to equilibrium. Usually, this interaction can be described by simple Michaelis kinetics as if a semienzymatic reaction were studied. By mass action, the equilibrium can be expressed as

$$K_a = \{RH\}/\{H\}\{R\} = k_{+1}/k_{-1}$$

where the first expression refers to the equilibrium concentrations of the reaction components and the second expression to the ratio of the forward and reverse rate constants, k_{+1} being known as the *on-rate* and k_{-1} being known as the *off-rate*. Equilibrium can be determined experimentally with a progress curve. A saturating amount of ligand must first be determined, as shown in Fig. 1-28.

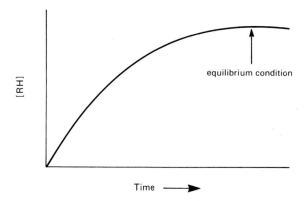

Figure 1-29. Progress curve of specific binding at saturating ligand concentration.

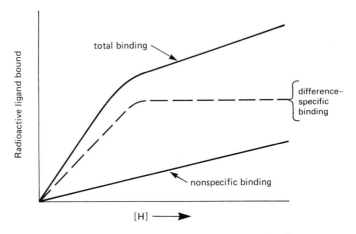

Figure 1-30. Determination of specific ligand binding.

As a rule, the receptor should be saturated by 20-fold the K_d (dissociation constant). With a saturating amount of ligand, it is possible to perform a progress curve of binding, as exemplified by Fig. 1-29. Thus, under these conditions (Fig. 1-29), the equilibrium concentrations of [H], [R], and [RH] can be measured. The starting amount of free hormone (radioactively labeled) is known and the specific binding, [RH], is measured. For the measurement of specific binding, the total nonspecific binding is measured. Nonspecific binding is determined by addition of unlabeled ligand at about 100–1000 times the concentration of the labeled ligand. Virtually all of the high-affinity binding to the receptor will be displaced, but the nonspecific (low-affinity) binding will not. Thus, specific binding as well as [RH] can be obtained as shown in Fig. 1-30. [H]$_{total}$ is known at t_0. The amount of hormone in [RH] is subtracted from [H]$_{t_0}$. Whether any unoccupied receptor is found at equilibrium is hard to deduce in a first approximation, so the K_d value is measured by the Scatchard plot from which the constant can be extracted. There may exist a pool of receptor [R] which is incapable of binding hormone due to lack of phosphorylation or for some other reason. Such a pool will pass undiscovered by this analysis. The Scatchard plot is visualized in Fig. 1-31. The examples in this figure are those most frequently encountered. A single class of binding sites assumes the form of a straight line, whereas two or more classes result in a composite of two or more curves with different slopes. The dissociation constant can be extracted from the slope of the line.

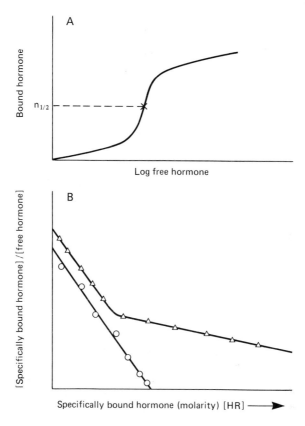

Figure 1-31. A typical model of a Scatchard plot for extraction of the dissociation constant (K_d) where $K_d = ([H][R]/[HR])$. (A) Semilogarithmic plot. (B) Linear plot.

A slightly more detailed analysis of the origin of the Scatchard plot is useful because of its application in describing hormone–receptor interactions. Basically, the Scatchard plot can be regarded as a manipulation of Michaelis-type kinetics. Thus, as shown, the direct binding plot in Fig. 1-28 conforms to the equation

$$\{RH\} = n/1 + 1/K_d\{H\}$$

which is in the form of the Michaelis–Menten expression for velocity of a simple enzymatic reaction in which A, the substrate, is converted to P, the product, with an initial velocity, v. The expression becomes

$$v = n/1 + 1/K_m\{A\}$$

where n is the number of sites. In the transformation to serve as an expression for binding, v is replaced by the concentration of the bound form of the hormone, [RH], and the K_m becomes the dissociation constant (K_d). Experimental observations must include those values of hormone concentration which clearly exceed the $n_{1/2}$ value, as shown in Fig. 1-31A, otherwise the level at which saturation occurs cannot be derived adequately and the extrapolation to give the number of binding sites (Fig. 1-31B) can be in considerable error. This stresses the importance, as in using Michaelis kinetics with enzymatic reactions, for using concentrations of free hormone in reasonable excess.

In the classical Lineweaver–Burk representation of Michaelis–Menten kinetics for a simple enzymatic reaction, the equation conforms to a straight line: $y = mx + b$, where y is the ordinate value, x the abscissa value, m the slope, and b the intercept on the ordinate. The equation for an enzymatic reaction is

$$1/v = 1/nk \ 1/\{A\} + 1/n$$
$$(y = m \quad x \quad + b)$$

This can be converted to hormone binding data:

$$1/\{RH\} = 1/nK_d \ 1/\{H\} + 1/n$$

and the plot would appear as in Fig. 1-32. The Scatchard plot conforms to the equation

$$\{RH\}/\{H\} = -K_d\{RH\} + nK_d$$
$$(y = m \quad x \quad + b)$$

which is a straight line equation for a single class of binding sites in Fig. 1-31.

Frequently, two classes of binding sites appear (Fig. 1-31B), one of higher affinity (upper part of curve) and one of lower affinity (lower part of curve). The line representing higher affinity is often the one of interest when the lower affinity curve represents nonspecific binding. In this case the upper part of the curve consists of the true line and the contribution from the lower affinity line as well. In order to obtain the true value of K_d [and thus, of the affinity constant, K_a (which is equal to $1/K_d$)], the contribution of the lower affinity line must be removed. Since the plot represents total binding, the true line of higher affinity may be calculated by subtracting nonspecific binding values from the values of total binding. This correction is shown in Fig. 1-33.

Another potential problem refers to the range of concentrations of free hormone used to obtain the Scatchard plot. It has been emphasized recently that the lessons of enzyme kinetics must be applied to binding

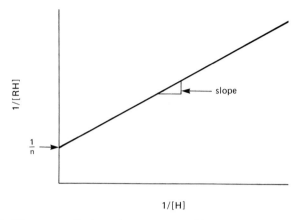

Figure 1-32. Lineweaver–Burk-type presentation of hormone–receptor binding data.

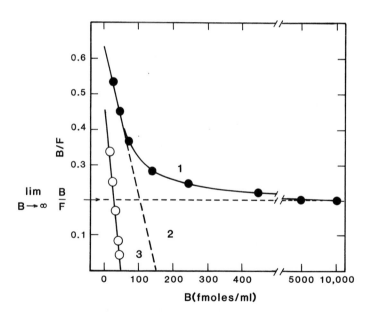

Figure 1-33. Scatchard plot showing correction of the high-affinity component by subtraction of nonspecific binding contributed from the low-affinity component. Curve 1: Scatchard plot of total binding. Curve 2: Linear extrapolation of descending portion (incorrect). Curve 3: Scatchard plot of B_{sp} after subtraction of nonspecific binding (correct). Reproduced from G. C. Chamness and W. L. McGuire, Scatchard plots: Common errors in correction and interpretation. *Steroids* **26,** 538–542 (1975).

studies. Thus, it is imperative to use a wide range of hormone concentrations which fall on either side of the K_d value.

VI. NEWER DEVELOPMENTS IMPACTING ON THE UNDERSTANDING OF HORMONE ACTION

The application of a number of newer techniques and findings has raised the level of understanding of hormone receptor mechanisms. One of these has been the use of covalent ligands of the steroid, peptide, or other small molecule variety. Thus, in essence, a structure that can be recognized by the receptor as a true ligand will bear a reactive grouping or one that can be activated, such as with appropriate wavelengths of light. This will produce a highly reactive species of ligand which will form a covalent bond with the receptor. When such a ligand is labeled with radioactivity, the covalent complex can be purified to homogeneity, without loss of the radioactive ligand, and thus mark the resulting protein as the receptor. This technique has also made it possible to discover the subunit structures of several receptors. In addition to reactive ligands which lead to covalent complexes, a variety of new chemical analogs are becoming available, especially in the steroid and small molecule amine areas, which make it possible to separate similar receptors with overlapping ligand binding specificities.

Receptors have been prepared in pure enough form to develop useful polyclonal antibodies. More recently, monoclonal antibodies have become available, both of which have advanced our knowledge of receptor topology. Further application of these approaches promises to make possible the isolation of reactive sites, such as the ligand binding site and the DNA binding site, and their eventual primary sequences. With high-affinity antibodies, it should be possible to obtain the mRNA encoding a specific receptor, translate the receptor *in vitro*, and clone the gene for each receptor.

With the advent of cell culture techniques, it is now possible to label newly formed receptor molecules with heavy amino acids (labeled with ^{15}N, ^{13}C, and deuterium) and subsequently to separate by density gradient centrifugation the newly formed (heavy) receptor from the preexisting (light) receptor. By performing the experiment at various times after exposure to heavy amino acids, the half-life of the receptor molecule can be determined from the decay of the light, preexisting form. The receptor peak is visualized by its binding of radioactive ligand.

Recently, the nuclear matrix has been implicated as a possible site of steroid hormone–receptor action. Analysis of the nuclear matrix fraction may unveil the localization of hormone-stimulatable genes as well as the specific molecular sequences of those genes to which steroid–receptor complexes bind to affect their actions.

VII. SUMMARY

In this chapter, a topical view of the hormone action field has been attempted. Some background information has been included where it may be helpful to the understanding of a particular topic. For example, considerations of cell membrane structure have been included to facilitate the discussion of cell membrane hormone receptors. Topics have been covered which should provide an overview of many of the subjects in later chapters and in some cases, methodology has been discussed. In sum, the field of biochemical endocrinology has moved forward at a very rapid pace. Hormone receptors were just becoming visible in the 1960s, and in only 20 years we approach the certainty of the complete structures of most of them. Cloning of receptor genes is ongoing in several laboratories and before long the availability of many different receptor molecules in relatively large amounts when they can be used to probe the structure of chromatin (in the case of the steroid receptors) may become a reality. By this time a strategy may be found to employ pure receptors to cure a number of endocrine diseases.

References

A. Books

Goldberger, R. F., and Yamamoto, K. R., eds. (1982). "Biological Regulation and Development," Vol. 3A. Plenum, New York.
Lewin, B. (1983). "Genes." Wiley, New York.
Wald, F. (1971). "Macromolecules: Structure and Function." Prentice-Hall, Englewood Cliffs, New Jersey.
Watson, J. D. (1970). "Molecular Biology of the Gene," 2nd ed. Benjamin, New York.
Williams, R. H., ed. (1981). "Textbook of Endocrinology," 6th ed. Philadelphia, Pennsylvania.

B. Review Articles

Barrack, E. R., and Coffey, D. S. (1983). The role of the nuclear matrix in steroid hormone action. *In* "Biochemical Actions of Hormones" (G. Litwack, ed.), Vol. 10, pp. 23–90. Academic Press, New York.

48

Boon Chock, P., Rhee, S. G., and Stadtman, E. R. (1981). Interconvertible enzyme cascades in cellular regulation. *Annu. Rev. Biochem.* **49,** 813–843.

Cohen, P. (1982). The role of protein phosphorylation in neural hormonal control of cellular activity. *Nature (London)* **296,** 613–620.

Kaplan, J. (1981). Polypeptide binding receptors: Analysis and classification. *Science* **212,** 14–20.

Katzenellenbogen, B. S. (1980). Dynamics of steroid hormone receptor action. *Annu. Rev. Physiol.* **42,** 17–35.

Klee, C. B., Crouch, T. H., and Richman, P. G. (1980). Calmodulin. *Annu. Rev. Biochem.* **49,** 489–515.

Pearse, B. M. F., and Bretscher, M. S. (1981). Membrane recycling by coated vesicles. *Annu. Rev. Biochem.* **50,** 85–101.

Rodbell, M. (1980). The role of hormone receptors and GTP regulatory proteins in membrane transduction. *Nature (London)* **284,** 17–22.

Rubenstein, R. (1982). Diseases caused by impaired communication among cells. *Sci. Am.* **127,** 102–121.

Shapiro, D. J., and Brock, M. L. (1985). Messenger RNA stabilization and gene transcription in the estrogen induction of vitellogenin mRNA. *In* "Biochemical Actions of Hormones" (G. Litwack, ed.), Vol. 12, pp. 139–172. Academic Press, New York.

Sheridan, P. J., Buchanan, J. M., Anselmo, V. C., and Martin, P. M. (1979). Equilibrium: The intracellular distribution of steroid receptors. *Nature (London)* **282,** 579–582.

Tomkins, G. M. (1975). The metabolic code. *Science* **189,** 760–763.

C. Research Papers

Compton, J. G., Schrader, W. T., and O'Malley, B. W. (1983). DNA sequence preference of the progesterone receptor. *Proc. Natl. Acad. Sci. U.S.A.* **80,** 16–20.

Faye, J.-C., Jozan, S., Redeuilh, G., Baulieu, E.-E., and Bayard, F. (1983). Physicochemical and genetic evidence for specific antiestrogen binding sites. *Proc. Natl. Acad. Sci. U.S.A.* **80,** 3158–3162.

Green, S., and Chambon, P. (1986). A superfamily of potentially oncogenic hormone receptors. *Nature (London)* **324,** 615–617.

King, W. J., and Greene, G. L. (1984). Monoclonal antibodies localize estrogen receptor in the nuclei of target cells. *Nature (London)* **307,** 745–747.

Klotz, I. M. (1982). Numbers of receptor sites from Scatchard graphs: Facts and fantasies. *Science* **217,** 1247–1249.

Mulvihill, E. R., LePennec, J-P., and Chambon, P. (1982). Chicken oviduct progesterone receptor: Location of specific regions of high-affinity binding in cloned DNA fragments of hormone-responsive genes. *Cell* **24,** 621–632.

Payvar, F., Wrange, O., Carlstedt-Duke, J., Okret, S., Gustafsson, J.-A., and Yamamoto, K. R. (1981). Purified glucocorticoid receptors bind selectively *in vitro* to a cloned DNA fragment whose transcription is regulated by glucocorticoids *in vivo*. *Proc. Natl. Acad. Sci. U.S.A.* **78,** 6628–6632.

Scatchard, G. (1949). The attractions of protein for small molecules and ions. *Ann. N.Y. Acad. Sci.* **51,** 660–682.

Welshons, W. V., Krummel, B. M., and Gorski, J. (1985). Nuclear localization of unoccupied receptors for glucocorticoids, estrogens, and progesterone in GH$_3$ cells. *Endocrinology* **117,** 2140–2147.

Chapter 2

Steroid Hormones: Chemistry, Biosynthesis, and Metabolism

49

I. INTRODUCTION

This chapter deals with the structural chemistry and biosynthetic pathways proven or presumptive of the major classes of steroid hormones. All have a complicated structure of fused rings which can be modified by functional group substitution at many points. Furthermore, the presence of asymmetric carbon atoms introduces steric modifications and isomeric possibilities. The reader will find it prudent first to grasp the essential features of the steroid structures and steroid relationships before attempting to delve into the discussion of specific hormonal activities in later chapters. Then, when so doing, it may be helpful to turn back to the appropriate portion of this chapter to heighten understanding of the structures of the hormones under review.

A. General Comments

The first steroid hormone, estrone, was isolated in 1929 at a time before the characteristic ring structure of the steroid nucleus had been elucidated. Today well over 225 naturally occurring steroids have been isolated and chemically characterized. In addition, an uncountable number of additional steroids and steroid analogs have been chemically synthesized.

All steroids belong to the chemical class of substances known as terpenoids or terpenes. Other biologically important terpenoid compounds include the plant hormones gibberellic acid and abscisic acid, the insect hormone (juvenile hormone), farnesol (a plant oil), the plant-produced isoprenoids which include carotene (a precursor of vitamin A), ubiquinone (a vitamin K analog), the plastoquinones (participants in photosynthesis), and natural rubber. All terpenoids have in common the same two C_5H_8 isoprene precursors employed for their biosynthesis, namely, isopentenyl pyrophosphate and dimethylallyl pyrophosphate. These structural relationships are summarized in Fig. 2-1.

B. Historical Perspective

The development of our modern understanding of hormones and the science of endocrinology has closely paralleled studies on isolation,

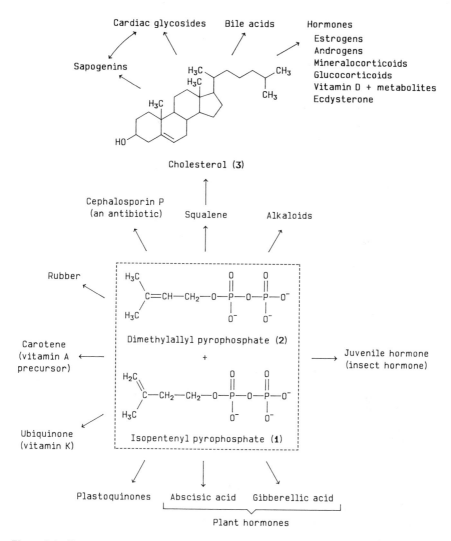

Figure 2-1. Representative isoprenoids which may be derived from isopentenyl pyrophosphate and dimethylallyl pyrophosphate.

chemical characterization, and synthesis of steroids and subsequent elucidation of their pathways of biosynthesis and catabolism. However, the foundation of many of these developments on steroid hormones is to be found in a lengthy series of papers which appeared in the late 1920s and early 1930s from Professor A. Windaus's laboratory in Göttingen, Germany and led to the structural determination of cholesterol. This was an extraordinarily challenging problem given the limitation that at that time the techniques of nuclear magnetic resonance spectroscopy (NMR), mass spectrometry, and ultraviolet (UV) and infrared (IR) spectroscopy were not available. Instead the structure was determined through elaborate classical organic chemistry manipulations which involved conversion of the compound under study to known reference compounds. At the present time the application of the powerful separation techniques of high-performance liquid chromatography (HPLC) or gas chromatography combined with the use of continuous on-line monitoring by mass spectrometry with computer-assisted data storage and analysis frequently permit unequivocal structural determinations on impure samples that contain less than 1 μg of the steroid of interest.

An equally important contribution to our present understanding of the biochemistry of steroids was the introduction and general availability of radioactively labeled compounds. Radioactive steroids offer two major advantages: The presence of the radioactive label (1) provides a significant increase in sensitivity of detection of the steroid under study (prior to the advent of radioactive steroids, investigators relied upon colorimetric or bioassay procedures to quantitate the steroid of interest), and (2) allows the investigator to detect, either from *in vivo* whole animal experiments or *in vitro* experiments with perfused organs, tissue slices, cell suspensions, cell homogenates, or purified enzyme preparations, the presence of new compounds which would otherwise be unappreciated. Thus, it was through the application of radioisotope techniques, modern procedures of chromatography, and structure determination that whole categories of new steroid hormones have been recently discovered, for example, vitamin D metabolites (Chapter 9) and catechol estrogens (Chapter 13).

II. CHEMISTRY OF STEROIDS

A. Basic Ring Structure

Steroids are derived from a phenanthrene ring structure (structure **4**) to which a pentano ring has been attached; this yields in the completely hydrogenated form cyclopentanoperhydrophenanthrene or the sterane ring structure (structure **6**, Fig. 2-2).

Steroid structures are not normally written with all the carbon and hydrogen atoms as illustrated in **5** of Fig. 2-2; instead the shorthand notation as presented for sterane (**6**, Fig. 2-2) is usually employed. In this representation the hydrogen atoms are not indicated and unless

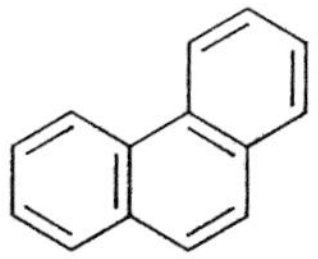

Phenanthrene (4)

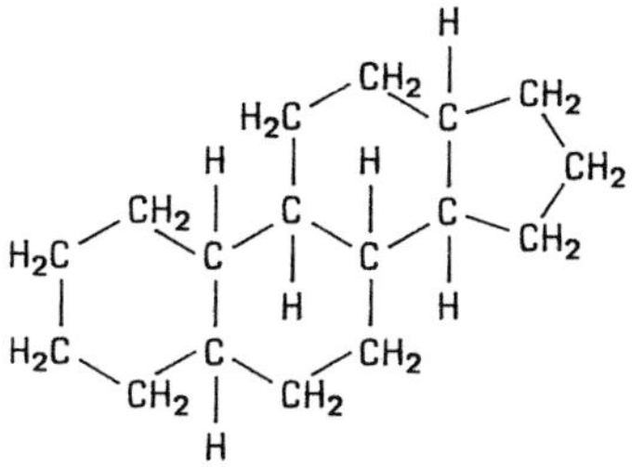

Cyclopentanoperhydrophenanthrene
(sterane) (5)

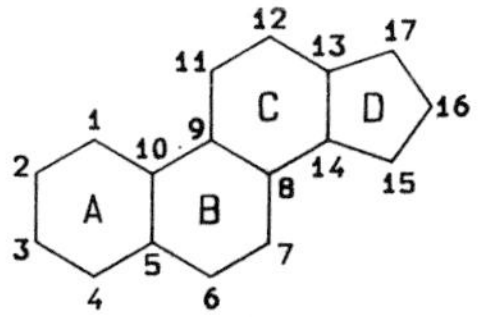

Sterane (6)

Figure 2-2. Parent ring structures of steroids.

specified otherwise it is assumed that the cyclohexane (A, B, C) or cyclo-pentane (D) ring is fully reduced, that is, each carbon has its full comple-ment of carbon and/or hydrogen bonds.

Also indicated in structure **6** is the standard numbering system for all the carbon atoms in the four rings. The three 6-carbon cyclohexane rings are respectively designated A, B, and C and the 5-carbon cyclopentane ring is notated as the D ring.

B. Classes of Steroids

In mammalian systems there are six families of steroid hormones that can be classified both on a structural and a biological (hormonal) basis. They are the estrogens (female sex steroids), the androgens (the male

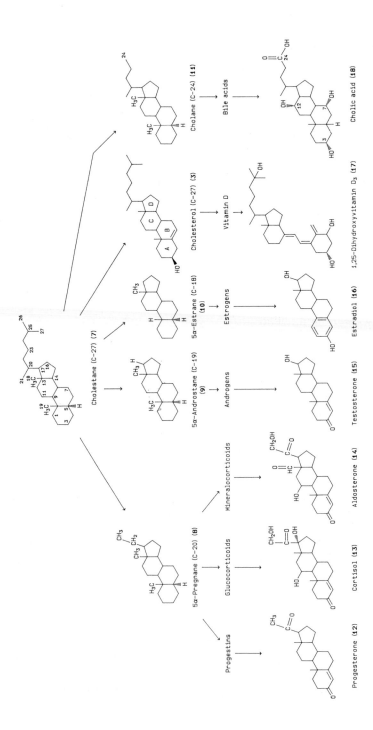

Figure 2-3. Family tree of seven principal classes of steroids (bottom row) which are structurally derived from the parent cholestane (top row).

Table 2–1. Classes of Steroids

Steroid class	Principal active steroid in man	Number of carbon atoms	Parent ring structure
Estrogens	Estradiol	17	Estrane
Androgens	Testosterone	18	Androstane
Progestins	Progesterone	19	Pregnane
Glucocorticoids	Cortisol	19	Pregnane
Mineralocorticoids	Aldosterone	19	Pregnane
Vitamin D steroids	1,25-Dihydroxyvitamin D_3	27	Cholestane
Bile acids	Cholic acid	24	Cholane

sex steroids), the progestins, the mineralocorticoids, the glucocorticoids, and vitamin D with its daughter metabolites. Also the bile acids are structurally related to cholesterol and thus constitute a seventh member of the steroid family. All of these steroids are biologically derived from cholesterol. Table 2-1 summarizes some fundamental relationships of these principal mammalian classes of steroids.

The parent ring structure for cholesterol is the fully saturated ring structure cholestane (**7,** Fig. 2-3). Cholestane, which has 27 carbons, differs from sterane (**6,** Fig. 2-2) by addition of an 8-carbon side chain on carbon-17 of ring D and the presence of two angular methyl groups at the juncture of the A:B ring (carbon-10) and C:D ring (carbon-13). The cholestane ring structure also gives rise to the parent ring structures for the six classes of mammalian steroids and the bile acids as summarized in Table 2-1. The parent ring compounds are the completely saturated ring structures pregnane (**8**), androstane (**9**), estrane (**10**), and cholane (**11**), each of which is structurally related to cholestane. These relationships are depicted in Fig. 2-3. The parent ring structures are used as the stem term in constructing the formal nomenclature of any steroid (see later).

The biosynthetic pathway of production of each of these general steroid classes will be separately presented later in this chapter. A discussion of their hormonal and biochemical aspects appears later in individual chapters.

C. Structural Modification

The basic ring structures presented in Fig. 2-3 can be subjected to a wide array of modifications by introduction of hydroxyl or carbonyl substituents and by introduction of unsaturation (double or triple

Table 2–2. Steroid Nomenclature Conventions

Modification	Prefix	Suffix
Hydroxyl group (—HO)	Hydroxy	-ol
Hydroxyl above plane of ring	β-OH	—
Hydroxyl below plane of ring	α-OH	—
Keto or carbonyl group (C=O)	Oxo-	-one
Aldehyde (—CHO)	—	-al
Carboxylic acid (COOH)	Carboxy	-oic acid
Double bond (—C=C—)		-ene
Triple bond (—C≡C—)	—	-yne
Saturated ring system	—	-ane
One less carbon atom	-Nor	—
One additional carbon atom	-Homo	—
One additional oxygenation	-Oxo	—
One less oxygen atom	-Deoxy	—
Two additional hydrogen atoms	-Dihydro	
Two less hydrogen atoms	-Dehydro-	—
Two groups on same sides of plane	Cis	—
Two groups on opposite sides of plane	Trans	—
Other ring forms (rings A and B trans, as in allopregnane)	Allo	
Opening of a ring (as in vitamin D)	Seco-	—
Conversion at a numbered carbon from conventional orientation (as in epicholesterol or 3α-cholesterol)	-Epi	—

bonds). In addition, heteroatoms such as nitrogen or sulfur can replace the ring carbons, and halogens and sulfhydryl or amino groups may replace steroid hydroxyl moieties. Furthermore, the ring size can be expanded or contracted by addition or removal or carbon atoms. The consequences of these structural modifications are designated by application of the standard organic nomenclature conventions of steroids. The pertinent aspects of this system are summarized in Table 2-2. Prefixes and suffixes are used to indicate the type of structural modification. Any number of prefixes may be employed (each with its own appropriate carbon number and specified in the order of decreasing preference of acid, lactone, ester, aldehyde, ketone, alcohol, amine, and ether); however, only one suffix is permitted.

Table 2-3 tabulates the systematic and trivial names of many common steroids. All these formal names are devised in accordance with the official nomenclature rules for steroids laid down by the International Union of Pure and Applied Chemistry (IUPAC).*

---

*The IUPAC definitive rules of steroid nomenclature are presented in full in *Pure Applied Chemistry* **31**, 285–322 (1972) or *Biochemistry* **10**, 4994–4995 (1971).

Table 2–3. Trivial and Systematic Names of Some Common Steroids

Trivial name	Systematic name
Aldosterone	18,11-Hemiacetal of 11β,21-dihydroxy-3,20-dioxo-pregn-4-ene-18-al
Androstenedione	Androst-4-ene-3,17-dione
Androsterone	3α-Hydroxy-5α-androstan-17-one
Cholecalciferol (vitamin D_3)	9,10-Secocholesta-5,7,10(19)-trien-3β-ol
Cholesterol	Cholest-5-ene-3β-ol
Cholic acid	3α,7α,12α-Trihydroxy-5β-cholan-24-oic acid
Corticosterone	11β,21-Dihydroxypregn-4-ene-3,20-dione
Cortisol	11β,17,21-Trihydroxypregn-4-ene-3,20-dione
Cortisone	17,21-Dihydroxypregn-4-ene-3,11,20-tricone
Dehydroepiandrosterone	3β-Hydroxy-5-androstene-17-one
Deoxycorticosterone	21-Hydroxypregn-4-ene-3,20-dione
Ergocalciferol (vitamin D_2)	9,10-Seco-5,7,10(19),22-ergostatetraen-3β-ol
Ergosterol	5,7,22-Ergostatrien-3β-ol
Estrone	3-Hydroxyestra-1,3,5(10)-triene-17-one
Estriol	Estra-1,3,5(10)-triene-3,16α,17β-triol
Etiocholanolone	3α-Hydroxy-5β-androstane-17-one
Lanosterol	8,24-Lanostadiene-3β-ol
Lithocholic acid	3α-Hydroxy-5β-cholan-24-oic acid
Progesterone	Pregn-4-ene-3,20-dione
Testosterone	17β-Hydroxyandrost-4-ene-3-one

D. Asymmetric Carbons

An important structural feature of any steroid is recognition of the presence of asymmetric carbon atoms and designation in the formal nomenclature of the structural isomer which is present. Thus, reduction of pregnane-3-one to the corresponding 3-alcohol will produce two epimeric steroids (see Fig. 2-4). The resulting hydroxyl may be above the plane of the A ring and is so designated on the structure by a solid line; it is referred to as a -3β-ol. The epimer or -3α-ol has the hydroxyl below the plane of the A ring and is so designated by a dotted line for the -C ···OH bond. If the α or β orientation of a substituent group is not known, it is designated with a wavy —C⌒OH line.

Another locus where asymmetric carbon atoms play an important role in steroid structure determination is the junction between each of the A, B, C, and D rings. Figure 2-5 illustrates these relationships for cholestanol and coprostanol. Thus, in the 5α form the 19-methyl and the α-hydrogen on carbon-5 are on opposite sides of the plane of the A:B ring; this is referred to as a *trans* fusion. When the 19-methyl and β-hydrogen

58

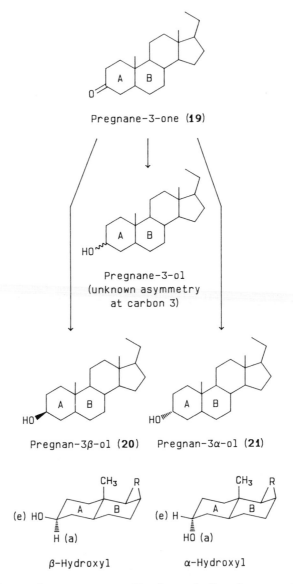

Pregnane–3–one (**19**)

Pregnane–3–ol
(unknown asymmetry
at carbon 3)

Pregnan–3β–ol (**20**)   Pregnan–3α–ol (**21**)

β–Hydroxyl   α–Hydroxyl

Figure 2-4. Structural consequences resulting from reduction of pregnane-3-one. The orientations of α- and β-hydroxyls of compounds (**20**) and (**21**) as equatorial (e) or axial (a) substituents, respectively, on the chair version of the A rings are shown in the bottom row.

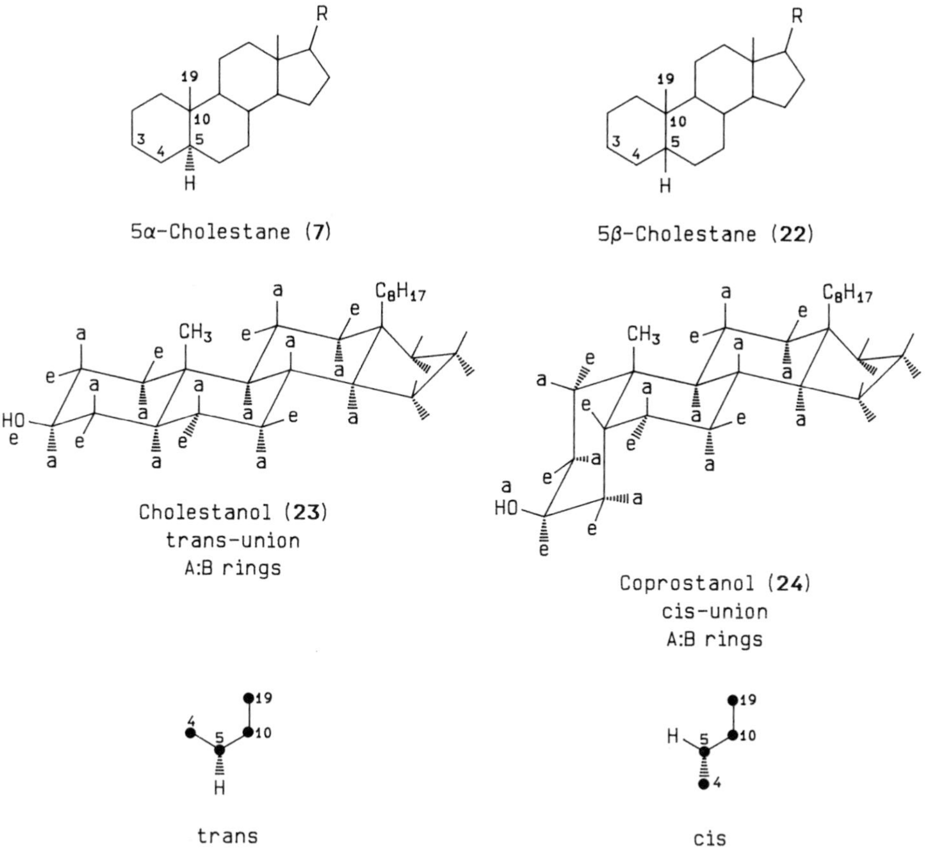

5α-Cholestane (7)

5β-Cholestane (22)

Cholestanol (23)
trans-union
A:B rings

Coprostanol (24)
cis-union
A:B rings

trans

cis

Figure 2-5. Structural relationships resulting from cis or trans A:B ring fusion in two typical steroids. In 5α-cholestane and cholestanol the A:B ring fusion is trans while in 5β-cholestane and coprostanol the A:B ring fusion is cis. The orientation of substituents around carbon-5 for the cis and trans circumstances are illustrated in the bottom row (●—● indicate carbon–carbon bonds).

on carbon-5 are on the same side of the A:B ring fusion, this is denoted *cis* fusion. In the instance of cis fusion of the A:B rings, the steroid structure can no longer be drawn in one plane (as in **24**); thus, in all 5β steroid structures which have cis fusion between rings A:B, the A ring is bent into a second plane which is approximately at right angles to the B:C:D rings (see **24** of Fig. 2-5). Although there are two families of naturally occurring steroids with either cis or trans fusion of the A:B rings, it is known that the ring fusions of B:C and C:D in virtually all naturally occurring steroids are trans. Thus, each of the ring junction

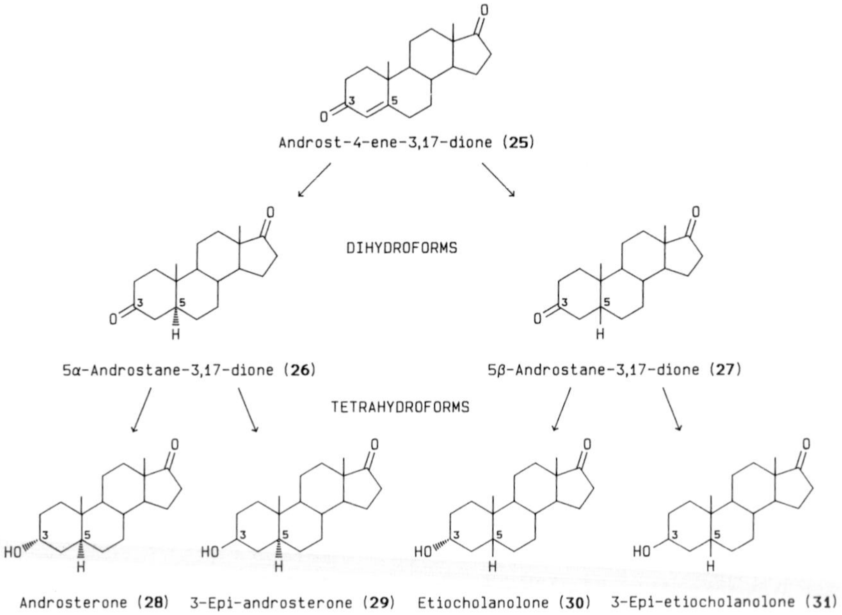

Androst-4-ene-3,17-dione **(25)**

DIHYDROFORMS

5α-Androstane-3,17-dione **(26)**   5β-Androstane-3,17-dione **(27)**

TETRAHYDROFORMS

Androsterone **(28)**   3-Epi-androsterone **(29)**   Etiocholanolone **(30)**   3-Epi-etiocholanolone **(31)**

Figure 2-6. Structural isomers derived by reduction of the $\triangle^{4,5}$ double bond and the 3-oxo function of androst-4-ene-3,17-dione.

carbons is potentially asymmetric and the naturally occurring steroid will have only one of the two possible orientations at each ring junction.

In the estrogen steroid series in which the A ring is aromatic, there is no cis–trans isomerism possible at carbon-5 and -10. Also, as will become apparent upon consideration of the metabolism of many of the steroids that contain a 4-ene-3-one structure in ring A (see **12–15**, Fig. 2-3) a family of structural isomers may be produced. Thus, when biological reduction of the 4-ene occurs, two dihydro products will arise, one with A:B cis and one with A:B trans fusion. A further two steroids will be generated by reduction of the 3-oxo group, giving rise to a total of four possible tetrahydro products of the 3-oxo-4-ene. Under normal biological circumstances, all four structural isomers can be detected. These relationships are summarized in Fig. 2-6 for the male sex steroid androst-4-ene-3,17-dione.

The side chain is a third domain of the steroid structure where asymmetry considerations are important. Historically, interest first centered on carbon-20 of the cholesterol side chain, although side chain asymmetry is also now known to be crucial for ecdysterone, for a number of vitamin D metabolites, as well as in the production of many bile acids. While the α, β notation is satisfactory for designation of substituents on the A, B, C, and D ring structure, this terminology is not applicable to the side chain. This is because there is free rotation of the side chain at the carbon-17, carbon-20 bond, and thus the side chain may assume a number of orientations in relation to the ring structure.

The chemical determination and designation of the absolute configuration of asymmetric carbon atoms on the side chain according to formal rules of nomenclature is complex. The "sequence rules" of Cahn* must be applied. These rules describe operational procedures to generate an unambiguous nomenclature specification of the absolute configuration of all chemical compounds whether they be steroids, sugars, amino acids, thiopolymers, etc. A detailed consideration of these rules is beyond the scope of this book; however, a brief consideration applicable to the steroid side chain is now given.

Asymmetric carbon atoms joined to four different substituents can be designated as $C_{a,b,c,d}$. Application of the sequence rule requires determination of the a, b, c, and d groups joined to the carbon atom under consideration. The steps of application of the sequence rule are summarized in the following:

1. The determination of priority is first based on the atomic weights of the four atoms attached to the asymmetric carbon, with higher atomic weights having priority over lower atomic weights (e.g., $^{16}O > {}^{14}C > {}^{12}C > H$). Thus, for asymmetric carbon atom-20 on the cholesterol side chain, the three carbons, 17, 21, and 22, have priority over the hydrogen atom.

2. In instances where identical atoms are bonded to the asymmetric carbon atom (e.g., carbon-17, -21, and -22 to the asymmetric carbon-20 of the steroid side chain), the determination of priority is made by reference to the next atoms in each radical and evaluation of the sum of the atomic weights directly bonded to it. Again the carbon with higher atomic weight claims a higher priority. In some instances it may be necessary to evaluate the substituents on a third atom distal to the asymmetric carbon.

3. The chirality or right- or left-handedness of the asymmetric carbon is determined by visualizing the tetrahedron comprised of the four substituent atoms bonded to the asymmetric carbon. The chirality is determined by looking at the atom with lowest priority (atom d) through the

---

*The sequence rule is described in detail by R. S. Cahn, C. K. Ingold, and V. Prelog, *Angew. Chem. Int. Ed. Engl.* **5**, 385 (1960); a simplified description is given by R. S. Cahn, *J. Chem. Educ.* **41**, 116 (1964).

62

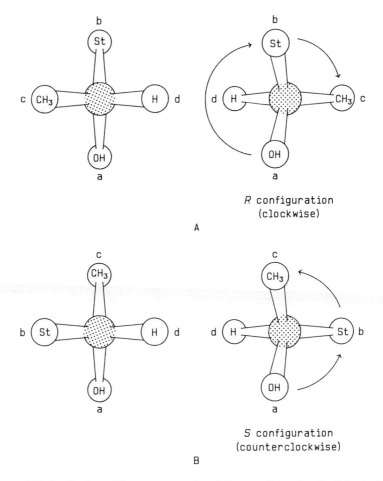

Figure 2-7. Application of the sequence rules of Cahn to determine the *R* (rectus) and *S* (sinister) asymmetry for carbon atoms of the steroid side chain.

center of the opposite triangular face (see example in Fig. 2-7). Thus, the tetrahedron around the asymmetric carbon under consideration should be oriented so that group of lowest priority (d) points away from the viewer. Then if the other three atoms, a, b, and c, are arranged in clockwise order, the asymmetry is designated rectus (*R*) or right or right-handed. Conversely, if the a, b, and c atoms are arranged in counterclockwise order, the asymmetry is designated sinister (*S*) or left-handed. Two examples of the application of the sequence rule are provided in Fig. 2-7.

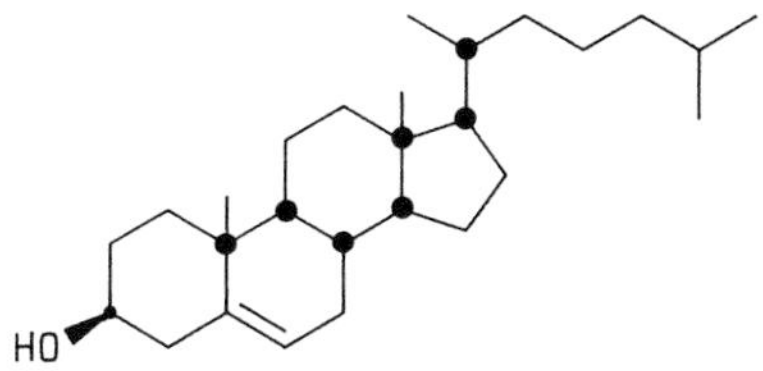

Cholesterol (3)

Figure 2-8. Asymmetric carbons of cholesterol. The asymmetric carbons are indicated by (●). There are 2^8 or 256 isomers of cholesterol.

Figure 2-8 identifies all the asymmetric carbon atoms of cholesterol. In the parent sterane ring structure (6, Fig. 2-2) there are six asymmetric carbons. Introduction of the $\Delta^{5,6}$ double bond deletes one asymmetric center, whereas addition of the 8-carbon side chain adds one asymmetric carbon at position 17. Carbon-20 of the side chain is also asymmetric. Finally, introduction of a hydroxyl group on carbon-3 creates still another asymmetric center. Thus, there are a total of eight asymmetric carbons or $2^8 = 256$ possible structural isomers. Considering that cholesterol is the most prevalent naturally occurring steroid, it is an impressive testament to evolutionary events and to the specificity of the many enzymes involved in the biosynthesis of cholesterol that only one major sterol product is present in mammalian systems.

E. Conformation of Steroids

The steroid nucleus, sterane, is composed of three cyclohexane rings and one cyclopentane ring. The six carbon atoms of a cyclohexane ring are not rigidly fixed in space but are capable of interchanging through turning and twisting between several structural arrangements in space called conformations. The two principal conformations of a cyclohexane ring are the chair (32) and boat (33) forms (see Fig. 2-9).

Each of the two substituent groups on the six carbon atoms of the cyclohexane ring may exist either in the general plane of the ring and are designated as equatorial (e) or in a plane perpendicular to the ring plane and are designated as axial (a). For the equatorial bonds, it is possible to superimpose on the equatorial notation an indication of whether they are below (α) or above (β) the general plane of the ring. Cyclohexane is highly conformationally mobile, interchanging between the boat and chair forms many thousands of times per second. The most stable form of the cyclohexane ring is the chair form; in this conformer there is a

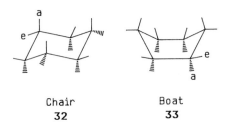

Chair
32

Boat
33

Figure 2-9. Principal conformational representations of cyclohexane.

greater interatomic distance between the equatorial and axial hydrogens than in the boat form. Figure 2-5 illustrates the nature of all the equatorial (e) and axial (a) hydrogens on the cholestane and coprostane ring structures.

As indicated, the B and C rings of both cholestane and coprostane are locked into a chair conformation (see Fig. 2-5). Although in principle the A ring of both these steroids is free to interchange between the boat and chair representations, the chair form is believed to be much more favored. In the case of vitamin D steroids which do not have an intact B ring due to the breakage of the carbon-9, carbon-10 bond (they are termed seco steroids), the A ring is much more conformationally mobile than that of the usual cholesterol-derived steroids (see Chapter 9).

An important point for the reader to consider is that the usual structural representation given for steroids (e.g., see Fig. 2-2, 2-3, and 2-4) provides no clear designation of either the three-dimensional geometry or space-filling aspects of the electron orbitals associated with each atom involved in the formation of the requisite bonds. A comparison for cholestanol is given in Fig. 2-10 of the planar representation (A), planar conformational model (B), a Dreiding three-dimensional model emphasizing bond angles (C), and a Corey–Pauling three-dimensional space-filling model (D). Certainly the space-filling molecular representation most closely approximates the biologically relevant form of the steroid.

The approach of steroid conformational analysis has been of extreme value to the organic chemist as a tool to predict or understand the course of synthetic organic chemical reactions. It is also to be expected that conformational considerations will play an increasingly useful role in the understanding of steroid hormone–receptor interactions. Steroid receptors are known to have very high ligand specificities. It would be surprising therefore if the intimate local structure of the receptor's ligand binding site did not have the capability of distinguishing and discriminating between the various conformational forms of the same steroid hormone.

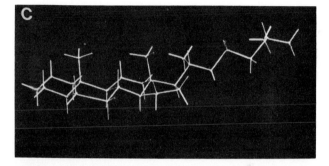

(A)
Cholestanol
5α- or A/B-trans
allo series (stanols)
(34)

(B)
Cholestanol (34)

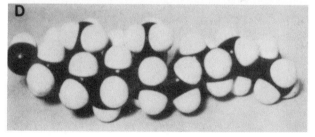

Figure 2-10. Structural representations of cholestanol. (A) Typical two-dimensional structure. (B) Planar conformational model. (C) A Dreiding model emphasizing bond angles and interatomic distances. (D) A Corey–Pauling space-filling model.

F. Other Steroid Structures

Figure 2-11 illustrates the structures of several other biologically significant steroids. Ecdysone (**35**) is the principal insect steroid hormone. Dexamethasone (**36**) is a potent artificial glucocorticoid. The presently employed orally active contraceptive steroids do not contain any naturally occurring estrogens or progestins. Two major classes of synthetic

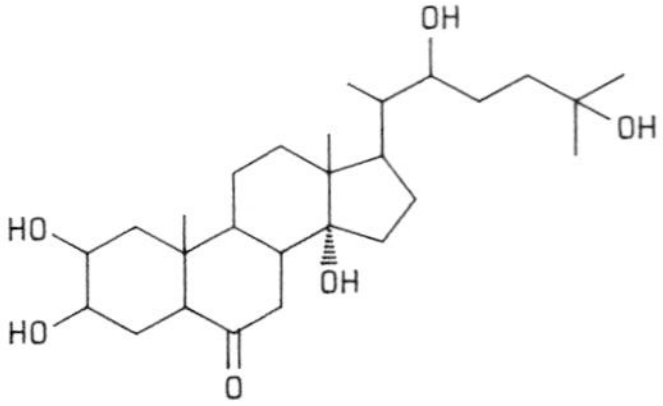

CH$_2$OH
C=O
OH
Prednisone (**38**)

CH$_2$OH
C=O
OH
OH
Triamcinolone (**37**)

CH$_2$OH
C=O
OH
CH$_3$
HO
F
Dexamethasone (**36**)

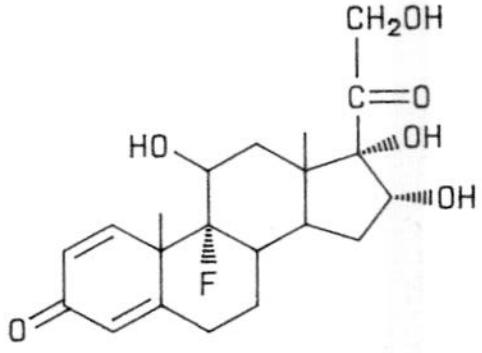

OH
OH
OH
HO
HO
O
Ecdysone (**35**)
(insect hormone)

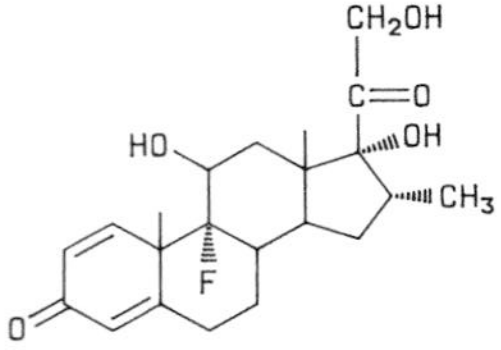

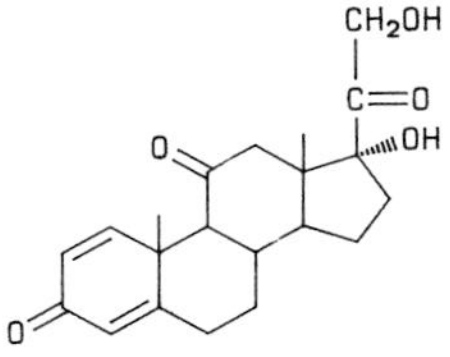

Nonsteroid
estrogenic
compounds

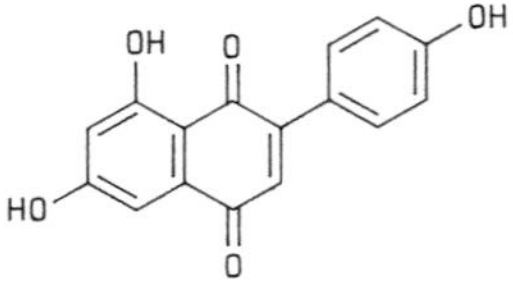

OH
OH
O
O
HO
Genistein (**39**)

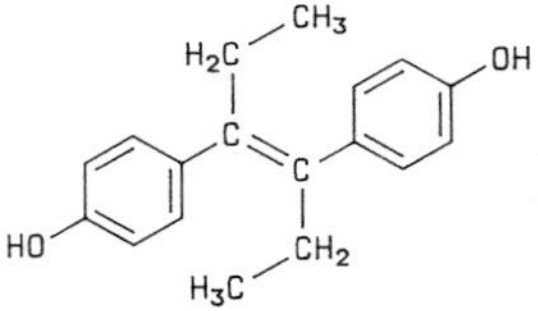

H$_2$C—CH$_3$
CH
CH
H$_3$C—CH$_2$
HO
OH
Hexoestrol (**41**)

H$_2$C—CH$_3$
C=C
H$_3$C—CH$_2$
HO
OH
Diethylstilbestrol (**40**)

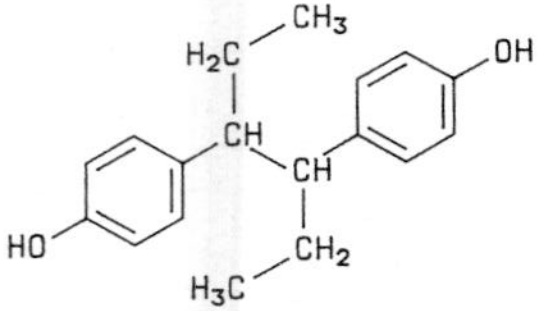

OH
C≡CH
H$_3$CO
Mestranol (**45**)

CH$_2$OH
C=O
OAC
CH$_3$
O
Medroxyprogesterone
acetate (**44**)

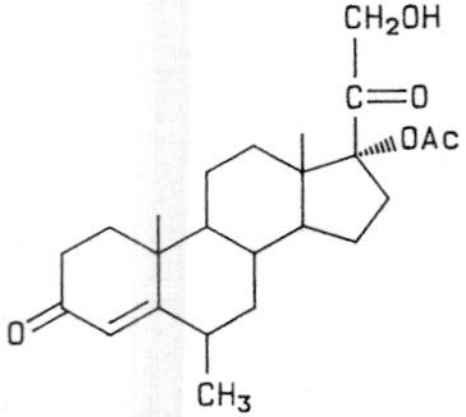

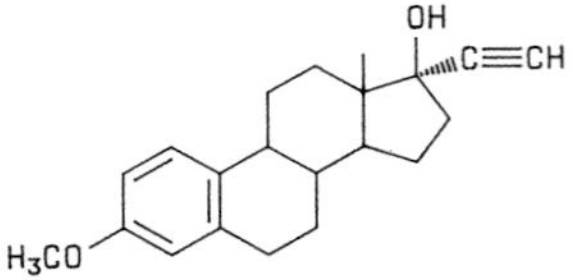

OH
C≡CH
O
Norethynodrel (**43**)

OH
C≡CH
O
Norethindrone (norlutin) (**42**)

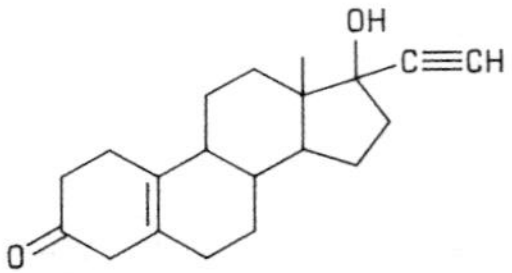

Orally active
contraceptive
steroids

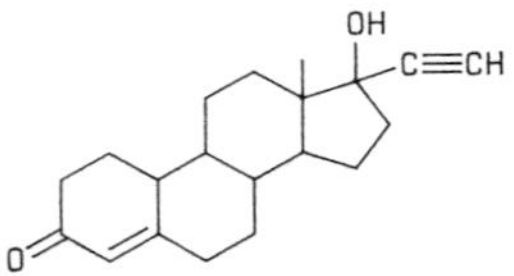

COOH
HO
H
Lithocholic acid (**46**)

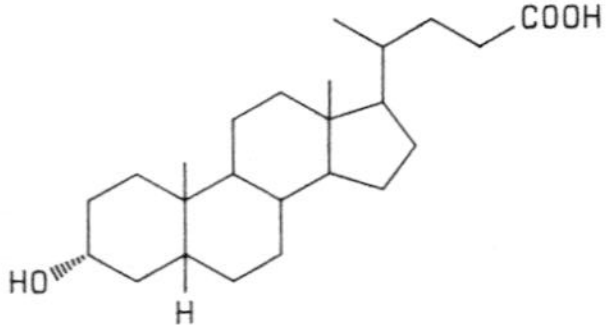

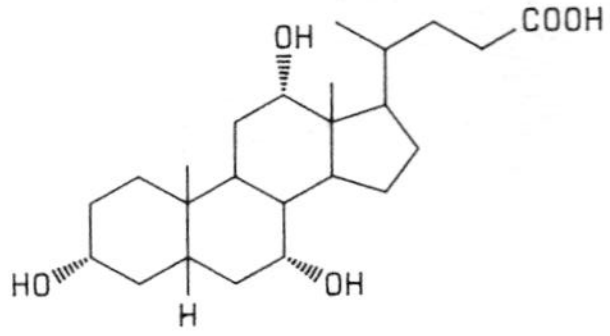

COOH
OH
HO
H
Cholic acid (**47**)

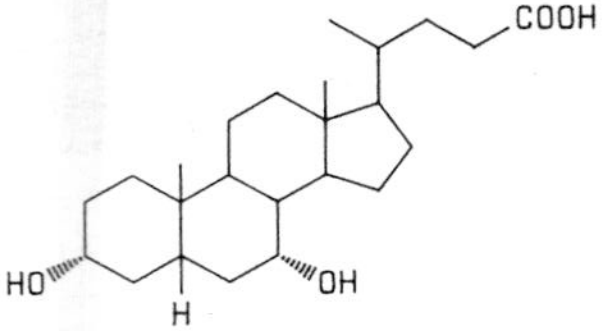

COOH
OH
HO
H
Chenodeoxycholic acid (**48**)

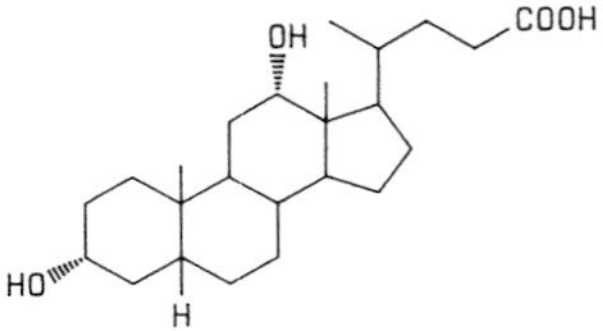

COOH
OH
HO
H
Deoxycholic acid (**49**)

Bile acids

progestins are employed: (1) derivatives of 19-nor-testosterone such as norethindrone (**42**) or norethynodrel (**43**), and (2) derivatives of 17α-actyoxyprogesterone such as medroxyprogesterone acetate (**44**). These progestens are administered in combination with varying doses of two synthetic estrogens—either ethinyl estradiol or ethinyl estradiol-3-methyl ether (**45**). Each of these compounds has an ethinyl group on carbon-17 which enhances their oral activity. The bile acid structures in Fig. 2-11 are those of the principal forms present in man.

III. BIOSYNTHESIS OF CHOLESTEROL

A. General Comments

The most commonly occurring steroid is cholesterol (**3**). Cholesterol is present in practically all living organisms including blue-green algae and bacteria. The levels of cholesterol in plant tissues are low, except in some pollen and seed oil. Animal products are rich sources of cholesterol; cholesterol is present in high concentrations in the myelin sheath and in almost pure form in gallstones. Above-average levels can be found in the skin, sperm cells, and egg yolk. Virtually all cell membranes in higher animals include cholesterol as an integral component.

A range of 180–260 mg of total cholesterol per 100 ml of serum is generally accepted as the normal level for the American adult. Although there is little esterified cholesterol in the peripheral tissues, 70–75% of the cholesterol of plasma is esterified.

Most organisms have an enzymatic capability to biosynthesize cholesterol. Notable exceptions include protozoa, fungi, arthropods, annelids, mollusks, sea urchins, and sharks. However, many organisms will incorporate cholesterol in their cellular membranes if it is provided as a dietary source. In mammalian tissues the principal sites of production of cholesterol are the skin, liver, and intestinal mucosa; measurable biosynthetic activity is also detectable in lung, kidney, adrenals, gonads, muscle, brain, and adipose tissue.

B. Pathway of Production

Because cholesterol is the precursor of the seven classes of steroids summarized in Table 2-1, it is necessary to consider the biosynthetic

---

Figure 2-11. Structures of other biologically significant steroids. Top row: The insect hormone, ecdysone and three synthetic glucocorticoids; second row: nonsteroid estrogenic compounds; third row: orally active contraceptive steroids; bottom row: bile acids.

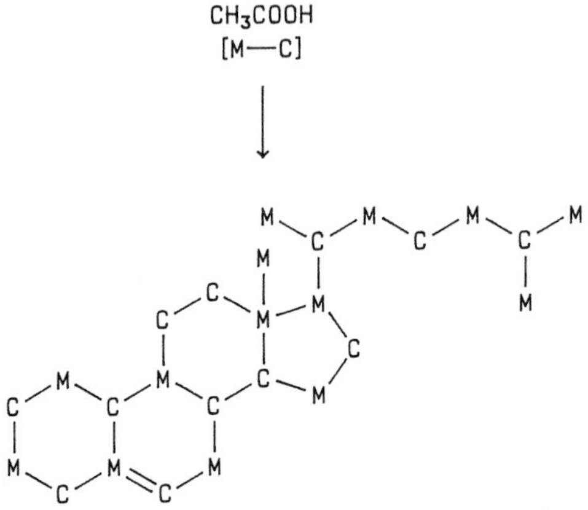

$$CH_3COOH$$
$$[M\!-\!C]$$

Figure 2-12. Source of the carbon atoms of cholesterol. The different carbon atoms are shown to be derived from either the methyl (M) carbon atom or the carboxyl (C) group of acetate.

pathway of production of cholesterol. The pioneering work of R. Scho-enheimer, D. R. Rittenburg, and K. Bloch established that all 27 carbons of cholesterol are derived from acetate. In this remarkable biosynthetic process, 18 molecules of acetate are processed by at least 27 enzymes to produce the final product, cholesterol. The source of all the carbon atoms of cholesterol in relation to the carboxyl and methyl carbons of the starting acetate is given in Fig. 2-12.

The overall biosynthetic pathway of cholesterol can be subdivided into four steps: (1) the formation of mevalonic acid (6 carbons) from three molecules of acetate; (2) the conversion of six molecules of mevalo-nic acid through a series of phosphorylated intermediates into the hy-drocarbon squalene (30 carbons); (3) the oxidation and cyclization of squalene into lanosterol, the first cyclic sterol precursor; and (4) the processing of lanosterol (to remove three methyl groups and rearrange-ment of double bonds) to yield cholesterol (27 carbons).

These steps are outlined in the following section.

1. Conversion of Acetate to Mevalonate

As summarized in Fig. 2-13, mevalonic acid is derived by the conden-sation of three molecules of acetyl-CoA which pass through the key intermediate of 3-hydroxy-3-methylglutaryl-CoA (HMG-CoA). This lat-ter compound is reduced by NADPH to yield mevalonic acid. As will be discussed later, the enzyme HMG-CoA-reductase is an important con-trol point in regulating the biosynthesis of cholesterol. Once the prod-

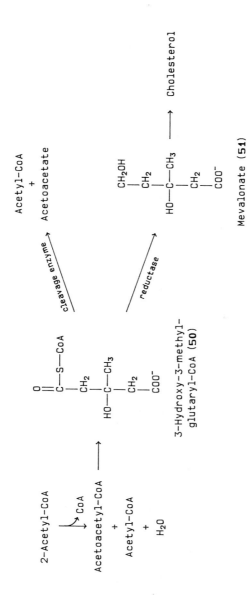

Figure 2-13. Biosynthesis of 3-hydroxy-3-methylglutaryl-CoA and indication of its metabolic fates.

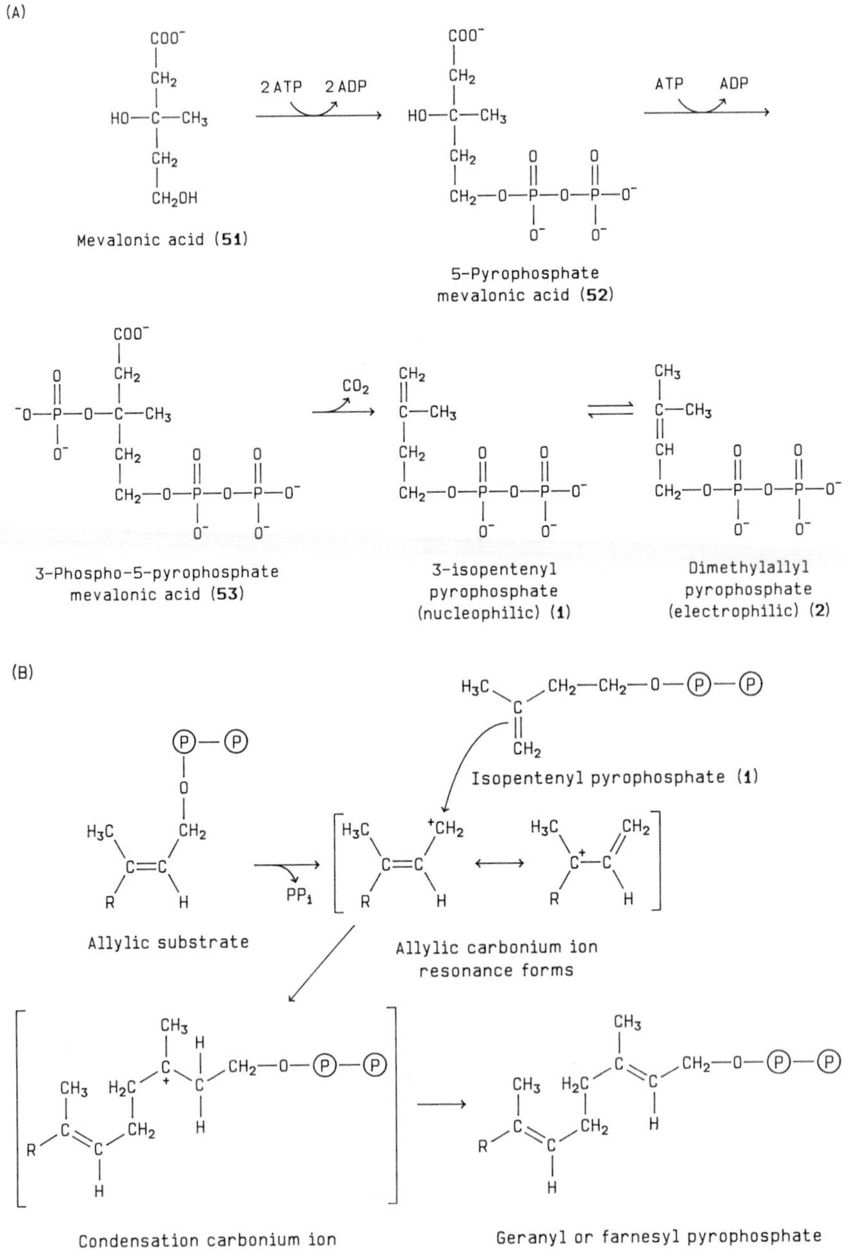

(A)

COO^-
|
CH_2
|
$HO-C-CH_3$ $\xrightarrow{\text{2 ATP} \quad \text{2 ADP}}$
|
CH_2
|
CH_2OH

Mevalonic acid (51)

COO^-
|
CH_2
|
$HO-C-CH_3$ $\xrightarrow{\text{ATP} \quad \text{ADP}}$
|
CH_2 O   O
| ‖   ‖
$CH_2-O-P-O-P-O^-$
           | |
           O^- O^-

5-Pyrophosphate
mevalonic acid (52)

COO^-
|
O CH_2
‖ |
$^-O-P-O-C-CH_3$ $\xrightarrow{CO_2}$
   | |
   O^- CH_2 O   O
              | ‖   ‖
              $CH_2-O-P-O-P-O^-$
                         | |
                         O^- O^-

3-Phospho-5-pyrophosphate
mevalonic acid (53)

CH_2
‖
$C-CH_3$
|
CH_2 O   O $\rightleftharpoons$
| ‖   ‖
$CH_2-O-P-O-P-O^-$
           | |
           O^- O^-

3-isopentenyl
pyrophosphate
(nucleophilic) (1)

CH_3
|
$C-CH_3$
‖
CH
|
$CH_2-O-P-O-P-O^-$
           O   O
           ‖   ‖
           | |
           O^- O^-

Dimethylallyl
pyrophosphate
(electrophilic) (2)

(B)

H_3C $CH_2-CH_2-O-\textcircled{P}-\textcircled{P}$
     \   /
      C
      ‖
      CH_2

Isopentenyl pyrophosphate (1)

$\textcircled{P}-\textcircled{P}$
|
O
|
H_3C CH_2
     \   /
      $C=C$
     /   \
    R H

Allylic substrate

$\xrightarrow{PP_i}$

$\left[\begin{array}{c} H_3C \quad ^+CH_2 \\ \diagdown \diagup \\ C=C \\ \diagup \diagdown \\ R \quad\quad H \end{array} \longleftrightarrow \begin{array}{c} H_3C \quad CH_2 \\ \diagdown \diagup \\ C^+{-}C \\ \diagup \diagdown \\ R \quad\quad H \end{array}\right]$

Allylic carbonium ion
resonance forms

$\left[\begin{array}{c} CH_3 \\ | \quad H \\ C \quad | \\ CH_3 \quad H_2C \diagup ^+{\diagdown} C{-}CH_2-O-\textcircled{P}-\textcircled{P} \\ \diagdown \diagup \quad\quad | \\ C=C \quad CH_2 \quad H \\ \diagup \diagdown \diagup \\ R \quad\quad C \\ | \\ H \end{array}\right]$

$\longrightarrow$

$\begin{array}{c} CH_3 \\ | \\ C{-}CH_2-O-\textcircled{P}-\textcircled{P} \\ CH_3 \quad H_2C \diagup \diagdown \diagup \\ \diagdown \diagup \quad C \quad H \\ C=C \quad \| \\ \diagup \diagdown \quad CH_2 \\ R \quad\quad C \\ | \\ H \end{array}$

Condensation carbonium ion   Geranyl or farnesyl pyrophosphate

Figure 2-14 (A and B). See legend on p. 72.

70

(C)

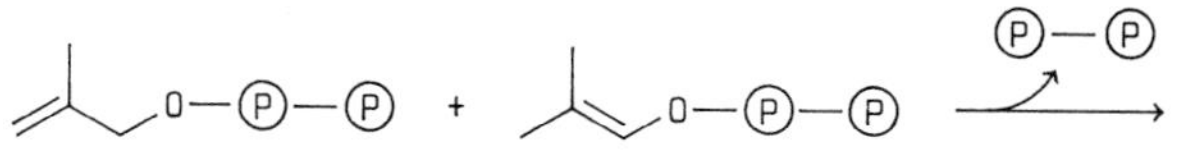

1   2

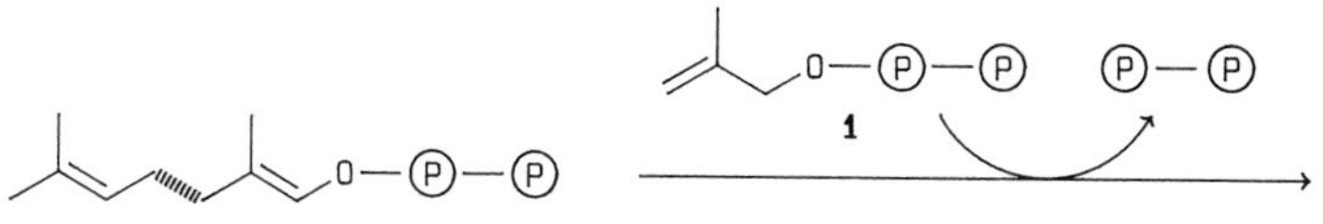

trans-Geranyl pyrophosphate (53A)

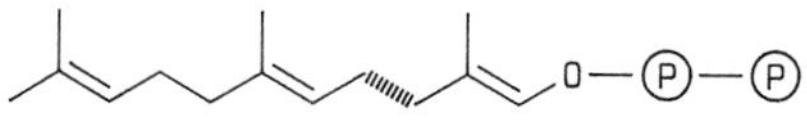

trans-trans-Farnesyl pyrophosphate (54)

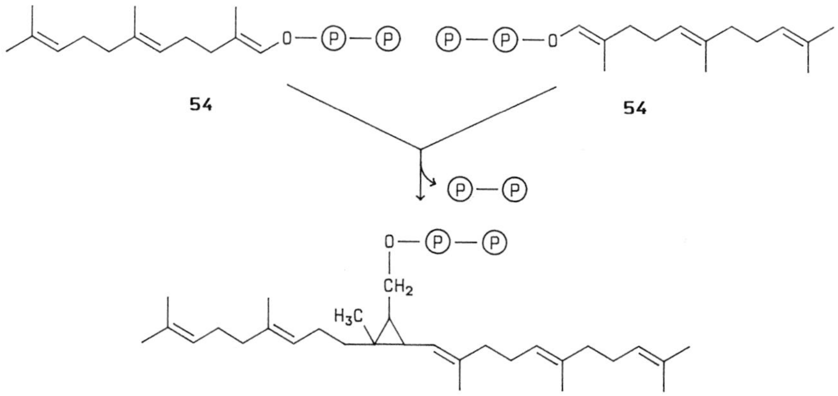

54   54

Presqualene pyrophosphate (55)

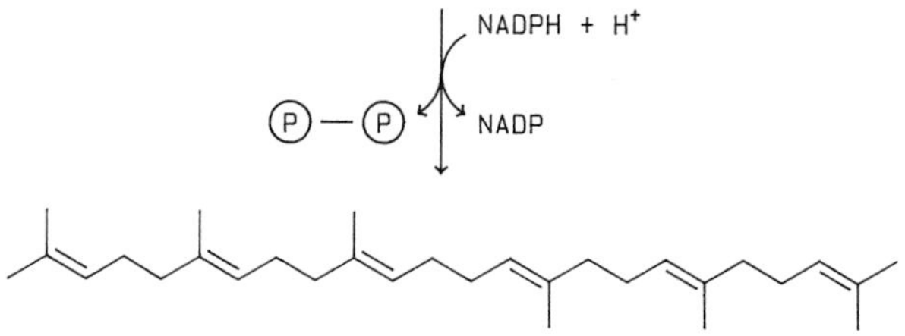

NADPH + H+

NADP

Squalene (56)

Figure 2-14 (C).

71

uct, mevalonic acid, is produced, it is virtually irreversibly committed to conversion to cholesterol.

2. Conversion of Mevalonic Acid into Squalene

Figure 2-14 summarizes the series of steps necessary to convert six molecules of mevalonic acid into the 30-carbon squalene + 6 CO_2. Mevalonic acid is sequentially phosphorylated by 3 mol of ATP and then decarboxylated to yield the key isoprene building block, 3-isopentenyl pyrophosphate. The nucleophilic reagent, isopentenyl pyrophosphate, is then subject to isomerization into the electrophilic (as a consequence of its double-bond position and its esterification with a strong acid) dimethylallyl pyrophosphate. These latter two 5-carbon units are then condensed by a "head-to-tail" mechanism yielding the 10-carbon intermediate geranyl pyrophosphate. Geranyl pyrophosphate is then condensed in a second head-to-tail step with isopentenyl pyrophosphate, yielding the 15-carbon farnesyl pyrophosphate. Finally, two farnesyl pyrophosphate units are reductively condensed in a "nose-to-nose" mechanism to yield first presqualene pyrophosphate (which contains a cyclopropane ring) and then finally, after reduction by NADPH, the symmetric squalene (**56**).

3. Conversion of Squalene into Lanosterol

As summarized in Fig. 2-15, the final steps of cholesterol biosynthesis involve the conversion of squalene into lanosterol. E. E. van Tamelen has chemically synthesized 2, 3-oxidosqualene and studied its spontaneous (nonenzymatic) cyclization into lanosterol. The initial step starts with the reactive species squalene epoxide where the double bond between carbon-6 and -7 attacks the epoxide to form the first ring and generate a carbonium ion at carbon-6. This ion is attacked by the double bond between carbon-10 and -11 to form the second ring and generate a new carbonium ion at carbon-10. This sequence continues until all four rings are formed; this is then followed by migration of the methyl car-

---

Figure 2-14. (A) Conversion of mevalonic acid (**51**) into the intermediate 3-phospho-5-pyrophosphate mevalonic acid (**53**), which is then decarboxylated to yield the nucleophilic 3-isopentenyl pyrophosphate (**1**). Structure (**1**) is then isomerized into equivalent amounts of the electrophilic dimethylallyl pyrophosphate (**2**). (B) A proposed mechanism for the key "head-to-tail" joining of the nucleophilic isopentenyl pyrophosphate to the allylic electrophilic "acceptor," which may be either dimethylallyl pyrophosphate (**2**) or geranyl pyrophosphate (**53A**). P, Phosphate. (C) Pathway of reactions leading from isopentenyl pyrophosphate + dimethylallyl pyrophosphate to squalene (**56**). A key reaction is the "nose-to-nose" reaction of trans-trans-farnesyl pyrophosphate (**54**) to yield presqualene pyrophosphate (**55**) which, after reduction by NADPH, produces squalene (**56**).

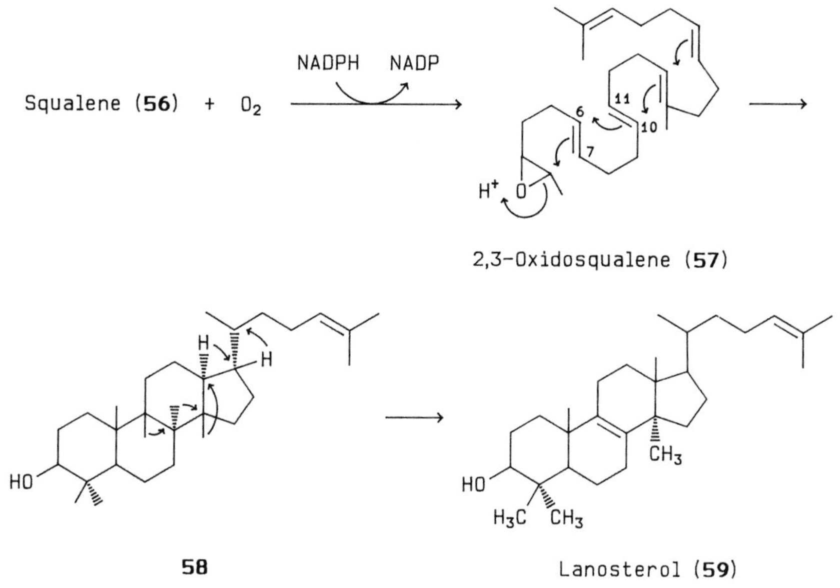

Squalene (56) + O_2 $\xrightarrow{\text{NADPH} \quad \text{NADP}}$

2,3-Oxidosqualene (57)

58

Lanosterol (59)

Figure 2-15. A proposed mechanism for the cyclization of 2,3-oxidosqualene (57) to produce lanosterol (59). This mechanism is postulated from model organic reactions.

bons on carbon-13 and carbon-14 to yield the first steroid product, lanosterol (59).

4. Metabolism of Lanosterol to Cholesterol

Three separate enzyme-catalyzed steps are required to convert lanosterol into cholesterol. These include (1) the oxidative removal of the two methyl groups at carbon-4 and the single methyl at carbon-14 (see Fig. 2-16 for possible mechanisms of demethylation); (2) reduction of the side chain carbon-24 double bond; and (3) movement of the Δ^8 double bond to the Δ^4 position. Many possible intermediates between lanosterol and cholesterol have been detected in homogenates of various animal tissues; this may reflect that there is more than one precise pathway of cholesterol biosynthesis. Figure 2-17 presents one possible route of transformation of lanosterol into cholesterol.

C. Role of Sterol Carrier Protein

The early precursors of sterol biosynthesis are all water soluble, but after the production of squalene the cholesterol precursors become

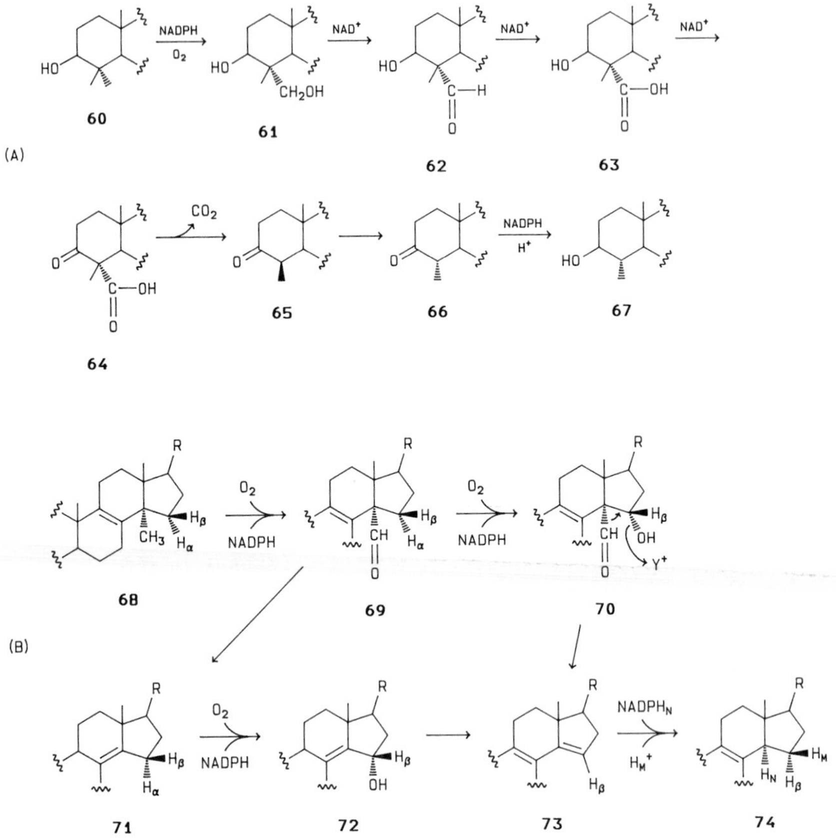

Figure 2-16. Suggested mechanisms for carbon-4 and carbon-14 demethylation of lanosterol. (A) Carbon-4 of the A ring of lanosterol (**60**) has two dimethyl groups which are eliminated in the conversion of lanosterol (**59**) to cholesterol (**3**). Each methyl group on carbon-4 (**60**) is believed to be removed via a separate series of transformations illustrated by (**60**) → → → (**67**). In this sequence, the elimination of a methyl group is preceded by the oxidation of the 3β-hydroxyl to an oxo group and the methyl group to a carboxylic acid, followed by methyl group elimination as CO_2 and reduction of the 3-oxo group to a 3β-alcohol. (B) The methyl group on carbon-14 (**68**) is removed by the series of reactions summarized by (**68**) → → → (**74**). In this instance, the methyl group is believed to be oxidized to an aldehyde followed by its removal as formic acid. H_N, Proton donated from the nucleotide $NADPH_N$; H_M, proton donated from the medium. Modified from a similar figure by L. H. Goad, *in* "Biochemistry of Steroid Hormones" (H. L. J. Makin, ed.), pp. 28–29. Blackwell, Oxford, 1975.

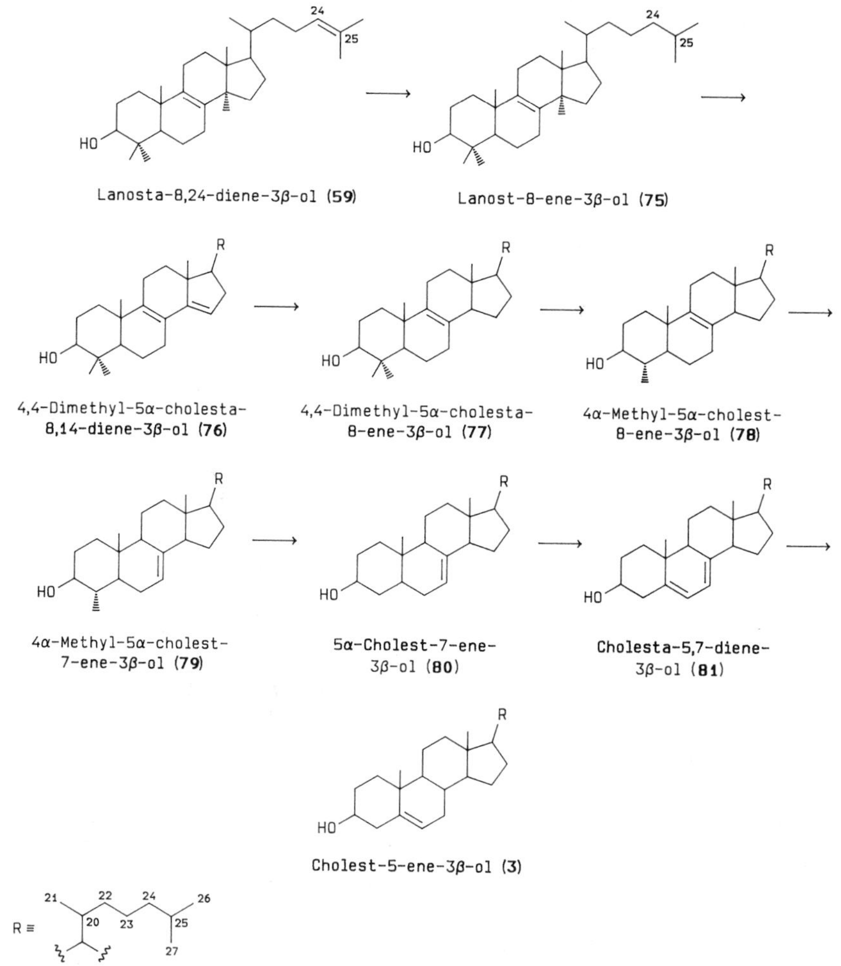

Lanosta-8,24-diene-3β-ol (**59**)   Lanost-8-ene-3β-ol (**75**)

4,4-Dimethyl-5α-cholesta-
8,14-diene-3β-ol (**76**)

4,4-Dimethyl-5α-cholesta-
8-ene-3β-ol (**77**)

4α-Methyl-5α-cholest-
8-ene-3β-ol (**78**)

4α-Methyl-5α-cholest-
7-ene-3β-ol (**79**)

5α-Cholest-7-ene-
3β-ol (**80**)

Cholesta-5,7-diene-
3β-ol (**81**)

Cholest-5-ene-3β-ol (**3**)

$R \equiv$

Figure 2-17. One possible pathway for conversion of lanosta-8,24-diene-3β-ol (lanosterol) (**59**) into cholesterol (**3**).

markedly water insoluble. The activity of the microsomal enzymes between squalene and cholesterol has been found to be stimulated by the
addition of a 105,000 g soluble supernatant protein. This protein has
been isolated, purified, characterized, and named sterol carrier protein
(SCP). SCP proteins are heat stable, with molecular weights in the range
of 16,000.

To date, three sterol carrier proteins have been isolated. SCP_1 enhances the conversion of squalene, but not cholesta-4,7-diene-3β-ol (7-dehydrocholesterol) to cholesterol. SCP_2 is active in the conversion of 7-dehydrocholesterol to cholesterol, but is inactive with squalene. SCP_3 is required for the conversion of 4,4-dimethylcholest-8-ene-3β-ol to polar precursors of cholesterol.

D. Regulation of Cholesterol Biosynthesis

The level of total body cholesterol is determined by a complex interplay of dietarily available cholesterol, the *de novo* synthesis of cholesterol, and the excretion of cholesterol and bile salts. These relationships are summarized in Fig. 2-18.

In an average 70-kg man, ~0.8–1.4 g of cholesterol are turned over per day. The daily ingestion of cholesterol in Western countries is 0.5–2.0 g; the efficiency of intestinal absorption ranges from 30 to 50%. However, it is known that dietary cholesterol is not the exclusive source of the bodily pool of cholesterol. The liver and intestine together account for more than 60% of the body's daily synthesis of this sterol. When considering the turnover of body cholesterol, it has been suggested that there are two principal compartments. Pool A, which comprises 30–35% of the total body cholesterol, consists of the cholesterol in liver, bile, plasma, erythrocytes, and intestine. Pool B constitutes the remaining 65–70% of the exchangeable body cholesterol and is principally comprised of the cholesterol in the skin, adipose tissue, and skeleton.

It is now well established that hepatic cholesterol biosynthesis can be greatly reduced by the feeding of a cholesterol-rich diet. This prevents excessive cholesterol accumulation through feedback mechanisms operative at the level of the HMG-CoA reductase enzyme. HMG-CoA reductase is the rate-limiting step in the conversion of acetate into cholesterol and thus is a logical site for feedback regulation. Dietary cholesterol does not function as an allosteric modulator directly on the HMG-CoA reductase; instead it lowers the steady-state level of the HMG-CoA reductase by decreasing the rate of biosynthesis of the enzyme without affecting its rate of enzyme degradation. Cholesterol SCP also may affect the HMG-CoA reductase by a similar mechanism. The rate of hepatic cholesterol biosynthesis exhibits a marked diurnal variation caused by changes in the level of the HMG-CoA reductase.

A wide variety of hormones and some dietary factors have been shown to modulate the biosynthesis of cholesterol (see Table 2-4). Most of these agents are believed to act through actions on the HMG-CoA reductase. The steady-state level of the HMG-CoA reductase is affected by a complex interplay between insulin, glucagon, triiodothyronine (T_3),

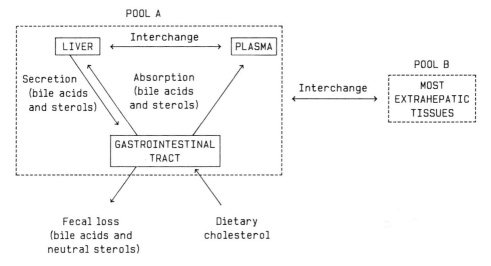

POOL A

Figure 2-18. Diagrammatic representation of body pools of cholesterol. Modified from a similar figure by L. J. Goad, *in* "Biochemistry of Steroid Hormones" (H. L. J. Makin, ed.), p. 34. Blackwell, Oxford, 1975.

and growth hormone. A precise understanding of the mechanisms whereby all these hormones modulate sterol biosynthesis is not yet available, yet these effects certainly emphasize an intriguing interplay between many hormone systems and the production of cholesterol, which is the central precursor of the steroid hormones.

Table 2–4. Factors Influencing Cholesterol Synthesis in the Liver

Decrease synthesis	Increase synthesis
Hypophysectomy	Growth hormone
Diabetes	Insulin
Glucocorticoids	Thyroid hormone
Glucagon	Catecholamines
Estrogen	—
Male	Female
Fasting	Feeding
Low-fat diet	Dietary fat
Cholesterol	Cholestyramine
Bile acids	

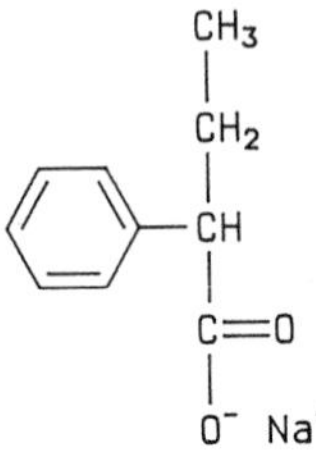

Sodium
2-phenylbutyrate
(**82**)

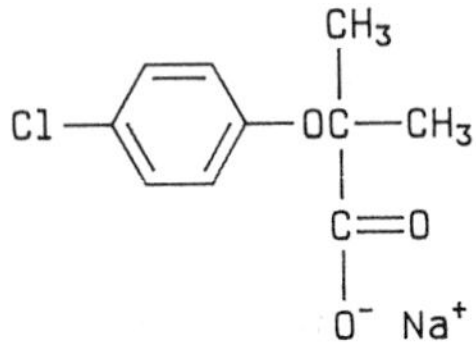

Sodium
p-chlorophenoxy-
isobutyrate
(**83**)

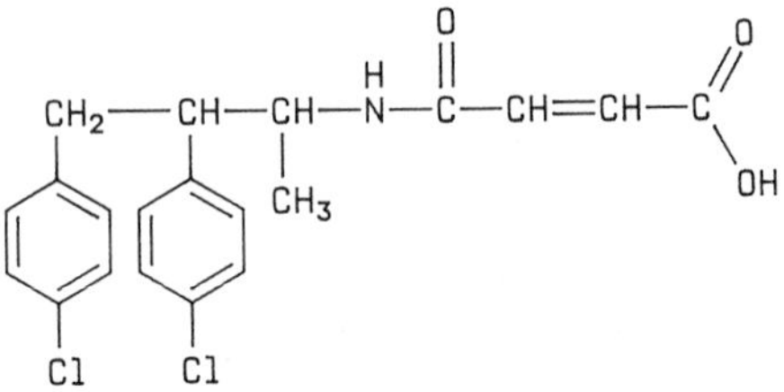

Benzmalacene (**84**)

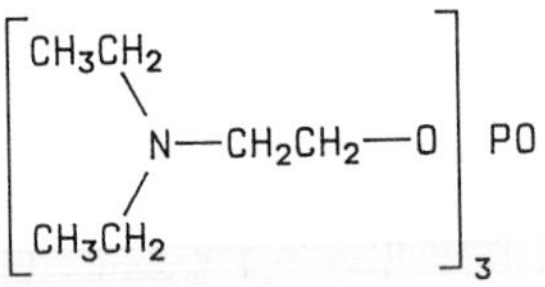

SKF-7997 (**85**)

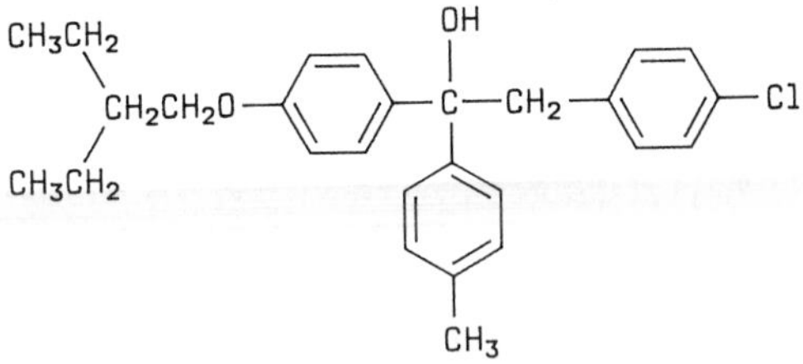

MER-29 (**86**)

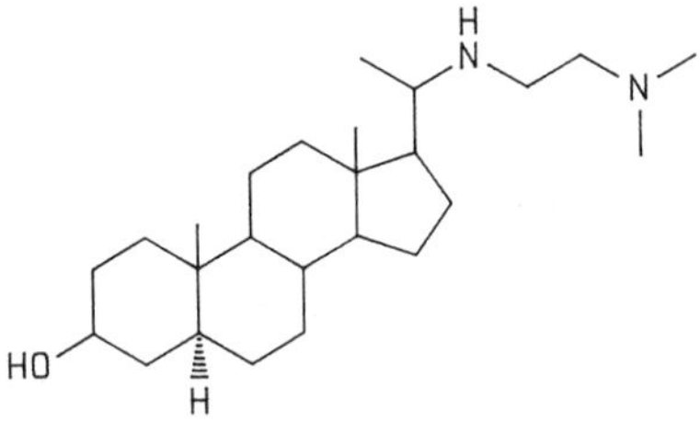

22,25-Diazacholestanol (**87**)

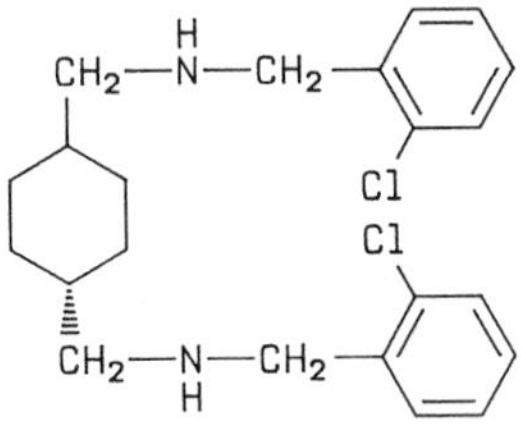

AY-9944 (**88**)

Figure 2-19. Inhibitors of cholesterol biosynthesis.

E. Inhibitors of Cholesterol Biosynthesis

Figure 2-19 presents the structures of some known inhibitors of cholesterol metabolism. These compounds have been developed in an effort to control clinically the biosynthesis of cholesterol, particularly in hypercholesterolemia, which is a familial disorder of lipid metabolism.

Sodium 2-phenylbutyrate (compound **82**) and sodium-*p*-chlorophen-oxyisobutyrate or clofibrate (compound **83**) are both aryl-substituted short-chain fatty acids which interfere with the acylation of coenzyme A and block the initiation of cholesterol synthesis. Benzmalacene (**84**) blocks sterol synthesis somewhere between isopentenyl pyrophosphate and farnesyl pyrophosphate. Analogs of tris(2-diethylaminoethyl)phosphate-trihydrochloride, such as SKF-7997 (**85**), effectively block the cyclization of the 2,3 epoxide of squalene. Both MER-29 (**86**) and 22,25-diazacholestanol (**87**) block the reduction of desmosterol to cholesterol while AY-9944 (**88**) blocks the conversion of 7-dehydrocholesterol to cholesterol.

IV. BIOSYNTHESIS OF STEROIDS

A. Introduction

The principal tissues of synthesis of the five classes of steroid hormones (estrogens, androgens, progestins, glucocorticoids, and mineralocorticoids) are the adrenal cortex, ovaries, and testes. Also during pregnancy, the fetal–placental unit can serve as a source of estrogen and some other hormones. The sites of synthesis of the sixth class of steroid hormones, those derived from vitamin D, are the skin, liver, and kidney (see Section IV,E). The bile acids, which are a seventh important structural class of mammalian steroids, have no known hormonal activity; they are principally synthesized in the liver (see Section IV,F).

Figure 2-20 outlines the general framework of the metabolic pathways which are used to convert cholesterol into these steroid hormones. The purpose of this section is only to review the metabolic pathways by which the six classes of steroid hormones are produced. All discussions of the endocrine systems for each of the steroid hormone classes as well as their biological properties and mode of action are deferred to subsequent chapters in this book.

B. Biosynthesis of Pregnenolone and Progestins

As indicated in Fig. 2-20, the conversion of cholesterol into pregnenolone and then progesterone is a common pathway to the production of five classes of steroids. Figure 2-21 illustrates the various steps involved in the production of progesterone.

The principal progestational steroid in man is progesterone. It is produced by both the corpus luteum of the ovary and the placenta. The physiological actions of progesterone will be described in Chapter 13.

(A)

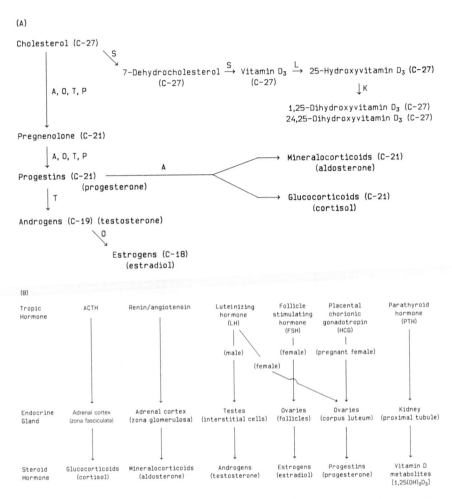

Cholesterol (C-27)

7-Dehydrocholesterol $\xrightarrow{S}$ Vitamin D$_3$ $\xrightarrow{L}$ 25-Hydroxyvitamin D$_3$ (C-27)
(C-27)　　　　　(C-27)

$\downarrow$ K

1,25-Dihydroxyvitamin D$_3$ (C-27)
24,25-Dihydroxyvitamin D$_3$ (C-27)

A, O, T, P

Pregnenolone (C-21)

A, O, T, P

Progestins (C-21)　　　　　　A

(progesterone)

Mineralocorticoids (C-21)
(aldosterone)

Glucocorticoids (C-21)
(cortisol)

T

Androgens (C-19) (testosterone)

O

Estrogens (C-18)
(estradiol)

(B)

Tropic Hormone	ACTH	Renin/angiotensin	Luteinizing hormone (LH)	Follicle stimulating hormone (FSH)	Placental chorionic gonadotropin (HCG)	Parathyroid hormone (PTH)
			(male)	(female)	(pregnant female)	
			(female)			
Endocrine Gland	Adrenal cortex (zona fasciculata)	Adrenal cortex (zona glomerulosa)	Testes (interstitial cells)	Ovaries (follicles)	Ovaries (corpus luteum)	Kidney (proximal tubule)
Steroid Hormone	Glucocorticoids (cortisol)	Mineralocorticoids (aldosterone)	Androgens (testosterone)	Estrogens (estradiol)	Progestins (progesterone)	Vitamin D metabolites [1,25(OH)$_2$D$_3$]

Figure 2-20. (A) Summary of pathway of biosynthesis of the six classes of mammalian steroid hormones. Numbers in parentheses, e.g., (C-27), indicate the number of carbons of that steroid. A, Adrenals; O, ovaries; T, testes; P, placenta; S, skin; L, liver; K, kidney. (B) Summary of tropic hormones and their endocrine gland(s) as site of production of the indicated active steroid hormones.

C. Biosynthesis of Glucocorticoids and Mineralocorticoids

Over 45 steroids have been isolated and chemically characterized from adrenal gland extracts. The 21-carbon corticosteroids include the gluco-corticoids and the mineralocorticoids; both subclasses are produced by

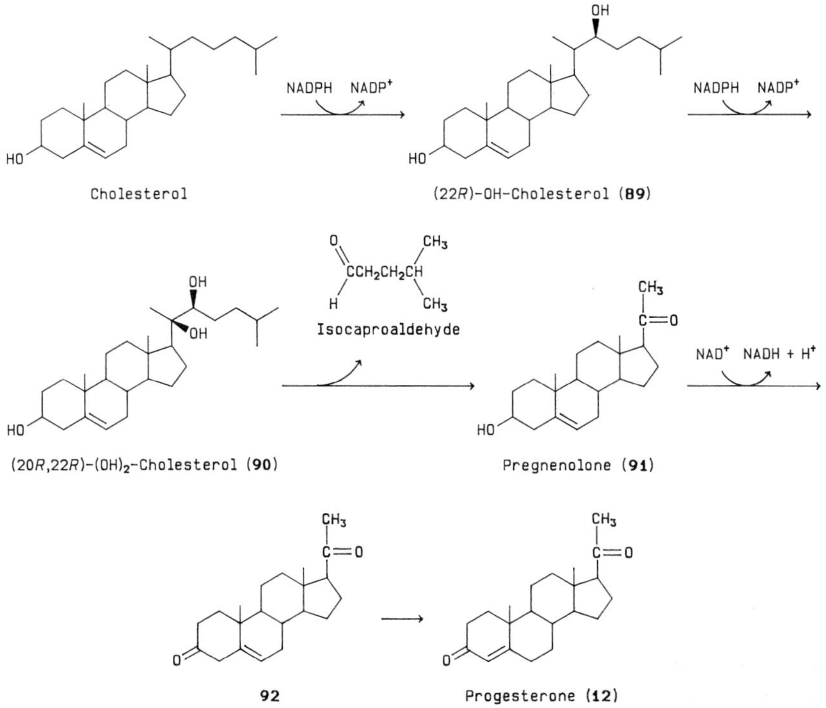

Figure 2-21. Biosynthesis of pregnenolone and progesterone.

the adrenal cortex (see Chapter 10). They are characterized by (1) an oxo group at carbon-3 and a double bond at carbon-4; (2) a 2-carbon side chain on carbon-17; (3) an oxo group at carbon-20 and hydroxyl on carbon-21. Glucocorticoids are characterized by (4) the presence or absence of hydroxyls both at carbon-11 and carbon-17. The principal glucocorticoid in man is cortisol.

Mineralocorticoids are characterized by (5) a hydroxyl at carbon-11, and (6) having carbon-18 oxidized to an aldehyde. The principal mineralocorticoid in man is aldosterone. As a consequence of its carbon-18 aldehyde moiety, it can form a five-membered hemiacetal ring with the carbon-11 hydroxyl or a six-membered hemiacetal with the carbon-21 hydroxyl.

The structures of many corticosteroids and the metabolic pathways for their interconversion are summarized in Fig. 2-22.

As indicated in Fig. 2-20, the adrenal cortex, particularly the *zona reticularis*, also has the enzymatic capability to produce steroids with mild androgenic activity. The principal adrenal androgens are an-

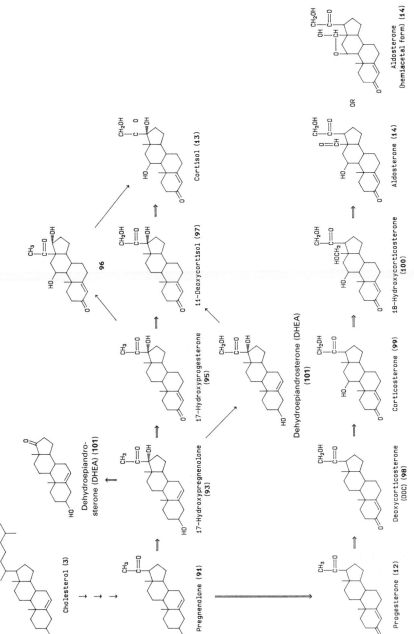

Figure 2-22. Pathways of glucocorticoid, mineralocorticoid, and dehydroepiandrosterone (DHEA) biosynthesis in the adrenal cortex. The boldface arrows indicate the major pathway of biosynthesis of cortisol and aldosterone; however, there is no single exclusive pathway; the alternate possibilities are indicated by regular arrows. Under some circumstances, the androgen DHEA can also be produced by the adrenals (see Chapter 10).

drosterone, 4-androstene-3,17-dione, dehydroepiandrosterone (**101**), and 4-androstene-3β,11β-diol-17-one. The production of these and related steroids may increase in some instances of adrenal tumors; women with such tumors may develop secondary male characteristics, including growth of beards and hirsutism.

D. Biosynthesis of Androgens and Estrogens

The androgens are all carbon-19 steroids. They are produced in the male in the testes and in the female by the ovaries and placenta. Also, as mentioned, the adrenal cortex can under some circumstances produce steroids with weak, but physiologically significant androgen activity. The androgens in man are characterized by (1) absence of the 2-carbon side chain on carbon-17, and (2) presence of an oxygen function on both carbon-3 and carbon-17. The major naturally occurring steroids with androgenic activity (in decreasing order of relative potency) are 5α-dihydrotestosterone (150–200%), testosterone (100%), androstanediol (65%), androst-4-ene-3,17-dione (25%), androsterone (10%), and dehydroepiandrosterone (10%).

Two general metabolic pathways lead from pregnenolone to testosterone; they are, respectively, either the Δ^5 or Δ^4 pathway (see Fig. 2-23). Steroid intermediates on the Δ^5 pathway can be converted to the corresponding steroid on the Δ^4 pathway by oxidation of the 3β-hydroxyl to a (oxo) ketone (3β-steroid dehydrogenase) followed by migration of the double bond from C_{5-6} to C_{4-5} (Δ^5-Δ^4-isomerase).

The hormonally active form of testosterone in the male is believed to be 5α-dihydrotestosterone (5α-DHT). There is evidence for the production of 5α-DHT by the testes, skin, and submaxillary glands, but it is formed especially in androgen target glands such as the prostate. The physiological actions of the androgens will be discussed in Chapter 12.

In the female in the follicular tissue there is evidence for both the Δ^5 and Δ^4 pathways of androgen production (as outlined on Fig. 2-24). Pregnenolone is apparently a more efficient precursor of carbon-19 steroids than progesterone in ovaries without corpora lutea.

In the human adrenal cortex there is also evidence for both the Δ^5 and Δ^4 pathways. However, the principal pathway appears to be a combination of both.

Pregnenolone → 17-α-OH-pregnenolone → 17-α-OH-progesterone → → androst-4-ene-3,17-dione → testosterone

The estrogens are all 18-carbon steroids. They are produced in the female in the ovaries (both the follicle and corpus luteum) and fetal–

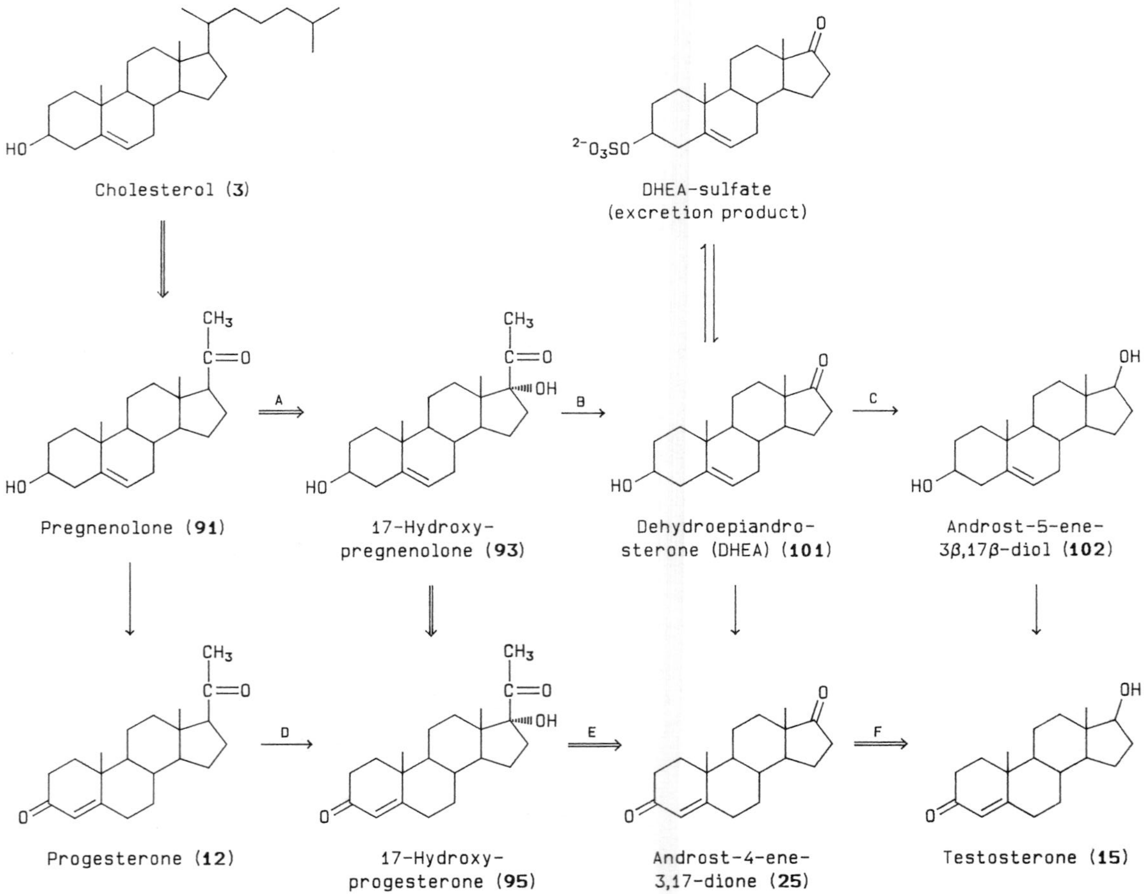

Cholesterol (3)

2^-O_3SO

DHEA-sulfate
(excretion product)

CH_3 C=O

Pregnenolone (91)

HO

CH_3 C=O ''''OH

17-Hydroxy-
pregnenolone (93)

HO

A

B

Dehydroepiandro-
sterone (DHEA) (101)

HO

C

OH

Androst-5-ene-
3β,17β-diol (102)

HO

Testosterone (15)

OH

CH_3 C=O

Progesterone (12)

CH_3 C=O ''''OH

17-Hydroxy-
progesterone (95)

D

E

F

Androst-4-ene-
3,17-dione (25)

placental unit. In males, the testes under some circumstances can produce estradiol. In both males and females the adrenal cortex can generate small quantities of estrone from androst-4-ene-3,17-dione. The estrogens in man are characterized by (1) loss of a carbon-19, (2) an aromatic A ring, (3) absence of the 2-carbon side chain on carbon-17, and (4) presence of an oxygen function at both carbon-3 and carbon-17 and, in the instance of estriol, a third oxygen at carbon-16. Intriguingly, estrogenic activity is not restricted to the steroid structure; compounds such as diethylstilbestrol (see Fig. 2-11) have potent estrogenic activity. The major naturally occurring steroids with estrogenic activity are estra-3,17β-diol (**16**), estra-3,16α,17β-triol (**106**), and estrone (**104**) (see Fig. 2-24).

The several metabolic pathways for the conversion of either androst-4-ene-3,17-dione (**25**) or testosterone (**15**) into estrogens are summarized in Fig. 2-24 (a unique feature of this conversion is the loss of carbon-19).

Pregnancy is characterized in humans by a massive increase in the production of both progesterone and estrogen. In contrast to the nonpregnant woman, the principal active estrogen of pregnancy is estriol. The increase in progesterone production occurs only in the placenta, whereas the production of estriol is dependent on the combined activity of the placenta and the fetal adrenals and liver. These relationships are summarized in Fig. 14-9, 14-10, and 14-11. The important role of the fetal adrenal gland as a source of dehydroepiandrosterone sulfate (DHEA sulfate), which acts as a precursor for the estriol of both the placenta and mother, is discussed in Chapters 10 and 14.

A new chapter of estrogen metabolism has recently been discovered with the appreciation that estradiol-17β may be hydroxylated by brain tissue either carbon-2 or carbon-4 to yield a family of steroids with vicinal phenolic hydroxyl moieties. These steroids are referred to as the catechol estrogens because of their structural similarity in the A ring to the catecholamines, epinephrine, and norepinephrine (see Chapter 11). Figure 2-25 summarizes the known pathways of metabolism for the production and breakdown of the catechol estrogens. It is to be anticipated that the near future shall provide an insight into the biological role of this interesting new class of biological substances.

Figure 2-23. Pathways of androgen biosynthesis in the testis. The pathway of conversion of steroid (**91**) → (**93**) → (**101**) → (**102**) is known as the Δ⁵ pathway, while (**12**) → (**95**) → (**25**) → (**15**) is known as the Δ⁴ pathway. Any steroid on the Δ⁵ pathway may be converted to its corresponding steroid on the Δ⁴ pathway by the sequential action of the two enzymes, the 3β-steroid dehydrogenase and the Δ⁵,Δ⁴ isomerase.

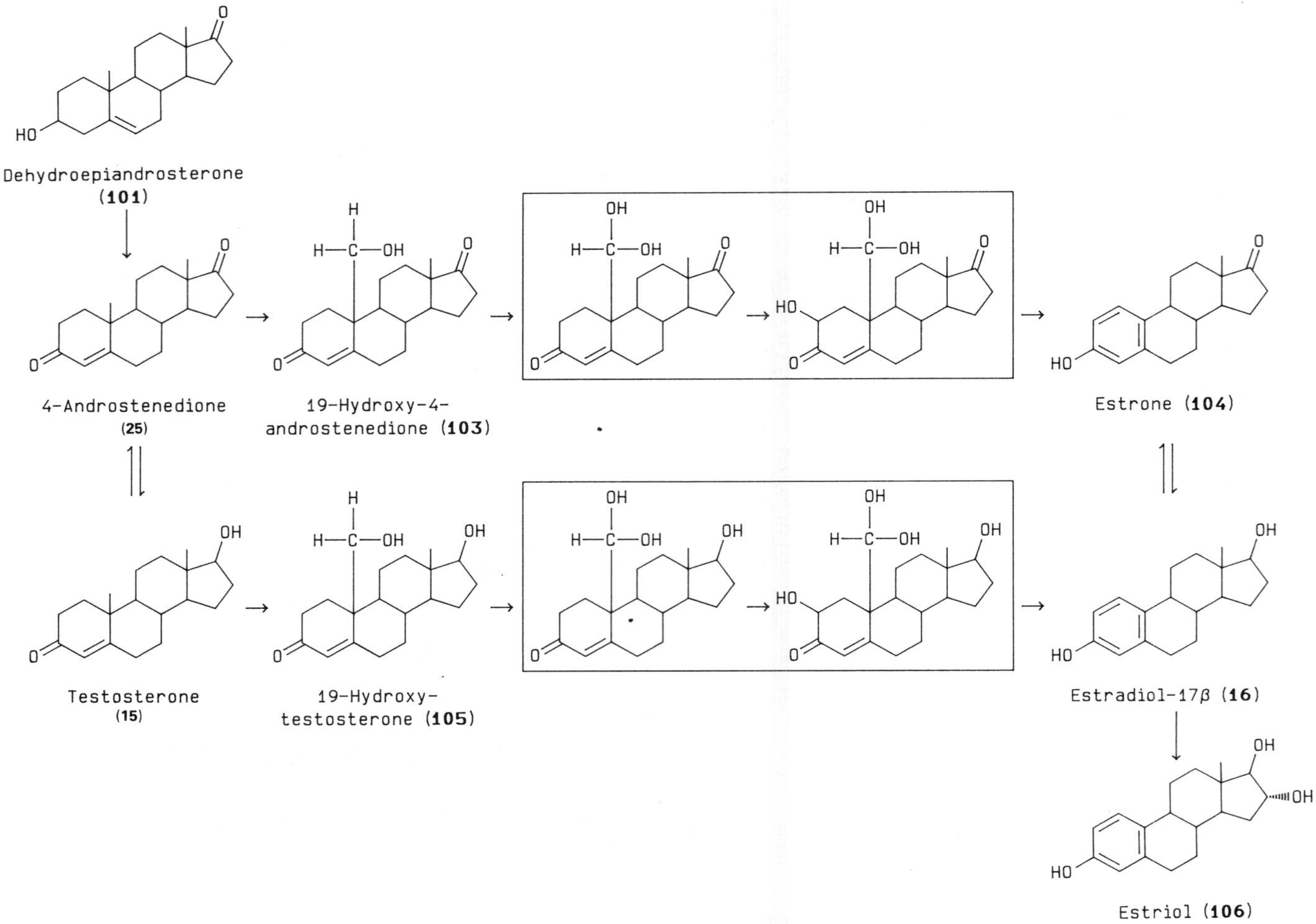

Dehydroepiandrosterone (**101**)

4-Androstenedione (**25**)

19-Hydroxy-4-androstenedione (**103**)

Estrone (**104**)

Testosterone (**15**)

19-Hydroxy-testosterone (**105**)

Estradiol-17β (**16**)

Estriol (**106**)

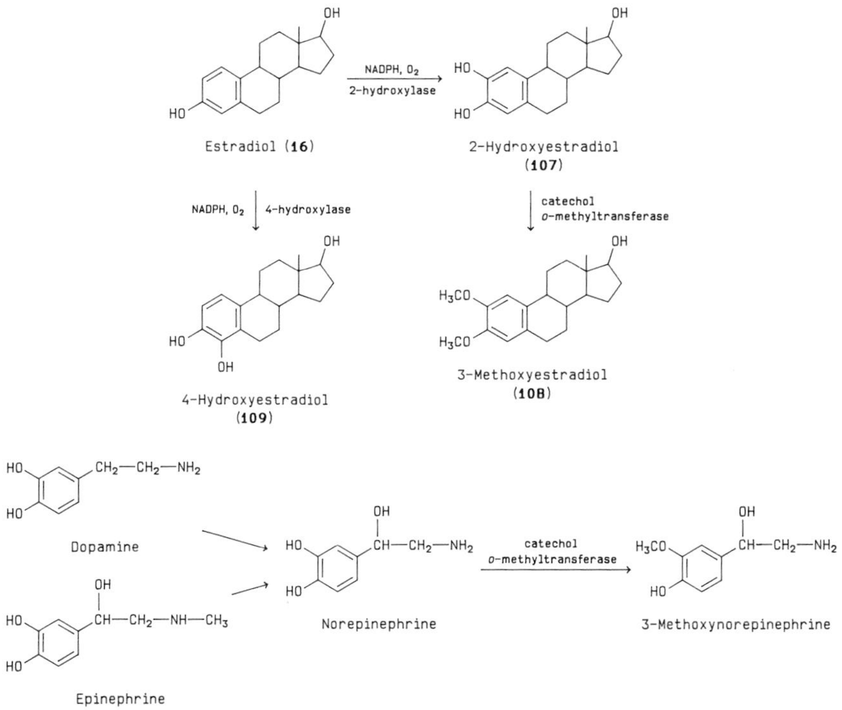

Figure 2-25. Metabolic pathways for biosynthesis of the catechol estrogens (top panel) and their structural similarity to the catecholamines (bottom panel).

E. Biosynthesis of Vitamin D Metabolites

Vitamin D_3 is chemically closely allied to the classical steroid hormones. Technically it is a seco-steroid; that is, due to the breakage of the carbon-9, carbon-10 carbon–carbon bond, the B ring is opened up so that only the A, C, and D rings are intact. As discussed in Chapter 9, there are several families of vitamin D steroids (i.e., vitamin D_2, vitamin D_3, vitamin D_4) which depend on the structure of the seco-steroid side chain. When the side chain is identical to that of cholesterol, then it is naturally occurring and belongs to the vitamin D_3 family.

Vitamin D_3 can be obtained dietarily or be produced photochemically by sunlight from a precursor, 7-dehydrocholesterol, present in the skin.

Figure 2-24. Pathway of estrogen biosynthesis. The structures shown in the boxes have not been unequivocally identified as free, i.e., not bound to the active site of the enzyme(s).

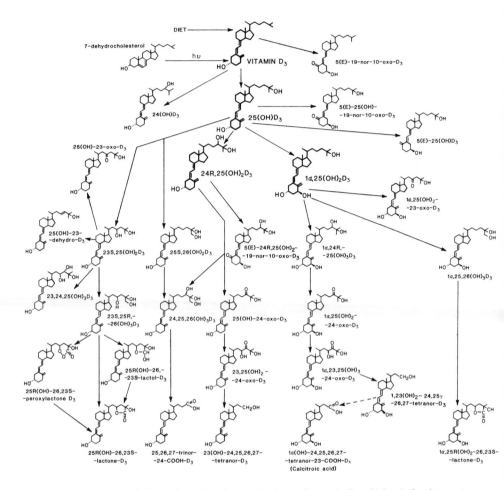

Figure 2-26. Metabolic pathway for the metabolism of vitamin D$_3$ (cholecalciferol) into its daughter metabolites. The seco-steroids presented in boldface are the physiologically relevant vitamin D compounds, while the other structures are believed to be catabolites of vitamin D$_3$ (see Chapter 9).

As documented in Fig. 2-26, vitamin D$_3$ is now known to be metabolized into a family of daughter metabolites. The hormonally active forms which produce the spectrum of biological responses attributable to vitamin D$_3$ are 1,25-dihydroxyvitamin D$_3$ [1,25(OH)$_2$D$_3$] and 24,25-dihydroxyvitamin D$_3$ [24,25(OH)$_2$D$_3$]. The principal form of vitamin D$_3$ present in blood is 25-hydroxyvitamin D$_3$ [25(OH)D$_3$]. The enzymes in the liver which convert vitamin D$_3$ into 25 (OH)D$_3$ are localized in the mitochondria, while the enzymes in the kidney which catalyze the conversion of 25(OH)D$_3$ into 1,25(OH)$_2$D$_3$ or 24,25(OH)$_2$D$_3$ are located in the mitochondria of the proximal kidney tubule. All three enzymes contain cytochrome *P*-450-type mixed-function oxidases. The other metabolites shown in Fig. 2-26 are believed to be catabolites of the hormonally active forms.

F. Biosynthesis of Bile Acids

The conversion of cholesterol into bile acids takes place largely in the liver. In most mammals cholic acid and chenodeoxycholic acid (see Fig. 2-11) are the principal products. Before excretion into the bile, the carbon-24 carboxyl of both steroids is conjugated with the amino group of the amino acids taurine or glycine. A key step in the production of the bile acids is the cleavage of the hydrocarbon side chain between carbon-24 and carbon-25. This occurs not by the lyase-type reactions associated with cholesterol side chain cleavage or production of androst-4-ene-3,17-dione (**25**). Instead the removal of the three terminal carbon atoms is believed to proceed by a β oxidation mechanism similar to that occurring in fatty acid catabolism. Additional key steps involve (1) microsomal-mediated hydroxylations at carbon-7 and carbon-12, (2) epimerization of the 3β-hydroxyl to a 3α orientation, and (3) reduction of the Δ^5 double bond so that the A:B ring junction is cis, as in 5β-cholestane (see Fig. 2-5).

V. PROPERTIES OF ENZYMES INVOLVED IN STEROID METABOLISM

A. Lyases

The two enzymes which respectively catalyze the cleavage of the side chain of cholesterol (to yield pregnenolone) and of 17α-OH-pregnenolone (to yield androst-4-ene-3,17-dione) are known as lyases. Lyases are enzymes which rupture carbon–carbon bonds bearing vicinal hydroxyls. The hydroxylations of these carbons will now be discussed.

B. Enzymes Concerned with Conversion of 5-ene-3β Steroids to 4-ene-3-oxo Steroids

A key enzymatic transformation in the biosynthetic pathway of five steroid hormones is the conversion of the 5-ene-3β hydroxysteroid to a

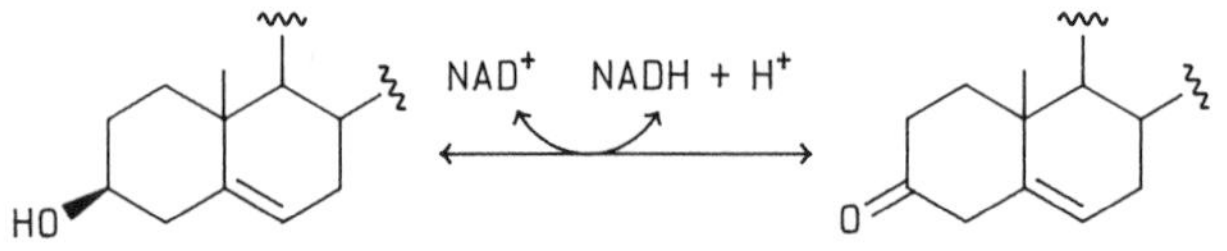

Figure 2-27. Reaction catalyzed by the 3β-hydroxysteroid dehydrogenase.

4-ene-3-oxo steroid. This transformation is mediated successively by a 5-ene-3β-OH-steroid dehydrogenase and Δ^5,Δ^4-steroid isomerase enzymes. Both enzymes are localized in the microsomes of all steroid-metabolizing tissues (i.e., adrenals, ovary, testes, and placenta). Some evidence suggests that these two enzymes may exist as a functional complex.

The 3β-OH-steroid dehydrogenase has as an obligatory cofactor NAD$^+$ and catalyzes the reaction (see Fig. 2-27).

The second reaction is immediately catalyzed by the Δ^5, Δ^4-steroid isomerase. A proposed mechanism is given in Fig. 2-28. The net effect of the enzyme reaction is to effect an intramolecular transfer of the 4β proton to the 6β position, which has the consequence of moving the Δ^5 double bond to the Δ^4 position.

C. Enzymes Associated with A Ring Aromatase

A key feature of estrogens is the presence of an aromatic A ring with a phenolic 3-hydroxyl group. The enzymes required for this transformation which utilize either testosterone or androst-4-ene-3,17-dione as sub-

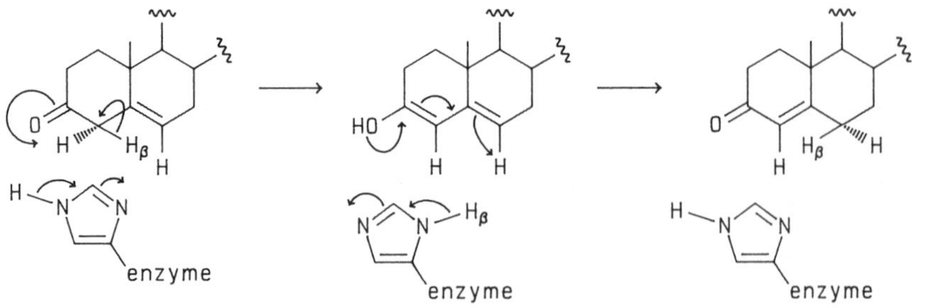

5-Ene-3-oxosteroid   4-Ene-3-oxosteroid

Figure 2-28. Proposed mechanism for the enzyme-mediated Δ^5,Δ^4 isomerase. Reproduced with permission from P. Talalay, *Proc. Int. Cong. Endocrinol. 2nd, 1964* Vol. 2, p. 1096 (1965).

strates occur in the microsomes of the placenta and ovaries and to a limited extent also in brain and adipose tissue; all the enzymes require NADPH and O_2 for activity. Figure 2-24 presents a proposed pathway for A ring aromatization. The accumulated evidence indicates that the biological aromatization steps in the placenta consist of an initial hydroxylation on carbon-19, followed immediately by a second hydroxylation at carbon-19 pro R (likely present either as the carbon-19 gem diol or aldehyde); the third hydroxylation is proposed to occur on carbon-2 with a β orientation. The product of this last hydroxylation then rapidly and spontaneously (nonenzymatically) collapses to yield an aromatic A ring. It is not yet certain whether the products of the first two hydroxylations of carbon-19 are released from the enzyme-catalytic center to give discrete products.

D. Steroid Hydroxylases

Hydroxylation reactions play an important role in the metabolic pathways of many steroids, both those producing hormones as well as those generating bile acids. The cleavage of the cholesterol side chain necessitates the sequential hydroxylation of carbon-22 and carbon-20 while the production of testosterone necessitates hydroxylation at carbon-17.

In the biosynthesis of cortisol three hydroxylases, the 17α, the 21-, and 11β-hydroxylases, are required. In addition, for aldosterone production an 18-hydroxylase and an 18-hydroxydehydrogenase are required. Also, as discussed in Chapter 9, many of the metabolic transformations of vitamin D involve selective addition of hydroxyl groups. All of these seemingly diverse hydroxylase reactions are mediated by a family of homologous enzymes known as the cytochrome *P*-450 hydroxylases. In each hydroxylase enzyme the general reaction catalyzed is as shown in Fig. 2-29.

In principle the oxygen atom of the hydroxyl group could be derived from either H_2O or molecular oxygen. But as indicated in the equation, it is known that the hydroxyl oxygen is derived exclusively in all steroid cytochrome *P*-450-containing hydroxylases from molecular oxygen. As a class these enzymes are designated as "mixed-function" oxidases. The term mixed function indicates that one atom of the diatomic substrate oxygen ends up in the steroid (as part of the hydroxyl) and the other as part of water. This result has been confirmed by utilization of $^{18}O_2$ and the subsequent appearance of ^{18}O in the steroid.

The key family of enzymes mediating the introduction of the oxygen atom into the steroid nucleus are proteins which have at their catalytic center a cytochrome moiety as a prosthetic group. This cytochrome

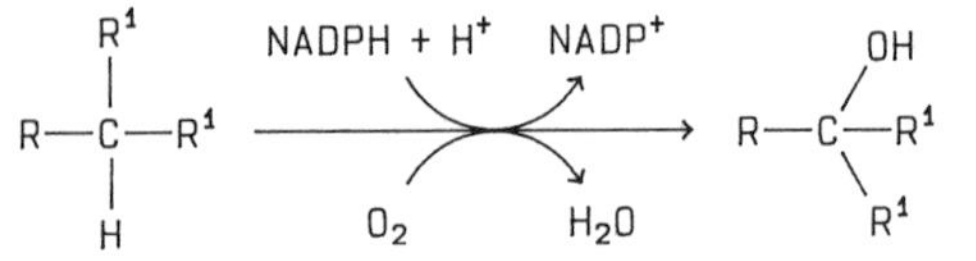

Figure 2-29. General reaction of cytochrome P-450-catalyzed steroid hydroxylases.

moiety is structurally analogous to the hemoprotein cytochromes of the electron transport chain present in mitochondria or hemoglobin; all contain some kind of covalently bound protoporphyrin ring coordinately bound to one atom of iron which can be reversibly oxidized and reduced (Fe^{2+}/Fe^{3+}). Many cytochrome P-450 enzymes have been isolated and purified; their molecular weights are around 50–60K. The terminology P-450 is uniquely characteristic of cytochromes which mediate steroid and other alkyl hydroxylation reactions. As a class, most of these enzymes are subject to inhibition by the presence of carbon monoxide. The CO coordinates to the Fe^{2+} thus blocking the essential cyclical oxidation and reduction which is associated with electron transfer. The P-450 notation is reflective of the fact that this CO binding alters the absorption spectrum of the heme pigment so that it absorbs light with a peak at 450 nm; the inhibition can then be selectively reversed by light with a wavelength of 450 nm. Cytochrome P-450 enzymes are known to be present in the liver, adrenal cortex, ovary, testis, kidney, placenta, lungs, and intestinal mucosa.

The class of reaction catalyzed by the cytochrome P-450 enzymes is one of oxidation/reduction; Fig. 2-29 describes the general reaction.

Virtually all steroid hydroxylases are membrane bound and are present either in the mitochondria or microsomes of the cell. Table 2-5 tabulates the subcellular localization of the cytochrome P-450 steroid hydroxylases. Comparison of the subcellular localization of the various hydroxylase enzymes with the sequence of steroid movement through a metabolic pathway indicates the important role of cellular compartmentalization. Thus, in the conversion of cholesterol into cortisol in the adrenal cortex, the steroid nucleus must move sequentially from the mitochondria (side chain cleavage) to the microsomes (17α and 21 hydroxylation) and then back to the mitochondria (11β hydroxylation).

Depending upon whether the cytochrome P-450-hydroxylase is localized in the mitchondria or microsomes, there are two slightly different electron transport chains which function to transfer a pair of electrons from NADPH to the cytochrome P-450 enzyme. These are presented in Fig. 2-30. In the mitochondrial system there are at least

Table 2–5. Steroid-Transforming Enzymes Requiring Cytochrome *P*-450[a]

Enzyme	Location	Steroid
Lyases		
C-20,22-	Adrenal, testis, corpus luteum, and placenta mitochondria	Pregnenolone
C-17,20-	Adrenal, testis, and ovarian microsomes	Testosterone
C-10,19-	Ovarian and placental microsomes	Estrogens
Hydroxylases		
24R	Kidney mitochondria	$24R,25(OH)_2$-Vitamin D_3
18α	Adrenal glomerulosa mitochondria	Aldosterone
17α	Adrenal, testis microsomes	17α-OH-Progesterone
16α	Testicular microsomes, liver	16α-OH-Testosterone
12α	Liver microsomes	Bile acids
11β	Adrenal mitochondria	Cortisol, corticosterone
7α	Liver microsomes	Bile acids
6β	Liver microsomes	Bile acids
1α	Kidney mitochondria	$1,25(OH)_2$-Vitamin D_3

[a] Only those enzymes for which a definite requirement for cytochrome *P*-450 has been demonstrated are included.

three separate components: (1) a flavoprotein dehydrogenase which accepts the electrons from NADPH; (2) a nonheme iron protein, termed adrenodoxin (molecular weight 13,000), which accepts the electrons from the flavoprotein and transfers them to (3) the cytochrome *P*-450 protein. The microsomal system lacks an adrenodoxin component; thus, the flavoprotein dehydrogenase transfers electrons directly to the cytochrome *P*-450 enzyme.

The most important component of the electron transport chain is the cytochrome *P*-450 protein in that it determines the substrate specificity and dictates the precise site of hydroxylation. It is believed that each hydroxylase has its own cytochrome *P*-450 protein, although there is some emerging evidence that the activity and possible substrate specificity can be modulated through an adenyl cyclase–phosphokinase–phosphatase system which operates on the cytochrome protein.

The process of binding of the substrates, a steroid and molecular O_2, by the cytochrome *P*-450 enzyme complex and transfer of the electrons is complex. The key participant is the hexacoordinate iron ion which is bound to the planar tetrapyrrolic heme prosthetic group. Four of the iron valencies are taken up by binding with the four nitrogen atoms of the tetrapyrrole; the remaining two valencies are utilized to coordinate with other ligands (cysteinate and molecular oxygen) at right angles to the plane of the pyrrole ring structure. The strength or weakness of the

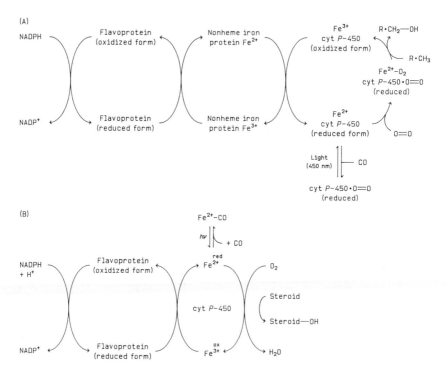

Figure 2-30. Electron transport chains for sterol hydroxylases. (A) Mitochondrial hydroxylases. (B) Microsomal hydroxylases.

bound ligands with respect to the nature of the uncharged or charged moiety bonding to the metal ion can greatly alter the physical properties of the hemoprotein. This alteration has been termed "low-spin" or "high-spin" state. In a weak ligand field the Fe^{2+}–Fe^{3+} complex has 4 or 5 unpaired electrons (high spin, $S = 2$ or $S/2$), whereas in a strong ligand field the unpaired electrons are paired into the lower energy "nonbinding" orbitals, creating the low-spin ($S = 0$ or $1/2$) state. Figure 2-31 presents a scheme for a complex series of steps associated with electron transfer and hydroxylation of steroids.

VI. CATABOLISM AND EXCRETION OF STEROID HORMONES

A. General Comments

The hormonally active form of most steroids is generally the molecular species released from the endocrine gland and transported systemically

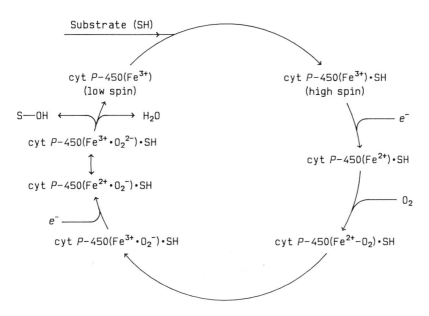

Figure 2-31. Proposed scheme for the cyclic reduction and oxidation of cytochrome *P*-450 in biological hydroxylations. Modified from G. S. Boyd, *in* "Biological Hydroxylation Mechanisms" G. S. Boyd and R. M. S. Smellie, eds.), p. 1. Academic Press, New York, 1973. © 1973 The Biochemical Society, London.

to various distal target tissues. A target tissue is defined as one that has stereospecific receptors permitting accumulation of the steroid in the target tissue against a concentration gradient. This in turn permits generation of the appropriate biological response in that target tissue for the specific steroid in question. Thus, a key determinant of the ability of a target tissue to bind the steroid hormone is the hormone's actual blood concentration. The concentration of a steroid in the plasma at any particular time depends on three factors: (1) the rate at which the steroid is biosynthesized and enters the body pools; (2) the rate at which the steroid is biologically inactivated by catabolism and removed from body pools; and (3) the "tightness" of binding of the steroid to its plasma carrier protein.

Previous sections of this chapter have considered in detail the metabolic pathways of production of many steroid hormones; subsequent chapters will discuss in detail the regulation of steroid metabolism. The remaining section of this chapter will briefly consider general pathways of steroid hormone inactivation and excretion. An extensive discussion of this subject is beyond the scope of this book.

Figure 2-32. Excretion pathways for steroid hormones.

Steroid class	Starting steroid	Inactivation steps	A:B ring junction	Steriod structure representations of excreted product	Principal conjugate present[a]
Progestins	Progesterone	1. Reduction of C-20 2a. Reduction of 4-ene-3-one or 2b. 3β-steriod dehydrogenase	(cis)	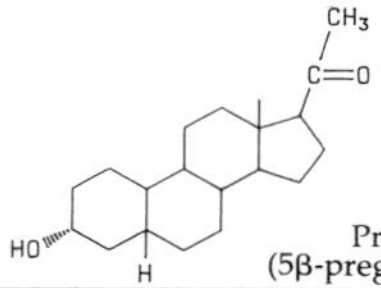 Pregnanediol (5β-pregnane-3α,20-diol)	G[a]
Estrogens	Estradiol	1. Oxidation of 17β-OH 2. Hydroxylation at C-2 with subsequent methylation 3. Further hydroxylation or ketone formation at a variety of positions, e.g., C-6, C-7, C-14, C-15, C-16, C-18		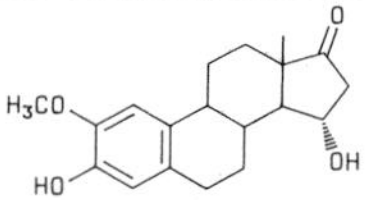 One of many possible compounds	G
Androgens	Testosterone	1. Reduction of 4-ene-3-one 2. Oxidation of C-17 oxo	(cis and trans)	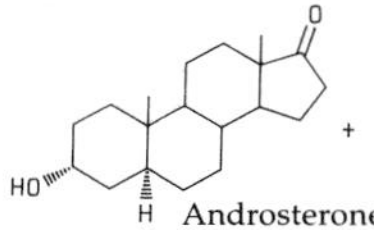 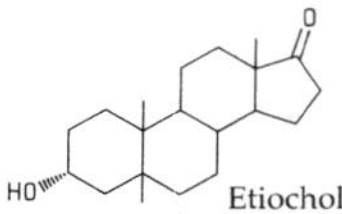 Etiocholanolone + Androsterone	G, S[i]
Glucocorticoids	Cortisol	1. Reduction of 4-ene-3-one 2. Reduction of 20-oxo group 3. Side chain cleavage	(trans)	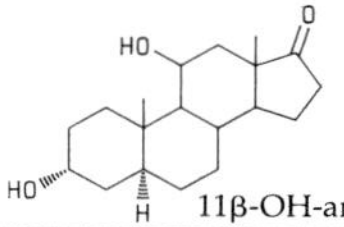 Allo tetrahydrocortisone + 11β-OH-androsterone 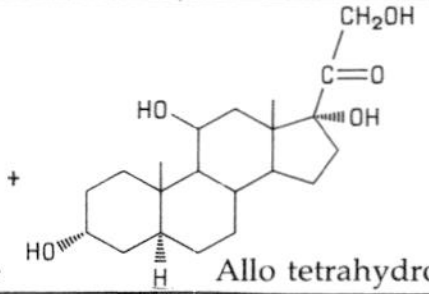	G
Mineralocorticoids	Aldosterone	1. Reduction of 4-ene-3-one	(trans)	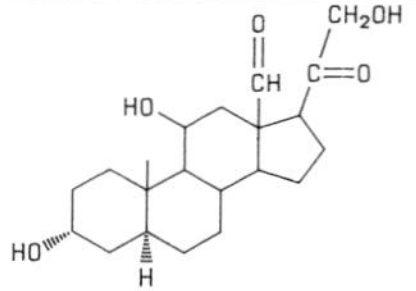 3α,11β,21-(OH)₃-20-oxo-5β-pregnane-18-al	G
Vitamin D metabolites	1,25(OH)₂D₃	1. Side chain cleavage between C-23 and C-24	—	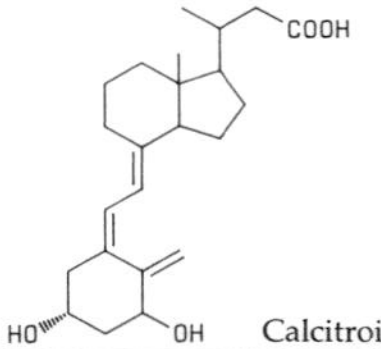 Calcitroic acid	?

B. Inactivation of Steroid Hormones

Steroids are quite hydrophobic compounds and many of the catabolic mechanisms not only inactivate the steroid hormone [i.e., markedly reduce its affinity for its receptor(s)], but also make the molecule more hydrophilic, thereby increasing its water solubility. The catabolic reactions occur mainly although not exclusively in the liver and are reductive in nature. A significant increase in water solubility is effected by conjugation of the steroids with either sulfate or glucuronides; these steroid conjugates are excreted in large quantities in the urine.

Figure 2-32 summarizes for the six classes of steroids some of the major excretory forms of these hormones. The excreted species is a mixture of polyhydroxyl forms and the indicated glucuronide or sulfate. The sulfokinase enzymes have been shown to be present in the cytoplasm of the placenta, testes, adrenal cortex, as well as the liver. These enzymes utilize "active sulfate" or phosphoadenosine phosphosulfate (PAPS) as substrate and catalyze reactions (shown in Fig. 2-33).

The glucuronyl transferases which are localized in the liver microsomes use as a substrate uridinediphosphoglucuronic acid (UDPGA) and catalyze the reaction:

$$UDPGA + sterol \rightarrow steroid\ glucuronide + UDP$$

C. Measurements of Rates of Secretion and Metabolic Clearance

The plasma concentration of a steroid is determined by the balance between biosynthesis and bioinactivation. With the ready availability of radioactively labeled steroids it has been possible to devise techniques of "compartmental" analysis which permit determination of both the secretion rates of steroids as well as their disappearance from the plasma. The interested reader should consult Tait and Horten (1966) for a detailed discussion of these methods.

(a) $SO_4^{2-} + ATP \xrightarrow[\text{sulfurylase}]{\text{ATP}} APS$ (adenosine 5'-phosphate) + pyrophosphate

(b) $APS + ATP \xrightarrow{\text{APS kinase}} PAPS + ADP$

(c) $PAPS + steroid—OH \longrightarrow steroid—O—SO_3^- + H^+ + PAP$ (3',5'-phosphoadenosine)

Figure 2-33. Enzymatic steps involved with the production of "active" sulfate (PAPS).

The metabolic clearance rate of a steroid (MCR) is the rate at which it is irreversibly removed by inactivation. Frequently the MCR for steroids approximates the plasma flow through the liver (~1500 liters/day in man).

Table 2-6 summarizes for a number of important steroid hormones their blood concentration, secretion rate, as well as metabolic clearance rate. These data emphasize the complex interplay between biosynthesis and biodegradation which permit an organism to regulate the blood concentrations of these potent hormonal agents.

Table 2-6. Mean Secretion Rates, Plasma Concentrations, and Metabolic Clearance Rates (MCR) of Various Steroids[a]

Steroid	Secretion rate (mg/day)		Plasma concentration (μg/100 ml)		MCR (liters plasma/day)	
	Men	Women	Men	Women	Men	Women
Cortisol	20	17	12		200	
Deoxycorticosterone (DOC)	0.24	0.5	0.024			
Aldosterone	0.19	0.14	0.0068			1630
Pregnenolone	9				1050	
Progesterone	0.6	2.9	0.03	0.14, 1.05	2920	
Testosterone	6.9	0.35	0.7	0.05	980	760
5α-Dihydrotestosterone (DHT)	0.32	0.075			500	
Androst-4-ene-3,17-dione	1.9	3.4	0.08	0.2	2300	
Dehydroepiandrosterone (DHEA)	3.0	0.7	0.50	0.48	950	
Dehydroepiandrosterone sulfate (DHEA)	15	10				
Estrone	0.11	0.11 (FP)[b] 0.15 (LP)	0.036	0.004 (FP) 0.015 (Ov)	2300	1750
Estrone sulfate	0.077	0.10 (FP)	0.072	0.05 (FP) 0.31 (Ov) 0.22 (LP₂)	167	146
Estradiol-17β	0.06	0.12 (FP) 0.20 (LP)	0.0023	0.003 (FP) 0.057 (Ov) 0.04 (LP₂)	1700	1055

[a] This table was abstracted from H. L. Makin, ed., "Biochemistry of Steroid Hormones." William Clowes & Sons, Ltd., London, 1975.

[b] FP, Follicular phase; Ov, ovulatory peak; LP, luteal phase; LP₂, secondary rise in LP following fall from value at Ov.

References

A. Books

Dorfman, R. I., and Ungar, F. (1965). "Metabolism of Steroid Hormones." Academic Press, New York.

Fieser, L., and Fieser, M. (1959). "Steroids." Van Nostrand-Reinhold, Princeton, New Jersey.

Heftmann, E. (1969). "Steroid Biochemistry." Academic Press, New York.

Makin, H. L., (1975). "Biochemistry of Steroid Hormones." Blackwell, Oxford.

B. Review Articles

Barton, D. H. R., and Cookson, R. C. (1956). Steroid conformational analysis. *Q. Rev., Chem. Soc.* **10,** 44–53.

Bloch, K. (1965). The biological synthesis of cholesterol. *Science* **150,** 19–23.

Brown, M. S., and Goldstein, J. L. (1976). Receptor-mediated control of cholesterol metabolism. *Science* **191,** 150–154.

Dempsey, M. A. (1974). Role of sterol carrier proteins. *Annu. Rev. Biochem.* **43,** 967–990.

Dugan, R. E., and Porter, J. W. (1977). Hormonal regulation of cholesterol synthesis. *In* "Biochemical Actions of Hormones" (G. Litwack, ed.), Vol. 4, pp. 197–247. Academic Press, New York.

New, M. I., and Levine, L. S. (1983). Recent advances in 21-hydroxylase deficiency. *Annu. Rev. Med.* **35,** 649–663.

Popjak, G., and Cornforth, J. W. (1960). The biosynthesis of cholesterol. *Adv. Enzymol.* **22,** 281–335.

IUPAC Rules of Steroid Nomenclature (1972). *Pure Appl. Chem.* **31,** 285–322.

Schroepfer, G. F., Jr. (1982). Sterol biosynthesis. *Annu. Rev. Biochem.* **51,** 555–586.

Simpson, E. R. (1979). Cholesterol side-chain cleavage, cytochrome *P*-450, and the control of steroidogenesis. *Mol. Cell. Endocrinol.* **13,** 213–227.

Siperstein, M. D. (1970). Regulation of cholesterol biosynthesis in normal and malignant tissues. *Curr. Top. Cell Regul.* **2,** 65–100.

Tait, J. F. (1963). The use of isotopic steroids for the measurement of production rates *in vivo. J. Clin. Endocrinol. Metab.* **23,** 1285–1297.

Tait, J. F., and Horton, R. (1966). Steroid compartmental analysis. *In* "Steroid Dynamics" (G. Pincus, J. F. Tait, and T. Nakao, eds.), p. 393. Academic Press, New York.

C. Research Papers

Cahn, R. S., Ingold, C. K., and Prelog, V. (1966). Specification of molecular chirality. *Angew. Chem., Int. Ed. Engl.* **5,** 385–415. (This paper describes the "sequence rule" for determination of *R* vs. *S* asymmetry.)

Caspi, E., Arunachalam, T., and Nelson, P. A. (1983). Biosynthesis of estrogens: The steric mode of the initial C-19 hydroxylation of androgens by human placental aromatase. *J. Am. Chem. Soc.* **105,** 6787–6989.

Caspi, E., Wicha, J., Arunachalam, T., Nelson, P., and Spiteller, G. (1984). Estrogen biosynthesis: Concerning the obligatory intermediacy of 2α-hydroxy-10α-formylandrost-4-ene-3,17-dione. *J. Am. Chem. Soc.* **106,** 7282–7283.

Gil, G., Goldstein, J. L., Slaughter, C. A., and Brown, M. S. (1986). Cytoplasmic 3-hydroxy-3-methylglutaryl coenzyme A synthase from the hamster. I. Isolation and sequencing of the full-length cDNA. *J. Biol. Chem.* **261,** 3710–3716.

Gil, G., Goldstein, J. L., and Slaughter, C. A. (1986). Cytoplasmic 3-hydroxyl-3-methylglutaryl coenzyme A synthase from the hamster. II. Isolation of the gene and characterization of the 5' flanking region. *J. Biol. Chem.* **261,** 3717–3724.

Heyl, B. L., Tyrrell, D. G., and Lambeth, J. D. (1986). Cytochrome *P*-450 substrate interactions. Role of the 3β- and side chain hydroxyls in binding to oxidized and reduced forms of the enzyme. *J. Biol. Chem.* **261,** 2743–2749.

Kellis, J. T., and Vickery, L. E. (1984). Inhibition of estrogen synthetase (aromatase) by 4-cyclohexylaniline. *Endocrinology (Baltimore)* **114,** 2128–2137.

Van Tamelen, E. E., Leopold, E. J., Marason, S. A., and Walspe, H. R. (1982). Action of 2,3-oxidosqualene-lanosterol cyclase on 15-nor-18,19-dihydro-2,3-oxidosqualene. *J. Am. Chem. Soc.* **104,** 6479–6480.

Chapter 3

Hypothalamic Regulating Hormones

I. INTRODUCTION

Releasing hormones are produced in various regions of the hypothalamus. In general, the releasing hormones may be thought of as the linkage between electrical/chemical activity of associated regions of the central nervous system (CNS) (the limbic system) and the beginning of a chemical (hormonal) cascade of messages connecting the hypothalamus, the pituitary, and other organs which secrete the final hormones of the system. Many of these are less than 10 amino acids in length, with short

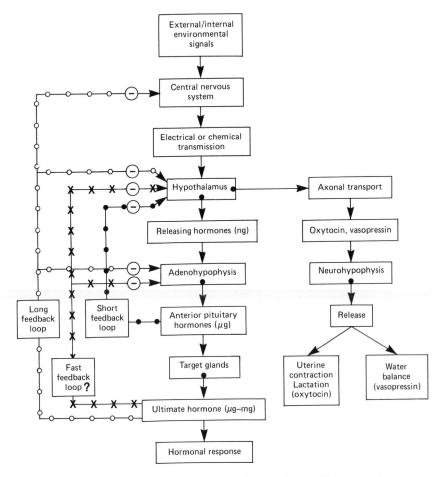

Figure 3-1. Many hormonal systems involve the hypothalamus. This figure shows a cascade of hormonal signals starting with an external or internal environmental signal. This is transmitted first to the central nervous system and may involve components of the limbic system, such as the hippocampus and amygdala. These structures innervate the hypothalamus in a specific region which responds with secretion of a specific releasing hormone, usually in nanogram amounts. Releasing hormones are transported down a closed portal system connecting the hypothalamus and the anterior pituitary. Peptide releasing hormones pass the blood–brain barrier at either end through fenestrations. A specific releasing hormone binds to a specific anterior pituitary cell membrane receptor and causes the secretion of specific anterior pituitary hormones, usually in microgram amounts. These access the general circulation through fenestrated local capillaries and bind to specific target gland receptors. The interactions trigger release of ultimate hormone in microgram to milligram daily amounts which cause the hormonal response by binding to receptors in several target tissues. In effect, this overall system is an amplifying cascade. Releasing

half-lives in serum. Newly characterized releasing hormones have higher molecular weights. A few others may be amino acid derivatives. The final hormones in a cascade bring about the systemic effects associated with hormone action at the level of the whole organism. The pathway of an overall system is pictured in Fig. 3-1.

An external or an internal signal starts the chain of events. An example of an external signal could be a sudden, loud noise which might activate the stress mechanism. An example of an internal signal might be the end of gestation and the beginning of parturition. This process could be started by a "biological clock" mechanism commencing with the release of a specific releasing hormone from the fetal hypothalamus. A subsequent chain of events would culminate in the release of fetal cortisol from the fetal adrenal cortex, the target gland. This ultimate hormone is responsible for a host of actions which lead to contractions of the uterus and expulsion of the fetus.

External or internal signals are often mediated by the limbic system or some other system of the brain and may result in generation of electrical or chemical signals to the hypothalamus. Such signals may produce depolarization of nerve endings affecting the secretion of releasing hormones. These hormones gain access to the local blood circulation through fenestrations (thin walls) in small vessels and are carried to the adenohypophysis (anterior pituitary) by the hypothalamic–hypophyseal portal system shown in Fig. 3-2. The releasing hormone binds to a specific receptor on a particular cell membrane in the anterior pituitary. The binding sets off a chain of events culminating in an elevation of intracellular calcium ions. There follows a release of preformed anterior pituitary hormone. This hormone is released into the bloodstream, gaining access to the circulation through fenestrations in nearby blood vessels. Subsequently, it binds to a specific receptor on the cell membrane

---

hormones are secreted in nanogram amounts and they have short half-lives of the order of a few minutes. Anterior pituitary hormones are produced often in microgram amounts and have longer half-lives than releasing hormones. Ultimate hormones can be produced in milligram amounts daily with much longer half-lives. Thus, the products of mass × half-life constitute an enormous cascade mechanism. With respect to differences in mass of hormone produced from hypothalamus to target gland, the range is nanogram to milligram, or as much as a millionfold. When the ultimate hormone has receptors in nearly every cell type, it is possible to affect the body chemistry of virtually every cell by a single environmental signal. Consequently, the organism is in intimate association with the external environment, a fact which we tend to underemphasize. Arrows with a black dot at the origin indicate a secretory process.

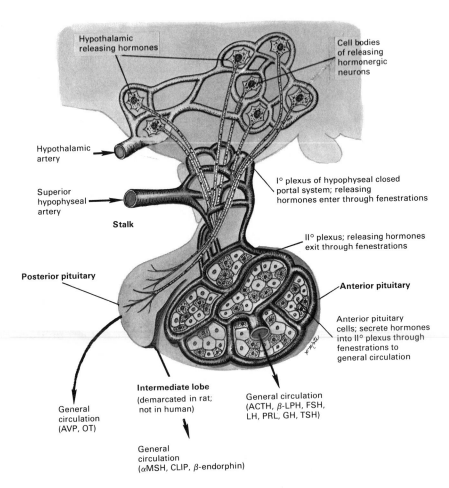

Figure 3-2. Diagram showing the hypothalamus with nuclei in various places in which the hypothalamic releasing hormones are synthesized. Also shown is the major vascular network consisting of a primary plexus where releasing hormones enter its circulation through fenestrated vessels and the secondary plexus in the anterior pituitary where the releasing hormones are transported out of the circulation again through fenestrations in the vessels to the region of the anterior pituitary target cells. This figure also shows the resultant effects of the actions of the hypothalamic releasing hormones causing the release into the general circulation of the anterior pituitary hormones.

of a target gland cell. Within the target cell a chain of events, similar to those following binding of releasing hormone to anterior pituitary cell, occurs culminating in the release of the ultimate hormone. The ultimate hormone has receptors in many tissues and produces the systemic hormonal response.

When maximal secretion of the ultimate hormone occurs in response to the initial signal, a set of negative feedback reactions takes place which operate at nearly every level of the cascade mechanism. In general, the anterior pituitary hormones feed back on the cells of the hypothalamus secreting the releasing hormone and inhibiting its further release. This mechanism operates by a hypothalamic cell membrane receptor to regulate the anterior pituitary hormone. Following the ligand binding event, a series of reactions occur which result in shutting down further secretion of the hypothalamic releasing hormone. This feedback link between the anterior pituitary and hypothalamus is called the "short feedback loop." Other important negative feedback mechanisms occur between the ultimate hormone and the structures higher up in the cascade (Fig. 3-1). These are "long-loop" negative feedback systems operating at the levels of anterior pituitary, hypothalamus, and CNS and mediated by receptors for the ultimate hormone. After ligand binding, the ultimate hormone shuts down further secretion of hormones from the anterior pituitary and hypothalamus and, in some cases, neutralizes signals emanating from the CNS. In addition to this long-loop negative feedback system which depends upon receptors, there is growing evidence of a rapid long-loop negative feedback system whose action occurs too quickly to allow for transcriptional mediation by a receptor specific for the ultimate hormone. In such cases an ultimate hormone may be expected to exert its effects on the nerve endings of hypothalamic neurons to reduce secretion of releasing hormone by some fast action, such as alteration of membrane ion flux. It will be interesting to learn more about exceptional nonreceptor mechanisms.

As indicated in Fig. 3-1, the hormones of the posterior pituitary are synthesized in the cell bodies of hypothalamic neurons and are transported in long axons to the nerve endings where they are stored, awaiting signals for release.

The system described here is applicable to a number of hormonal mechanisms, all of which are covered in this book. Consequently, the releasing hormones of the hypothalamus are critically important as they are required to set the anterior pituitary hormones in motion. The anterior pituitary is referred to as the "master gland" and is responsible for maintaining a large array of essential bodily functions.

II. ANATOMICAL, MORPHOLOGICAL, AND PHYSIOLOGICAL RELATIONSHIPS

A. Hypothalamus

As seen from Fig. 3-3, the hypothalamus is located below the third ventricle of the brain just above the median eminence. The functions of

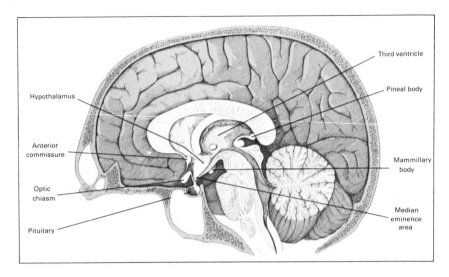

Figure 3-3. Lateral view of the brain showing the relationship of the pituitary gland to the hypothalamus. Reproduced from D. T. Krieger, The hypothalamus and neuroendocrinology. *In* "Neuroendocrinology" (D. T. Krieger and J. C. Hughes, eds.), pp. 3–12. Sinauer Associates, Sunderland, Massachusetts, 1980.

the hypothalamus are intimately connected to the pituitary which lies below the hypothalamus at the end of the delicate infundibular stalk.

In the process of development of the brain, a structure known as the diencephalon appears. It is referred to as the second division of the brain and is a relay center for the cerebral hemispheres. It has a central cavity known as the third ventricle (Fig. 3-3). The diencephalon can be divided into a dorsal epithalamus, a middle thalamus, and a ventral hypothalamus. The lateral walls of the diencephalon, the thalamus, are a relay center for tracts connecting the cerebral hemispheres. The hypothalamus contains optic chiasma where the optic nerves cross at their entrance to the brain, tuber cinerium, infundibulum, hypophysis, and mammillary region. The tuber cinerium contains gray matter behind the optic chiasma involved with olfaction. It continues ventrally as the infundibular stalk whose cavity is an extension of the third ventricle connecting the pituitary (see Chapter 5).

B. Blood Supply of Hypothalamus

Small branches of the anterior cerebral artery and the posterior communicating artery extend to form a network within the hypothalamic

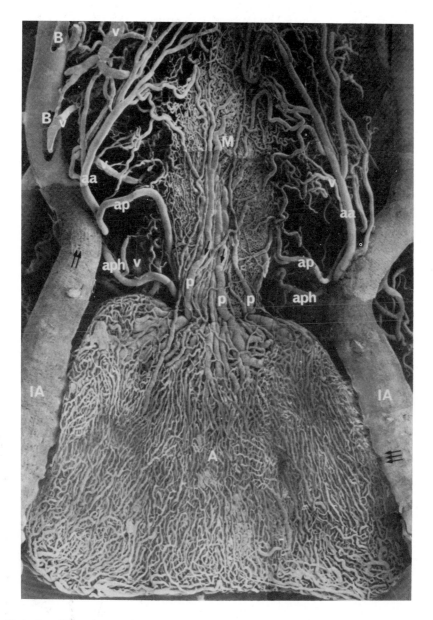

Figure 3-4. Ventral view of an isolated and osmium-stained hypophyseal block of a pliable replica obtained by injection of semipolymerized methyl methacrylate and mixed with hydroxypropyl methacrylate monomer which polymerizes with methyl methacrylate. The plexus of the median eminence (M) is supplied by the anterior hypophyseal (aa), peduncular (ap), and accessory peduncular (aph) arteries which converge into the portal venules

region. The supraoptic and paraventricular nuclei are situated in a dense capillary network supplied by branches of the supraoptic–paraventricular arteries. Small branches from the superior hypophyseal artery also serve the supraoptic nucleus. The nuclei of the tuber cinerium have a less dense vasculature supplied partly by the posterior communicating arteries. Thus, two large pairs of arteries supply this region. There are no direct connections between vessels of the hypothalamic nuclei and the pituitary. The hypophysis is supplied by the superior and inferior hypophyseal arteries which are branches of the internal carotid (Fig. 3-2). The vasculature of the hypothalamus and pituitary is shown vividly in Fig. 3-4.

C. The Electrical Connections from the Brain to the Hypothalamus

The systems and circuitry between the brain and the hypothalamus (afferent) and the electrical connections from the hypothalamus to other structures (efferent) are extremely complex and probably unnecessary to the subject matter of this book. Naturally, many of the electrical signals conducted by these fibers will either stimulate or depress the release of releasing hormones from the nerve endings of the peptidergic nerve terminals in which they are stored.

D. The Neuron

Neurons, whether they manufacture small molecule neurotransmitters such as norepinephrine or polypeptides, have the general structure as diagrammed in Figs. 3-5 and 3-6. The cell body is the site of synthesis and packaging of the releasing hormones. Some of the amine neurotransmitters may be synthesized in the nerve endings. The secretory granules are transported down the axon, which in some cases may be extremely long, into the nerve ending where a signal will cause the exocytotic release of the granules, defined in Chapter 4. The signal can be electrical, presumably transmitted through fibers traveling the length of the axon and causing depolarization at the nerve ending and Ca^{2+} uptake there, which appears to be essential in the exocytosis process.

(p) to supply the anterior lobe (A) of the pituitary. The plexus of the median eminence (M) drains directly at its periphery into the systemic venus twigs (v) surrounding the eminence. Reproduced from T. Murakami, Pliable methacrylate cast of blood vessels: Use in scanning electron microscope study of the microcirculation in rat hypophysis. *Arch. Histol. Jpn.* **38**, 151–168 (1975).

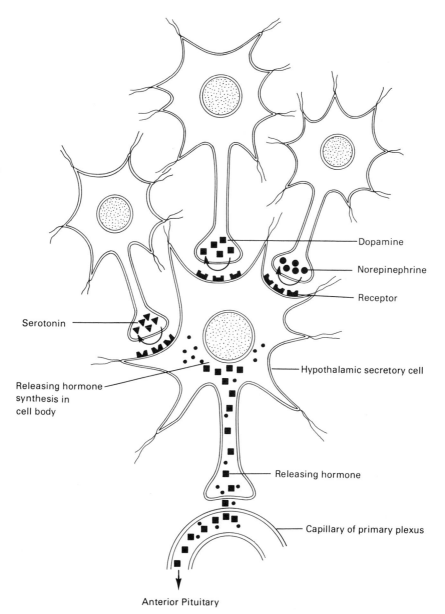

Figure 3-5. Drawing of a neuron (center) which is synthesizing and secreting a releasing hormone and its regulation by aminergic neurons (interneurons), in this case which secrete serotonin, dopamine, and norepinephrine. The regulatory interneurons synapse with the cell body in this illustration. The catecholamines are usually synthesized in the nerve ending. The releasing hormones and precursors are synthesized in the cell body and

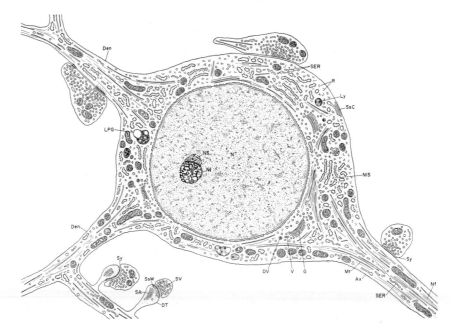

Figure 3-6. Drawing of a neuron showing the cell body with a number of branching dendrites (Den). The axon (Ax) extends from the pole opposite to that giving rise to dendrites. It has a large, round nucleus (N) with a nucleolus (Nl). The rough endoplasmic reticulum is organized into aggregation of cisternae studded with ribosomes (R) known as Nissl substance (NiS). Smooth-surfaced endoplasmic reticulum (SER) is extensive and tubular. The Golgi apparatus (G) is a short stack of flattened cisternae with small vesicles (V): Dense core vesicles (DV) may contain catecholamines. Lysosomes (Ly) are numerous. Intermediate stages between lysosomes and lipofuscin granules (LPG) are found. Microtubules (Mt) course from the perikaryon into the axon (Ax). Neurofilaments (Nf) and smooth endoplasmic reticulum run into the axon. Sy, Synapse; SV, synaptic vesicle; SA, spine apparatus; SsW, subsynaptic web; SsC, subsurface cisternae. Reproduced from T. L. Lentz, "Cell Fine Structure." Saunders, Philadelphia, Pennsylvania, 1971.

transported down the axon to the nerve terminal where the signal is awaited for release. Afterward, the releasing hormone enters the closed portal circulation through capillary fenestrations in the primary plexus. After transport down the portal vessel, the hormone empties from the secondary plexus into the anterior pituitary. This figure was redrawn and modified from L. A. Frohman, Neurotransmitters as regulators of endocrine function. *In* "Neuroendocrinology" (D. T. Krieger and J. C. Hughes, eds.), pp. 44–58. Sinauer Associates, Sunderland, Massachusetts, 1980.

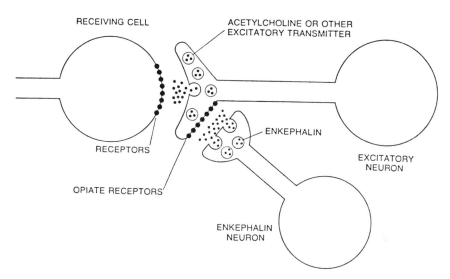

Figure 3-7. Diagram of a neuron (in this case, cholinergic) whose secretion is regulated by an enkephalinergic interneuron interacting at the nerve ending to modify secretion as mediated by opiate receptors. Reproduced from D. Agnew, *City Hope Q.* **8**, 6–10 (1970).

The nerve endings may also be regulated by an interneuron forming a synapse with the nerve ending, as shown in Fig. 3-7. In this case, receptors for the neurotransmitter, such as enkephalin in this example, would be located on the surface of the nerve ending in the synaptic region. Through a second messenger, an action would occur in the nerve ending which influences, positively or negatively, the release of the secretory material stored there.

The targets of the releasing hormones are the cells of the adenohypophysis in the anterior pituitary which secrete the anterior pituitary hormones. The anatomy and cellular characteristics of the anterior pituitary are presented in Chapter 5.

III. CHEMISTRY

Because only a few of the releasing hormones have been sequenced, these will be referred to as hormones, whereas the others, whose activities are measurable but whose primary structure is unknown, will be referred to as "factors." There are two kinds of releasing hormone systems in the hypothalamus, one in which a single releasing hormone appears to control positively the secretion of a given anterior pituitary hormone and the other in which a pair of releasing hormones, one

112

Table 3–1. Well-Characterized Hypothalamic Releasing Hormones/Factors[a]

Hypothalamic positive-acting single hormone	Releases anterior pituitary hormone(s)	Inhibits release of anterior pituitary hormone(s)
Thyrotropin releasing hormone (TRH)	TSH,PRL	
Gonadotropin releasing hormone (GnRH)	LH,FSH	
Corticotropin releasing hormone (CRH or CRF)	ACTH, β-lipotropin, β-endorphin (MSH)	
Dual-acting releasing hormone		
Growth hormone releasing hormone (somatocrinin, GRH)	GH	
Growth hormone release-inhibiting hormone (somatostatin, GIH, SRIF)		GH
Prolactin releasing factor (PRF)	PRL	
Prolactin release-inhibiting factor (PIF)		PRL
Melanocyte-stimulating hormone releasing factor (MRF)[a]	MSH	
Melanocyte-stimulating hormone release-inhibiting factor (MIF)[a]		MSH

[a] Evidence is weak for existence of this hormone in higher animals.

acting positively and one acting negatively, modulate the secretion of a specific anterior pituitary hormone (Table 3-1).

In the single controlling set are thyrotropin releasing hormone (TRH), gonadotropin releasing hormone (GnRH), and corticotropin releasing hormone (CRH). All of these act positively on the release of thyroid-stimulating hormone from thyrotrophic cells of the anterior pituitary (TRH) and prolactin from lactotrophic cells of the anterior pituitary (TRH), luteinizing hormone (LH) from luteotrophic cells of the anterior pituitary (GnRH) and follicle-stimulating hormone (FSH) from folliculotrophic cells of the anterior pituitary (GnRH), and finally adrenocorticotropin from corticotrophic cells of the anterior pituitary (CRH). Some evidence suggests that LH and FSH can be secreted from the same cell, that is, that luteotrophs and folliculotrophs may be one and the same, or that there may exist both types of cells. In the set of dual-controlling releasing hormones there are growth hormone releasing hor-

Figure 3-8. Sequences of known hypothalamic releasing and releasing-inhibiting hormones.

SEQUENCES OF KNOWN HYPOTHALAMIC RELEASING
AND RELEASING INHIBITING HORMONES

TRH (Thyrotropin releasing hormone; releases TSH and PRL; it is
not yet clear whether PRF is different from TRH, if so there
would be 2 positive releasers of PRL and one or more negative
releasers: PIF which may be dopamine or some other hormone).

pGLU*-HIS-PRO-NH₂**

GnRH (Gonadotropic releasing hormone; releases LH and FSH; residue 3, Trp, is important in association with receptor).

```
1        3                      10
pGlu-His-Trp-Ser-Tyr-Gly-Leu-Arg-Pro-Gly-NH₂
```

GIH or SRIF (somatotropin release-inhibiting factor); or somatostatin
inhibits release of GH and affects release of pancreatic and other hormones.

```
1       ┌─────────────────────────────────────┐ 14
Ala-Gly-Cys-Lys-Asn-Phe-Phe-Trp-Lys-Thr-Phe-Thr-Ser-Cys
```

CRH (corticotropin releasing hormone; releases ACTH,
β-lipotropin); some β-LPH may form β-endorphin; ACTH usually
degraded to αMSH in intermediate lobe of pituitary.

```
1
Ser-Gln-Glu-Pro-Pro-Ile-Ser-Leu-Asp-Leu-Thr-Phe-His-
                        20
Leu-Leu-Arg-Glu-Val-Leu-Glu-Met-Thr-Lys-Ala-Asp-Gln-
                  30
Leu-Ala-Gln-Gln-Ala-His-Ser-Asn-Arg-Lys-Leu-Leu-Asp-
40  41
Ile-Ala-NH₂.
```

GRH (growth hormone releasing hormone; somatocrinin; releases
growth hormone).

```
1                             10
Tyr-Ala-Asp-Ala-Ile-Phe-Thr-Asn-Ser-Tyr-Arg-
                      20
Lys-Val-Leu-Gly-Gln-Leu-Ser-Ala-Arg-Lys-Leu-
                  30
Leu-Gln-Asp-Ile-Met-Ser-Arg-Gln-Gln-Gly-Glu-
                    40        44
Ser-Asn-Gln-Glu-Arg-Gly-Ala-Arg-Ala-Arg-Leu-NH₂.
```

*Denotes pyroglutamyl-

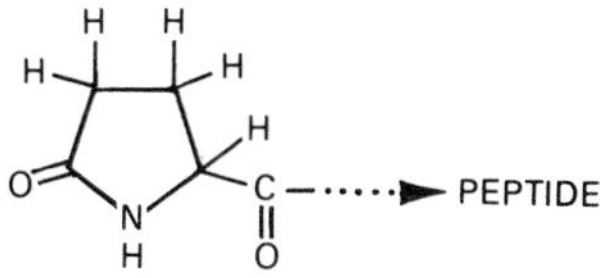

**Denotes amide of C-terminal amino acid, thus prolinamide in TRH,
glycinamide in GnRH, alanylamide in CRH or leucinamide in GRH.

mone (GRH) and growth hormone release-inhibiting hormone (GIH or somatostatin), and prolactin releasing factor (PRF) and prolactin release-inhibiting factor (PIF). The structures of the releasing hormones with known sequences are shown in Fig. 3-8.

GRH is a polypeptide. β-Endorphin is active in causing the release of growth hormone and PRL, and in inhibiting the release of gonadotropins and TSH. β-Endorphin arises from the proopiomelanocortin precursor in corticotrophic cells of the anterior pituitary. It is a cleavage product of β-lipotropin which is directly translated to proopiomelanocortin. It is possible that β-endorphin could stimulate GH release indirectly by increasing the release of GRH or inhibiting the release of somatostatin. Recently, a peptide and its partial degradation products have been discovered by the R. Guillemin group in human pancreatic carcinoma. This 44 amino acid peptide possesses growth hormone releasing activity and appears to be human GRH. Its structure is shown in Fig. 3-8.

PIF is closely related to dopamine and this neurotransmitter may be identical to PRF. However, there is some evidence that not all PIF activity in the hypothalamus can be attributed to dopamine. Again, however, dopamine could be acting to modify (stimulate) the secretion of another unique PIF. The structure of dopamine is

$$HO-\text{\textcircled{}}-CH_2-CH_2-NH_2$$

CRH, the corticotrophic releasing hormone, is a polypeptide, and there may be an auxiliary hormone to CRH which appears to be vasopressin. Vasopressin is synthesized in the hypothalamus and can release ACTH when injected directly into the brain but depends upon CRH; it stimulates the activity of CRH. The structure of vasopressin is given in Chapter 4.

Although the releasing factors controlling the release of melanocyte-stimulating hormone presumably from the corticotrophic cells of the anterior pituitary are not well substantiated for man, peptide structures have been described which possess specific activities of release and release inhibition, particularly in amphibians. These factors may be produced from oxytocin, also synthesized in the hypothalamus (see Chapter 4). Production of MRF and MIF is summarized in Fig. 3-9, although there is considerable skepticism about the existence of MRF and MIF in higher forms. Very recently, other proteolytic cleavage products of oxytocin and vasopressin have been shown to result from the action of proteolytic enzymes present in brain synaptic membrane preparations.

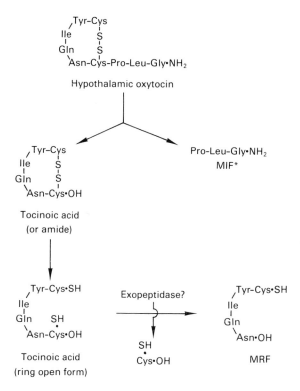

Figure 3-9. Processing of oxytocin to form peptides with reported activities of MIF and MRF. (*), In animal models, this MIF acts like an anti-Parkinsonian agent and an anti-depressive, although rather little recent research supports claims of MIF and MRF in higher animals.

The products and sites of attack on these molecules are reviewed in Fig. 3-10. It is presumed that some or all of these products will have neuro-transmitter or other direct functions in the CNS. In contrast to known brain aminopeptidases, synaptic (nerve ending) membrane-associated enzymes can cleave oxytocin or vasopressin without a prior requirement for reduction of the disulfide bridge. Releasing hormones (excluding GRH and CRH which need more information) are not synthesized from mRNAs directly on polysomes, but rather evolve through cleavage of proproteins of considerably larger size. This is also true of some anterior pituitary hormones, such as ACTH, MSH, and β-lipotropin, all of which derive from a single protein precursor, proopiomelanocortin. In higher forms, MSH derives from the intermediate pituitary under controls separate from CRH.

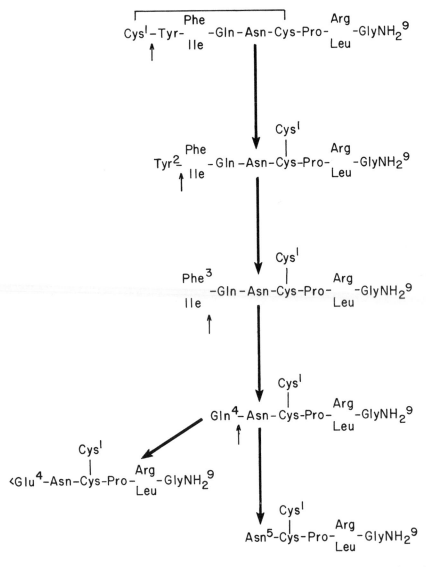

Figure 3-10. Sequence of proteolytic events during exposure of arginine-vasopressin and oxytocin to brain synaptic membranes. The pathway is based on time course studies. (↑), Cleavage sites. Reproduced from J. P. H. Burbach and J. L. M. Lebouille, Proteolytic conversion of arginine-vasopressin and oxytocin by brain synaptic membranes. *J. Biol Chem.* **258**, 1487–1494 (1983).

IV. BIOCHEMISTRY

A. Location of Releasing Hormones in the Central Nervous System

The location of the releasing hormones in various cells of the CNS has been accomplished frequently by the use of fluorescent-labeled mono-specific antibodies and microscopic detection of fluorescence. The localization of TRH by this method is to the nerve terminals of the hypothalamic nuclei of the dorsomedial nucleus, the paraventricular nucleus, and the perifornical region. There are some other locations for TRH outside of the hypothalamus, suggesting a more diversified role for this peptide. Thus, the TRH neuroendocrine system has its cell bodies in the periventricular region, and these neurons extend to the median eminence. The cell bodies are located in an area described as the thyrotropic area.

GnRH has been more difficult to localize. It is present in neurons located in the external layer of the median eminence closest to the stalk. It is located caudally from this area of the median eminence as well. TRH-positive locations also exist in other regions of the brain.

Somatostatin (GIH)-containing neurons reside in the median eminence, periventricular nuclei of the hypothalamus, the peripheral nervous system, and the gut. It has been located as well in cells of the gastroenteropancreatic endocrine system (see Chapter 7) and in the thyroid as well as several areas of the CNS. GRH has been localized to the arcuate nucleus of the hypothalamus.

CRH also appears to be located elsewhere in addition to the hypothalamic–hypophyseal axis. It has been found in the central nucleus of the amygdala (of the limbic system) and in polar neurons and dendrites in the cortex as well as in some cells of the reticular formation. The dorsal motor nucleus has some fibers which may contain CRH. Some CRH-positive fibers terminate in the posterior pituitary and hypothalamic regions in addition to the median eminence.

Polypeptides other than the releasing hormones are produced by neurons. These are substance P (hypothalamus, gut, and various regions of the CNS), enkephalins (CNS, hypothalamic nuclei, including periventricular nucleus, medial preoptic nucleus, ventromedial nucleus, dorsal and ventral premammillary nuclei, the prefornical area and the arcuate nucleus, and in 20 other regions outside the hypothalamus, including the adrenal medulla) and gastrin (heterogeneously distributed in the nervous system, including the periventricular, dorso-, and ventromedial nuclei of the hypothalamus and in the external layer of the median eminence, it is present in the cerebral cortex, the hippocampus, and of course has long been known to be located in the stomach). Angiotensin II is located in the CNS in the paraventricular nucleus and prefornical area. In the hypothalamus, angiotensin II-containing nerve terminals are located in the external layer of the median eminence, the dorsomedial nucleus, and the ventral portions. Angiotensin II is also located outside the hypothalamus in other brain areas. There appear to be many other active hormones as well, in addition to the releasing hormones.

B. Secretion of Releasing Hormones and General Actions

Neurons synthesize and package releasing hormone precursors in their cell bodies, and these products are transported down the length of their axons to the nerve terminals (nerve endings) where a signal is awaited for secretion. Since most of the cell bodies of these peptidergic neurons are located in various areas of the hypothalamus, signals for secretion come from higher levels, usually from aminergic or cholinergic neurons in various parts of the brain. The hippocampus (and amygdala) of the limbic system may signal releasing hormone-containing neurons by changes in firing rates of electric signals or chemically by inter-neuronal contacts (Fig. 3-11). The specificity of the overall process is a function of the unique structure of the releasing hormone (Fig. 3-8) which interacts with the specific receptor in the target cell membrane. For example, a hypophyseal cell (folliculotroph) producing FSH contains receptors for GnRH just as a producing LH cell (luteotroph) since both anterior pituitary hormones are released by the same releasing hormone, GnRH. In fact, it is questioned whether one cell produces both hormones. TRH interacts with receptors on membranes of the thyrotroph, producing TSH and the lactotroph, producing PRL. Somatostatin has receptors on somatotrophic cell membranes which also contain GRH receptors, since the control of GH secretion is under the influence of both releasing hormones. In addition, there are other regulators of anterior pituitary secretion, such as the aminergic hormones. A particular anterior pituitary cell membrane should contain all of the different receptors necessary for hormonal control.

The aminergic neurons exert similar kinds of control at the level of hypothalamic neurons which manufacture releasing hormones. Figure 3-11 shows possible mechanisms by which neurons synthesizing releasing hormones are regulated. The primary signal may be to the cell body

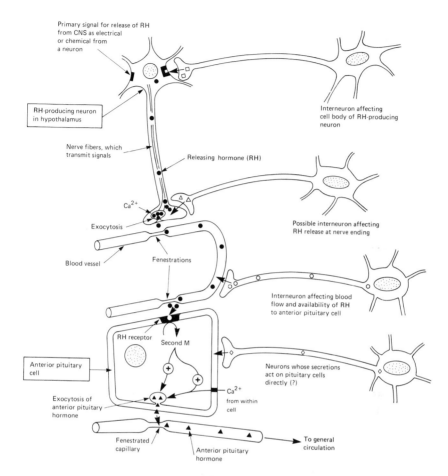

Figure 3-11. Neuronal controls of secretion of releasing hormones. The pathway of synthesis and secretion of releasing hormone (RH) is shown in vertical array at the left. The peptidergic neuron synthesizes RH which is released in response to electrical or chemical signals delivered by neurons probably at the level of the cell body. RH is released by exocytosis from the nerve ending where Ca^{2+} uptake plays a role in the process of exocytosis. RH, released from the nerve ending, enters the total hypothalamic–hypophyseal portal system by way of fenestrations in blood vessels (thin–walled capillaries). RH is transported to anterior pituitary cell exiting the portal system through fenestrations. RH binds to specific anterior pituitary cell membrane receptor to produce a second messenger (second M) which enhances Ca^{2+} uptake and exocytosis of specific anterior pituitary hormone. Shown on the right are hypothetical interneurons that can act positively or negatively on RH release and transport at a variety of levels of the overall system.

Extracellular space

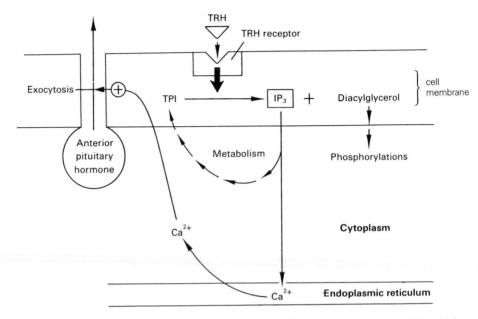

Figure 3-12. Suggestion for the mode of action of the releasing hormone, TRH, which relates the stimulation of phospholipid metabolism, calcium mobilization, and anterior pituitary hormone (prolactin) secretion. In this model, TRH binds to its receptor in the cell membrane, causing a stimulation of the conversion of phosphatidylinositol-4,5-diphosphate (TPI) to inositol triphosphate (IP$_3$) and diacylglycerol. The mechanism by which the receptor complex accomplishes this stimulation is unclear. IP$_3$ stimulates the release of calcium ions from the endoplasmic reticulum to the cytoplasm where it further stimulates the exocytotic release of the anterior pituitary hormone. This figure with modifications was generated from M. J. Rebecci, R. N. Kolesnick, and M. C. Gershengorn, Thyrotropin releasing hormone stimulates rapid loss of phosphatidylinositol and its conversion to 1,2-diacylglycerol and phosphatidic acid in rat mammotropic pituitary cells. *J. Biol. Chem.* **258,** 227–234 (1983).

of the neuron producing a particular releasing hormone. The signal is chemical (e.g., serotonin or other amine; in such cases, synthesis of the amine is likely to occur in the nerve ending rather than in the cell body) or electrical from an interneuron. The secreted releasing hormone passes through fenestrations (thin walls or openings) in the ends of the closed portal system connecting the median eminence with the anterior pituitary cells. Fenestrations overcome the blood–brain barrier which otherwise might not allow polypeptides to be translocated. The releasing hormones enter the neighborhood of the anterior pituitary cells through fenestrations at the terminus of the portal system (secondary plexus) and then bind to specific plasma membrane receptors of target cells. This interaction produces a second messenger (second M) which directly or indirectly opens the calcium channel so that Ca^{2+} ions accumulate in the cytoplasm (Fig. 3-11). The specific anterior pituitary hormone is secreted and enters the general circulation via fenestrations in local capillaries. These hormones then are transported to distant target cells which contain specific membrane receptors. Various interneurons regulate specific processes (Fig. 3-11), such as events in the cell body of the releasing hormone-producing cell, secretion of releasing hormone, and blood flow in the closed portal system connecting hypothalamus (median eminence) with anterior pituitary.

Speculations on the mechanism by which a specific releasing hormone operates on an anterior pituitary cell are given in Fig. 3-12. Following the interaction of membrane receptor with releasing hormone, in this case TRH, there is an increase in phospholipid metabolism culminating in increased cytoplasmic calcium ion concentration. Increased Ca^{2+} levels lead to exocytosis of preformed anterior pituitary hormones.

Specific Regulators of Releasing Hormones and Anterior Pituitary Hormone Release

The regulators of anterior pituitary hormone release are shown in Table 3-2. Table 3-2 is incomplete and information on regulation of releasing hormones and of anterior pituitary hormones is still developing. In some cases, a regulator has one effect *in vitro* and an opposite effect *in vivo*. This table exemplifies complexities of regulating the secretion of releasing hormones and anterior pituitary hormones (see Fig. 3-11).

C. Actions of Releasing and Release-Inhibiting Hormones and Their Receptors

1. TRH

Recent evidence is suggestive of an activation mechanism of the TRH–receptor complex. TRH in cultures of rat pituitary cells binds to a form of the receptor from which the ligand is rapidly dissociable. The ligand–receptor complex is converted in a temperature-dependent fashion to a more stable form with slow dissociation kinetics. This process can occur in whole cells as well as in isolated cell membranes. At elevated temperatures within 10 min of hormone binding, TRH–receptor complex is

Table 3–2. Regulators of Release of Anterior Pituitary Hormones

Anterior pituitary hormone	Releasing factors		Other regulators	
	+	−	+	−
Growth hormone (GH)	GRH (somatocrinin)	GIH (somatostatin)	Insulin β-Endorphin Serotonin PGE$_1$ PGE$_2$ Acetylcholine (lowers GIH) Hypoglycemia (mediated by norepinephrine or serotonin)	Melatonin Dopamine Norepinephrine (releases GIH) Neurotensin (releases GIH)
Thyrotropin-stimulating hormone (TSH)	TRH		Histamine (stimulates TRH release) Norepinephrine (stimulates TRH release) Dopamine (stimulates TRH release)	Serotonin (inhibits TRH release) GIH (inhibits TRH release)
Adrenocorticotropic hormone (ACTH)	CRH		Serotonin (stimulates CRH release) Epinephrine	Melatonin GABA[a] Norepinephrine

Hormone			
Follicle-stimulating hormone (FSH)	GnRH	GnRIF(?) (dopamine?)	Melatonin (stimulates GnRH release), Norepinephrine (stimulates GnRH release), Acetylcholine (stimulates GnRH release), Thymosin (stimulates GnRH release), Serotonin (may act on anterior pituitary), GABA[a], GIH (inhibits TRH release)
Luteinizing hormone (LH)	GnRH	GnRIF(?) (dopamine?)	Norepinephrine (releases GnRH), Thymosin (stimulates GnRH release)
Prolactin (PRL)	TRH(?)	PIF(?) (dopamine?)	β-Endorphin, Suckling (mediated by serotonin), Hypoglycemia (mediated by serotonin)
β-Lipotropin (β-LPH) and β-endorphin	CRH (same regulation as for ACTH)		
Melanocyte-stimulating hormone (MSH)	CRH (same regulation as for ACTH)[b]		

[a] γ-Aminobutyric acid.
[b] MSH usually is secreted from intermediate pituitary under controls different from CRH.

altered further to become resistant to salt or acid. These reactions, taking place in the cell membrane, can be summarized as follows:

Unoccupied receptor	Occupied receptor	First conformational change (?)	Second conformational change (?)
	0–37°C	>20°C	>20°C
TRH + R $\longrightarrow$	TRH – R $\longrightarrow$	TRH – R′ $\longrightarrow$	TRH – R*
	cells or	cells or	cells
	membranes	membranes	

These reactions indicate that there are at least three forms of modified receptor (R*) or ligand–receptor complexes. The transitions in the cell membrane are reminiscent of the activation mechanism of steroid receptors which may take place in the cell cytoplasm (e.g., see Chapter 10). Some of the physical changes of the occupied receptor might relate to potential movements in the membrane having to do with aggregation of receptors and their ultimate internalization. After activation has transpired, the receptor complex may facilitate alterations in membrane phospholipids (Fig. 3-12). The breakdown of phosphatidylinositol to (diacylglycerol and) inositoltriphosphate could avail Ca^{2+} directly from stores in the endoplasmic reticulum. The action of TRH–receptor complex may thus generate increased cytoplasmic Ca^{2+}. Phosphorylation of a 97,000 molecular weight protein (S97) is stimulated by Ca^{2+} and blocked by a calcium channel blocker. Treatments causing release of mitochondrial Ca^{2+} also stimulated phosphorylation of S97. Calmodulin enhanced this reaction at low Ca^{2+} concentrations. Many of the actions of TRH on protein phosphorylation can be accounted for by a Ca^{2+}-dependent pathway. Thus, the mechanism of action of TRH may involve Ca^{2+} as the second or third messenger. It is not clear to what extent cyclic AMP is a direct second message of releasing hormone action. Some work on TRH emphasizes the stimulation by Ca^{2+} of an unknown direct second messenger to cause the activation of cyclic AMP-independent protein kinase. The second message could be restricted to the cell membrane and involve alterations in phospholipid metabolism.

TRH–receptor complexes stimulate PRL synthesis in cultures of anterior pituitary cells. This stimulation aligns with increases in levels of cytoplasmic mRNA translating prolactin sequences.

2. GIH (Somatostatin)

Somatostatin (GIH) receptors have been measured and partially characterized in some tissues. The mode of action of this releasing hormone, besides its recognized function in inhibiting the release of growth hormone in the anterior pituitary, is unclear. An extra role(s) seems evident

Table 3–3. Locations of Somatostatin[a]

Pancreatic islets
D cells and D-like cells in gut (somatostatin inhibits secretions of neighboring cell types)
Median eminence (neurons producing somatostatin)
Nerve fibers of the posterior pituitary
Brain in several regions
Vagus nerve
Sympathetic ganglia
Intrinsic nerves of several organs
Nerves in wall of gut
Intrinsic nerves of the gut
Peptidergic and adrenergic nerve fibers (but not cholinergic nerves)
Proximal duodenum
Parafollicular region of thyroid gland

[a] Compiled from information in R. H. Williams, ed., "Textbook of Endocrinology," 6th ed. Saunders, Philadelphia, Pennsylvania, 1981.

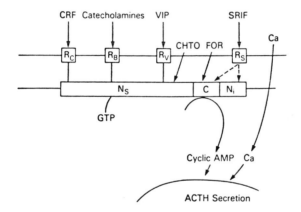

Figure 3-13. Multireceptor regulation of ACTH secretion. Regulation of ACTH secretion may involve the following molecular and cellular events: CRF, catecholamines (β_2 agonists), and VIP bind to their respective receptors (R_C, R_B, and R_V), allowing the guanyl nucleotide unit (N_S) of the adenylate cyclase system, along with GTP, to stimulate the catalytic unit (C). This leads to the production of intracellular cyclic AMP and, in the presence of calcium, an enhanced release of ACTH. (For simplicity, a single N_S unit is depicted for all three agonists.) Cholera toxin (CHTO) and forskolin (FOR) bypass surface receptors and activate adenylate cyclase at the N_S and C units, respectively. SRIF binds to a specific receptor (R_S), possibly allowing a different guanyl nucleotide unit (N_i) to inhibit adenylate cyclase activity in the presence of agonist and GTP. Alternatively, SRIF may directly inhibit the C unit of adenylate cyclase. Reproduced from S. Heisler, T. D. Reisine, V. Y. H. Hook, and J. Axelrod, Somatostatin inhibits multireceptor stimulation of cyclic AMP formation and corticotropin secretion in mouse pituitary tumor cells. *Proc. Natl. Acad. Sci. U.S.A.* **79,** 6502–6506 (1982).

in view of the extrahypothalamic production of somatostatin. Table 3-3 lists several of the locations in which somatostatin has been found.

Secretion of somatostatin from pancreatic D cells is stimulated by norepinephrine and inhibited by acetylcholine. Somatostatin may bind to specific receptors on the pancreatic β cell which in turn can affect the α receptor (histamine). The second messenger of the somatostatin receptor might act on the Ca^{2+}-stimulated release of insulin in the β cell.

More specific conclusions on the mode of action of somatostatin have been drawn recently in the laboratory of J. Axelrod from mouse anterior pituitary tumor cells (At T-20/D16-16) which secrete ACTH in response to CRH, isoproterenol, and vasoactive intestinal peptide (VIP). GIH or SRIF (somatotropin release inhibitory factor, GIH) was shown to decrease intracellular levels of cyclic AMP elevated by CRH, isoproterenol, or VIP. GIH does not decrease basal levels of cyclic AMP in cells, suggesting that GIH operates only in the presence of stimulating agents. GIH does not appear to block binding of β agonists or increase the activity of phosphodiesterase. Consequently, it was concluded that GIH may act directly on the catalytic subunit of adenylate cyclase (Fig. 3-13). This could occur by direct interaction with the GIH–receptor complex or through some unknown second messenger. Regulation of adenylate cyclase has been studied more from the aspect of interactions with regulatory subunits of the membrane complex (including receptor) rather than from the point of view of direct interaction with the catalytic subunit of the complex.

3. GnRH

GnRH acts on the gonadotropic cells of the anterior pituitary to stimulate the release of LH and FSH (see Chapter 5). This polypeptide hormone must interact with a similar or identical receptor on two different cell types in the anterior pituitary, one which secretes primarily LH and the other FSH. On the other hand, there is evidence that both FSH and LH may be secreted from the same cell in response to GnRH. A period occurs in the ovarian cycle during which the estrogen from the developing follicle is usually high in blood and feeds back positively (rather than negatively) on the release of LH and FSH, but more intensively in terms of LH release. GnRH receptors may be more plentiful on the LH-containing cells than on the FSH-containing cells. There are other possible explanations, such as ovarian elaboration of inhibin, which is a specific inhibitor of FSH but not LH secretion. Ovarian estrogen could operate at the level of the anterior pituitary cell or on the release of GnRH.

A speculative mode of action of GnRH is shown in Fig. 3-14. P. Conn's laboratory has shown that ability to microaggregate receptors, presum-

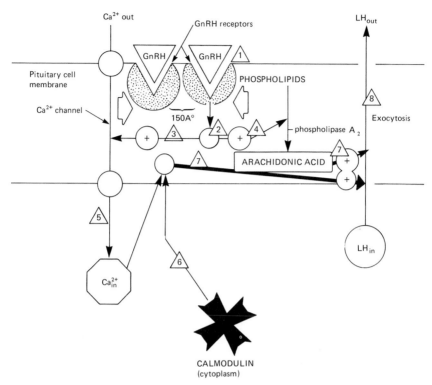

Figure 3-14. A possible mechanism of action of the releasing hormone, GnRH. At the top, two molecules of GnRH have bound to their membrane receptors on a luteotrophic cell. The liganded receptors move toward each other or "cap" (1). Some change occurs when two receptor complexes move within 150 Å of each other (2). The alteration or "second messenger" leads to the opening of a calcium channel (3,5), permitting an increase in cytoplasmic Ca^{2+} level. Ca^{2+} may derive from intracellular sources as well. Cytoplasmic calmodulin is translocated to the plasma membrane (6), but the timing of this process with respect to Ca^{2+} uptake is not yet clear. A stimulation of the appearance of arachidonic acid from membrane phospholipids mediated by phospholipase a_2 occurs (4). Arachidonic acid may have some direct role in the exocytosis process (7), together with Ca^{2+}–calmodulin complex, of LH (8). Presumably a similar mechanism would operate for the GnRH stimulation of FSH secretion.

ably a minimum of 2 to within about 150 Å distance, even if accomplished by means other than using GnRH, is sufficient to promote GnRH agonist activity. GnRH–receptor complexes could thus move in the membrane to within a critical distance as a first step in hormone action following receptor occupation. This hypothetical movement is indicated by the opposing arrows in Fig. 3-14. Receptor internalization and turnover may follow. However, large-scale patching and capping or internalization may not be required for gonadotropin release. Prostaglandins do not seem to be implicated in the process of exocytosis, according to K. Catt's laboratory, so either arachidonic acid or some nonprostagladin product may be involved. Note that the mechanism of GnRH action proposed here differs from the one proposed for TRH action (Fig. 3-12).

There may be receptor sites for GnRH on gonadal cells. GnRH, in low concentrations *in vitro*, can alter responses of these cells to gonadotropes such as FSH so as to inhibit cyclic nucleotide accumulation. Such experiments would suggest an extrahypothalamic production of this releasing hormone, reflecting the well-known situation with somatostatin. Extrahypothalamic actions of GnRH, especially on the testis, are discussed in Chapter 12.

GnRH is released, perhaps indirectly, by Met-enkephalin, and it may be that Met-enkephalin operates through dopamine (Table 3-2) from dopaminergic neurons. GnRH suppresses dopamine synthesis in the rat, suggesting a negative feedback effect, and the fact that the dopaminergic neuron and the GnRH-secreting cell are adjacent geographically renders dopamine a possible candidate for a GnRIF. The number of GnRH receptors on gonadotrophic cells of the anterior pituitary is positively controlled by the level of GnRH itself. This is of significance in the middle of the ovarian cycle (see Chapter 13). There is a dramatic increase in LH ("LH spike"), which is initiated by high levels of estrogen from the developing ovarian follicle. Estrogen probably operates on the CNS to make GnRH more effective or increase its secretion by acting at the anterior pituitary level, or both.

4. CRH

Corticotropin-releasing hormone, a newly characterized 41 amino acid polypeptide, releases the products of the proopiomelanocortin, ACTH, (MSH), and β-lipotropin, from the corticotrophic cells of the anterior pituitary. Since all of these products are encoded on the same gene and included within the same proprotein, they are released simultaneously in response to CRH, the rate of release differing only minutely as a result of variable processing by trypsin-like proteases to the ultimate hormones. CRH has been separated into two size classes by the W. Vale laboratory. One form is CRH, as shown in Fig. 3-8, and the second form may be similar to vasopressin, which has long been known to induce release of ACTH. CRH possesses homologies with an amphibian skin hormone, sauvagine, which can release ACTH experimentally in mammals, and with urotensin I from the hypophysis of fish. Some homolo-

gies also exist with calmodulin and with angiotensin, especially in the
—Phe—His—Leu—Leu renin cleavage site. CRH stimulates levels of cyclic
AMP, which is the probable second messenger in the release of ACTH.
The 41 amino acid-containing CRH is large compared to the earlier characterized releasing hormones. Fragments of CRH are less active, suggesting that the 41 amino acid factor is the native form and not a precursor. Removal of the first 3 amino acids from the N terminal does not
reduce ACTH releasing activity, but removal of the first 5 N-terminal
amino acids destroys activity. Apparently the pituitary can secrete more
ACTH than the adrenal gland is able to respond to. As much as 500 pM
CRH is present in hypothalamic–hypophyseal portal blood, representing physiologically active concentrations. Vasopressin is weakly active
in causing secretion of ACTH, but is synergistic with CRH in this action.
Oxytocin also potentiates CRH and may act by eliciting its release. CRH
is capable of stimulating ACTH release even at high glucocorticoid levels. The action of CRH, in addition to releasing ACTH and other hormones, stimulates the synthesis of proopiomelanocortin mRNA. Epinephrine and norepinephrine potentiate CRH and may bring about
CRH secretion (see Table 3-2), but epinephrine by itself does not cause
release of ACTH. On the other hand, glucocorticoids and prostaglandins exert negative effects on ACTH release, the former through the
well-known long feedback loop.

The intermediate lobe of the pituitary (*pars intermedia*) in animals below man produces acetylated β-endorphin in large amounts in response
to CRH, whereas dopamine antagonizes the release of products of the
pars intermedia. ACTH, β-lipotropin, and β-endorphin are major secretions of the anterior pituitary, while ACTH, α-MSH, CLIP (a cleavage
product representing amino acids 18–39 of ACTH), β-lipotropin, and β-
endorphin are released predominantly in the *pars intermedia* in the rat.
The defined *pars intermedia* in the rat (but not necessarily in the human)
may be under a different control than corticotrophic cells of the anterior
pituitary. CRH stimulates secretion of somatostatin by brain cells and
can modify the acquisition of learned behavior.

V. CLINICAL ASPECTS

Malfunction of the hypothalamus will be as far ranging as malfunction
of the anterior pituitary gland. The symptoms will be similar, since the
hypothalamic releasing hormones occur early in a chain of events that
lead to the ultimate activities of a final hormone in the series (Fig. 3-1).
Damage leading to failure of secretion or passage through the portal

system of releasing hormones may result from trauma to the head producing damage to the stalk and/or scarring of the system, tumors, etc. This general syndrome is known as "panhypopituitarism" and may include the failure of all of the anterior pituitary hormones. After careful diagnosis, therapy usually takes the form of supplying the missing terminal hormones where necessary, for example, glucocorticoids, thyroid hormone, and sex hormones. A method to determine whether the hypothalamus or pituitary is involved in problems of this kind is based on an evocator assay analogous to a glucose tolerance test where purified GnRH is injected and blood samples are tested subsequently for elevated levels of LH. If a normal response in LH concentration is found and the terminal hormone production is responsive to the pituitary hormone, the damage is likely to be at the level of the hypothalamus or stalk.

References

A. Books

Ganong, W. F. (1977). "The Nervous System." Lange Medical Publications, Los Altos, California.

Krieger, D. T., and Hughes, J. C. eds. (1980). "Neuroendocrinology." Sinauer Associates, Sunderland, Massachusetts.

Labhart, ed. (1976). "Clinical Endocrinology." Springer-Verlag, Berlin and New York.

B. Review Articles

Boss, B., Vale, W., and Grant, G. (1975). Hypothalamic hormones. In "Biochemical Actions of Hormones" (G. Litwack, ed.), Vol. 3, pp. 87–118. Academic Press, New York.

Conn, P. M., McMillian, J. M. M., Stern, J., Rogers, D., Hamby, M., Penna, A., and Grant, E. (1981). Gonadotropin-releasing hormone action in the pituitary: A three-step mechanism. Endocr. Rev. 2, 174–185.

Elde, R., and Hokfelt, T. (1978). Distribution of hypothalamic hormones and other peptides in the brain. In "Frontiers in Neuroendocrinology" Vol. 5, pp. 1–33. Raven Press, New York.

Jackson, I. M. D., and Mueller, G. P. (1982). Neuroendocrine interrelationships. In "Biological Regulation and Development (R. F. Goldberger and K. R. Yamamoto, eds.), Vol. 3A, pp. 127–202. Plenum, New York.

Krieger, D. T., and Martin, J. B. (1981). Brain peptides, N. Engl. J. Med. 304, 876–885, 944–951.

Meites, J., and Sonntag, W. E. (1981). Hypothalamic hypophysiotropic hormones and neurotransmitter regulation: Current views. Annu. Rev. Pharmacol. Toxicol. 21, 295–322.

Negro-Vilar, A., Ojeda, S. R., and McCann S. M. (1980). Hypothalamic control of LHRH and somatostatin: Role of central neurotransmitters and intracellular messengers. In "Biochemical Actions of Hormones" (G. Litwack, ed.), Vol. 7, pp. 246–285. Academic Press, New York.

Schally, A. V., Arimura, A., and Kastin, A. J. (1973). Hypothalamic regulatory hormones. *Science* **179**, 341–350.

Schally, A. V., Kastin, A. J., and Arimura, A. (1977). Hypothalamic hormones: The link between brain and body. *Am. Sci.* **65**, 712–719.

Schally, A. V., Coy, D. H., and Meyers, C. A. (1978). Hypothalamic regulatory hormones. *Annu. Rev. Biochem.* **47**, 89–128.

Terry, L. C., and Martin, J. B. (1977). Hypothalamic hormones: Subcellular distribution and mechanisms of release. *Annu. Rev. Pharmacol. Toxicol.* **18**, 111–123.

Weiner, R. I., and Ganong, W. F. (1978). Role of brain monoamines and histamine in regulation of anterior pituitary secretion. *Physiol. Rev.* **58**, 905–976.

C. Research Papers

Baird, A., Wehrenberg, W. B., Shibasaki, T., Benoit, R., Chong-Li, Z., Esch, F., and Ling, N. (1982). Ovine corticotropin-releasing factor stimulates the concomitant secretion of corticotropin, β-lipotropin, β-endorphin, and γ-lipotropin by the bovine adenohypophysis *in vitro*. *Biochem. Biophys. Res. Commun.* **108**, 959–964.

Blum, J. J., and Conn, P. M. (1982). Gonadotropin-releasing hormone stimulation of luteinizing hormone release: A ligand receptor-effector model. *Proc. Natl. Acad. Sci. U.S.A.* **79**, 7307–7311.

Drust, D. S., and Martin, T. F. J. (1982). Thyrotropin-releasing hormone rapidly and transiently stimulates cytosolic calcium-dependent protein phosphorylation in GH_3 pituitary cells. *J. Biol. Chem.* **257**, 7566–7573.

Esch, F. S., Bohlen, P., Ling, N. C., Brazeau, P. E., Wehrenberg, W. B., and Guillemin, R. (1983). Primary structures of three human pancreas peptides with growth hormone-releasing activity. *J. Biol. Chem.* **258**, 1806–1812.

Giguere, V., and Labrie, F. (1983). Additive effects of epinephrine and corticotropin-releasing factor (CRF) on adrenocorticotropin release in rat anterior pituitary cells. *Biochem. Biophys. Res. Commun.* **110**, 456–462.

Heisler, S., Reisine, T. D., Hook, V. Y. H., and Axelrod, J. (1982). Somatostatin inhibits multireceptor stimulation of cyclic AMP formation and corticotropin secretion in mouse pituitary tumor cells. *Proc. Natl. Acad. Sci. U.S.A.* **79**, 6502–6506.

Hinkle, P. M., and Kinsella, P. A. (1982). Rapid temperature-dependent transformation of the thyrotropin-releasing hormone receptor complex in rat pituitary tumor cells. *J. Biol. Chem.* **257**, 5462–5470.

Miller, W. L., Kaplan, S. L., and Grumbach, M. M. (1980). Child abuse as a cause of post-traumatic hypopituitarism. *N. Engl. J. Med.* **302**, 724–728.

Naor, Z., and Catt, K. J. (1982). Mechanism of action of gonadotropin-releasing hormone in the rat. *Nature (London)* **296**, 354.

Pieper, D. R., Gala, R. R., Regiani, S. R., and Marshall, J. C. (1982). Dependence of pituitary gonadotropin-releasing hormone (GnRH) receptors on GnRH secretion from the hypothalamus. *Endocrinology (Baltimore)* **110**, 749–753.

Rebecci, M. J., Kolesnick, R. N., and Gershengorn, M. C. (1983). Thyrotropin-releasing hormone stimulates rapid loss of phosphatidylinositol and its conversion to 1,2-diacylglycerol and phosphatidic acid in rat mammotropic pituitary cells. *J. Biol. Chem.* **258**, 227–234.

Richardson, S. B., Prasad, J. A., and Hollander, C. S. (1982). Acetylcholine. melatonin and potassium depolarization stimulate release of luteinizing hormone-releasing hormone from rat hypothalamus *in vitro*. *Proc. Natl. Acad. Sci. U.S.A.* **79**, 2686–2689.

Rivier, C., Brownstein, M., Spiess, J., Rivier, J., and Vale, W. (1982). *In vivo* corticotropin releasing factor-induced secretion of adrenocorticotropin, β-endorphin, and corticosterone. *Endocrinology (Baltimore)* **110**, 272–278.

Spiess, J., Rivier, J., Rivier, C., and Vale, W. (1981). Primary structure of corticotropin-releasing factor from ovine hypothalamus. *Proc. Natl. Acad. Sci. U.S.A.* **78**, 6517–6521.

Wang, W.-K., Jeng, L. S., Chiang, Y., and Chien, N. K. (1982). Inhibition of dopamine biosynthesis by gonadotropin releasing hormone in the rat. *Nature (London)* **296**, 354.

Chapter **4**

Posterior Pituitary Hormones

I. INTRODUCTION

Two important hormones are secreted from the posterior pituitary in both males and females. These are vasopressin (VP), the antidiuretic hormone, and oxytocin (OT), which in females acts as the milk ejection factor. Both are nonapeptides, closely related in structure and apparently derived from the same ancestral gene.

The primary recognized function of VP is to stimulate reabsorption of water from the distal tubular kidney. This is clearly established because in the absence of VP up to as much as 25 liters of diluted urine can be excreted each day. Accordingly, the release of VP is generated by the need to maintain the blood osmolarity of plasma within strict limits (homeostasis), especially with reference to increased Na^+ concentrations in blood produced by ingestion of NaCl. VP secretion is also increased when blood volume or blood pressure is decreased. The sites of VP synthesis in the hypothalamus appear to be close to the osmoreceptor sites, which sense changes in electrolyte (solute) concentrations in the circulation, and signal release of the hormone from the neuronal terminals in the posterior pituitary. The osmoreceptor is close to the thirst center in the hypothalamus and also interacts with the renin–angiotensin system. Collectively, these systems appear to be the primary elements for regulation of water balance (see also Chapter 15). The role of OT is less clear.

In females, OT plays a major role in milk letdown for nourishing the suckling infant (see also Chapter 14). Obviously there is no corresponding role for OT in the male. In addition, oxytocin action on the uterine myometrium may play an important role in inducing the uterine contractions leading to the normal termination of pregnancy. Consequently, it is important to ensure that OT not be released prematurely during pregnancy; and indeed there are safeguards to ensure this does not occur.

Some responses are elicited both by VP and OT. Thus, VP also stimulates uterine contractions in humans and can also stimulate the milk ejection to a slight degree. However, the stimuli for the release of each hormone are different, ensuring, to a certain extent, that only one of the hormones is released in response to a specific need. Similar biological activities can be expected from homologies in the molecular structure of VP and OT, and the homologous regions may be involved in the responses generated in common. Some functions are affected oppositely by the two hormones. While VP, in pharmacological amounts, elevates blood pressure, OT slightly lowers it, and the same trend is evident in constriction of the coronary arteries by VP and their dilation by OT.

In its major action, VP inhibits water diuresis, and OT can also produce this effect. Of interest is the possible precursor status of OT for the formation of CNS-active peptides. If indeed VP is actually involved in ACTH secretion and OT produces MIF and MRF in some species (probably not in higher mammals), then there may be regulatory systems to partition the fates of VP and OT between the formation of releasing factors or other biological products active in the CNS and storage in the terminals of the neurohypophysis. As new actions of OT become apparent in tissues common to the male and female, the role of this hormone in the male may emerge.

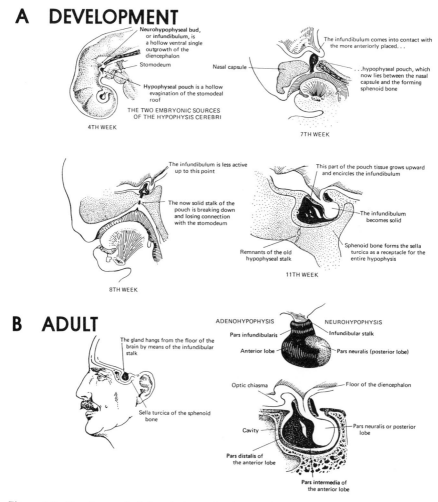

Figure 4-1. Development of the pituitary gland. Reproduced by permission from D. A. Langebartel, "The Anatomical Primer." University Park Press, Baltimore, Maryland, 1977.

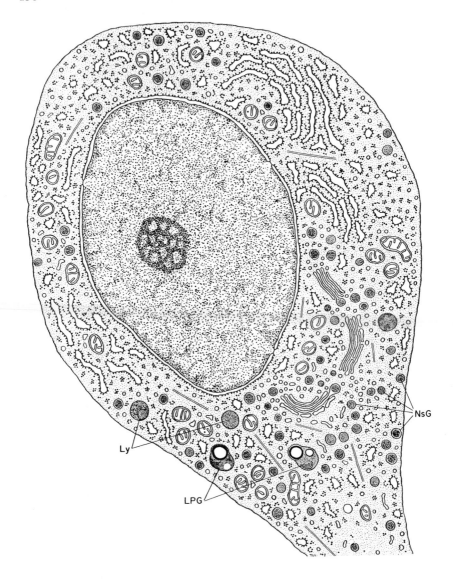

Figure 4-2. Drawing of a neurosecretory cell body of the pituitary. Ly, Lysosomes; LPG, lipofuscin pigment bodies; NsG, neurosecretory granule. Smooth endoplasmic reticulum and Golgi apparatuses are evident. The lower portion of the cell would extend into an axon. Cell bodies of the hormone-producing neurons are located in the hypothalamus and the long axons of these cells (beginning at the lower right in the figure) extend through the median eminence to the terminus of the posterior pituitary. A well-developed Golgi apparatus is visible close to the nucleus. Neurosecretory granules are 1200–2000 Å in diameter, are usually seen near the Golgi apparatus, and may originate in that structure. The endo-

II. ANATOMY, DEVELOPMENT,
AND FINE STRUCTURE
OF THE POSTERIOR PITUITARY

The posterior pituitary or neurohypophysis or *pars neuralis* derives as a hollow ventral outgrowth of the diencephalon of the developing brain. Thus, by the fourth week of human development this outgrowth (neurohypophyseal bud or infundibulum) of the diencephalon becomes apparent (Fig. 4-1A). At this stage a hypophyseal pouch, also hollow, evaginates from the stomodeal roof (Fig. 4-1A). These two outgrowths will form the pituitary while that of the diencephalon will form the posterior pituitary. By the seventh week, both buds have grown steadily and have come into close contact (Fig. 4-1A) with the hypophyseal pouch anterior to the infundibulum. By the eighth week the stalk of the pouch has become solid and begins to deteriorate within the sphenoid bone. The precursor of the posterior pituitary, the outpocket of the brain, remains hollow. Some of the tissue of the hypophyseal pouch encircles the infundibular stalk. The sphenoid bone remodels into the *sella turcica*, which serves as a receptacle for the gland, and this process is accomplished by the eleventh week. The surface and cross section of the finished gland are shown in Fig. 4-1B as well as its gross anatomical location in the adult. The fine structure of the hormone neurosecretory cell is shown in Fig. 4-2. The nerve endings containing the neurosecretory granules may end on a pituicyte (Fig. 4-3).

III. CHEMISTRY

A. Structures of Active and Substituted
Posterior Pituitary Hormones

Shown in Fig. 4-4 are the structures of active and substituted posterior pituitary hormones. The free amino terminal (amino acid 1) is not important for activity, as deaminooxytocin is more biologically active than OT.

---

plasmic reticulum is abundant, consisting of short, rough-surfaced cisternae often aggregated into Nissl bodies. There are numerous clusters of free ribosomes. Small mitochondria are present in the cytoplasm. Lysosomes and lipofuscin pigment bodies are distinguished from neurosecretory granules. The neurosecretory granules are transmitted from the cell body, shown here, down the long axons and are stored in their terminations in the *pars nervosa*. From T. L. Lentz, "Cell Fine Structure." Saunders, Philadelphia, Pennsylvania, 1971.

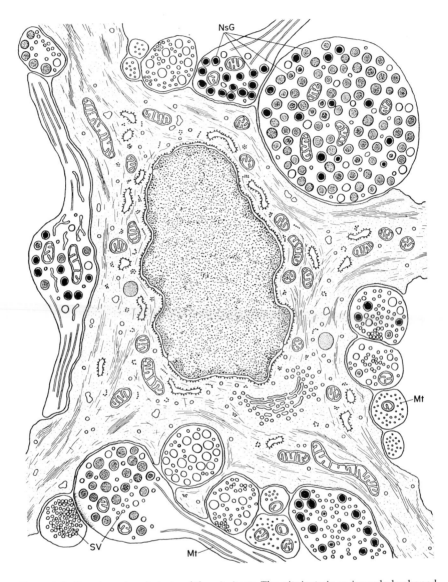

Figure 4-3. Drawing of a pituicyte of the pituitary. The pituicyte is an irregularly shaped cell with long cytoplasmic processes which relate to axons of neurons; consequently nerve fibers often appear to be partially embedded in this cell (top and bottom). Mt, Microtubules; SV, synaptic vesicles; NsG, neurosecretory granules. Reproduced from T. L. Lentz, "Cell Fine Structure." Saunders, Philadelphia, Pennsylvania, 1971.

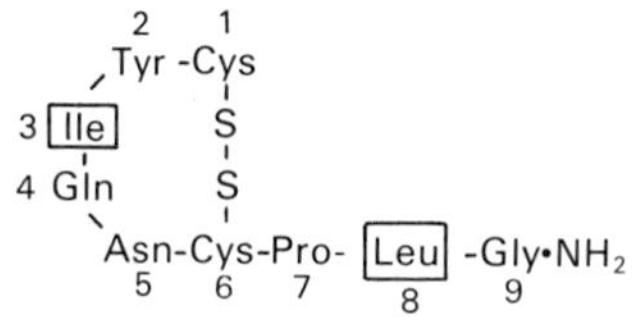

```
        2   1
      ,Tyr -Cys
   3 [Ile]    S
              |
   4 Gln      S
       \      |
        Asn-Cys-Pro- [Leu] -Gly•NH2
         5   6   7     8    9
```

OXYTOCIN (50 mU/mg in supraoptic nucleus or paraventricular
nucleus; 1 mg OXYTOCIN= 400-500 units of activity
compared to USP posterior pituitary reference standards)

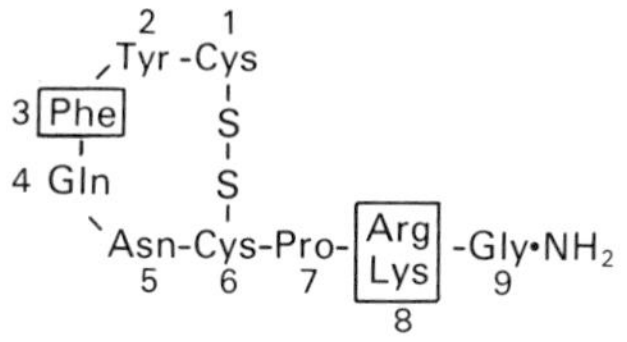

```
        2   1
      ,Tyr -Cys
   3 [Phe]    S
              |
   4 Gln      S
       \      |
        Asn-Cys-Pro- [Arg]  -Gly•NH2
         5   6   7   [Lys]   9
                       8
```

Arg/Lys **VASOPRESSIN** ($\sim$200 mU/mg in supraoptic nucleus;
85 mU/mg in paraventricular nucleus)

```
        2   1
      , Tyr -Cys
   3 [Ile]    S
              |
   4 Gln      S
       \      |
        Asn-Cys-Pro- [Arg] -Gly•NH2
         5   6   7     8    9
```

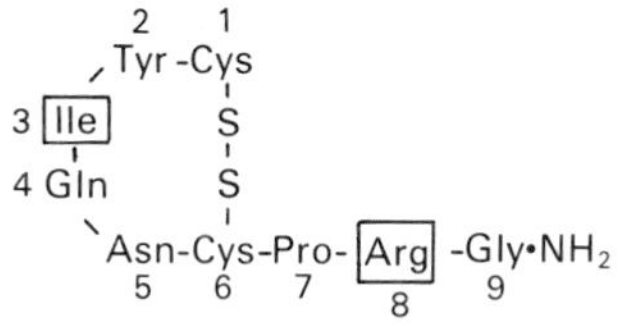

Arg **VASOTOCIN** (ancient structure; questionable whether
it is in pineal gland)

Figure 4-4. Structures of OT and arginine or lysine VP and arginine vasotocin.

Replacement of Leu_8 with Ile reduces activity. If Gln_4 is replaced by Glu,
the hormone is inactivated. In Arg-vasopressin (AVP), the basic side
chain (Arg_8) is essential for antidiuretic activity and explains the lack of
crossover effect of OT. Another point of difference is the amino acid
residue at position 3.

The structure of arginine vasotocin (AVT), present in the pineal gland,
also is shown in Fig. 4-4. AVT reflects the structure of OT at position 3
(Ile) and of VP at position 8 (Arg). AVT is a very active hormone, especially in the control of developing reproductive functions. More information will appear on this interesting hormone in the chapter on the
pineal gland (Chapter 18). AVT appears to be the ancestral precursor of
both VP and OT. A scheme showing the evolution of these hormones
appears in Fig. 4-5. Recently, two neurophysins (NPs) have been reported in the pineal gland. NPs are proteins derived from the same gene
product as either VP or OT in the hypothalamus.

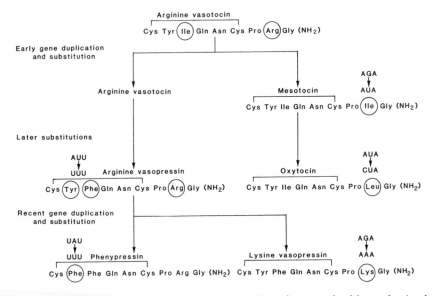

Figure 4-5. Evolution of posterior pituitary peptides of mammals. Mammals simultaneously produce two posterior pituitary hormones by gene duplication. Point mutations account for individual amino acid substitutions. Possible changes in nucleotide sequences accounting for point mutations are shown and substituted amino acids are circled. Reproduced from D. W. Lincoln and R. V. Short, eds., "Reproduction in Mammals. Book III. Hormonal Control of Reproduction," 2nd ed. Cambridge Univ. Press, London and New York, 1984.

B. Interaction of Posterior Pituitary Hormones with Active Sites of NPs

The posterior pituitary hormones are transported down the long axons of the cell bodies of the neurons responsible for their synthesis. During transport, a preprotein product of a single gene is processed into VP or OT (Fig. 4-6) and the NP protein with which it complexes. NP I is associated with OT and NP II is associated with VP. The preprotein (Fig. 4-7) is about 20,000 molecular weight and is cleaved by proteases to an NP of about 9,500–10,000 molecular weight (Fig. 4-8).

The two NPs are very similar in structure and either OT or VP can form a complex with either NP *in vitro*. In some cases, it has been reported that NPs contain lipids, bonded noncovalently, such as cholesterol, phosphatidylcholine, phosphatidylethanolamine, phosphatidyl-

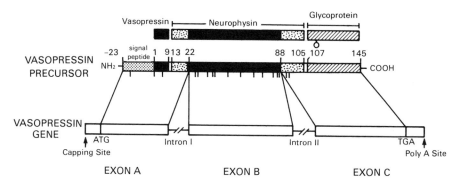

Figure 4-6. Proposed structure of the VP gene, its translation product, and the matured peptides. The gene codes for arginine VP, NP, and glycoprotein and contains two introns. The gene product, provasopressin, is indicated in the middle. Negative numbers indicate amino acid sequence of the signal sequence while the positive numbers indicate the prohormone sequence. The attached open circle on the matured glycoprotein product at the top right stands for carbohydrate. Reproduced from D. Richter, VP and OT are expressed as polyproteins. *Trends Biochem. Sci.* **8,** 278–281 (1983).

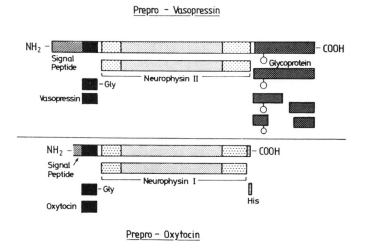

Figure 4-7. Prepro-vasopressin and prepro-oxytocin. Proteolytic maturation proceeds from top to bottom for each precursor. The organization of the gene translation products is similar in either case except that a glycoprotein is included in the proprotein of VP in the C-terminal region. Heavily stippled bars of the NPs represent conserved amino acid regions; lightly stippled bars represent variable C and N termini. Reproduced from D. Richter, VP and OT are expressed as polyproteins. *Trends Biochem. Sci.* **8,** 278–281 (1983).

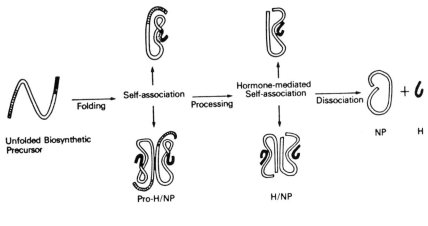

Unfolded Biosynthetic
Precursor

Folding → Self-association → Processing → Hormone-mediated Self-association → Dissociation → NP + H

Pro-H/NP

H/NP

Biosynthesis-Packaging   Transport-Storage   Exocytosis

Figure 4-8. Relationship of biosynthetic precursor structure to molecular events occurring in neurohypophyseal hormone/NP biosynthesis. The filled and open lines denote hormone and NP segments, respectively. The hatched line represents the COOH-terminal glycopeptide occurring in pro-AVP/NP II. Folding of the precursors is visualized to lead to self-association through the NP domains of the precursors. The NP–NP and H–NP interaction surfaces are retained after enzymatic processing, the latter of which leads to formation of noncovalent complexes between hormone (H) and NP as well as dimers in secretory granules until released by exocytosis. Biosynthesis occurs in the cell body followed by folding of the precursor. These are packaged in granules in the Golgi apparatus and the granules (neurosecretory vesicles) are transported down the axon (the hormone is bound to NP in the vesicles). Finally, the granules are stored in the nerve terminals of the posterior pituitary until the signal for secretion occurs, after which H and NP may rapidly dissociate, producing the hormone free in the blood. Reproduced from T. Kanmera and I. M. Chaiken, Molecular properties of the oxytocin/bovine neurophysin biosynthetic precursor. *J. Biol. Chem.* **260,** 8474–8482 (1985). © 1985 by The American Society of Biological Chemists, Inc.

serine, and sphingomyelin. The significance of lipids in these proteins is not clear.

The half-life of VP or OT is increased dramatically from about 3 min to about 10–20 min when it is complexed with NP in blood. The hormone–NP complex probably stabilizes the hormone within the neurosecretory granules, but following release from the secretory granule, it is unlikely that the complex survives in the bloodstream.

The first three amino acids of either hormone are active in binding to the NP molecule, as shown for OT in Fig. 4-9. Binding of the hormone with the NP probably involves a conformational change in the latter. Cysteine$_1$ of the hormone incorporates its free amino group in an elec-

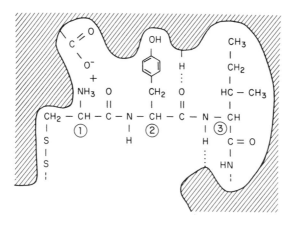

Figure 4-9. Interactions of the first three residues of OT with the strong site of NP. The shaded area represents the protein. The first three residues of VP are the same as those of OT with the exception of phenylanine in position 3. Residues 4–9 are not shown. Note that the peptide bond between residues 2 and 3 contributes to the hormonal interaction with NP through hydrogen bonding. Reproduced with permission from E. Breslow, *in* "Cell Biology of the Secretory Process" (M. Cantin ed.), pp. 276–308. Karger, Basel (1984).

trostatic linkage to a charged carboxyl group of the NP binding site (Fig. 4-9). This carboxyl group could be on a glutamate residue. Amino acid 2, Tyr, and 3, Phe, of VP (Ile in OT) participate in hydrophobic interactions at the NP binding site. The peptide bond between amino acid residues 2 and 3 appears to hydrogen bond to NP (Fig. 4-9).

The amino acid sequences of NP I and II are shown in Fig. 4-10. There is extensive homology between NP I and NP II. Recently, it has been shown that posterior pituitary hormones can be methylated (Arg or Lys residues are most likely), and it is surmised that the modified hormones will have altered biological activities. Apparently NP serves only a stabilizing role insofar as the activities of the posterior pituitary hormones are concerned. Although NP is undoubtedly released in free form in the blood, a distinct activity of uncomplexed NP has not been found.

IV. BIOCHEMISTRY

Formation and Neurosecretion of Posterior Pituitary Hormones

VP and OT are formed in the cell bodies of neurons located in the hypothalamus. Separate neurons probably synthesize each type of hor-

	1	2	3	4	5	6	7	8	9	10	11	12	13	14	15	16	17	18	19	20
Bovine II	Ala	Met	Ser	Asp	Leu	Glu	Leu	Arg	Gln	Cys	Leu	PRO	CYS	GLY	PRO	GLY	GLY	LYS	GLY	ARG
Porcine III																				
Porcine I																				
Bovine I		Val	Leu		Asp	Val		Thr												
Porcine II		Val	Leu		Asp	Val		Lys												

	21	22	23	24	25	26	27	28	29	30	31	32	33	34	35	36	37	38	39	40
Bovine II	CYS	PHE	GLY	PRO	SER	ILE	CYS	CYS	GLY	ASP	GLU	Leu	Gly	Cys	Phe	Val	Gly	Thr	Ala	Glu
Porcine III																				
Porcine I																				
Bovine I																				
Porcine II																				

	41	42	43	44	45	46	47	48	49	50	51	52	53	54	55	56	57	58	59	60
Bovine II	Ala	Leu	Arg	Cys	Gln	Glu	Glu	Asn	Tyr	Leu	Pro	Ser	Pro	Cys	Gln	Ser	Gly	Gln	Lys	PRO
Porcine III																				
Porcine I																				
Bovine I																				
Porcine II																				

	61	62	63	64	65	66	67	68	69	70	71	72	73	74	75	76	77	78	79	80
Bovine II	CYS	GLY	SER	GLY	GLY	ARG	CYS	ALA	ALA	ALA	GLY	ILE	CYS	CYS	ASN	ASP	GLU	Ser	Cys	Val
Porcine III																				
Porcine I																				
Bovine I															Ser	Pro	Asp	Gly		His
Porcine II			Glu													Pro	Asp	Gly		Arg

	81	82	83	84	85	86	87	88	89	90	91	92	93	94	95
Bovine II	Thr	Glu	Pro	Glu	Cys	Arg	Glu	Gly	Ile / Val	Gly	Phe	Pro	Arg	Arg	Val
Porcine III								Ala	Ser		Leu			Ala	
Porcine I								Ala	Ser		Leu				
Bovine I	Glu	Asp		Ala		Asp	Pro	Glu	Ala	Ala		Ser	Leu / Gln		
Porcine II	Phe	Asp		Ala		Asp	Pro	Glu	Ala	Thr		Ser	Gln		

Figure 4-10. Amino acid sequences of representative NPs. The complete sequence of only bovine NP II is shown. The sequences of the other NPs differ from that of bovine NP II only as indicated. All Cys residues are half-cystines. The duplicated segments are capitalized and should be compared by considering the Gly–Lys sequence deleted from the second duplicated segment. Where two residues are identified at the same position, this indicates microheterogeneity (bovine NP II) or ambiguity (bovine NP I). There is a large extent of homology between NP I and NP II. Reproduced from E. Breslow, "Neurophysin: Cell Biology of the Secretory Process," pp. 276–308. Karger, Basel, 1984.

mone and its accompanying NP. Neuronal cell bodies synthesizing OT are located primarily, but not exclusively, in the paraventricular nucleus, whereas neuronal cell bodies synthesizing VP are located primarily, but not exclusively, in the supraoptic nucleus. There are claims that the same cell can synthesize both types of hormones; however, this seems unlikely in view of separate interneuronal stimulation of either secretion product. Figure 4-11A shows a concept of the VP-producing neuron and how the neurosecretion may be signaled and controlled by interneurons, including the osmoreceptor which represents the primary positive signaling mechanism. Electrical signals from the osmoreceptor will be either on or off depending on the osmolarity of the extracellular fluids. From this figure, we can see that the hormone is synthesized in the cell body and moves down the long axon extending from the hypothalamus to the nerve ending. VP–NP II secretion is stimulated exclusive of OT–NP I release using the drug nicotine mediated by stimulation of a cholinergic receptor. OT–NP I can be released specifically through the action of estradiol.

The VP–NP I complex is released by the osmoreceptor, probably via an interneuron which senses the Na^+ concentration in surrounding fluids. Its own cellular volume shrinks at elevated salt concentrations, and the ionic changes induce receptor deformation that generates an electrical or chemical signal which is transmitted to the vasopressinergic neuron. This signal, if electrical, may be transmitted down the axon of the vasopressinergic neuron (possibly along axonal nerve fibers) and in the nerve ending the electrical signal depolarizes the membrane, causing exocytosis of VP–NP II (Fig. 4-11B). Other interneurons may convey signals from baroreceptors located in the carotid sinus, aortic arch, and in the left atrium. The signals impinging on the vasopressinergic neuron may be either electrical or chemical, but in Fig. 4-11A, they have been pictured for convenience as electrical signals. The VP–NP II complex permeates local fenestrated capillaries in order to research the general circulation.

At some point, the VP/NP complex dissociates and free VP in the circulation binds to its membrane receptors. An analogous situation can be pictured for neurons synthesizing oxytocin–NP complexes, except that such neurons are more abundant in paraventricular nuclei than in supraoptic nuclei, although they are present in both locations in the hypothalamus.

An aspect of this overall process of neurosecretion which has not been discussed up to this point is the fact that the membrane of the neurosecretory granule is retrieved by the nerve ending following exocytosis and presumably supplies starting materials for subsequently

A

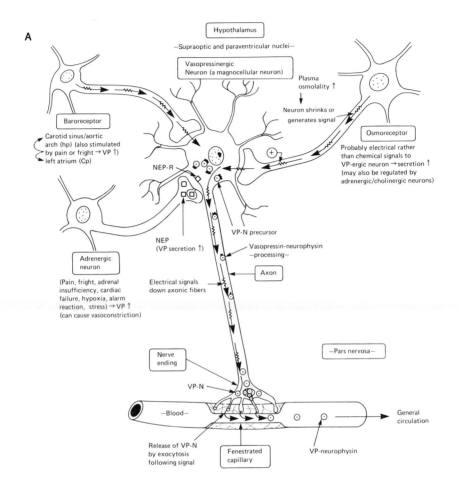

Figure 4-11. Vasopressinergic magnocellular neuron and its regulation. (A) Speculative concept of vasopressinergic neuron and interneurons which provide positive and negative stimuli for secretion of posterior pituitary hormone. The vasopressinergic neuron in the center has a cell body in the hypothalamus with a long axon extending to the terminal region of the posterior pituitary. The osmoreceptor is a neuron pictured at the right. When plasma osmolality increases, the cell volume of the osmoreceptor neuron shrinks or ionic changes conformationally alter a receptor to a point where the cell sends an electrical or chemical signal down its axon to the cell body of the vasopressinergic neuron. This signal would generate an action potential, or via a receptor for a chemical signal, generate a second messenger whose information would be transmitted down the axon of the vasopressinergic cell to cause release of the VP–NP complex from the nerve ending by exocytosis. The complex passes through fenestrations in local capillaries and reaches the general circulation. Other interneurons that regulate VP secretion are pictured on the left: Some aminergic neurons restrict neurotransmitter synthesis to the nerve ending. In the

146

B

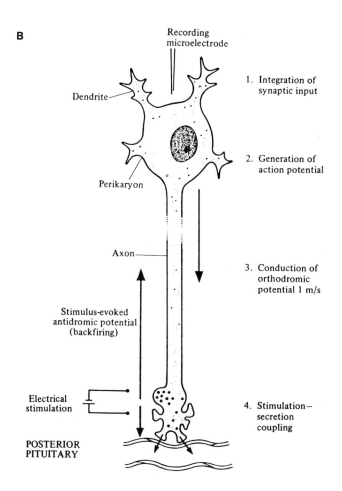

Recording
microelectrode

Dendrite

Perikaryon

Axon

Stimulus-evoked
antidromic potential
(backfiring)

Electrical
stimulation

POSTERIOR
PITUITARY

1. Integration of
synaptic input

2. Generation of
action potential

3. Conduction of
orthodromic
potential 1 m/s

4. Stimulation—
secretion
coupling

cell body, synthesis of prohormones occurs and the products are packaged into granules. These are moved by fast axonal transport (2 mm/hr) down the axon and the prohormone is cleaved during this process to the mature products. These are stored in the nerve ending awaiting a signal, as described above. After exocytosis, there is retrograde transport of the granule membrane for reuse. (B) Electrophysiological properties of the magnocellular neuron. The numbered right-hand column describes the stages in the production of an action potential (the electrical signal) and its conduction along the axon to the nerve ending in the posterior pituitary. This results in depolarization, influx of calcium ions, and hormone release by exocytosis. Hormone release can be induced by electrical stimulation of the posterior pituitary using an implanted electrode as indicated in the bottom left. Reproduced from D. W. Lincoln, The posterior pituitary. In "Reproduction in Mammals. Book III. Hormonal Control of Reproduction" (C. R. Austin and R. V. Short, eds.), 2nd ed., pp. 21–50. Cambridge Univ. Press, London and New York, 1984. Reproduced by copyright permission of Cambridge University Press.

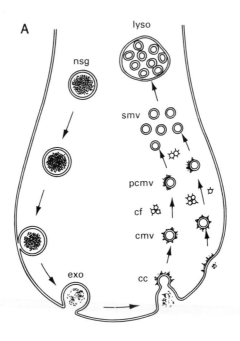

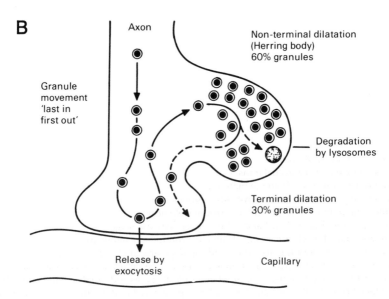

Figure 4-12. Mechanism of secretion of posterior pituitary hormones. (A) Scheme showing exocytosis–vesiculation sequence operating in neurohypophyseal terminals. Contents of the neurosecretory granules (nsg) are emptied into the extracellular space by exocytosis

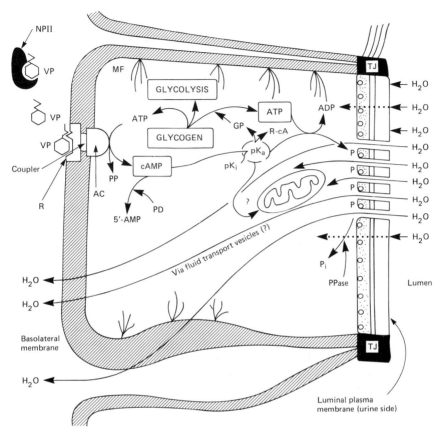

Figure 4-14. Model of VP action on water reabsorption in distal tubule. NPII, Neurophysin II; VP, vasopressin; R, receptor; AC, adenylate cyclase; MF, myofibril; PP, pyrophosphate; cAMP, cyclic AMP; GP, glycogen phosphorylase; PK_i, inactive protein kinase; PK_a, active protein kinase; R–cA, regulatory subunit–cyclic AMP complex; TJ, tight junction; PD, phosphodiesterase; PPase, pyrophosphatase. Vasopressin–neurophysin complex dissociates at some point and free VP binds to its cell membrane receptor in the plasma membrane surface. Perhaps through a transducing agent (coupler) adenylate cyclase is stimulated on the cytoplasmic side of the cell membrane, generating increased levels of cyclic AMP from ATP. Cyclic AMP-dependent protein kinases are stimulated and phosphorylate various proteins (perhaps including microtubular subunits) which, through aggregation, insert as water channels in the luminal plasma membrane, thus increasing the reabsorption of water by free diffusion. Reproduced with permission from T. P. Dousa and H. Valtin, Cellular actions of vasopressin in the mammalian kidney. *Kidney Int.* **10,** 45–63 (1975).

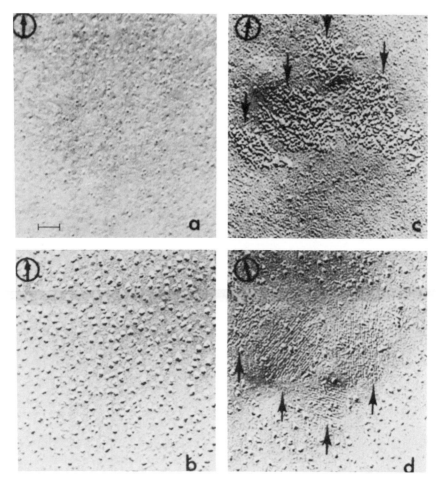

Figure 4-15. Effects of VP on toad bladder granular cell luminal membrane by freeze-fracture and electron microscopy. (a and b) Freeze-fracture faces in the absence of VP. (c and d) Freeze-fracture faces in the presence of VP. Apparent aggregation of membrane particles occurs after VP stimulation. In (c), the uncircled arrows point to separate sites of aggregated particles, and in (d) they point to linear arrays of depressions corresponding to the aggregation shown in (c). The circled arrows indicate the shadowing direction. The scale marker (in a) denotes 0.1 μm. Reproduced with permission from R. M. Hays, Antidiuretic hormone. *N. Engl. J. Med.* **295,** 659–665 (1976).

reaches the extracellular space and binds to the VP receptors on the basolateral membrane of the cell. It is required that VP is released from the VP–NP complex prior to associating with its receptor, since the specificity of ligand binding shows that Tyr_2 and Asn_5 play critical roles in the interaction with receptor. Since Tyr_2 is also involved in the interaction with NP, the hormone must be in the free form to interact with receptor. Through this interaction, there is a stimulation of adenylate cyclase activity on the cytoplasmic side of the membrane. This process involves the transducing guanine nucleotide regulatory protein (Fig. 4-16). ATP is converted to cyclic AMP on the cytoplasmic side of the cell membrane by the activated cyclase. Thyroid hormone may affect VP-sensitive adenylate cyclase. Thus, in hypothyroid rats both the basal activity as well as the VP-stimulated activity of adenylate cyclase is decreased. Treatment with thyroxine restored the activity to normal levels. The elevated level of cyclic AMP, produced by VP, combines with the regulatory subunits (R) of inactive protein kinase (PK_i or R_2C_2) to release the catalytically active subunit (C):

$$R_2C_2 + 4 \text{ cAMP} \rightarrow R_2 \cdot 4 \text{ cyclic AMP} + 2C$$

The active protein kinase (PK_a or C) is thought by some to catalyze the phosphorylation of tubulin which aggregates into microtubules. These insert into the apical membrane forming channels for water uptake which occurs by a process of free diffusion. Thus, the tight epithelial cell takes up little water in the unstimulated state and takes up a considerable amount of water in the VP-stimulated state owing to a profusion of water channels created in the apical membrane.

Electron micrographs from toad bladder granular cell luminal membrane untreated or treated with VP show aggregation of membrane particles after stimulation with VP (Fig. 4-15). These observations suggest the possibility that water channels are being inserted into the membrane under the influence of the hormone.

D. Nature of Kidney VP-Sensitive Adenylate Cyclase, a Receptor Preparation

The VP receptor has been studied extensively in beef renal medullary membrane preparations which contain the receptor and the coupled hormone-sensitive adenylate cyclase. Isolated membrane particles retain nearly all of the specificity of binding and the affinity of the receptor for VP, characteristic of the whole cell, enabling evaluation of ligand binding and consequences for adenylate cyclase activity. In essence, the system can be summarized as shown in Fig. 4-16. The binding of the hormone to the membrane receptor results in the activation of adenylate cyclase so that the intracellular level of cyclic AMP can be raised effectively. The rate-limiting step in the activation of adenylate cyclase is the formation of the hormone–receptor complex. As in other hormone–receptor systems, there appears to be one ligand binding site per recep-

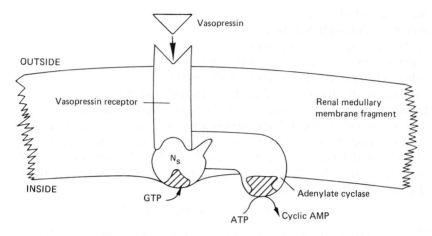

Figure 4-16. Speculative structure of the vasopressin (VP) receptor and coupled adenylate cyclase in the kidney. N_s, Guanylate nucleotide stimulatory factor.

tor molecule. The transducing action coupling ligand interaction with receptor to activation of adenylate cyclase is a linear function.

In the analysis of the interaction of [³H]AVP with this receptor preparation according to

$$VP + receptor \underset{k_{-1}}{\overset{k_{+1}}{\rightleftharpoons}} VP\text{–receptor complex}$$

k_{+1}, the association rate constant, is $3 \times 10^6 \, M^{-1} \, sec^{-1}$ and k_{-1}, the dissociation rate constant, is $7 \times 10^{-3} \, sec^{-1}$. Thus, the affinity of VP for receptor is

$$k_{+1}/k_{-1} = 0.5 \times 10^9 \, M^{-1} \, (K_a)$$

and the dissociation constant is

$$k_{-1}/k_{+1} = 1/K_a = 2 \times 10^{-9} \, M \, (K_d)$$

Similar analysis of OT binding to this receptor preparation produces a k_{+1} of about $9 \times 10^4 \, M^{-1} \, sec^{-1}$, a k_{-1} of $12 \times 10^{-3} \, sec^{-1}$, a K_d in the range of $10^{-7} M$, and a K_a of about $1 \times 10^7 \, M^{-1}$. Thus, as shown in Table 4-1, VP associates with its receptor about 30 times faster than OT and the receptor has about 100 times the affinity for VP compared to OT.

GTP accelerates the rate at which VP stimulates adenylate cyclase activity. GTP may accomplish this by binding to an allosteric site (guanine nucleotide binding protein, N_s) on adenylate cyclase, which

Table 4–1. Physical Measurements of Ligand Interactions with VP Receptor (Kidney Distal Tubule) and OT Receptor (Mammary Gland Myoepithelial Cell)

Measurement	VP receptor		OT receptor for OT
	For VP	For OT	
k_{+1}, association rate constant	$3 \times 10^6 \ M^{-1} \ sec^{-1}$	$9 \times 10^4 \ M^{-1} \ sec^{-1}$	$2 \times 10^5 \ M^{-1} \ sec^{-1}$
k_{-1}, dissociation rate constant	$7 \times 10^{-3} \ sec^{-1}$	$11 \times 10^{-3} \ sec^{-1}$	$6 \times 10^{-4} \ sec^{-1}$
K_a, affinity	$0.5 \times 10^9 \ M^{-1}$	$10^7 \ M^{-1}$	$\sim 10^8 \ M^{-1}$
K_d, dissociation constant	$2 \times 10^{-9} \ M$	$10^{-7} \ M$	$1–5 \times 10^{-9} \ M$

ultimately stimulates the rate at which the hormone interacts with the receptor. An allosteric change may be communicated in the reverse direction from the inner cell membrane to affect receptor conformation. At $10^{-5} \ M$, GTP also stimulates the catalytic rate of adenylate cyclase by producing a conformational change directly in the enzyme. The effect of GTP is independent of phosphorylation activity. It is possible that the conformational change in the enzyme induced by GTP is the one which subsequently affects the rate of interaction between limiting amounts of VP and the receptor. Consequently, the availability of GTP or nucleoside triphosphates, such as ATP, acting similarly is important for the production of this effect in the cell. Under certain conditions nucleoside triphosphates can inhibit this process.

E. Effects of VP on the Liver

VP, like α-adrenergic agonists, acts on the hepatocyte to promote glycogenolysis; however, the physiological importance of this action is not well understood. In this effect, VP, like angiotensin II and phenylephrine (see Chapter 11), via increase in cytoplasmic Ca^{2+}, releases glucose from the liver while promoting the uptake of K^+. Release of glucose is accomplished by stimulating the breakdown of glycogen. These actions of VP can be blocked by phentolamine, an α-blocking agent whose structure is shown in Fig. 4-17.

Glycogenolysis is stimulated by VP in liver by mobilizing intracellular stores of Ca^{2+} (mitochondrial and/or endoplasmic reticulum) which results in an increase of cytosolic Ca^{2+}. Increased cytosolic Ca^{2+} stimulates phosphorylase b kinase, hence phosphorylase activation (conversion of phosphorylase b to a) extrusion of Ca^{2+} and uptake of K^+. VP

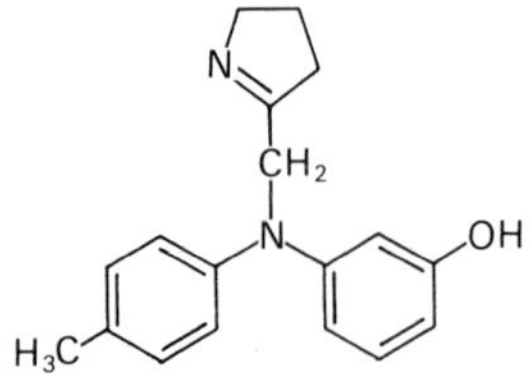

Figure 4-17. Structure of phentolamine, an α-blocking agent.

interacts with a receptor in the hepatocyte cell membrane, resulting in generation of a second messenger causing Ca^{2+} mobilization. Ca^{2+} released from the intracellular storage sites (e.g., mitochondrion) is expelled in part from the cell by a specific mechanism in the cell membrane. VP also stimulates phosphorylation of about a dozen proteins in hepatocyte cytosol, including pyruvate kinase in addition to phosphorylase. Cyclic AMP, a second messenger in β-receptor reactions, is not involved in the effects of VP. VP appears to stimulate the turnover of phosphatidylinositol in hepatocytes, and this effect is either linked to the VP–receptor interaction or to the process of extrusion of intracellular Ca^{2+} and the uptake of extracellular Ca^{2+}.

F. VP and ACTH Release

It has been known for some time that VP injected at a point where it could rapidly gain access to the hypothalamic–pituitary axis could stimulate the release of ACTH and indeed, VP seems to be a releasing factor for ACTH in addition to CRH (see Chapters 3 and 10). The most likely biological role for VP in this context is to function to potentiate the release of ACTH by CRH. CRH has now been shown to produce a rapid stimulation of cyclic AMP in rat anterior pituitary cells. Although VP agonists cause an increase in CRH-induced ACTH release from rat anterior pituitary cells in culture, VP alone has no effect on cyclic AMP levels in these cells. However, when combined with CRH, VP causes a twofold increase in CRH-induced accumulation of cyclic AMP; thus VP acts by enhancing effectiveness of CRH. The second messenger produced by VP apparently results from an interaction of VP with a receptor that is different from the CRH receptor.

G. Behavioral Effects of VP

Lysine and arginine-VP have been shown in model systems to affect positively the consolidation of memory and learning. Whereas puromycin induces amnesia, VP attenuates the puromycin effect by a process distinct from that by which puromycin exerts its effects on the cell. A single subcutaneous injection of VP increases resistance to extinction of a pole-jumping avoidance response in the rat, confirming the positive effects of the hormone on conditioned behavior. So far, the structural requirements for the behavioral effects of VP are less stringent than for hormonal activities (e.g., stimulation of renal adenylate cyclase activity). This suggests that the VP receptors in kidney and brain are different. The Brattleboro rat has been used to assess the effects of VP deficiency. These animals are homozygous in their inability to synthesize VP and they have diabetes insipidus. Recent work suggests a single base deletion in the VP gene which predicts a hormone precursor having a different C terminus, indicating the possibility of faulty transcription/translation. Norepinephrine levels are elevated in the dorsal septal nucleus and in the supraoptic nucleus compared to homozygous nondiabetic rats. Catecholamine levels are lower in the paraventricular nucleus of the diabetic rats compared to controls. These results and other studies suggest that VP modulates catecholamine neurotransmission in specific brain regions and may be related to the effects of VP on behavior, learning, and memory.

H. Overview of Regulation of OT Secretion from the Posterior Pituitary

A summary of secretion of OT from the posterior pituitary is shown in Fig. 4-18. Two major functions are milk ejection in the lactating female and participation in signaling uterine contractions at termination of pregnancy. Some experiments suggest that OT may cause inhibition of androgen synthesis in the testis, but knowledge of the regulation of secretion of OT in the male is not clear. Suckling and related stimuli (auditory, visual) result in milk ejection from the mammary gland of the nursing female and are transmitted rapidly over a spinal reflex arc to the paraventricular nucleus of the hypothalamus (see also Chapter 14). This stimulus appears to be cholinergic and is transmitted to nerve endings in the posterior pituitary, resulting in Ca^{2+} uptake, depolarization, and exocytosis of OT–NP into the circulation. The OT–NP complex is probably rapidly dissociated after exocytosis.

Transmission of the suckling stimulus to the paraventricular nucleus of the hypothalamus by way of a spinal arc reflex is accomplished in milliseconds. The oxytocinergic neuron is stimulated by acetylcholine and repressed by norepinephrine; thus, it can be envisioned as being positively regulated by a cholinergic interneuron and negatively regu-

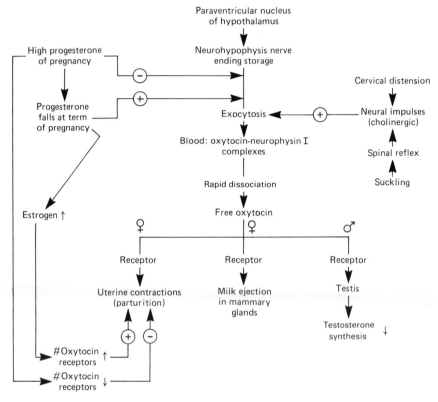

Figure 4-18. Secretion of OT from the posterior pituitary. The effect of OT in the testis appears to lower androgen levels and elevate pregnenolone and progesterone.

lated by an adrenergic interneuron. Visual stimuli (e.g., the sight of a hungry infant) or auditory stimuli (e.g., sound of a baby's cry) can lead to dripping of milk from the breast. These signals are transmitted to the hypothalamus and result in the release of some OT. Only a few seconds are required for OT to reach its target in the mammary gland. After dissociation of the NP, OT binds to a specific cell membrane receptor on myoepithelial cells and causes Ca^{2+} uptake in these cells which derepresses the contractile mechanism. Consequently, ductules and ducts contract and milk is ejected from the gland through the nipple into the infant's mouth. It is not known whether any activities can be ascribed to NP once they have been dissociated from the hormonal complex in the blood.

In the case of terminal uterine contractions at birth, the primary signal for OT release from the posterior pituitary is a marked decline in the

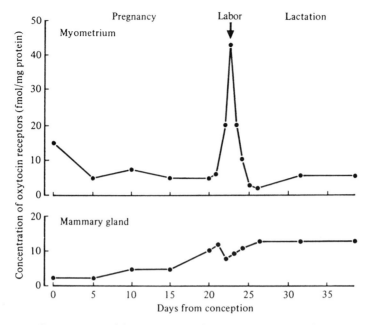

Figure 4-19. Concentration of OT receptors in the rat myometrium and mammary gland during pregnancy and lactation. Receptor number is expressed as the specific binding of tritiated OT to particulate fractions (fmol/mg protein). Reproduced from D. W. Lincoln, The posterior pituitary. *In* "Reproduction in Mammals. Book III. Hormonal Control of Reproduction" (C. R. Austin and R. V. Short, eds.), 2nd ed., pp. 21–50. Cambridge Univ. Press, London and New York, 1984. Reproduced by copyright permission of Cambridge University Press.

level of circulating free progesterone which was being produced at high levels from the placenta during the latter course of pregnancy. At term, there is a surge of estradiol production with the dramatic decline of free progesterone. Estradiol stimulates the uterine myometrium to become more sensitive to OT, perhaps by inducing the formation of new OT receptors (Fig. 4-19). At the same time estrogen causes the release of OT–NP from the posterior pituitary. The immature uterus is not stimulated to contract by OT. Experimentally, estrogen treatment in normal male subjects caused dramatic increases in estrogen-stimulated NP (for OT) plasma levels, but had no significant effect on nicotine (for VP)-stimulated NP secretion.

I. Mechanism of Action of OT

1. Mammary Myoepithelium

The anatomy and morphology of the breast myoepithelial cells are the sites of action of OT are presented in Chapter 14. Released OT–NP

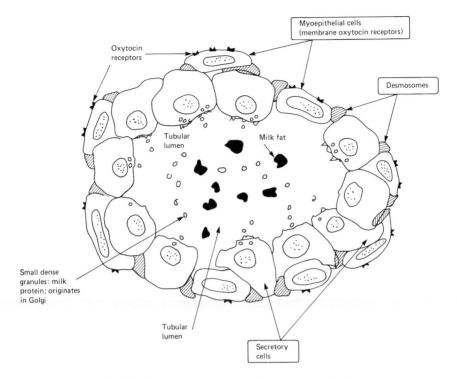

Figure 4-20. Drawing of a cross section of a mammary tubular gland.

complex dissociates in the blood and free oxytocin binds to its receptor located on the membrane of the myoepithelial cell. Although the second messenger of this interaction is unknown, it probably regulates increased intracellular Ca^{2+}, since it is required for depression of the contractile system. Contraction occurs, the tubular lumen is narrowed by contraction, and milk is ejected (Figs. 4-20 and 4-21).

2. Uterine Myometrium

Some reports suggest that OT stimulates the release of $PGF_{2\alpha}$ from the ovine endometrium *in vitro* and from the rat uterus. A direct effect of receptor-bound OT could lead to regulation of membrane phospholipase to release arachidonic acid, the precursor of $PGF_{2\alpha}$. This prostaglandin seems to be produced by OT in the uterine myometrium as part of its effect on initiation of labor. How $PGF_{2\alpha}$ would act to promote contractions is unclear. Synthesis of estrogen is stimulated at termination of pregnancy. This may increase the number of OT binding sites in

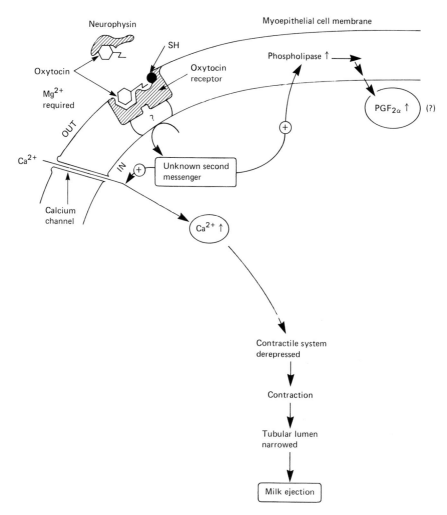

Figure 4-21. Speculative model of OT action on mammary gland.

uterine myometrium at this time. This could explain the sensitivity of the near-term uterus to OT coinciding with the burst of OT released from the posterior pituitary as availability of free progesterone falls dramatically near term. Recent evidence pertaining to the mechanism of OT-induced increase in intracellular Ca^{2+} is depicted in Fig. 4-22. These data were generated for the uterine myometrium. In this system the Ca^{2+} concentration in the cell cytosol is normally about 1/10,000 that of

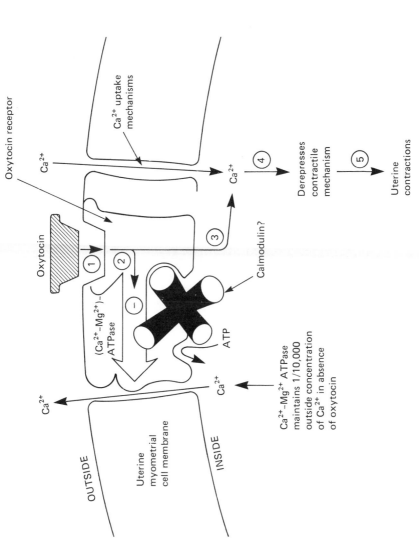

Figure 4-22. Theory that OT induces uterine contraction by receptor regulation of Ca^{2+}, Mg^{2+}-ATPase (outward pumping). Constructed from data reported by M. S. Soloff and P. Sweet, OT inhibition of Ca^{2+}, Mg^{2+}-ATPase activity in rat myometrial plasma membranes. *J. Biol. Chem.* **257**, 10687–10693 (1982).

Oxytocin receptor

Oxytocin

Ca²⁺ uptake mechanisms

Ca^{2+}

① ②

Ca^{2+}

④

Derepresses contractile mechanism

⑤

Uterine contractions

Calmodulin?

③

$(Ca^{2+}-Mg^{2+})$-ATPase

–

ATP

OUTSIDE

Uterine myometrial cell membrane

INSIDE

Ca^{2+}

Ca^{2+}

$Ca^{2+}-Mg^{2+}$ ATPase maintains 1/10,000 outside concentration of Ca^{2+} in absence of oxytocin

the outside concentration owing to the function of Ca^{2+}, Mg^{2+}-ATPase enzyme pump in the plasma membrane which pumps Ca^{2+} out of the cell. According to the work of M. Soloff and P. Sweet, the function of the OT receptor complex can be inferred to generate a conformational effect on the Ca^{2+}, Mg^{2+}-ATPase so as to lower its activity in the outward pumping of Ca^{2+}. This would result in a large increase of intracellular Ca^{2+} by mechanisms of uptake normally occurring. The enhanced Ca^{2+} in cytosol is now available to derepress the contractile mechanism to generate uterine contractions or possibly those of the mammary myoepithelial cells, as the case may be. Note that the model infers the function of calmodulin in this outward-pumping ATPase for which there is some evidence.

J. The OT Receptor

An enriched myoepithelial cell fraction can be obtained from mammary glands with collagenase treatment. The amount of [^{3}H-tyrosyl]oxytocin binding is proportional to the number of cells and the concentration of OT and is about 0.45 fmol/10^6 cells. The apparent dissociation constant in the reaction

$$[^3H]OT + \text{myoepithelial cell receptor} \underset{k_{-1}}{\overset{k_{+1}}{\rightleftharpoons}} [^3H]OT\text{--myoepithelial cell receptor complex}$$

is about 1–5 nM, giving an affinity constant, K_a, of 10^9 to 2×10^8 M^{-1} from equilibrium binding (see Table 4-1). The association rate, k_{+1}, is about 2×10^5 M^{+1} sec^{-1} and the dissociation rate, k_{-1}, is about 6×10^{-4} sec^{-1}, which produce a dissociation constant,

$$K_d = k_{-1}/k_{+1} = 6 \times 10^4 \text{ sec}^{-1}/2 \times 10^5 \, M^{-1} \text{ sec}^{-1} = 3 \text{ n}M$$

and the affinity constant

$$k_{+1}/k_{-1} = 2 \times 10^5 \, M^{-1} \text{ sec}^{-1}/6 \times 10^{-4} \text{ sec}^{-1} = 0.4 \times 10^9 \, M^{-1}$$

The equilibrium measurements are in good agreement with those obtained from rate constants, aligning with a single-step model for the ligand binding function in contrast to some other receptor systems. The subcellular localization of OT receptor in mammary tissue or in uterine smooth muscle is not well known. The K_d of [^{3}H]OT binding to particles is about 1 nM. The affinities of synthetic analogs paralleled milk-ejecting activities and are similar to the potency schedule outlined above with whole cell receptor. Binding was inhibited by millimolar amounts of ATP, but not by GTP or other nucleoside triphosphates. Susceptibility of the binding site to trypsin and *p*-hydroxymercuribenzoate but not to phospholipases and neuraminidase determined its nature as a protein. OT binding is potentiated by certain divalent metal ions, the most potent being divalent zinc, followed by magnesium, nickel, manganese, and cobalt. The binding of the metal ion is a fast step followed by the slow rate-limiting step of OT binding. One of the effects of the metal (Ni, Mg, Mn) is to increase the concentration of OT binding sites. Cobalt increases the affinity of the receptor for OT without changing the number of binding sites. It is postulated that there are two distinct regions for metal ion interaction on the basis of the above results.

In rat uterine smooth muscle, the OT receptor has been localized on the plasma membrane. The K_d of particulate receptor binding to [^{3}H]OT is in the nanomolar range, in agreement with the mammary myoepithelial system. The order of potency of analogs of OT resembles the mammary gland system. Other facets of receptor characterization are similar to the mammary system. The OT receptor remains to be purified extensively and studied.

K. Degradation of Posterior Pituitary Hormones

Two enzymes are involved in the breakdown of OT and VP, cystine aminopeptidase and glutathione transhydrogenase (with oxidized glutathione reductase coupled as a reduced glutathione regenerating system). The products of the reaction are shown in Fig. 4-23. The degrading enzymes, GSH transhydrogenase and cystine aminopeptidase, can operate in random order as shown. Other pathways of degradation, principally in brain or pituitary, are shown in Fig. 3-9. The reactions pictured in Fig. 4-23 take place in liver, in other tissues, and in blood, particularly during pregnancy.

VI. CLINICAL ASPECTS

Many of the clinical applications apply to those considered under releasing factors (Chapter 3), since both hypothalamic releasing factors as well as posterior pituitary hormones travel down the pituitary stalk. Consequently, damage by trauma or tumors also will impede the output of VP and OT. Water balance will be affected and frequency of urination will be controlled medically by administration of hormone or hormone analog to treat diabetes insipidus. Presumably the male will have less consequences to OT deficiency. This disease is somewhat rare in occurrence. In principle, a number of conditions can lead to the failure of VP expression from the posterior pituitary or of its effectiveness at the site

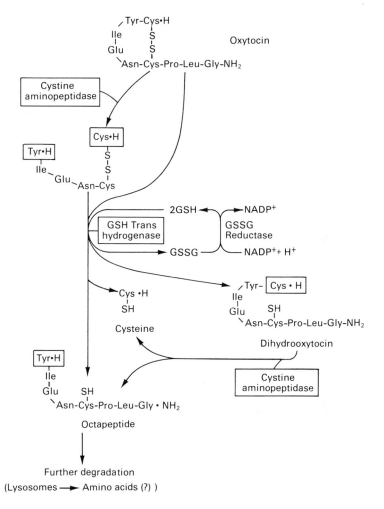

Figure 4-23. Degradation of posterior pituitary hormones: OT transhydrogenase (human placenta) similar to degrading enzymes of other tissues; also similar to enzymes degrading insulin. These enzymes presumably also degrade VP.

of action. Damage by tumors or cysts, encephalitis, granulomatous diseases such as tuberculosis, sarcoidosis, syphilis, as well as meningitis, and arteriosclerosis to the secretory apparatus or to the hypothalamohypophyseal portal system may occur. Vascular destruction may also occur to the portal system as a result of degenerative diseases. Brain tumors may be a most important factor. A major cause is trauma. Hereditary diseases may also play a role with abnormal functions at the level of the hypothalamus–pituitary or the kidney. The latter case is presumed to alter the expression or function of VP receptors. Other unsubstantiated possibilities are increased degradation of VP or development of autoimmune antibodies.

OT induces uterine contractions at the start of labor; however, OT in physiological doses does not induce labor during pregnancy. Hypophysectomized females can have a normal labor, indicating either that the important amounts of OT generate from the fetus or that other factors besides OT are involved. These have been discussed in this chapter and in Chapter 14. Excess or deficiency of OT has, so far, not been associated with a disease process.

References

A. Books

Goldberger, R. F., and Yamamoto, K. R., eds. (1982). "Biological Regulation and Development," Vol. 3A, pp. 253–298. Plenum, New York.

Greep, R. O., Astwood, E. B., Knobil, E., Sawyer, W. H., and Geiger, S. R., eds. (1974). "Handbook of Physiology," Sect. 7, Vol. IV, Part 2, pp. 103–394. Am. Physiol. Soc., Washington, D.C.

Krieger, D. T., and Hughes, J. C., eds. (1980). "Neuroendocrinology," pp. 149–155. Sinauer Associates, Sunderland, Massachusetts.

Williams, R. H., ed. (1981). "Textbook of Endocrinology," 6th ed., pp. 590–591. Saunders, Philadelphia, Pennsylvania.

B. Review Articles

Bie, P. (1980). Osmoreceptors, vasopressin, and control of renal water excretion. *Physiol. Rev.* **60,** 961–1048.

Breslow, E. (1984). Neurophysin: Biology and chemistry of its interactions. In "Cell Biology of the Secretory Process" (M. Cantin, ed.), pp. 276–308. S. Karger, Basel.

Brownstein, M. J., Russell, J. T., and Gainer, H. (1982). In "Frontiers in Neuroendocrinology" (W. F. Ganong and L. Martini, eds.), Vol. 7, pp. 31–43. Raven Press, New York.

Hays, R. M. (1976). Antidiuretic hormone. *Engl. J. Med.* **295,** 659–665.

Heap, R. B. (1983). New functions for oxytocin? *Nature (London)* **301,** 113.

C. Research Papers

Adashi, E. Y., Tucker, E. M., and Hsueh, A. W. W. (1984). Direct regulation of rat testicular steroidogenesis by neurohypophyseal hormones. *J. Biol. Chem.* **259,** 5440–5446.

Bicknell, R. J., and Leng, G. (1982). Endogenous opiates regulate oxytocin but not vasopressin secretion from the neurohypophysis. *Nature (London)* **298,** 161–162.

Capra, J. D., and Walter, R. (1975). Primary structure and evolution of neurophysins. *Ann. N.Y. Acad. Sci.* **248,** 397–407.

Drenth, J. (1981). The structure of neurophysin. *J. Biol. Chem.* **256,** 2601–2602.

Fuchs, A.-R., and Dawood, M. Y. (1980). Oxytocin release and uterine activation during parturition in rabbits. *Endocrinology (Baltimore)* **107**, 1117–1126.

Gainer, H., Sarne, Y., and Brownstein, M. J. (1977). Biosynthesis and axonal transport of rat neurohypophyseal proteins and peptides. *J. Cell Biol.* **73**, 366–381.

Garrison, J. C., and Wagner, J. D. (1982). Glucagon and the Ca^{2+}-linked hormones angiotensin II, norepinephrine, and vasopressin stimulate the phosphorylation of distinct substrates in intact hepatocytes. *J. Biol. Chem.* **257**, 13135–13143.

Giguere, V., and Labrie, F. (1982). Vasopressin potentiates cyclic AMP accumulation and ACTH release induced by corticotropin releasing factor (CRF) in rat anterior pituitary cells in culture. *Endocrinology (Baltimore)* **111**, 1752–1754.

Hechter, O., Terada, S., Spitsberg, V., Nakahara, T., Nakahara, S. H., and Flouret, G. (1978). Neurohypophyseal hormone-responsive renal adenylate cyclase. *J. Biol. Chem.* **253**, 3230–3237.

Muhlethaler, M., Dreifuss, J. J., and Gahwiler, B. H. (1982). Vasopressin excites hippocampal neurons. *Nature (London)* **296**, 749–751.

North, W. G., Walter, R., Schlessinger, D. H., Breslow, E., and Capra, D. J. (1975). Structural studies of bovine neurophysin. I. *Ann. N.Y. Acad. Sci.* **248**, 408–422.

Padfield, P. L., Brown, J. J., Lever, J. F., Morton, J. J., and Robertson, J. I. S. (1981). Blood pressure in acute and chronic vasopressin excess. *N. Engl. J. Med.* **304**, 1067–1070.

Prpic, V., Blackmore, P. F., and Exton, J. H. (1982). Phosphatidylinositol breakdown induced by vasopressin and epinephrine in hepatocytes is calcium-dependent. *J. Biol. Chem.* **257**, 11323–11331.

Roy, C., Hall, D., Karish, M., and Ausiello, D. A. (1981). Relationship of (8-lysine) vasopressin receptor transition to receptor functional properties in a pig kidney cell line (LLC-PK$_1$). *J. Biol. Chem.* **256**, 3423–3427.

Schmale, H., and Richter, D. (1981). Immunological identification of a common precursor to arginine vasopressin and neurophysin II synthesized by *in vitro* translation of bovine hypothalamic mRNA. *Proc. Natl. Acad. Sci. U.S.A.* **78**, 766–769.

Schmale, H., and Richter, D. (1984). Single base deletion in the vasopressin gene is the cause of diabetes insipidus in Bratteboro rats. *Nature (London)* **308**, 705–709.

Schwartz, J., Keil, L. C., Maselli, J., and Reid, I. A. (1983). Role of vasopressin in blood pressure regulation during adrenal insufficiency. *Endocrinology (Baltimore)* **112**, 234–238.

Soloff, M., and Sweet, P. (1982). Oxytocin inhibition of $(Ca^{2+} + Mg^{2+})$ATPase activity in rat myometrial plasma membranes. *J. Biol. Chem.* **257**, 10687–10693.

Zimmerman, E. A., and Robinson, A. G. (1976). Hypothalamic neurons secreting vasopressin and neurophysin. *Kidney Int.* **10**, 12–24.

Chapter **5**

Anterior Pituitary Hormones

I. INTRODUCTION

The anterior pituitary (adenohypophysis) which is the source of 10 polypeptide hormones is considered to be the "master gland." It is comprised by the *pars distalis* and the *pars intermedia*. The hormones of the anterior pituitary with their general actions as well as overall regulation are shown in Fig. 5-1.

In various cells within the anterior pituitary are expressed the following hormones which govern a wide variety of important bodily functions: (1) *growth hormone* (GH, somatotropin, STH), which stimulates the growth of bone, liver, and other tissues and in many cases may act through the agency of *somatomedins* produced in the liver and elsewhere; (2) *thyrotropic hormone* (thyrotropin, TSH), also known as thyroid-stimulating hormone, which stimulates the thyroid gland to release thyroxin (T_4) and triiodothyronine (T_3) into the bloodstream for circulation to the tissues, where they are required for cells to burn nutrients as fuels at adequate rates and also for differentiation and development; (3) *luteinizing hormone* (lutropin, LH) and (4) *follicle-stimulating hormone* (follitropin, FSH), which play major roles in reproductive activities; (5) *adrenocorticotropic hormone* (corticotropin, ACTH), which appears to be one of the principal mediators of the stress adaptation mechanism in its tropic stimulation of adrenocortical hormones; (6) *prolactin* (PRL), which is important for the synthesis of milk constituents during lactation and may have other actions somewhat similar to growth hormone as well as being secreted during stress; (7) *melanocyte-stimulating hormone* (melanotropin, MSH), which plays a role in skin-darkening reactions and influences important CNS functions, such as memory and learning;* (8) β-*lipotropin* (β-LPH), through its proteolytic products, (9) β-endorphin and (10) Met-enkephalin, may promote analgesia in stress and act as neurotransmitters in signaling the release of other hormones or affect ion flux. Thus, through the effects of all of these hormones in the anterior pituitary, the processes of somatic cell growth, metabolic rate, reproductive functions, stress adaptation, mammary gland development and function, skin darkening, and CNS reactions are regulated. The importance of these hormones is all too evident in cases of their inadequate production such as occurs when tumors or other physical pressures reduce the output of one or more of these hormones or during their overproduction when tumors may secrete them in large quantities ectopically. All of the anterior pituitary hormones are proteins or polypeptides. They are sub-

---

*Although MSH and ACTH derive from the same precursor polypeptide and share homologous sequences, they apparently act through distinct receptors.

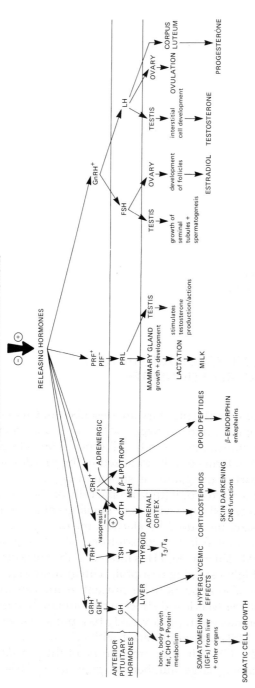

Figure 5-1. Overview of the anterior pituitary hormones showing the connections between the aminergic hormones and neurotransmitters of the CNS, the releasing hormones from the hypothalamus, and the anterior pituitary hormones together with the organs upon which they act and their general effects. GRH, Growth hormone releasing hormone, or somatocrinin; GIH, growth hormone release-inhibiting hormone, or somatostatin; TRH, thyroid-stimulating hormone releasing hormone; CRH, corticotropic releasing hormone; PRF, prolactin releasing factor; PIF, prolactin release-inhibiting factor; GnRH, gonadotropic releasing factor; GH, growth hormone; TSH, thyrotropic-stimulating hormone; ACTH, adrenocorticotropic hormone; MSH, melanocyte-stimulating hormone; PRL, prolactin; FSH, follicle-stimulating hormone; LH, luteotropic hormone; CHO, carbohydrate; IGFs, insulin-like growth factors; T_3, triiodothyronine; T_4, thyroxine. Superscript plus or minus signs or encircled plus or minus signs refer to positive or negative actions.

stantially larger (1500–35,000 Da) than many of the earlier recognized hypothalamic releasing hormones, but not larger than CRH and GRH. Anterior pituitary hormones seem to have longer half-lives in the bloodstream than the releasing hormones. As already indicated in Chapter 3, the secretion of these hormones is under the control of the releasing hormones and sometimes directly or indirectly under neuronal control. The secretion of anterior pituitary hormones also is regulated by an elaborate feedback control by terminal target gland hormones. Thus, for example, cortisol inhibits further output of ACTH and β-endorphin.

We then focus upon the explanation of the effects of the anterior pituitary hormones. Some mechanisms are better understood than others. The actions of ACTH and TSH are clearer at this point than the actions of the rest; prolactin, growth hormone, and MSH are less well understood and the actions of β-lipotropin cleavage products are so new as to require considerably more research effort. Accordingly, more emphasis will be allocated here to prolactin, growth hormone, and β-lipotropin, since ACTH actions are covered in Chapter 10, TSH actions are emphasized in Chapter 6, and LH and FSH actions are reported in Chapters 11 and 12.

II. ANATOMICAL, MORPHOLOGICAL, AND PHYSIOLOGICAL RELATIONSHIPS

Location and anatomy of the pituitary are described in Chapter 3 (see Fig. 3-2). It is appropriate here to begin with the localization of the anterior pituitary hormones into discrete cell types. The anterior pituitary can be discussed in terms of cells localized to the *pars distalis* which occupies the major part of the gland, as shown in Fig. 5-2.

TSH is located in the thyrotrope (thyrotropic cells of the *pars distalis*). This is a *basophilic* large cell type with very small granules of the hormone. The granule size, measured by electron microscopy, is 120–200 nm. LH and FSH are located in the gonadotrope, also basophilic, containing granules of 200–250 nm. ACTH is located in the corticotropic cell of the *pars distalis*, a highly staining basophil, with granules 100–200 nm in diameter. This cell also appears to be present in the *pars intermedia* (Fig. 5-2). The *pars intermedia* is less distinct in the human than in the rat. MSH is located in the melanotrope, a weakly basophilic cell with granules of 200–300 nm. MSH antisera interact with cells of the *pars distalis* and the *pars intermedia*. GH is in the somatotrope of the *pars distalis*, an acidophilic cell containing large numbers of granules of 300–400 nm.

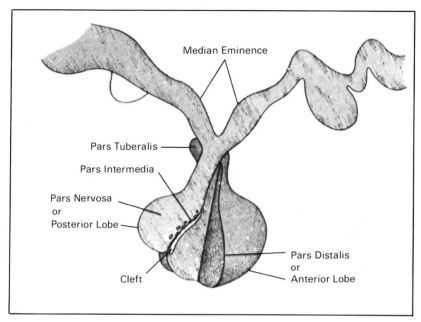

Figure 5-2. Pituitary and its structures. Reproduced from R. Guillemin, Beta-lipotropin and endorphins: Implications of current knowledge. *In* "Neuroendocrinology" (D. T. Krieger and J. C. Hughes, eds.), p. 70. Sinauer Associates, Sunderland, Massachusetts, 1980.

Prolactin is in the mammotrope, an acidophilic cell of the *pars distalis* containing large, dense, and variable secretory granules in the size range of 400–700 nm. β-Lipotropin is also in the *pars distalis,* presumably in corticotropes, and its processing to β-endorphin can also occur in these cells. Since ACTH, MSH, and β-endorphin derive from a single gene and ACTH and β-endorphin are secreted together in response to a stimulus, it seems possible that all three could, at least in theory, derive from the same cell type, and their secretion could respond to the same regulatory signals.* In fact, MSH is a breakdown product of ACTH, and this breakdown is not extensive when the corticotrope is stimulated by CRH, resulting in the primary release of ACTH and β-endorphin. The latter is derived from the enzymatic breakdown of β-lipotropin.

The cells of the *pars distalis* are recognized in the light microscope on

---

*It should be mentioned that LH has been found in the gonadotropic cell of the *pars tuberalis* in the rat, a basophilic cell. This derives from experiments with antisera to LH, but antisera to other *pars distalis* hormones were negative for this zone of the anterior pituitary.

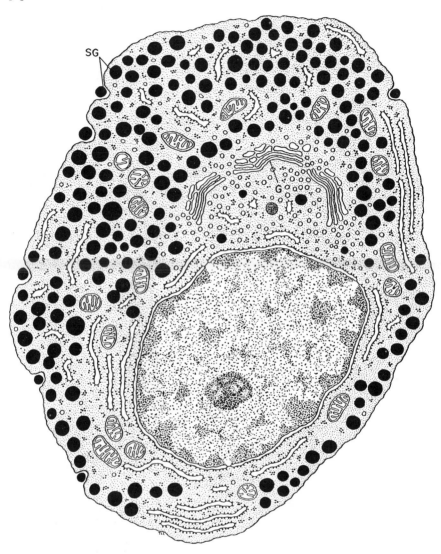

Figure 5-3. (A) Pituitary somatotrophic cell. SG, Secretion granules. Reproduced with permission from T. L. Lentz, "Cell Fine Structure," p. 307. Saunders, Philadelphia, Pennsylvania, 1971. (B) Pituitary mammotrophic cell. SG, Secretion granules; Ly, lysosomes. Reproduced with permission from T. L. Lentz, "Cell Fine Structure," p. 309. Saunders, Philadelphia, Pennsylvania, 1971. (C) Gonadotrophic cell (pituitary folliculotroph). SG, Secretion granules; ER, endoplasmic reticulum. Reproduced with permission from T. L.

B

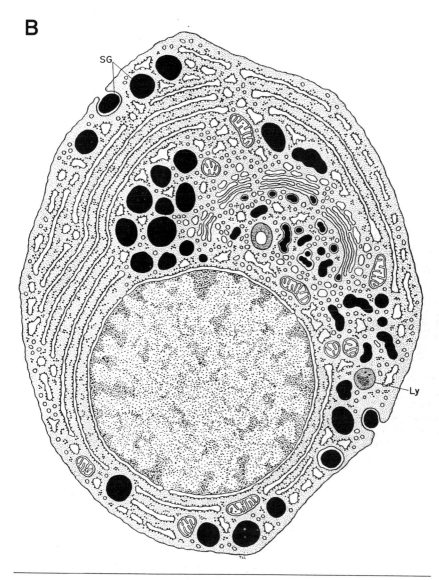

SG

Ly

Lentz, "Cell Fine Structure," p. 311. Saunders, Philadelphia, Pennsylvania, 1971. (D) Pituitary luteotrophic cell. Reproduced from T. L. Lentz, "Cell Fine Structure," p. 313. Saunders, Philadelphia, Pennsylvania, 1971. (E) Thyrotrophic cell. Reproduced with permission from T. L. Lentz, "Cell Fine Structure," p. 315. Saunders, Philadelphia, Pennsylvania, 1971. (F) Corticotrophic cell. Reproduced from T. L. Lentz, "Cell Fine Structure," p. 317. Saunders, Philadelphia, Pennsylvania, 1971. (G) Melanotrophic cell of the pituitary. Reproduced from T. L. Lentz, "Cell Fine Structure," p. 319. Saunders, Philadelphia, Pennsylvania, 1971.

178

C

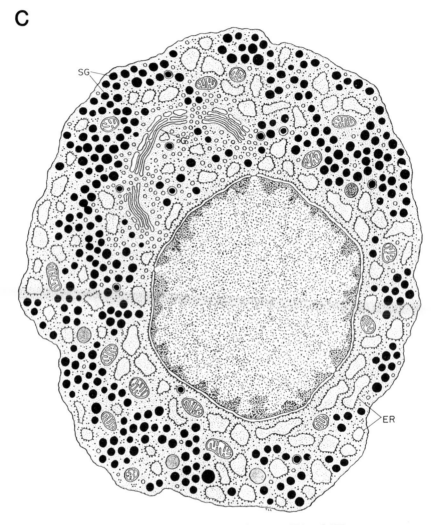

SG

ER

Figure 5-3 (cont'd.). See legend on pp. 176 and 177.

the basis of their affinity for stains. The two types already mentioned are acidophils (acid stainable) and basophils (base stainable) and are easily distinguished. Cells that are not stained by these procedures usually represent degranulated cells which are undergoing recovery after secretion of granular contents.

The adenohypophysis itself consists of three parts: the *pars distalis*, the *pars intermedia*, and the *pars tuberalis*, as shown in Fig. 5-2. Cells of the

D

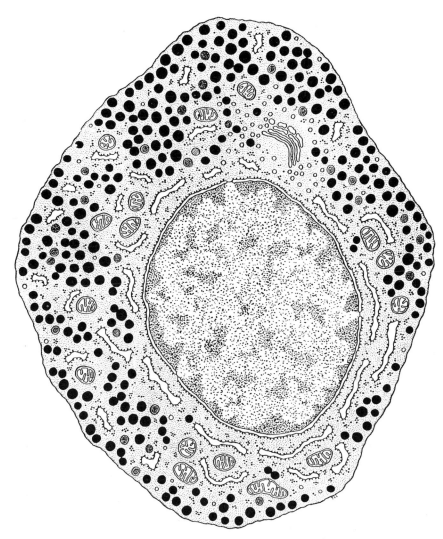

Figure 5-3 (cont'd.). See legend on pp. 176 and 177.

pars distalis are arranged in anastomosing cords close to fenestrated capillaries in the secondary capillary plexus of the hypophyseal portal system. The *pars intermedia,* a narrow region separating the *pars distalis* from the posterior pituitary (*pars nervosa*), consists of basophils with MSH and possibly some endorphins, with ACTH virtually absent. The situation in

180

E

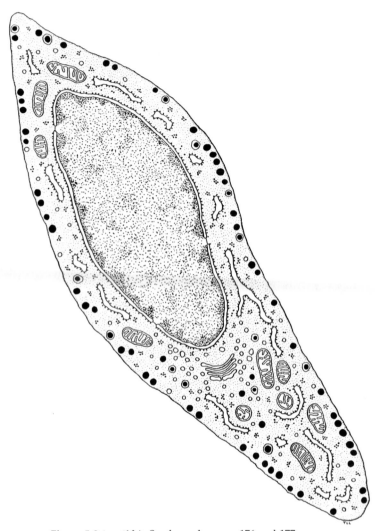

Figure 5-3 (cont'd.). See legend on pp. 176 and 177.

man is not completely clear in relation to the products of the *pars inter-media* which, itself, is not well defined anatomically in comparison with lower forms. The *pars tuberalis*, which is dorsal to the *pars distalis* and *intermedia*, has no specifically assigned function. The *pars distalis* has 30–35% acidophils, 15–20 μm in diameter, which contain GH and PRL. The basophils, 15–25 μm in diameter, make up about 10–15% of the cells and contain LH, FSH, TSH, and ACTH.

F

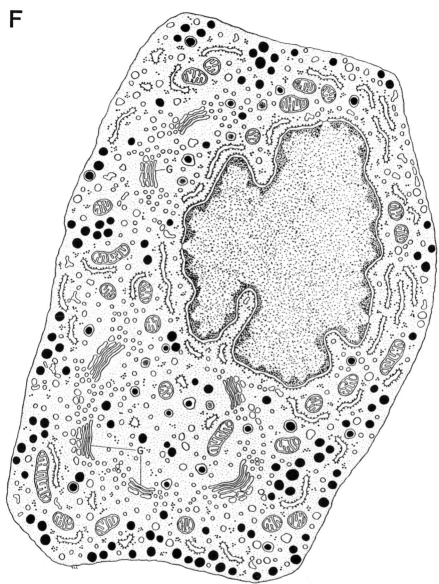

Figure 5-3 (cont'd.). See legend on pp. 176 and 177.

The release of *pars distalis* hormones is signaled by the action of releasing hormones, and the general mechanism is shown in Fig. 3-12. The synthesis of these hormones occurs on ribosomes which are transported within the rough endoplasmic reticulum cisternae and then concentrated into granules of the Golgi complex. Small granules arise from the

G

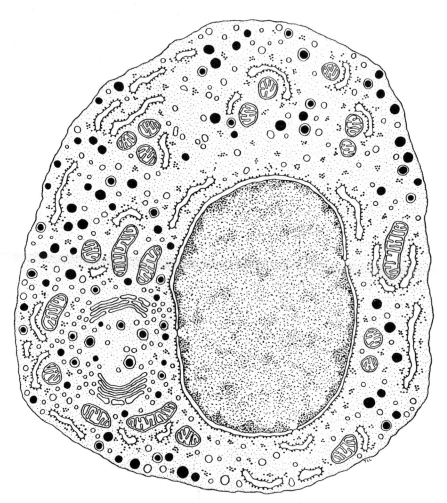

Figure 5-3 (cont'd.). See legend on pp. 176 and 177.

Golgi to fuse and form mature secretion granules. At this point the releasing hormones, when triggered, cause the granules to be released by exocytosis.

At the electron microscopic level, there appear to be separate cells for the secretion of each of the six major hormones of the anterior pituitary. However, the total picture is incomplete. One must remember that ACTH and β-LPH derive from the same gene and both of these peptides can be further degraded even within the anterior pituitary to the MSH hormones as well as β-endorphin and possibly to the enkephalins. However, there does appear to be some segregation in terms of one or two of these hormones being secreted while the others are not. The corticotroph secretes mainly ACTH and β-endorphin, while the cells in the rat *pars intermedia* secrete mainly β-endorphin, corticotropin-like intermediate lobe peptide (CLIP), with some MSH. It is not clear whether the cell types are identical but have divergent regulation or whether they contain proteases which specifically degrade some of the hormones produced but not others. Some work suggests that rat *pars intermedia* hormone secretion is controlled by the adrenergic system rather than by CRH. The situation with humans is less clear, since the *pars intermedia* is less well demarcated anatomically.

The cells of the anterior pituitary are pictured in Figs. 5-3A–G and distinguishing features are summarized in Table 5-1.

III. CHEMISTRY

A. Growth Hormone (GH)

In Table 5-2 is a summary of the molecular weights and biochemical properties of all of the peptide hormones of the anterior pituitary. The human growth hormone is about 21,500 molecular weight containing 191 amino acid residues. The gene for the human growth hormone has been sequenced and cloned and the corresponding nucleic acid and amino acid sequences appear in Figs. 5-4 and 5-5. Various enzymatically modified forms of human growth hormone have been described which may reflect enzymatic processing occurring *in vivo*. A 20,000 molecular weight form (1000–2000 molecular weight less than the normal hormone) appears to lack 15 amino acid residues occurring between positions 32 and 46, but otherwise the hormone is identical to the normal form. The deleted form has normal growth-promoting activity, but lacks the insulin-like activity usually associated with the hormone. It comprises about 15% of the total growth hormone content of the human pituitary. There are three introns (intervening sequences) in the gene encoding growth hormone messenger, and one of these starts at the same point (corresponding to amino acid residues 31 and 32) as the amino acid sequence deletion. Residue 46, corresponding to the end of the deleted amino acid sequence, contains AG in the mRNA, two bases which usually are found at the 3' end of an intervening sequence in the

Table 5–1. Summary of Properties of Secretory Cells of the Anterior Pituitary

Cell	Hormone secreted	Staining type	Diameter of secretory granules (μm)	Distinguishing features
Somatotroph[a] (Fig. 5–3A)	GH (STH)	Acidophilic (stains with acid dye)	300–350	Typical cell
Mammotroph (Fig. 5–3B)	PRL	Acidophilic	600–900	Large round, ovoid secretory granules. Cells vary in shape. Cell number increases in pregnancy and lactation. Lysosomes more prominent when secretion is suppressed.
Gonadotroph (Fig. 5–3C)	FSH	Basophilic (stains with basic dye)	~200	Large round cell body. Rough endoplasmic reticulum (RER) and Golgi probably play a role in synthesis of carbohydrate moiety of subunits.
Luteotroph (Fig. 5–3D)	LH	Basophilic	~250	Secretory granules slightly larger than FSH-containing cells. Granules tend to accumulate in one

184

				pole of cell near periphery. Golgi apparatus less extensive than FSH cell.
Thyrotroph (Fig. 5–3E)	TSH	Basophilic	120–150	Smaller than other cell types. Irregular in shape. Flattened nucleus. Smaller granules than in other cell types.
Corticotroph (Fig. 5–3F)	ACTH	Basophilic	~200	Large cell with irregular shape. Granules associated with Golgi. Gastrin has been reported to occur in these cells.
Melanocyte-stimulating hormone cell (Fig. 5–3G)	MSH	Basophilic	—	A few layers of cells between *pars distalis* and *pars nervosa*. In human cells may extend into neural lobe. Cells of *pars intermedia* are polygonal. Morphologically similar to corticotroph. Also possible that corticotroph can produce MSH.

[a] The suffix troph is used here to connote a growth function. The suffix trope (e.g., gonadotrope) is used to connote a cell containing a substance which produces change rather than growth. There is some confusion in the usage of these terms since at one stage an anterior pituitary hormone may cause a target cell to grow (act as a mitogen), whereas at another stage the same hormone may cause the same cell to alter its metabolism or produce some change other than growth. Most of the information in this table is summarized from descriptions by T.L. Lentz, "Cell Fine Structure." Saunders, Philadelphia, Pennsylvania, 1971.

Table 5-2. Properties of Adenohypophyseal Hormones

Hormone		$t_{1/2}$ in blood (min)	Molecular weight (K = 1000)	Comments on structure
GH	Structurally related	30	21.5K (191 amino acids in human)	Single chain; 2 S–S bonds
PRL		—	23K (199 amino acids in ovine)	Single chain; 3 S–S bonds
TSH	Structurally related / GTH	30	28.3K (211 amino acids in human)	Glycoprotein: 16% carbohydrate, 2 subunits $(\alpha\text{-}\beta_1)^a$
FSH		240	34K (210 amino acids in human)	16% carbohydrate, 2 subunits $(\alpha\text{-}\beta_2)^a$; contains S–S bonds
LH		30	28.5K (204 amino acids in human)	15.5% carbohydrate, 2 subunits $(\alpha\text{-}\beta_3)^a$, contains S–S bonds
ACTH		15	4.5K (39 amino acids in human)	Open chain; homology with β-LPH and MSH
MSH	$\begin{cases} \alpha \\ \beta \end{cases}$ Structurally related	—	— (13 amino acids in human)	Linear change; heptapeptide common to α- and β-MSH, ACTH, β-LPH, and γ-LPH
		—	3K (22 amino acids in human)	
β-LPH	$\begin{cases} \beta \\ \gamma \end{cases}$	—	9.5K (91 amino acids in human)	Open chain; β-LPH is precursor of β-endorphin, enkephalins (ACTH + β-LPH encoded by same mRNA)

a α subunits are similar or identical and can be interchanged experimentally with α subunits of TSH, FSH, or LH. The β subunit determines hormonal activity; it is the major immunological determinant and is involved in recognizing specific binding (receptor) site; α subunit is involved in penetrating membrane and stimulation of adenylate cyclase. The β subunit appears to cover most of the surface of the hormones.

```
       1                                              10                                                   20
     Met Phe Pro Thr Ile Pro Leu Ser Arg Leu Phe Asp Asn Ala Met Leu Arg Ala His Arg Leu
AATTCT ATG TTC CCA ACT ATA CCA CTA TCT CGT CTA TTC GAT AAC GCT ATG CTT CGT GCT CAT CGT CTT
                                              30                                                   40
     His Gln Leu Ala Phe Asp Thr Tyr Gln Glu Phe Glu Glu Ala Tyr Ile Pro Lys Glu Gln
     CAT CAG CTG GCC UUU GAC ACC UAC CAG GAG UUU GAA GAA GCC UAU AUC CCA AAG GAA CAG
                                              50                                                   60
     Lys Tyr Ser Phe Leu Gln Asn Pro Gln Thr Ser Leu Cys Phe Ser Glu Ser Ile Pro Thr
     AAG UAU UCA UUC CUG CAG AAC CCC CAG ACC UCC CUC UGU UUC UCA GAG UCU AUU CCG ACA
                                              70                                                   80
     Pro Ser Asn Arg Glu Glu Thr Gln Gln Lys Ser Asn Leu Glu Leu Leu Arg Ile Ser Leu
     CCC UCC AAC AGG GAG GAA ACA CAA CAG AAA UCC AAC CUA GAG CUG CUC CGC AUC UCC CUG
                                              90                                                   100
     Leu Leu Ile Gln Ser Trp Leu Glu Pro Val Gln Phe Leu Arg Ser Val Phe Ala Asn Ser
     CUG CUC AUC CAG UCG UGG CUG GAG CCC GUG CAG UUC CUC AGG AGU GUC UUC GCC AAC AGC
                                              110                                                  120
     Leu Val Tyr Gly Ala Ser Asp Ser Asn Val Tyr Asp Leu Leu Lys Asp Leu Glu Glu Gly
     CUA GUG UAC GGC GCC UCU GAC AGC AAC GUC UAU GAC CUC CUA AAG GAC CUA GAG GAA GGC
                                              130                                                  140
     Ile Gln Thr Leu Met Gly Arg Leu Glu Asp Gly Ser Pro Arg Thr Gly Gln Ile Phe Lys
     AUC CAA ACG CUG AUG GGG AGG CUG GAA GAU GGC AGC CCC CGG ACU GGG CAG AUC UUC AAG
                                              150                                                  160
     Gln Thr Tyr Ser Lys Phe Asp Thr Asn Ser His Asn Asp Asp Ala Leu Leu Lys Asn Tyr
     CAG ACC UAC AGC AAG UUC GAC ACA AAC UCA CAC AAC GAU GAC GCA CUA CUC AAG AAC UAC
                                              170                                                  180
     Gly Leu Leu Tyr Cys Phe Arg Lys Asp Met Asp Lys Val Glu Thr Phe Leu Arg Ile Val
     GGG CUG CUC UAC UGC UUC AGG AAG GAC AUG GAC AAG GUC GAG ACA UUC CUG CGC AUC GUG
                                              190
     Gln Cys Arg Ser Val Glu Gly Ser Cys Gly Phe Stop
     CAG UGC CGC UCU GUG GAG GGC AGC UGU GGC UUC UAG CUGCCCGGGUGGCAUCCCUGUGACCCUCCC
     CAGUGCCUCUCCUGGCC
```

Figure 5-4. The amino acid and mRNA sequences of HGH from DNA sequencing of pHGH31. Reproduced from D. V. Goeddel, H. L. Heyneker, T. Hozumi, R. Arentzen, K. Itakura, D. G. Yansura, M. J. Ross, G. Miozzari, R. Crea, and P. H. Seeburg, *Nature (London)* **281,** 544–548 (1979). © 1979 Macmillan Journals Limited.

Phe Pro Thr Ile Pro Leu Ser Arg Leu Phe Asp Asn Ala Met Leu Arg Ala

His Arg Leu His Gln Leu Ala Phe Asp Thr Tyr Gln Glu Phe Glu Glu Ala

Tyr Ile Pro Lys Glu Gln Lys Tyr Ser Phe Leu Gln Asn Pro Gln Thr Ser

Leu Cys Phe Ser Glu Ser Ile Pro Thr Pro Ser Asn Arg Glu Glu Thr Gln

Gln Lys Ser Asn Leu Gln Leu Leu Arg Ile Ser Leu Leu Leu Ile Gln Ser

Trp Leu Glu Pro Val Gln Phe Leu Arg Ser Val Phe Ala Asn Ser Leu Val

Tyr Gly Ala Ser Asn Ser Asp Val Tyr Asp Leu Leu Lys Asp Leu Glu Glu

Gly Ile Gln Thr Leu Met Gly Arg Leu Glu Asp Gly Ser Pro Arg Thr Gly

Gln Ile Phe Lys Gln Thr Tyr Ser Lys Phe Asp Thr Asn Ser His Asn Asp

Asp Ala Leu Leu Lys Asn Tyr Gly Leu Leu Tyr Cys Phe Arg Lys Asp Met

Asp Lys Val Glu Thr Phe Leu Arg Ile Val Gln Cys Arg Ser Val Glu Gly

Ser Cys Gly Phe

Figure 5-5. Amino acid sequence of the HGH molecule reproduced from several illustrations by C. H. Li. The N-terminal two-thirds of the molecule is supposed to contain the active core, while the C-terminal one-third is to stabilize or protect the structure. Various sources indicate activities traceable to portions of the molecule: Residues 32–46 possess glucose uptake and lipolysis activities; residues 98–128 are involved in binding to the GH receptor; a slightly larger fragment, residues 96–133, has somatomedin-like activities and insulin competition for receptor binding. C-terminal peptide (177–191) could be cleaved and act at the cell surface possibly to lower insulin binding to the insulin receptor.

Thr Pro Val Cys Pro Asn Gly Pro Gly Asp Cys Gln Val Ser Leu Arg Asp

Leu Phe Asp Arg Ala Val Met Val Ser His Tyr Ile His Asn Leu Ser Ser

Glu Met Phe Asn Glu Phe Asp Lys Arg Tyr Ala Gln Gly Lys Gly Phe Ile

Thr Met Ala Leu Asn Ser Cys His Thr Ser Ser Leu Pro Thr Pro Glu Asp

Lys Glu Gln Ala Gln Gln Thr His His Glu Val Leu Met Ser Leu Ile Leu

Gly Leu Leu Arg Ser Trp Asn Asp Pro Leu Tyr His Leu Val Thr Glu Val

Arg Gly Met Lys Gly Val Pro Asp Ala Ile Leu Ser Arg Ala Ile Glu Ile

Glu Glu Glu Asn Lys Arg Leu Leu Glu Gly Met Glu Met Ile Phe Gly Gln

Val Ile Pro Gly Ala Lys Glu Thr Glu Pro Tyr Pro Val Trp Ser Gly Leu

Pro Ser Leu Gln Thr Lys Asp Glu Asp Ala Arg His Ser Ala Phe Tyr Asn

Leu Leu His Cys Leu Arg Arg Asp Ser Ser Lys Ile Asp Thr Tyr Leu Lys

Leu Leu Asn Cys Arg Ile Ile Tyr Asn Asn Asn Cys

Figure 5-6. Amino acid sequence of ovine prolactin reproduced from several illustrations of C. H. Li.

```
     Met Asn Ile Lys Gly Ser Pro Trp Lys Gly Ser Leu Leu Leu Leu Leu Val
AAAC AUG AAC AUC UCG CCA UGG AAA GGG UCC CUC CUG CUG CUG CUG CUG CUG GUG
                                       1
Ser Asn Leu Leu Leu Cys Gln Ser Val Ala Pro Leu Pro Ile Cys Pro Gly Gly
UCA AAC CUG CUG CUG UGC CAG AGC GUG GCC CCC UUG CCC AUC UGU CCC GGC GGG
                                            20
Ala Ala Arg Cys Gln Val Thr Leu Arg Asp Leu Phe Asp Arg Ala Val Val Leu
GCU GCC CGA UGC CAG GUG ACC CUU CGA GAC CUG UUU GAC CGC GCC GUC GUC CUG
             30                                         40
Ser His Tyr Ile His Asn Leu Ser Ser Glu Met Phe Ser Glu Phe Asp Lys Arg
UCC CAC UAC AUC CAU AAC CUC UCC UCA GAA AUG UUC AGC GAA UUC GAU AAA CGG
                 50                                             60
Tyr Thr His Gly Arg Gly Phe Ile Thr Lys Ala Ile Asn Ser Cys His Thr Ser
UAU ACC CAU GGC CGG GGG UUC AUU ACC AAG GGC AUC AAC AGC UGC CAC ACU UCU
70
Ser Leu Ala Thr Pro Glu Asp Lys Glu Gln Ala Gln Gln Met Asn Gln Lys Asp
UCC CUU GCC ACC CCC GAA GAC AAG GAG CAA GCC CAA CAG AUG AAU CAA AAA GAC
80                                          90
Phe Leu Ser Leu Ile Val Ser Ile Leu Arg Ser Trp Asn Glu Pro Leu Tyr His
UUU CUG AGC CUG AUA GUC AGC AUA UUG CGA UCC UGG AAU GAG CCU CUG UAU CAU
            100                                         110
Leu Val Thr Glu Val Arg Gly Met Gln Glu Ala Pro Glu Ala Ile Leu Ser Lys
CUG GUC ACG GAA GUA CGU GGU AUG CAA GAA GCC CCG GAG GCU AUC CU. UCC AAA
             120                                        130
Ala Val Glu Ile Glu Glu Gln Thr Lys Arg Leu Leu Glu Gly Met Glu Leu Ile
GCU GUA GAG AUU GAG GAG CAA ACC AAA CGG CUU CUA GAG GGC AUG GAG CUG AUA
                 140                                            150
Val Ser Gln Val His Pro Glu Thr Lys Glu Asn Glu Ile Tyr Pro Val Trp Ser
GUC AGC CAG GUU CAU CCU GAA ACC AAA GAA AAU GAG AUC UAC CCU GUC UGG UCG
                     160
Gly Leu Pro Ser Leu Gln Met Ala Asp Glu Glu Ser Arg Leu Ser Ala Tyr Tyr
GGA CCU CCA UCC CUG CAG AUG GCU GAU GAA GAG UCU CGC CUU UCU GCU UAU UAU
170                                     180
Asn Leu Leu His Cys Leu Arg Arg Asp Ser His Lys Ile Asp Asn Tyr Leu Lys
AAC CUG CUC CAC UGC CUA CGC AGG GAU UCA CAU AAA AUC GAC AAU UAU CUC AAG
            190                                     199
Leu Leu Lys Cys Arg Ile Ile His Asn Asn Asn Cys
CUC CUG AAG UGC CGA AUC AUC CAC AAC AAC AAC UGC
```

Figure 5-7. Nucleotide sequence and predicted amino acid sequence of the mRNA coding for human prolactin. Reproduced from N. E. Cooke, D. Coit, J. Shine, J. D. Baxter, and J. A. Martial, *J. Biol. Chem.* **256,** 4007–4016 (1981).

precursor RNA transcribed from the gene. Thus, processing differences or separate genes account for the appearance of these two forms of human growth hormone. Animal GH sequences are now being produced in bacteria by recombinant DNA technology involving a link between the β-lactamase gene of a plasmid and the cloned gene for rat growth hormone.

B. Prolactin (PRL)

Ovine prolactin is about 23,000 molecular weight and is comprised of 199 amino acids in the sequence. The sequence is shown in Fig. 5-6. GH and PRL are structurally related and seem to have some similar activities. Human PRL sequence has been deduced from mRNA sequences

190

```
                                              8
α                        NH₂-Phe Pro Asp Gly Glu Phe Thr Met
                                                          13
TSH-β               NH₂-Phe Cys Ile Pro Thr Glu Tyr Met Met His Val Glu Arg
                                    CHO
                                                          20
LH-β    Acyl-Ser Arg Gly Pro Leu Arg Pro Leu Cys Glu Pro Ile Asn Ala Thr Leu Ala Ala Gln Lys

        9                                                 28
α       Glx Gly Cys Pro Gly Cys Lys Leu Lys Glu Asn Lys Tyr Phe Ser Lys Pro Asx Ala Pro
                                                                              CHO
        14                                                23
TSH-β   Lys Glu Cys Ala Tyr Cys                        Leu Thr Ile Asn
        21                                                30
LH-β    Glu Ala Cys Pro Val Cys                        Ile Thr Phe Thr

        29                                                48
α       Ile Tyr Gln Cys Met Gly Cys Cys Phe Ser Arg Ala Tyr Pro Thr Pro Ala Arg Ser Lys
        24                                                43
TSH-β   Thr Thr Val Cys Ala Gly Tyr Cys Met Thr Arg Asx Val Asx Gly Lys Leu Phe Leu Pro
        31                                                50
LH-β    Thr Ser Ile Cys Ala Gly Tyr Cys Pro Ser Met Lys Arg Val Leu Pro Val Ile Leu Pro
                                CHO

        49                                                67
α       Lys Thr Met Leu     Val Pro Lys Asn Ile Thr Ser Glx Ala Thr Cys Cys Val Ala Lys
        44                                                63
TSH-β   Lys Tyr Ala Leu Ser Gln Asp Val Cys Thr Tyr Arg Asp Phe Met Tyr Lys Thr Ala Glu
        51                                                69
LH-β    Pro Pro Met Pro     Gln Arg Val Cys Thr Tyr His Glu Leu Arg Phe Ala Ser Val Arg
                                                                  CHO

        68                                                86
α       Ala Phe Thr     Lys Ala Thr Val Met Gly Asn Val Arg Val Glx Asn His Thr Glx Cys
        64                                                83
TSH-β   Ile Pro Gly Cys Pro Arg His Val Thr Pro Tyr Phe Ser Tyr Pro Val Ala Ile Ser Cys
        70                                                89
LH-β    Leu Pro Gly Cys Pro Pro Gly Val Asp Pro Met Val Ser Phe Pro Val Ala Leu Ser Cys

        87                          96
α       His Cys Ser Thr Cys Tyr Tyr His Lys Ser-COOH
        84                                                103
TSH-β   Lys Cys Gly Lys Cys Asx Thr Asx Tyr Ser Asx Cys Ile His Glu Ala Ile Lys Thr Asn
        90                                                109
LH-β    His Cys Gly Pro Cys Arg Leu Ser Ser Thr Asp Cys Gly Pro Gly Arg Thr Glu Pro Leu

        104                         113
TSH-β   Tyr Cys Thr Lys Pro Gln Lys Ser Tyr Met-COOH
        110                                120
LH-β    Ala Cys Asp His Pro Pro Leu Pro Asp Ile Leu-COOH
```

Figure 5-8. Alignment of the chains of TSH and LH to show maximum homology. CHO indicates the position at which the carbohydrate chains are attached. Reproduced from J. G. Pierce, T. H. Liao, and R. B. Carlsen, *In* "Hormonal Proteins and Peptides" (C. H. Li, ed.), Vol. 1, pp. 17–57. Academic Press, New York, 1973.

as shown in Fig. 5-7. Studies with chemical probes suggest that His-27 and His-30 are involved in the interaction of PRL with its receptor.

C. Thyroid-Stimulating Hormone (TSH)

Human TSH is 28,300 molecular weight, containing two subunits and 211 amino acid residues. It is structurally related to LH and FSH (and HCG). Its sequence is shown in Fig. 5-8. There is a high degree of structural homology between the gonadotropic hormones, LH, FSH,

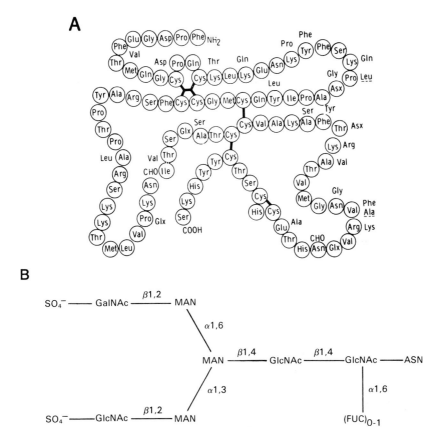

Figure 5-9. (A) Amino acid sequence of the α subunit of ovine–bovine LH. The residues outside the circles show the substitutions reported in human and porcine α chains. Those underlined are substitutions in porcine LH-α. The LH-α is similar to FSH-α and to TSH-α. Reproduced from J. G. Pierce, M. R. Faith, L. C. Guidice, and J. R. Reeve, *Ciba Found. Symp. (Excerpta Medica)* **41**, 225–250 (1976). (B) General structure of the carbohydrate units of ovine luteotropin (OLH) and bovine TSH. Carbohydrate structures of other anterior pituitary hormones (FSH) are similar. These structures are important, since they play a role in the biological function of glycoprotein hormones, although they may not be critical for interaction of the hormone with its receptor. Reprinted by permission from G. S. Bedi, W. C. French, and O. P. Bahl, Structure of carbohydrate units of ovine luteinizing hormone. *J. Biol. Chem.* **257**, 4345–4355 (1982). © 1982 by The American Society of Biological Chemists, Inc.

hCG, and one other anterior pituitary hormone, TSH (see Table 13-3 and Chapter 5). They all are composed of two noncovalently linked subunits, designated α and β. The α subunits of LH, hCG, TSH, and FSH are of identical structure (MW 13,000). The binding activity of each hormone is determined by the β subunit. Each of these four peptide hor-

```
                                    10                              20
hTSH-β                        Phe — Ile — Thr-Glx-Tyr-(Met, Thr, His, Val,— )Arg-Arg-Glx — Ala-
pTSH-β                        Phe — Ile — Thr-Glu-Tyr-Met-Met-His-Val — Arg-Lys-Glu — Ala-
bTSH-β                        Phe — Ile — Thr-Glu-Tyr-Met-Met-His-Val — Arg-Lys-Glu — Ala-
b, oLH-β     Ser-Arg-Gly-Pro-Leu-Arg-Pro-Leu-Cys-Gln-Pro-Ile-Asn-Ala-Thr-Leu-Ala-Ala-Glu-Lys-Glu-Ala-Cys-Pro-
pLH-β        — — — — — — — — — Arg — — — — — — — — — Asp — — — —
hLH-β        — — Glx — — — — — Trp — Glx — — Asx -Ala-Ile — — — Val — — — — Gly — —
hCG-β        — Lys-Gln — — — — — Arg — Arg — — — —. — — — Val — — — Gly — — —
hFSH-β       —(Asx-Ser) — Glu-Leu-Thr — Ile — Ile — Ile — — — — Glu — Arg-

                      30                      40
hTSH-β       Tyr — Leu — Ile-Asn — Thr — —( — — — — Met, Thr)Arg-Asx-Ile-Asx-Gly-Lys-Leu-Phe-
pTSH-β       Tyr — Leu — Val-Asn-Ser — — — — .— — — Met-Thr-Arg-Asx-Phe-Asx-Gly-Lys-Leu-Phe-
bTSH-β       Tyr — Leu — Ile- Asn-Thr-Thr-Val — — — — — Met-Thr-Arg-Asx-Val-Asx-Gly-Lys-Leu-Phe-
b, oLH-β     Val-Cys-Ile-Thr-Phe-Thr-Thr-Ser-Ile-Cys-Ala-Gly-Tyr-Cys-Pro-Ser-Met-Lys-Arg-Val-Leu-Pro-Val-Ile-
pLH-β        — — — — — — — — — — — — — — — Arg — — — — Ala-Ala-
hLH-β        — — — — Val-Asx — Thr — — — — — — Thr — Arg(Met)Leu — Glx-Ala-Val-
hCG-β        — — — — Val-Asn — Thr — — — — — — Thr — Thr — — — Gln-Gly-Val-
hFSH-β       Phe — — Ser-Ile -Asn — Thr( †) — — — — — Tyr-Thr-Arg-Asp-Leu — Tyr-Lys-Asp-Pro-

             50                      60                      70
hTSH-β       — — Lys-Tyr-Ala-Leu-Ser — Asx — — — — Arg-Asp-Phe-Ile-Tyr-Arg-Thr — Glx-Ile —
pTSH-β       — — Lys-Tyr-Ala-Leu-Ser — Asx — — — — Arg-Asp-Phe-Met-Tyr-Lys-Thr-Val-Glx-Ile —
bTSH-β       — — Lys-Tyr-Ala-Leu-Ser — Asp — — — — Arg-Asp-Phe-Met-Tyr-Lys-Thr-Ala-Glu-Ile —
b, oLH-β     Leu-Pro-Pro   Met-Pro   Gln-Arg-Val-Cys-Thr-Tyr-His-Glu-Leu-Arg-Phe-Ala-Ser-Val-Arg-Leu-Pro-
pLH-β        — — — Val — — Pro — — — Arg-Glu — Ile — — — Ser — — —
hLH-β        — — — Val — — Pro — — — Arg-Asx-Val — — Glx — Ile — — —
hCG-β        — — Ala   Leu — Leu — — Asn — Arg-Asp-Val — — Glu — Ile — — —
hFSH-β       Ala-Lys-Pro-Arg-Ile — Lys-Thr — Phe-Lys-Glu — Val-Tyr-Glu-Thr — — Val —

                      80                      90
hTSH-β       — — — Leu-His — (Ala, —, Tyr) Phe — Tyr — —( —, —, —, —)Lys — — Lys — Asx-
pTSH-β       — — — His-His — Thr — Tyr- Phe — Tyr — — — Ile . — — Lys — Lys — Asx-
bTSH-β       — — — Arg-His — Thr — Tyr- Phe — Tyr — — — Ile — — Lys — Lys — Asx-
b, oLH-β     Gly-Cys-Pro-Pro-Gly-Val-Asp-Pro-Met-Val-Ser-Phe-Pro-Val-Ala-Leu-Ser-Cys-His-Cys-Gly-Pro-Cys-Arg-
pLH-β        — — — — — — — — Thr — — — — — — — — — — — —
hLH-β        — — Arg — — Val — — — — — — — — Arg — — — —
hCG-β        — — — Arg — — Asn — Val — — Tyr-Ala — — — — — Gln — , Ala-Leu — Arg-
hFSH-β       — — Ala-His-His-Ala — Ser-Leu-Tyr-Thr-Tyr — — — Thr-Gln — — — — Lys — Asp-

             100                     110
hTSH-β       Thr-Asx-Tyr-Ser — — Ile-His (Glu, Ala, Ile) Lys-Thr-Asx-Tyr — Thr-Lys — Glx-Lys-Ser-Tyr-COOH
pTSH-β       Thr-Asx-Tyr-Ser — — Ile-His-Glx- Ala- Ile- Lys-Thr-Asx-Tyr — Thr-Lys — Glx-Lys-Ser-Tyr-COOH
bTSH-β       Thr-Asx-Tyr-Ser — — Ile-His-Glu-Ala- Ile- Lys-Thr-Asn-Tyr — Thr-Lys — Gln-Lys-Ser-Tyr-Met-COOH
b, oLH-β     Leu-Ser-Ser-Thr-Asp-Cys-Gly-Pro-Gly-Arg-Thr-Glx-Pro-Leu-Ala-Cys-Asx-His-Pro-Pro-Leu-Pro-Asp-Ile-
pLH-β        — — — Ser — — — — — — Ala-Gln — — — — — Arg- — — — — -Gly-Leu-
hLH-β        (Arg) — Thr-Ser — — — -Gly-Pro-Lys-Asx(His) — Thr — —(Glx -Asx-Ser-Lys-)Gly — -COOH
hCG-β        (Arg) — Thr — — — — Gly-Pro-Lys-Asp-His — Thr — Asp — Arg-Phe-Gln-Asp-Ser
hFSH-β       Ser-Asp — — — — Thr-Val-Arg-Gly-Leu-Gly — Ser-Tyr — Ser-Phe-Gly-Glu-Met-(Glx Lys)COOH


bTSH-β
b, oLH-β     Leu-COOH
pLH-β        Leu
hLH-β
hCG-β        Ser-Ser-Lys-Ala-Pro-Pro-Pro-Ser-Leu-Pro-Ser-Pro-Ser-Arg-Leu-Pro-Gly-Pro-Pro-Asx-Thr-Pro-Ile-Leu-


hCG-β        Pro-Gln-Ser-Leu-Pro-COOH
```

Figure 5-10. Comparative sequences of β subunits of glycoprotein hormones, including human FSH (hFSH). Reproduced from J. G. Pierce, M. R. Faith, L. C. Guidice, and J. R. Reeve, *Ciba Found. Symp. (Excerpta Medica)* **41**, 225–250 (1976).

```
                         10                                              20
H₂N-Ala Pro Asx Val Glx Asx Cys Pro Glx Cys Thr Leu Glx Glx Asx Pro Phe Phe Ser Glx


 21                              30                                      40
Pro Gly Ala Pro Ile Leu Gln Cys Met Gly Cys Cys Phe Ser Arg Ala Tyr Pro Thr Pro


 41                              50                                      60
Leu Arg Ser Lys Lys Thr Met Leu Val Gln Lys Asn(CHO) Val Thr Ser Glx Ser Thr Cys Cys


 61                              70                                      80
Val Ala Lys Ser Tyr Asn Arg Val Thr Val Met Gly Gly Phe Lys Val Glx Asn(CHO) His Thr


 81                              90
Ala Cys His Cys Ser Thr Cys Tyr Tyr His Lys Ser-COOH
```

Figure 5-11. Linear amino acid sequence of hCG-α. Reproduced from O. P. Bahl, *Fed. Proc., Fed. Am. Soc. Exp. Biol.* **36,** 2119–2127 (1977).

mones has a significant number of carbohydrate moieties covalently linked to the peptide chain (Fig. 5-9B). These relationships are summarized in Table 5-2.

D. Follicle-Stimulating Hormone (FSH)

Human FSH is a 34,000 molecular weight protein with two subunits consisting of 210 amino acid residues. Its amino acid sequence is presented in Figs. 5-9A and 5-10 for the α and β subunits, respectively.

```
                        10                                              20
H-Ser-Lys-Gln-Pro-Leu-Arg-Pro-Arg-Cys-Arg-Pro-Ile-Asn(CHO)-Ala-Thr-Leu-Ala-Val-Glu-Lys-
                        30                                              40
Glu-Gly-Cys-Pro-Val-Cys-Ile-Thr-Val-Asn(CHO)-Thr-Thr-Ile-Cys-Ala-Gly-Tyr-Cys-Pro-Thr-
                        50                                              60
Met-Thr-Arg-Val-Leu-Gln-Gly-Val-Leu-Pro-Ala-Leu-Pro-Glx-Leu-Val-Cys-Asn-Tyr-Arg-
                        70                                              80
Asp-Val-Arg-Phe-Glu-Ser-Ile-Arg-Leu-Pro-Gly-Cys-Pro-Arg-Gly-Val-Asn-Pro-Val-Val-
                        90                                             100
Ser-Tyr-Ala-Val-Ala-Leu-Ser-Cys-Gln-Cys-Ala-Leu-Cys-Arg-(Arg)-Ser-Thr-Thr-Asp-Cys-
                       110                                             120
Gly-Gly-Pro-Lys-Asp-His-Pro-Leu-Thr-Cys-Asp-Asp-Pro-Arg-Phe-Gln-Asp-Ser-Ser-Ser-
                              130
Ser(CHO) - Lys-Ala-Pro-Pro-Pro-Ser(CHO)-Leu-Pro-Ser-Pro-Ser(CHO)-Arg-Leu-Pro-Gly-Pro-
          140            145
Ser(CHO)-Asx-Thr-Pro- Ile-Leu-Pro-Gln-OH
```

Figure 5-12. Linear amino acid sequence of hCG-β subunit. Reproduced from O. P. Bahl, *Fed. Proc., Fed. Am. Soc. Exp. Biol.* **36,** 2119–2127 (1977).

194

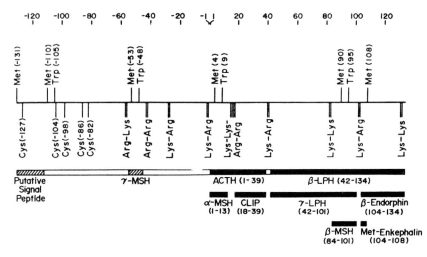

Figure 5-13. Schematic representation of the structure of bovine ACTH-β-LPH precursor. Characteristic amino acid residues are shown and the positions of the Met, Trp, and Cys residues are given in parentheses. The location of the translational initiation site at the Met residue at position 131 is assumed. The closed bars represent known amino acid sequence regions and open and shaded bars represent predicted regions of amino acid sequence from the nucleotide sequence of the precursor mRNA. The locations of known component peptides are shown by closed bars; the amino acid numbers are given in parentheses. The locations of γ-MSH and the putative signal peptide are indicated by shaded bars; the termini of these peptides are not definitive. Reproduced from S. Nakanishi, A. Inoue, T. Kita, M. Nakamura, A. C. Y. Chang, S. N. Cohen, and S. Numa, *Nature (London)* **278,** 423–427 (1979). © 1979 Macmillan Journals Limited.

E. Luteinizing Hormone (LH)

Human LH is 28,500 molecular weight consisting of two subunits and sequences of 204 amino acid residues. The sequence of the ovine α subunit is shown in Fig. 5-9A and the β subunit in Fig. 5-10. Human chorionic gonadotropin (hCG), which has strong homology with LH, is produced during pregnancy by the trophoblast in order to provide the hormonal stimulus for progesterone production (see Chapter 14). Interestingly, it is rather similar to LH, but is distinct from FSH (see Fig. 5-10) and its antibody cross-reacts with LH. Consequently, a radioimmunoassay of circulating LH has been developed with the anti-hCG antibody. The sequences of the α and β subunits of hCG are shown in Figs. 5-11 and 5-12.

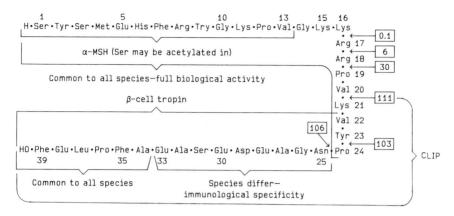

Figure 5-14. Linear sequence of human ACTH. Arrows point to hydrolytic cleavage and residual activity is denoted in boxes as a percentage of activity of the native structure after cleavage at specific linkage. α-MSH comprises the first 13 amino acid sequence from the N terminus. β-Cell tropin has the same sequence as ACTH 22–39. Immunological specificity is conferred by sequence 25–33 and the invariable C-terminal sequence is 34–39. CLIP, Corticotropin-like intermediary peptide. These data are a summary from a number of different literature sources.

F. Adrenocorticotropic Hormone (ACTH)

Human ACTH is 4500 molecular weight in a single chain consisting of 39 amino acids. It is structurally related to MSH and β-lipotropin. All three hormones derive from the same gene product (see Fig. 5-13). The sequence of human ACTH is given in Fig. 5-14. Note that α-MSH is contained in the first 13 amino acid residues of ACTH.

Human pituitary extracts appear to contain a corticotropin-inhibiting peptide which consists of 32 amino acids with a sequence probably identical to residues 7–38 of ACTH. It cannot stimulate the synthesis of corticosteroids, but inhibits ACTH-stimulated corticosterone production in isolated rat adrenal cells. Its structure is shown in Fig. 5-15. It has been shown that in genetically obese mice (*ob/ob*) a hormone is located in the neurointermediate lobe of the pituitary (*pars intermedia*) which stimulates insulin release. It cross-reacts with an antiserum directed against the C-terminal portion of ACTH, suggesting that it may be related to CLIP, the 18–39 fragment of ACTH (see Fig. 5-13). This hormone has been named β-cell tropin and is present in the plasma of *ob/ob* mice. It potentiates glucose-induced insulin secretion. It appears to have identical properties to $ACTH_{22-39}$ prepared from ACTH (Fig. 5-14).

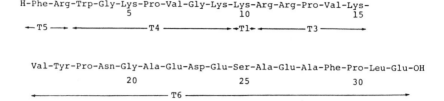

```
H-Phe-Arg-Trp-Gly-Lys-Pro-Val-Gly-Lys-Lys-Arg-Arg-Pro-Val-Lys-
            5                  10                    15
←─T5──→  ←────────────T4────────────→ ←─T1─← ←──────T3──────→
```

```
Val-Tyr-Pro-Asn-Gly-Ala-Glu-Asp-Glu-Ser-Ala-Glu-Ala-Phe-Pro-Leu-Glu-OH
        20                  25                    30
←────────────────────────T6────────────────────────────→
```

Figure 5-15. A proposed amino acid sequence for adrenocorticotropin-inhibiting peptide. Reproduced from C. H. Li, D. Chung, D. Yamashiro, and C. Y. Lee, *Proc. Natl. Acad. Sci. U.S.A.* **75,** 4306–4309 (1978).

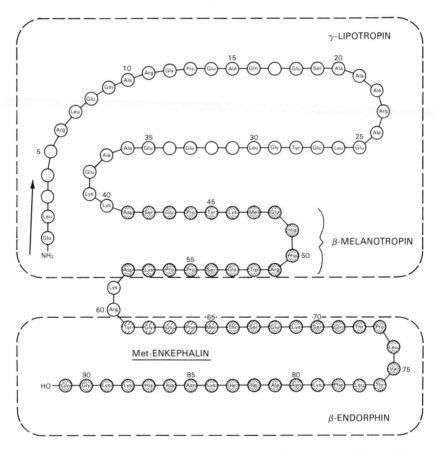

Figure 5-16. The structural relationship of γ-LPH, β-MSH, Met-enkephalin, and β-endorphin to the ovine β-LPH structure. Reproduced from C. H. Li, "Biochemical Actions of Hormones" (G. Litwack, ed.), Vol. 9, pp. 1–41. Academic Press, New York, 1982.

G. Melanocyte-Stimulating Hormone (MSH)

Human MSH occurs in two major forms, α-MSH and β-MSH. α-MSH is ~1500 molecular weight and consists of 13 amino acid residues. β-MSH is ~2600 molecular weight and consists of 22 amino acid residues. α-MSH is represented in residues 1–13 of the ACTH molecule (Fig. 5-14) and β-MSH is derived from a cleavage of β-lipotropin (42–134 of translation product; Fig. 5-13) to yield γ-lipotropin (42–101) and further cleavage to yield β-MSH (84–101). The sequence of human β-MSH is shown in Fig. 5-16.

H-Glu-Leu-Thr-Gly-Gln-Arg-Leu-Arg-Gln-Gly-
5   10

Asp-Gly-Pro-Asn-Ala-Gly-Ala-Asp-Asp-Gly-
15   20

Pro-Gly-Ala-Gln-Ala-Asp-Leu-Glu-His-Ser-
25   30

Leu-Leu-Val-Ala-Ala-Glu-Lys-Lys-Asp-Glu-
35   40

Gly-Pro-Tyr-Arg-Met-Glu-His-Phe-Arg-Trp-
45   50

Gly-Ser-Pro-Pro-Lys-Asp-Lys-Arg-Tyr-Gly-
55   60

Gly-Phe-Met-Thr-Ser-Glu-Lys-Ser-Gln-Thr-
65   70

Pro-Leu-Val-Thr-Leu-Phe-Lys-Asn-Ala-Ile-
75   80

Ile-Lys-Asn-Ala-Tyr-Lys-Lys-Gly-Glu-OH
85   89

Figure 5-17. Amino acid sequence of β-LPH. Reproduced from C. H. Li, "Biochemical Actions of Hormones" (G. Litwack, ed.), Vol. 9, pp. 1–41. Academic Press, New York, 1982.

$$5 \qquad\qquad 10$$
H-Tyr-Gly-Gly-Phe-Met-Thr-Ser-Glu-Lys-Ser-

$$15 \qquad\qquad 20$$
Gln-Thr-Pro-Leu-Val-Thr-Leu-Phe-Lys-Asn-

$$25 \qquad\qquad 31$$
Ala-Ile-Ile-Lys-Asn-Ala-Tyr-Lys-Lys-Gly-Glu-OH

Figure 5-18. Amino acid sequence of human β-endorphin. Reproduced from C. H. Li, "Biochemical Actions of Hormones" (G. Litwack, ed.), Vol. 9, pp. 1–41. Academic Press, New York, 1982.

H. Lipotropin (β-LPH)

There are two forms of lipotropin: β-LPH and γ-LPH. In Fig. 5-16 is shown the primary sequence of β-lipotropin (β-LPH). It contains sequences that become liberated by the actions of endopeptidases which cleave the chain at basic amino acid residues. These sequences are 1–58, which is γ-LPH, 41–58, which is β-MSH, and 61–91, which is β-endorphin. Thus, α-MSH derives from further cleavage of the ACTH molecule and β-MSH derives from cleavage of γ-LPH, which, in turn, is broken down from β-LPH. The sequence for human β-LPH is presented in Fig. 5-17 and for human β-endorphin in Fig. 5-18. β-LPH is 9500 molecular weight and consists of 91 amino acid residues. It is on the same translation product as ACTH. γ-LPH is a proteolytic cleavage product of β-LPH and consists of 58 amino acid residues. The maturation of these forms is shown in Fig. 5-13.

IV. BIOCHEMISTRY

A. Neural Controls

Central controls on the secretion of hormones of the *pars distalis* are comprised by hypothalamic releasing hormones and by neurotransmitters. A summary of some of the major controlling factors is presented in Fig. 5-19. In many cases it is unclear whether a neurotransmitter is acting through an interneuron to stimulate or inhibit the release of releasing hormone or acting directly at the anterior pituitary. Other possibilities for interaction with the closed portal circulation have been discussed in Chapter 3.

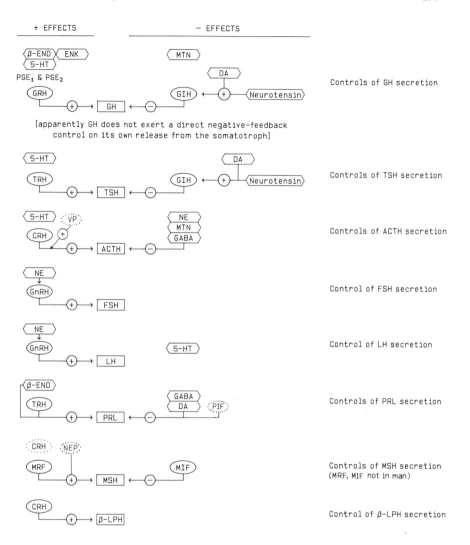

Figure 5-19. Summary of some of the major controlling factors on the secretion of hormones from the *pars distalis*. Factors encircled by ovals are releasing hormones/factors. Factors enclosed by hexagons are neurotransmitters. + effects are those that augment the secretion of the anterior pituitary hormone; − effects are those that decrease the secretion of the anterior pituitary hormone. ENK, Enkephalin; MTN, melatonin; DA, dopamine; 5-HT, serotonin; NE, norepinephrine; MRF, melanocyte hormone releasing factor; MIF, melanocyte hormone release-inhibiting factor. See text for other abbreviations.

200

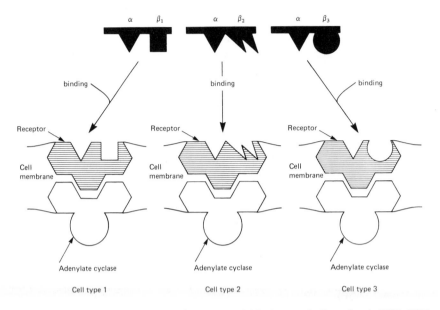

Figure 5-20. How anterior pituitary hormones which share a similar subunit (TSH, FSH, LH) specify receptors on different cell types.

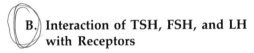

B. Interaction of TSH, FSH, and LH with Receptors

As shown in Table 5-2, these three hormones are very similar in that they each have two subunits and share a similar α subunit. How then must TSH specifically recognize its cellular target on the thyroid gland cell membrane apart from LH and FSH, which must individually recognize the Leydig cell membrane/ovarian follicle, respectively? Several possibilities are apparent and they must account for the similar or identical α subunit common to all three. Thus, in Fig. 5-20 is shown a hypothetical scheme in which this kind of selection can be incorporated and which allows the α subunit to play a role in facilitating binding while the antigenically unique β subunit could specify the binding site (see footnote to Table 5-2). Recently, the α and β subunits of human chorionic gonadotropin were deglycosylated with trifluoromethane sulfonic acid to remove most of the carbohydrate portions. The remaining protein core was unaffected in terms of amino acid analysis, molecular weight, and immunological activity. Deglycosylated subunits reassociated and interacted with receptor normally. Thus, the carbohydrate portions, as demonstrated by the O. P. Bahl laboratory, may not be required for these functions, but could play a role in some other function, such as in catabolism or hormonal transport (Fig. 5-9B). Furthermore, C. H. Li's laboratory has shown that the β subunits alone of hCG and LH have steroidogenic activity.

V. PROLACTIN

The most obvious role of prolactin is in the differentiation of the mammary gland cells and as a signal in the differentiated cells to produce milk proteins and other constituents. Prolactin may act like a secondary growth hormone, particularly on the liver, although this is not well understood. PRL also can act on the testis to stimulate the production of testosterone. It seems to have some role in stress adaptation as its release from the anterior pituitary is signaled, in this case, by the release of β-endorphin in response to stress and as a consequence of the action of CRH; β-endorphin then acts, apparently directly, on the mammotrope (lactotrope) to stimulate the release of PRL. It has been known for some time that nursing an infant on demand over a long period of time creates a period in which pregnancy rarely occurs. This is apparently the result of frequent release of PRL from the anterior pituitary in response to suckling which may have the effect of reducing GnRH release from the hypothalamus.

A. Inhibition of Prolactin Release

Inhibition of prolactin release by drugs is discussed in Chapter 14 in connection with lactation.

PIF, the endogenous inhibitor of PRL release, appears to be dopamine. Apparently, the dopamine may derive from the posterior pituitary rather than from the hypothalamus, which is typical of the releasing hormones. Posterior pituitary extracts contain high levels of dopamine. When the posterior pituitary is removed, there is a prompt and significant increase in the level of circulating prolactin. This is reversible specifically by dopamine. Thus, posterior pituitary dopamine (from a dopaminergic neuron?; see Fig. 5-21) appears to reach the anterior pituitary by way of the short hypophyseal portal vessels and participates in the regulation of prolactin secretion at the mammotrope. Recently, in the laboratory of P. H. Seeburg, the cloned DNA sequence encoding GnRH precursor protein contains an associated peptide called GAP (GnRH-

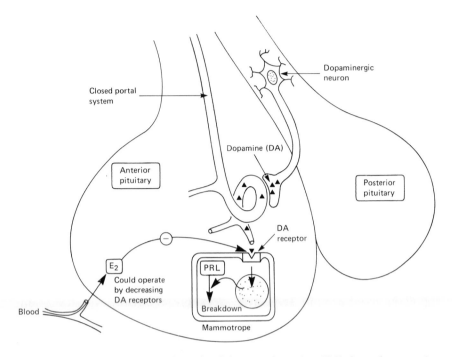

Figure 5-21. A possible morphology for delivering dopamine (DA) from the posterior pituitary to the mammotrope.

associated peptide).This peptide was found to be an inhibitor of PRL secretion and may be a candidate for PIF.

B. Stress-Induced Release of Prolactin

During stress ACTH, β-LPH and β-endorphin are released simultaneously from the corticotroph (see also Chapter 10). β-Endorphin appears to interact with a receptor which mediates the release of PRL from the mammotrope. GH probably is released in addition to PRL as a result of the action of β-endorphin. Morphine- or β-endorphin-induced release of PRL may operate through a neural site (receptor) of action and may involve dopaminergic but not serotonergic pathways. A serotonergic pathway may cause the stimulation of basal PRL levels in the anterior pituitary as diagnosed by *p*-chlorophenylalanine methyl ester, an inhibitor of serotonin biosynthesis, and by metoclopramide, which stimulates PRL release. The structures of these compounds are shown in Fig. 5-22.

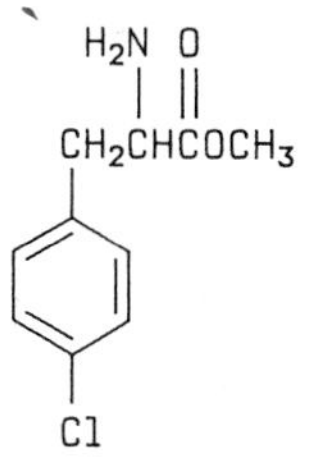

H$_2$N O
 | ||
CH$_2$CHCOCH$_3$

CONHCH$_2$CH$_2$N(C$_2$H$_5$)$_2$

OCH$_3$

Cl

NH$_2$

Cl

p-Chlorophenylalanine

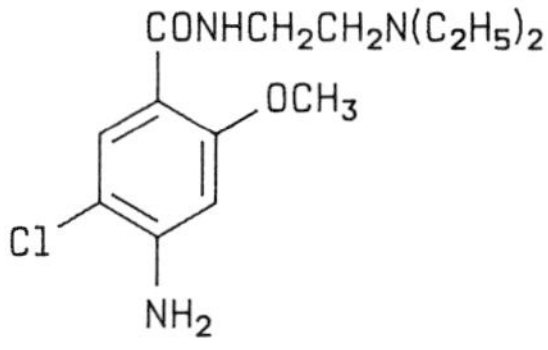

Metoclopramide
(4-amino-5-chloro-N-
[(2-diethylamino)ethyl]-
2-methoxybenzamide)

Figure 5-22. Structures of inhibitors of serotonin biosynthesis.

Thus, at least two pathways are possible for the regulation of PRL release. A positive pathway operates via a serotonergic mechanism and a negative pathway via a dopaminergic mechanism. A number of factors influence the secretion of PRL and GH. These are summarized in Table 5-3.

Table 5–3. Some Factors Affecting Human Prolactin and Growth Hormone Secretion[a]

Factor	Prolactin	Growth hormones
Physiologic		
Sleep	↑ ↑	↑ ↑
Nursing	↑ ↑ ↑	N
Breast stimulation (not postpartum)	↑	N
Stress	↑ ↑	↑ ↑
Hypoglycemia	↑	↑ ↑
Glucose	N or ↓	↓
Strenuous exercise	↑	↑
Sexual intercourse (women)	↑	N
Pregnancy	↑ ↑ ↑	N
Estrogens	↑	↑
Hypothyroidism	↑	N
Pharmacologic		
L-Dopa	↓ ↓	↑ ↑
Apomorphine	↓ ↓	↑ ↑
Ergot derivatives	↓ ↓	↑
Phenothiazines, butyrophenones	↑ ↑	N or ↓
Thyrotropin-releasing hormone	↑ ↑	N
Somatostatin	N	↓
Opiates[b]	↑	↑

[a] N denotes no change, ↑ increase and ↓ decrease. Reproduced from A.G. Frantz, *N. Engl. J. Med.* **298,** 201–207 (1978).

[b] May operate via α-adrenergic mechanism and/or GABA.

C. Prolactin Receptors in Nonmammary and Mammary Tissues

A large number of tissues appear to have membrane PRL receptors, such as liver, kidney, adrenal, testis, and brain.

In the animal testis, prolactin appears to enhance the effect of LH on the Leydig cell production of testosterone. Apparently PRL increases esterified cholesterol in the testis, suggesting its role in the transport of lipoprotein precursors for steroid biosynthesis. PRL also acts with testosterone to stimulate the growth and secretory activity of the prostate and seminal vesicles, although such actions have not been demonstrated yet in the human. The complete physiological role of prolactin in the human male is not clear.

Prolactin receptors on cell membranes of kidney and adrenal are regulated by glucocorticoids. Hypophysectomy reduces receptor number measured by ligand binding assays with ^{125}I-labeled PRL in kidney and adrenal. Glucocorticoid administration causes a further decrease.

Prolactin receptor has been purified from mammary gland, for example, of the rabbit, and characterized. Because of its location in the cell membrane as an integral rather than peripheral protein, a surface-active agent is used to solubilize specific PRL binding activity. The PRL receptor is clearly different from the GH receptor. The receptor thus solubilized retained specificity of PRL binding, but gave a higher affinity ($K_a = 16 \times 10^9 \, M^{-1}$) than the membrane-bound receptor ($K_a = 3 \times 10^9 \, M^{-1}$). About 0.5 mg of partially purified receptor is obtained from 100 g mammary gland. The molecular weight of the receptor is $\sim$220,000.

VI. GROWTH HORMONE

A. Growth Hormone Structure

The sequence of human GH is given in Fig. 5-4. The active core of the hormone involves the N-terminal two-thirds of the sequence; the remainder one-third of the sequence in the C terminal apparently stabilizes or protects the structure. In bovine GH, fragment 96–133 has the activity of a somatomedin in that it stimulates sulfation in bone and DNA synthesis in cells. Fragment 177–191 can be cleaved by extracellular endopeptidases and this fragment may have actions at the cell surface in *in vitro* experiments. It inhibits insulin binding to the insulin receptor at a concentration of $2.5 \times 10^{-10} \, M$. Although unknown, if GH is internalized like other polypeptide ligand–receptor complexes, such as the insulin–receptor complex, subsequent degradation in the lysosomal granule could avail a mitogenic cleavage product resembling the somatomedins. Somatomedins are thought to mediate the effects of GH on growth, as will be seen later. Much remains to be learned about GH action at the molecular level, especially in terms of its growth promotion of somatic cells.

B. Regulation of Growth Hormone Secretion

The overall regulation of GH secretion and its actions are summarized in Fig. 5-23 and Table 5-3. At the hypothalamic level a number of aminergic neurons can exert influences on GH secretion. These neurons are reviewed generally in Chapter 3. In Fig. 5-23 are shown catecholaminergic neurons, which may stimulate release of GRF from its neuron, and serotonergic as well as β-endorphinergic neurons, which could stimulate the release of TRH from its nerve ending. Although less certain, melatoninergic neurons or melatonin from the pineal gland could stimulate release of somatostatin from somatostatinergic neurons which inhibit release of GH from the somatotroph. These interneurons probably are linked to various conditions known to operate through the CNS: hypoglycemia (insulin?), exercise, and surgical stress. Once released from the somatotroph, GH circulates in the blood at levels greater than 3 ng/ml, with a total daily output of 1–4 mg.

GH has several major activities. It interacts with GH receptors in adipose cells and brings about an increase in free fatty acids by increasing lipolysis. Possibly phosphorylation of triglyceride lipase is involved in this mechanism. GH interacts with receptors on the cell membranes of liver, kidney, and muscle and causes the release of somatomedins into the circulation. The somatomedins are mitogenic (growth stimulatory) for many types of somatic cells and are of great importance in growth. GH also interacts with vascular walls, presumably containing a GH receptor also, resulting in the breakdown of vascular polysaccharides to glucose which enters the circulation. Finally, some older reports indicate that GH binds to a receptor in the cell membrane of the pancreatic A cell, an interaction resulting in the release of glucagon, an important hyperglycemic agent, although this last activity of GH is in doubt.

One form of dwarfism in man is caused by the defective production of pituitary GH. This condition appears from an autosomal recessive characteristic. Dwarfs in this category completely lack GH but not other pituitary hormones. Treating the condition with hGH causes prompt antibody reaction in that the dwarf recognized hGH as a xenobiotic. Through the use of cDNA probes of hGH, there appear to be several

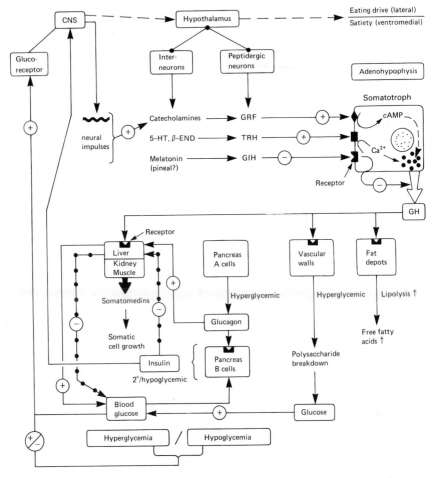

Figure 5-23. Control of secretion of growth hormone and its general actions. cAMP, Cyclic AMP. Solid lines ending in arrows indicate direct actions; beaded lines ending in arrows refer to feedback effects and encircled sign (+ or −) indicates whether the feedback effect is positive or negative. The same signs are used for direct actions to indicate positive or negative effects. Dashed lines refer to hypothetical stimulatory pathways.

hybridizing bands corresponding to this cDNA. The dwarfs lack one of these bands, however, and their immediate family members have this band but in less than normal amounts. There are probably two types of hGH gene, normal and variant (there are at least three types of gene for placental lactogen, which is closely related to GH). GH-deficient subjects may predominate in expression of a variant GH gene which is poorly functional. Other forms of short stature exist which do not result from a simple lack of GH. Such individuals have normal immunoreactive GH levels and no other obvious cause. A defective GH may be present indistinguishable by radioimmunoassay. Sometimes administration of hGH in these children may induce growth, but this is a very costly treatment. Further advances in molecular biology are bound to solve the problem of human dwarfism. Recent work has shown, by use of somatic cell hybridization and following the course of human genomic segregation, that the genes for GH, chorionic somatomammotropin (HCS), also known as placental lactogen, have been localized to chromosome 17 in humans. It appears that GH and chorionic somatomammotropin originated from the same ancestral gene that diverged 50–60 million years ago. PRL and GH diverged ~400 million years ago; probably all of these hormones were derived from the same ancestral gene.

C. Growth Hormone and Somatomedins

The relationship between GH and somatomedins is demonstrated in Fig. 5-24. Three somatomedins are formed in the human, A, B, and C. One of these (somatomedin C) is identical to IGF I. Once secreted into the bloodstream, GH binds to a specific receptor on the hepatocyte cell membrane and probably triggers an unknown second message. In response, the hepatocyte (see Chapter 10 for cell biology of the hepatocyte) either synthesizes or releases preformed somatomedins into the blood and the hepatocyte also produces a somatomedin binding protein of ~50,000 molecular weight. The somatomedins are ~7000 molecular weight and circulate mostly complexed to a binding protein. There seems to be specific somatomedin receptors on liver cells and cells of adipose, lymphocytes, bone, placental membrane, and others and these receptors are distinct from insulin receptors as revealed by competition experiments. The interaction of free somatomedin (not the somatomedin binding protein complex) with its receptor triggers an unknown second messenger, resulting in a mitogenic effect. The second messenger may occur through stimulation of a tyrosine kinase, which may be associated with the IGF receptor.

The sequence of a somatomedin is shown in Fig. 5-25. No distinctions are made here between somatomedins (SM-C), nonsuppressible insulin-like activities (NSILAs), cell multiplication factors, or insulin-like growth factors (IGFs) (see Chapter 19). It appears that a family of related polypeptides exists which have similar activities. Because of the rather extensive homology of somatomedins with insulin (see Fig. 7-6), it has been

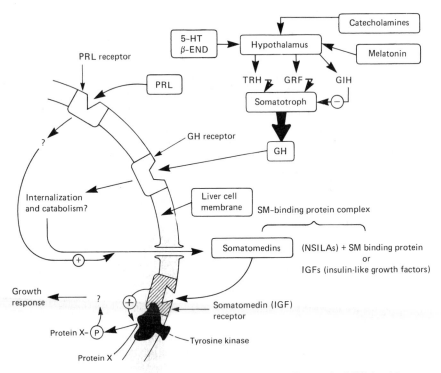

Figure 5-24. Somatomedins appear to mediate somatic cell growth. NSILAs, Nonsuppressible insulin-like activities; SM, somatomedin; these factors are now generally referred to as insulin-like growth factors, IGFs. Growth hormone is released from the somatotroph of the anterior pituitary whose regulation is suggested in this figure. After binding to the hepatocyte (in this illustration) GH receptor, reactions follow in the cell which stimulate the release of somatomedins, e.g., SM-C = IGF-I. IGFs bind to their receptors (one shown here) and tyrosine kinase activity is stimulated (this enzyme may be part of the receptor). It is hypothesized that a specific protein may be phosphorylated whose action, directly or indirectly, results in a growth response.

deduced that both hormones derive from the same ancestral gene. The growth-promoting activity of insulin itself may be due to its limited ability to bind to IGF receptors.

Interestingly, as shown in Fig. 5-26, the level of circulating somatomedin increases to a maximum until about 8 years of age when the human adult level is reached. Since growth continues on for many years beyond age 8, it is obvious that the amount of circulating somatomedins is not rate-limiting for growth. Thus, some other component of the overall system may limit growth, such as the development of somatomedin

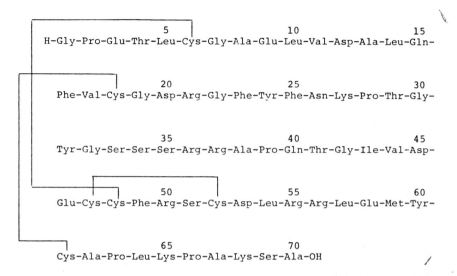

Figure 5-25. Primary structure of somatomedin-C (SM-C). Reproduced from C. H. Li, D. Yamoshiro, D. Gospodarowicz, S. L. Kaplan, and G. Van Vliet, *Proc. Natl. Acad. Sci. U.S.A.* **80,** 2216–2220 (1983).

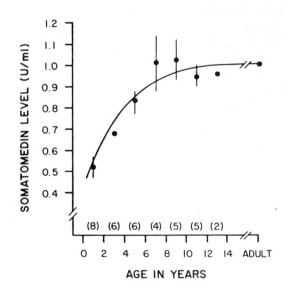

Figure 5-26. Levels of somatomedins and somatomedin activity in normal children of different ages. Figures in parentheses denote numbers of studies providing data in each age range; in each study, mean levels (+/− SEM) in normal; adults were defined as 1.00 U/ml and values in children were expressed accordingly. Reproduced by permission from L. S. Phillips and R. Vassilopoulou-Sellin, *N. Engl. J. Med.* **302,** 438–446 (1980).

receptors or some other factor involved in the utilization of these mitogens.

The effect of somatomedins on sulfation is important to bone growth. The mechanism by which somatomedins stimulate sulfation reactions is unclear.

D. Regulation of GH Gene Expression

An interesting model to study the regulation of growth hormone expression is the system of cultured pituitary cells which produce mRNAs encoding GH and PRL. From this model emerges information showing that both thyroid hormone and glucocorticoids are involved intimately in the expression of GH by these cells. Thyroid hormone appears to be an activator of the expression of the growth hormone gene. Thyroid hormone also controls the magnitude of the effect of glucocorticoids on GH mRNA; thus thyroid hormone may act as a permissive hormone in this system. It appears that the two hormones increase GH mRNA by different mechanisms.

VII. β-LIPOTROPIN

In recent years much excitement has developed around this hormone and its degradation products. The information showing that β-lipotropin and ACTH are encoded by the same gene product (see Fig. 5-13) soon was followed by evidence that ACTH and β-lipotropin are secreted from the anterior pituitary together in response to stress (see Chapter 10). More recently it has been shown that β-endorphin, and this hormone acts perhaps directly at the anterior pituitary level to stimulate the release of PRL which must have an as yet undisclosed role to play in stress adaptation (PRL may exert some hyperglycemic-like effects in the liver).

In purified neurosecretory granules from bovine pituitary glands proopiomelanocortin converting enzyme activity (an acid–thiol protease) has been found, making it likely that "maturing" activities operate within the granule itself.

A. β-Endorphin and Stress

β-Endorphin and ACTH were discovered to be secreted simultaneously from the anterior pituitary in response to stress. Long-term adrenalectomy also promoted the secretion of these two peptides indi-

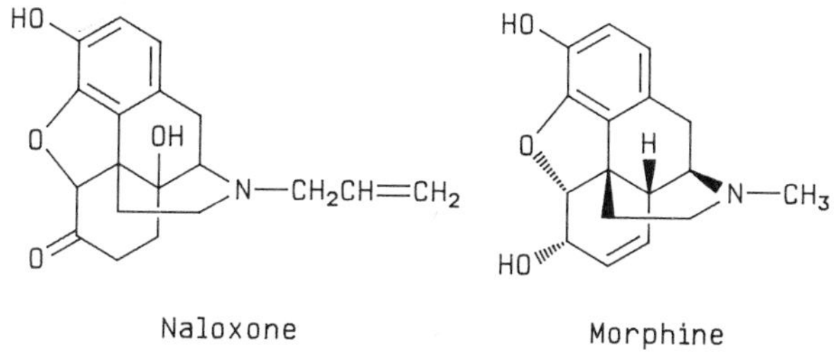

Figure 5-27. Structures of the opiate receptor antagonist, naloxone, and the opiate receptor agonist, morphine.

cating that cortisol might be a feedback inhibitor for both and therefore that β-endorphin may be involved, as well as ACTH, in the stress adaptation mechanism. Both of these hormones are secreted in response to corticotropin releasing hormone (CRH), a further confirmation of their relatedness in terms of mechanism of action and derivation from the same gene product. Administration of the synthetic glucocorticoid, dexamethasone, inhibited the secretion of both ACTH and β-endorphin. The glucocorticoid functions by reducing the level of translatable mRNA encoding both ACTH and endorphin. Processing of the precursor RNA is unaffected.

B. β-Endorphin Receptor

Interaction of β-endorphin with receptor in neuroblastoma–glioma hybrid cells has been studied by a number of investigators. In these experiments, human tritiated β-endorphin was used as ligand. The K_d value is 0.3 nM and $K_a = 1.8 \times 10^8\ M^{-1}\ min^{-1}$. β-Endorphin had 3 to 4 times as many binding sites as Leu-enkephalin which bound with an affinity of about 10% of that of β-endorphin. Monovalent and divalent cations inhibited binding. Trypsin, phospholipase A, and N-ethylmaleimide inhibit binding, indicating the protein and phospholipid nature of the receptor as well as a role for —SH groups in the ligand receptor interaction. Enkephalins, morphine, and naloxone, a specific inhibitor of analgesic action (see Fig. 5-27) were not as potent competitors as β-endorphin. From the point of view of the β-endorphin molecule, there are three binding sites, two of which could explain binding to distinct receptors. The δ receptor is located in the Met-enkephalin segment, as shown in Fig. 5-28. The μ receptor, specific for the morphine binding site, is in the carboxy terminus (Fig. 5-28). The middle

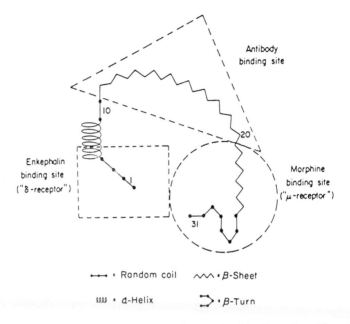

Antibody
binding site

Enkephalin
binding site
("δ-receptor")

Morphine
binding site
("μ-receptor")

●—● : Random coil   ∿∿ : β-Sheet

ɰɰ : α-Helix   ⟩ : β-Turn

Figure 5-28. Potential receptor binding sites for β-endorphin. Reproduced from C. H. Li, *Cell* **31**, 504–505 (1982).

segment is the antibody binding site. These conclusions are made by C. H. Li.

C. Processing of β-Endorphin

β-Endorphin is produced as a cleavage product of β-lipotropin, as shown previously (see Fig. 5-16). A model of the proadrenocorticotropin/endorphin is shown in Fig. 5-13. It appears that β-endorphin (1–31) is first formed and this molecule is rapidly N-acetylated on its amino terminal residue and then converted more slowly to α-N-acetyl-β-endorphin (1–27) and subsequently to α-N-acetyl-β-endorphin (1–27). This posttranslational processing is summarized in Fig. 5-29.

VIII. THYROTROPIC HORMONE

Thyrotropic Receptor

Like other polypeptide hormone receptors, TSH receptor is located in the cellular membrane of thyroid cells. A functional model of the TSH

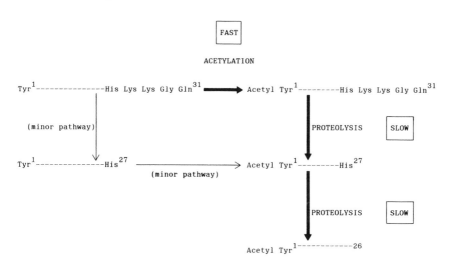

Figure 5-29. Posttranslational processing of β-endorphin in rat intermediate pituitary. Reproduced from B. A. Eipper and R. E. Mains, *J. Biol. Chem.* **256,** 5689–5695 (1981).

receptor has been hypothesized and is shown in Fig. 5-30. Recent work has shown that various lipids can affect the binding of ^{125}I-labeled TSH to bovine thyroid glands. Acidic phospholipids were potent inhibitors in the order cardiolipin > phosphatidylglycerol > phosphatidylinositol >> phosphatidylserine. Other phospholipids, neutral lipids, and neutral glycolipids were without activity. Gangliosides had some activity but were found to interact with the hormone, whereas the phospholipids interacted with the membrane. Phospholipase A treatment of the membrane enhanced the binding of ^{125}I-labeled TSH. Thus, the status of phospholipids in the membrane influences the ability of the receptor to bind TSH. Studies on cation uptake by cultured thyroid cells in the presence or absence of TSH indicate that a primary mode of action of the hormone may be an alteration in the electrical potential across the plasma membrane, which may be an activity shared in common with certain other polypeptide hormones acting on the cell membrane.

Monoclonal antibodies have been developed against the TSH receptor and they prevent binding of TSH to the ligand binding site. Since the antigenic specificity resides in the glycoprotein constituent of the receptor and not in the ganglioside portion, the antibody, when bound to receptor, fails to stimulate adenylate cyclase, in partial support of the view that the ganglioside is involved in the transmission of the signal that activates adenylate cyclase on the inner side of the membrane. Interestingly, the monoclonal antibody directed against TSH receptor

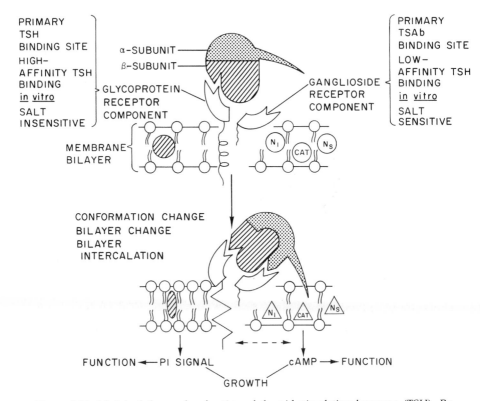

Figure 5-30. Model of the mode of action of thyroid-stimulating hormone (TSH). Reproduced from L. D. Kohn, "Cell Receptor Disorders" (T. Melnechuk, ed.). Western Behavioral Sciences Institute, La Jolla, California (1980).

was inhibited partially in its interaction with the receptor by cholera toxin, suggesting that the cholera toxin receptor shares common properties with the TSH receptor. The interaction of antibody and receptor is not prevented by insulin or human chorionic gonadotropin. In Graves' disease, autoantibodies are produced which prevent TSH binding, like the ones described above, but differ by stimulating adenylate cyclase and are thus thyroid stimulators. Perhaps these antibodies are directed against the ganglioside component of the TSH receptor rather than the glycoprotein component.

IX. ACTH

The principal biological action of ACTH is to stimulate corticosteroid production in adrenal cortical cells. This hormone interacts with receptors in membranes of the *zona fasciculata* and *zona reticularis*. A further discussion appears in Chapter 10.

An important aspect of ACTH action as well as for actions of other anterior pituitary hormones is that they undergo retrograde transport and redistribution within the CNS, especially the hypothalamus.

X. CLINICAL ASPECTS

Abnormalities of the anterior pituitary stem from a number of causes. Trauma to the anterior pituitary can occur often by mechanical pressure from tumors. The anterior pituitary may decline in function because there has been trauma to the delicate stalk connecting the pituitary to the hypothalamus and the releasing hormone concentrations in the pituitary become inadequate. Tumors of individual cell types may arise and produce high amounts of one or two anterior pituitary hormones, or hormones that act like them, ectopically. Detection of primary abnormal functioning at the pituitary level is easier now owing to the availability of many of the releasing hormones which make evocator tests possible (see Chapter 3). In cases of inadequate availability of a pituitary hormone the target gland hormone can be supplied (e.g., cortisol for inadequate ACTH supply).

Autoimmune diseases are an important consideration. In Graves' disease, an antibody is produced, apparently directed against the lipid component of the TSH receptor. In binding to the receptor, adenylate cyclase is activated and the thyroid responds as if TSH were there. Unfortunately, thyroid hormone does not feed back negatively on the autoantibody production as it does with TSH production and hyperthyroidism develops. Treatment usually involves ablating the function of the thyroid gland and maintaining normal subsequent hormone levels by replacement therapy.

Two situations will be discussed briefly: those resulting in hypofunction of the anterior pituitary and those resulting in hyperfunction of the anterior pituitary. Many anterior pituitary hormones may be affected in "panhypopituitarism." In this disease, the function or access of the pituitary to hypothalamic releasing hormones is destroyed by trauma, tumors, or vascular insufficiency. Such conditions are eventually corrected by surgical intervention, if a tumor, and by administration of the terminal hormones, whichever are required, such as the sex hormones, glucocorticoids, or thyroid hormone. Fortunately, evocator tests with purified releasing hormones (e.g., GnRH) and anterior pituitary hormones are available to localize the center of disturbance as being in the hypothalamus, pituitary, or terminal gland. A particular disease important to development is dwarfism, which can occur because of a deficiency of GH, often beginning at infancy. Other anterior pituitary hormones may be affected in this disease. Primary hypothyroidism, for example, can produce substantial inhibition of release of GH, resulting in dwarfism. Human growth hormone can be used to treat GH hyposecretion, but it is presently available in limited quantity. Presumably the cloned gene product will help in the treatment of dwarfism. Other conditions are associated with hypofunctions in ACTH and TSH, and in some cases the results are not severe. ACTH deficiency is substituted therapeutically.

Overproduction of pituitary hormones can occur when tumors ectopically produce a pituitary hormone(s). Disease states occur with excessive proplactin and growth hormone overproduction leads to gigantism during growth (epiphyseal cartilages are open) or to acromegaly if epiphyseal cartilages are fused. Overproduction of prolactin leads to galactorrhea and amenorrhea in the absence of acromegaly and pregnancy. Galactorrhea is often controlled by reducing prolactin secretion using a drug (bromocryptine) which inhibits prolactin formation and release.

Hyperproduction of growth hormone can result from a tumor of the somatotroph (acidophil pituitary adenoma) during growth and result in gigantism. The process of growth is accelerated under this condition, leading to giants. This form of GH overproduction is relatively rare. If left untreated, the tumor destroys the functional gland, impairing the other pituitary hormones and resulting in death. This disease usually involves enlargement of the sella, but principally manifests by unusually high circulating levels of GH. Therapy involves removal of acidophil tumor, but sometimes high levels of GH persist even after surgical intervention.

Acromegaly is also relatively uncommon. There are two metabolic types of acromegaly: those in which circulating GH levels fall after glucose administration and those whose GH levels are unaffected by glucose. The precise explanation of acromegaly is unknown and some views infer that humans can revert to a more primitive phase and resemble the Neanderthal man.

Recently, abnormal levels of brain opiates in the form of endorphins and enkephalins have been postulated as the cause of mental illness. This idea extends either to levels that are too high or too low. Analogies are drawn from clinical experiences with exogenous opiate drugs which act much like the endogenous normal counterparts. If this suggestion turns out to be correct, we can look forward to some rational, effective chemotherapy of mental disease.

References

A. Books

Krieger, D. T., and Hughes, J. C., eds. (1980). "Neuroendocrinology." Sinauer Associates, Sunderland, Massachusetts.
Li, C. H., ed. (1973). "Hormonal Proteins and Peptides," Vol. 1. Academic Press, New York.
Li, C. H., ed. (1975). "Hormonal Proteins and Peptides," Vol. 3. Academic Press, New York.
Litwack, G., ed. (1978). "Biochemical Actions of Hormones," Vol. 5. Academic Press, New York.
Litwack, G., ed. (1982). "Biochemical Actions of Hormones," Vol. 9. Academic Press, New York.
Williams, R. H., ed. (1981). "Textbook of Endocrinology." Saunders, Philadelphia, Pennsylvania.

B. Review Articles

Bahl, O. P. (1977). Human chorionic gonadotropin, its receptor and mechanism of action. *Fed. Proc., Fed. Am. Soc. Exp. Biol.* **36,** 2119–2127.
Frantz, A. G. (1978). Prolactin. *N. Engl. J. Med.* **298,** 201–207.
Li, C. H. (1978). Chemical messengers of the adenohypophysis from somatotropin to lipotropin. *Perspect. Biol. Med.* **21,** 447–465.
Li, C. H. (1982). β-Endorphin. *Cell* **31,** 504–505.
Li, C. H. (1982). The lipotropins. *In* "Biochemical Actions of Hormones" (G. Litwack, ed.), Vol. 9, pp. 1–41. Academic Press, New York.
Moore, D. D., Conkling, M. A., and Goodman, H. M. (1982). Human growth hormone: A multigene family. *Cell* **29,** 285–286.

C. Research Papers

Adelman, J. P., Masson, A. J., Hayflick, J. S., and Seeburg, P. (1986). Isolation of the gene and hypothalamic cDNA for the common precursor of gonadotropic-releasing hormone and prolactin release-inhibiting factor in human and rat. *Proc. Natl. Acad. Sci. USA* **83,** 179–183.
Beloff-Chain, A., Morton, J., Dunmore, S., Taylor, G. W., and Morris, H. R. (1983). Evidence that the insulin secretagogue, β-cell tropin, is $ACTH_{22-29}$. *Nature (London)* **301,** 255–258.
Birk, Y., and Li, C. H. (1978). Two fragments from fibrinolysin digests of ovine prolactin: Characterization and recombination to generate full immunoreactivity. *Proc. Natl. Acad. Sci. U.S.A.* **75,** 2155–2159.
Challis, J. R. G., and Torosis, J. D. (1977). Is α-MSH a trophic hormone to adrenal function in the fetus? *Nature (London)* **269,** 818–819.
Cooke, N. E., Coit, D., Shine, J., Baxter, J. D., and Martial, J. A. (1981). Human prolactin. cDNA structural analysis and evolutionary comparisons. *J. Biol. Chem.* **256,** 4007–4016.
Dannies, P. S., and Rudnick, M. S. (1980). 2-Bromo-α-ergocryptine causes degradation of prolactin in primary cultures of rat pituitary cells after chronic treatment. *J. Biol. Chem.* **255,** 2776–2781.

218

Dave, J. R., and Knazek, R. A. (1980). Prostaglandin I$_2$ modifies both prolactin binding capacity and fluidity of mouse liver membranes. *Proc. Natl. Acad. Sci. U.S.A.* **77**, 6597–6600.

Ealey, P. A., Kohn, L. D., Ekins, R. P., and Marshall, N. J. (1984). Characterization of monoclonal antibodies derived from lymphocytes from Graves' disease patients in a cytochemical bioassay for thyroid stimulators. *Endocrinology (Baltimore)* **58**, 909–914.

Eipper, B. A., and Mains, R. E. (1981). Further analysis of posttranslational processing of β-endorphin in rat intermediate pituitary. *J. Biol. Chem.* **256**, 5689–5699.

Fang, V. S., and Shian, L.-R. (1981). A serotonergic mechanism of the prolactin-stimulating action of metoclopramide. *Endocrinology (Baltimore)* **108**, 1622–1627.

Farley, J. R., and Baylink, D. J. (1982). Purification of the skeletal growth factor from human bone. *Biochemistry* **21**, 3502–3507.

Goeddel, D. V., Heyneker, H. L., Hozumi, T., Arentzen, R., Itakura, K., Yansura, D. G., Ross, M. J., Miozzari, G., Crea, R., and Seeburg, P. H. (1979). Direct expression in *Escherichia coli* of a DNA sequence coding for human growth hormone. *Nature (London)* **281**, 544–548.

Grollman, E. F., Lee, G., Ambesi-Impiombato, F. S., Meldolisi, M. F., Aloj, S. M., Coon, H. G., Kaback, H. R., and Kohn, L. D. (1977). Effects of thyrotropin on the thyroid cell membrane: Hyperpolarization induced by hormone–receptor interaction. *Proc. Natl. Acad. Sci. U.S.A.* **74**, 2352–2356.

Guillemin, R., Vargo, T., Rossier, J., Minick, S., Ling, N., Rivier, C., Vale, W., and Bloom, F. (1977). β-Endorphin and adrenocorticotropin are secreted concomitantly by the pituitary gland. *Science* **197**, 1368–1369.

Hammonds, R. G., Jr., Ferrara, P., and Li, C. H. (1981). β-endorphin: Characteristics of binding sites in a neuroblastoma–glioma hybrid cell. *Proc. Natl. Acad. Sci. U.S.A.* **78**, 2218–2220.

Josefsberg, Z., Posner, B. I., Patel, B., and Bergeron, J. J. M. (1979). The uptake of prolactin into female rat liver. Concentration of intact hormone in the Golgi apparatus. *J. Biol. Chem.* **254**, 209–214.

Kalyan, N. K., and Bahl, O. P. (1983). Role of carbohydrate in human chorionic gonadotropin. *J. Biol. Chem.* **258**, 67–74.

Keutmann, H. T., Lampman, G. W., Mains, R. E., and Eipper, B. A. (1981). Primary sequence of two regions of mouse proadrenocorticotropin/endorphin. *Biochemistry* **20**, 4148–4155.

Li, C. H. (1975). Human pituitary growth hormone: A biologically active hendekakaiheketon peptide fragment corresponding to amino acid residues 15–125 in the hormone molecule. *Proc. Natl. Acad. Sci. U.S.A.* **72**, 3878–3882.

Li, C. H., Chung, D., Yamashiro, D., and Lee, C. Y. (1978). Isolation, characterization and synthesis of a corticotropin-inhibiting peptide from human pituitary glands. *Proc. Natl. Acad. Sci. U.S.A.* **75**, 4306–4309.

Mains, R. E., and Eipper, B. A. (1981). Differences in the posttranslational processing of β-endorphin in rat anterior and intermediate pituitary. *J. Biol. Chem.* **256**, 5683–5688.

Manni, A., Chambers, M. J., and Pearson, O. H. (1978). Prolactin induces its own receptors in rat liver. *Endocrinology (Baltimore)* **103**, 2168–2171.

Marshall, S., Huang, H. H., Kledzik, G. S., Campbell, G. A., and Meites, J. (1978). Glucocorticoid regulation of prolactin receptors in kidneys and adrenals of male rats. *Endocrinology (Baltimore)* **102**, 869–875.

Martial, J. A., Seeburg, P. H., Guenzi, D., Goodman, H. M., and Baxter, J. D. (1977).

Regulation of growth hormone gene expression: Synergistic effects of thyroid and glucocorticoid hormones. *Proc. Natl. Acad. Sci. U.S.A.* **74,** 4293–4295.

Matsuoka, H., Mulrow, P. J., and Li, C. H. (1980). β-lipotropin: A new aldosterone-stimulating factor. *Science* **209,** 307–308.

Mode, A., Norstedt, G., Simic, B., Eneroth, P., and Gustafsson, J.-A. (1981). Continuous infusion of growth hormone feminizes hepatic steroid metabolism in the rat. *Endocrinology (Baltimore)* **108,** 2103–2108.

Morris, D. H., and Schalch, D. S. (1982). Structure of somatomedin-binding protein: Alkaline pH-induced dissociation of an acid-stable, 60,000 molecular weight complex into smaller components. *Endocrinology (Baltimore)* **111,** 801–805.

Moudgal, N. R., and Li, C. H. (1982). β-Subunits of human choriogonadotropin and ovine lutropin are biologically active. *Proc. Natl. Acad. Sci. U.S.A.* **79,** 2500–2503.

Nansel, D. D., Gudelshy, G. A., Reymond, M. J., and Porter, J. C. (1981). Estrogen alters the responsiveness of the anterior pituitary gland to the actions of dopamine on lysosomal enzyme activity and prolactin release. *Endocrinology (Baltimore)* **108,** 903–907.

Nikolics, K., Mason, A. J., Szonyi, E., Ramachandran, J., and Seeburg, P. H. (1985). A prolactin-inhibiting factor within the precursor for human gonadotropic-*releasing* hormone. *Nature (London)* **316,** 511–517.

Omodeo-Sale, F., Brady, R. O., and Fishman, P. H. (1978). Effect of thyroid phospholipids on the interaction of thyrotropin with thyroid membranes. *Proc. Natl. Acad. Sci. U.S.A.* **75,** 5301–5305.

Owerbach, D., Rutter, W. J., Martial, J. A., Baxter, J. D., and Shows, T. B. (1980). Genes for growth hormone, chorionic somatomammotropin and growth hormone-like gene on chromosome 17 in humans. *Science* **209,** 289–292.

Peters, L. L., Hoefer, M. J., and Ben-Jonathan, N. (1981). The posterior pituitary: Regulation of anterior pituitary prolactin secretion. *Science* **213,** 659–661.

Retegui, L. A., de Meyts, P., Pena, C., and Masson, P. L. (1982). The same region of human growth hormone is involved in its binding to various receptors. *Endocrinology (Baltimore)* **111,** 668–676.

Roberts, J. L., Budarf, M. L., Baxter, J. D., and Herbert, E. (1979). Selective reduction of proadrenocorticotropin/endorphin proteins and messenger ribonucleic acid activity in mouse pituitary tumor cells by glucocorticoids. *Biochemistry* **18,** 4907–4915.

Seeburg, P. H., Shine, J., Martial, J. A., Ivarie, R. D., Morris, J. A., Ullrich, A., Baxter, J. D., and Goodman, H. M. (1978). Synthesis of growth hormone by bacteria. *Nature (London)* **276,** 795–798.

Seidah, N. G., Rochemont, J., Hamelin, J., Lis, M., and Chrétien, M. (1981). Primary structure of the major pituitary pro-opiomelanocortin NH_2-terminal glycopeptide. *J. Biol. Chem.* **256,** 7977–7984.

Shiu, R. P. C., and Friesen, H. G. (1974). Solubilization and purification of a prolactin receptor from the rabbit mammary gland. *J. Biol. Chem.* **249,** 7902–7911.

Wallis, M. (1982). Molecular basis of growth hormone deficiency. *Nature (London)* **296,** 112–113.

Walsh, R. J., Posner, B. I., Kopriwa, B. M., and Brawer, J. R. (1978). Prolactin binding sites in the rat brain. *Science* **201,** 1041–1043.

Wehrenberg, W. B., McNicol, D., Wardlaw, S. L., Frantz, A. G., and Ferin, M. (1981). Dopaminergic and serotonergic involvement in opiate-induced prolactin release in monkeys. *Endocrinology (Baltimore)* **109,** 544–547.

Yavin, E., Yavin, Z., Schneider, M. D., and Kohn, L. D. (1981). Monoclonal antibodies to the thyrotropin receptor: Implications for receptor structure and the action of autoantibodies in Graves disease. *Proc. Natl. Acad. Sci. U.S.A.* **78,** 3180–3184.

Zanni, A., Giannattasio, G., Nussdorfer, G., Margolis, R. K., Margolis, R. U., and Meldolesi, J. (1980). Molecular organization of prolactin granules. II. Characterization of glycosaminoglycans and glycoproteins of the bovine prolactin matrix. *J. Cell Biol.* **86,** 260–272.

Thyroid Hormones

I. INTRODUCTION

A. Background

The thyroid gland and its hormonal products play an indispensible role affecting a variety of biochemical reactions at the level of the peripheral tissues which collectively control the basal metabolic activity of the organism. The principal target tissues of action of the thyroid hormones are skeletal muscle, cardiac muscle, liver, and kidney. The basal metabolic activity (BMR) of an intact organism is a measure of the energy expended after completion of the intestinal absorption of food; it is proportional both to the oxygen consumption and surface area (body volume) of the organism. The BMR is traditionally expressed in Calories* per square meter per hour (or day). The normal BMR for adult euthyroid males is 35–40 Cal/m² body surface/hr or 0.6 Cal/m²/min; for euthyroid women of the same age the BMR is 6–10% lower. In the hormonally deficient (hypothyroid) state the BMR can fall to 20–25 Cal/m²/hr, whereas in instances of hormone excess (thyrotoxicosis or hyperthyroidism) it may rise as high as 60–65 Cal/m²/hr. /

B. Iodine Metabolism

- The principal hormones produced by the thyroid are thyroxine (T_4) and triiodothyronine (T_3) which contain, respectively, four and three atoms of organically bound iodine-(see Section III). Accordingly, the normal functioning of the thyroid is dependent upon an adequate and regular dietary intake of iodine. For adults the recommended daily allowance (RDA) of iodine established by the U.S. National Research Council is 150–300 μg/day. In the United States the average daily intake of iodine by adults is in the range of 200–600 μg/day, largely as iodide. For technical reasons the dietary intake of iodine is normally assessed by measuring its urinary excretion; under circumstances of intake of the RDA of 150 μg/day, ~60–100 μg/day of iodine will be excreted in the urine. The main dietary source of iodine is iodized salt; present-day iodized salt contains 100 mg KI/kg of salt (0.01% KI).

In the absence of adequate dietary access to iodine, an individual will adaptively develop iodine deficiency or endemic goiter. The definition of endemic goiter is described in statistical terms and exists when 10–20% or more of preadolescent children in a given geographic or population grouping have enlarged, mildly hypertrophied thyroid glands. In most adults with endemic goiter, their intake of iodine will be below 25–75 μg/day and their urinary excretion can fall to 20–50 μg/day. Endemic goiter can be found in areas in which there is a suboptimal level of iodine in the soil and in food crops grown thereon. It has been clearly demonstrated that endemic goiter can be prevented by the oral administration of potassium iodide at 6-month intervals.

C. Metabolic Effects of Thyroid Hormones

- The thyroid hormones, depending upon whether they are present at elevated or reduced levels, have a wide range of effects in man which

Go to pg. 240.

*The C of calorie, when it is used to denote a kilocalorie, must be capitalized; thus, 1000 cal = 1 kcal = 1 Cal.

are evident at many different levels of organization; these range from behavioral changes, growth effects, changes in cardiac output, in gastrointestinal function, and in tissue oxygen consumption, muscle myopathy (weakness), and perturbations of the immune mechanism. ⁻

⤳ In instances of thyroid hormone excess the subject has an accelerated BMR and an elevated cardiac output associated with high body temperature, warm skin, and inappropriate sweating for the ambient temperature. Because the muscle mass of the body constitutes 50% of the body weight and because muscle tissue has a high rate of oxygen consumption, the increased muscular activity contributes substantially to the higher BMR. Although hyperthyroid subjects often increase their food intake, there is usually a concomitant weight loss related to the greater gastrointestinal activity and associated diarrhea. Such an individual is often hyperactive, with rapid movements and exaggerated reflexes, and often exhibits short attention spans. The muscle myopathy is attributable to both abnormal protein catabolism with negative nitrogen balance as well as to abnormal neuromuscular transmission. A prominent external physical feature of hyperthyroidism is exophthalmos or bulging of the eyeball.

In many respects the symptoms of a hypothyroid subject are the inverse of that described above for thyroid hormone excess. The BMR is reduced with an associated enlarged heart that has a reduced cardiac output. Accordingly, the body temperature is lowered, the skin is "cool," and sweating is reduced in relation to the ambient temperature. Also, the hypothyroid's appetite is poor and there is reduced gastrointestinal activity. Although the skeletal muscles are somewhat enlarged, there is an obvious myopathy. The principal external clinical features of hypothyroidism include a "myexdemic appearance." This describes the accumulation under the skin of mucoproteins and fluids which result in the subject having a "puffy" appearance as a consequence of alterations in electrolyte and water balances.

II. ANATOMICAL AND MORPHOLOGICAL RELATIONSHIPS

Thyroid Gland

1. Gross Level

Figure 6-1 shows the location and structure in man of the thyroid gland. In the adult the thyroid gland weighs 15–20 g. It consists of brownish-red right and left lobes. The two lobes are connected by an isthmus and lie on the lower part of the layrnx and the upper part of the

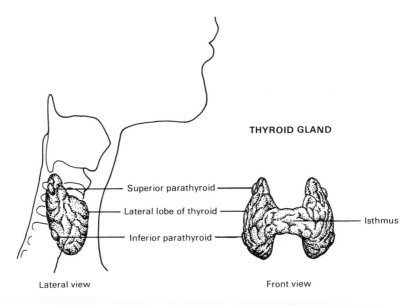

Figure 6-1. Location and structure of thyroid gland in man.

trachea. From the inner capsule of the thyroid, septa extend into the gland, dividing it into lobules of varying shape and size. The separate lobules are composed of follicles which are the main structural and functional unit of the thyroid parenchyma. In the human thyroid gland there are 20–30 million follicles.

2. Ultrastructure

The thyroid tissues are comprised of two principal cell types—the follicle cell and parafollicular cells or C cells. The C cells are found in the follicular wall or the interfollicular spaces and are responsible for the production of the polypeptide hormone, calcitonin (see Chapter 9).

The follicle that is the smallest functional unit of the thyroid is a cryptlike spheroidal structure varying between 0.05 and 0.5 mm. A follicle consists of a single layer of epithelial cells enclosing a cavity termed the follicle lumen. This lumen is filled with a viscous proteinaceous solution—the colloid. Each follicle is encased by a thin basement membrane (see Fig. 6-2).

The fresh colloid is clear in appearance and composed of homogeneous granules which are secretory products of the follicle cell, principally thyroglobulin, and a small proportion of larger cells. The colloid represents the storage form of the thyroid hormones.

The follicle cell contains a visible rough endoplasmic reticulum (RER)

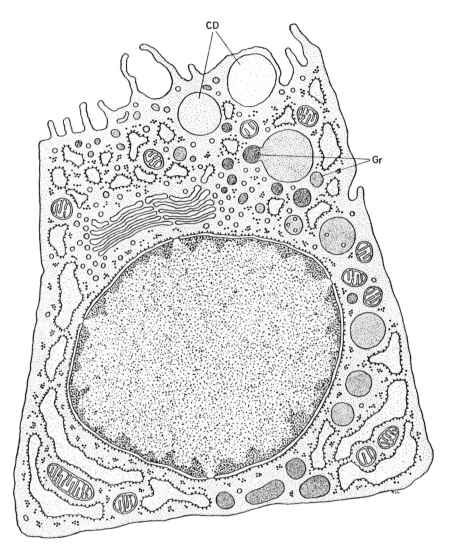

Figure 6-2. Thyroid follicular epithelial cell and its adjacent follicle lumen (Fl). The cells have a well-developed Golgi apparatus which is associated with the synthesis of thyroglobulin and its transport into the follicle lumen. Also, membrane-bounded dense granules (Gr) and colloid droplets (CD) are present in the cytoplasm. Reproduced with permission from T. L. Lentz, "Cell Fine Structure." Saunders, Philadelphia, Pennsylvania, 1971.

which occupies most of the space in the basal and paranuclear portions of the cell. The cisternae of the RER are of varying size and shape; most are dedicated to thyroglobulin synthesis. The Golgi apparatus in the follicle cells show a composition similar to that in many other secretory cells. It is normally located apically to the nucleus. Also visible in the follicle cell are the exocytic vesicles containing the thyroglobulin destined for the colloid.

A prerequisite for thyroid hormone release from the colloid is the degradation of the thyroglobulin. It is now generally accepted that the degradation of the thyroglobulin occurs after reentry of the colloid into the follicular cell by the process of endocytosis. The mechanism of reentry involves the appearance on the follicular cell luminal membrane of pseudopods which participate in the phagocytic reabsorption of a colloid droplet. It is also likely that a small proportion of colloid reabsorption occurs by micropinocytosis. Under certain basal or resting conditions there is a possibility that micropinocytosis plays a significant role in colloid reabsorption and subsequent release of thyroid hormone(s). In some cytological studies it is possible to observe the presence of microtubules in the follicular cell. They have been suggested as being associated with the endocytic process. Colchicine, a drug which blocks microtubule formation, is known to interfere with thyroid hormone release from the follicular cells. Lysosomes are often seen in close relation to the reabsorbed colloid droplets (see Fig. 6-2) and it seems likely that they play a role in release of the thyroid hormones from thyroglobulin.

III. CHEMISTRY

A. Endogenous Hormones

The mammalian thyroid gland biosynthesizes, stores, and secretes two molecular species of "thyroid hormones." They are thyroxine (T_4) or L-3,5,3′,5′-tetraiodothyronine and triiodothyronine (T_3) or L-3,5,3′-triiodothyronine (see Fig. 6-3). The parent compound for the iodinated series of thyroid-active hormones is thyronine. Thyronine is 4-(4′-hydroxyphenoxy)-L-phenylalanine; the conventional numbering system for the carbon atoms of the thyronine molecule is also indicated in Fig. 6-3.

B. Thyroid Hormone Analogs

A detailed study of the structural requirements for thyromimetic action suggests that thyroid hormone "active" compounds must have at a minimum a central lipophilic core containing bulky 3,5,3′ substituents (not necessarily iodine atoms) and two anion groups at each distal end of the molecule. Thus, extensive structural modification of the molecule

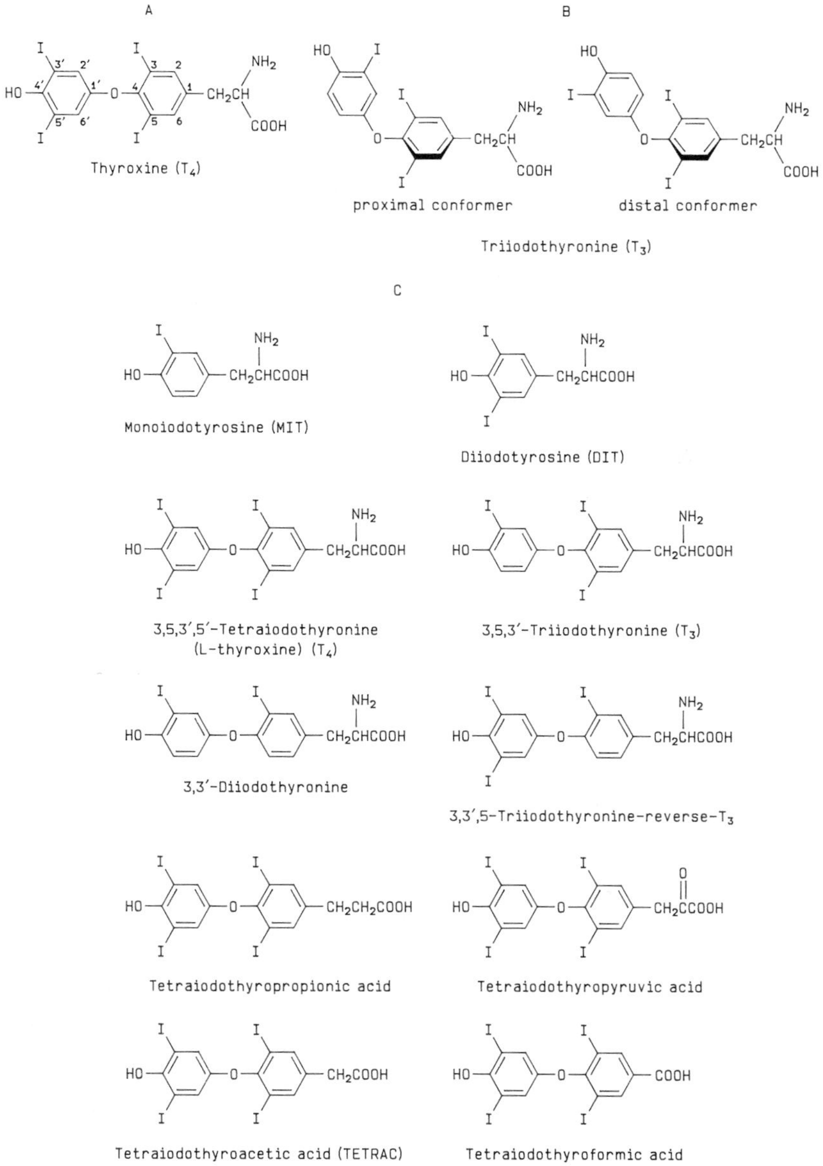

A

Thyroxine (T$_4$)

B

proximal conformer   distal conformer

Triiodothyronine (T$_3$)

C

Monoiodotyrosine (MIT)

Diiodotyrosine (DIT)

3,5,3',5'-Tetraiodothyronine
(L-thyroxine) (T$_4$)

3,5,3'-Triiodothyronine (T$_3$)

3,3'-Diiodothyronine

3,3',5-Triiodothyronine-reverse-T$_3$

Tetraiodothyropropionic acid

Tetraiodothyropyruvic acid

Tetraiodothyroacetic acid (TETRAC)

Tetraiodothyroformic acid

Figure 6-3. Structure of thyroxine, triiodothyronine, and precursors and analogs. (A) The numbering system of the carbons for the two aromatic rings of thyroxine or 3,5,3',5'-tetraiodothyronine (T$_4$) is indicated. (B) Schematic representation of the conformation of triiodothyronine (T$_3$), illustrating that the phenyl rings exist in planes that are normal to

Table 6–1. Biological Activity of Some Thyroxine Analogs[a]

Compound	Goiter prevention	Calorigenic	Other	Comments
	Percentage of thyroxine-like activity			
Iodinated thyronines				
L-Thyroxine	100	100		
3,5,3'-Triiodo-L-thyronine	500–800	300–500		
3,3',5'-Triiodo-L-thyronine	<1	<1		
3,3'-Diiodo-DL-thyronine	<1	<3		
3-Iodo-DL-thyronine	<2	<2		
3' or 5' position phenolic ring substituents				
3',5'-Dibromo-3,5-diiodothyronine	7–10			
3'-Bromo-3,5-diiodothyronine	130–200			
3',5'-Dichloro-3,5-diiodo-L-thyronine	15–27			
3'-Chloro-3,5-diiodo-L-thyronine	27			
3 or 5 position phenolic ring substituents				
3,5-Dibromo-3',5'-diiodo-DL-thyronine		12		
3,5-Dichloro-3',5'-diiodo-DL-thyronine		0.2		
Side chain alterations				
3,5,3',5'-Tetraiodothyroacetic acid	57	10–15		
3,5,3',5'-Tetraiodothyropyruvic acid	75	10–20		
4'-Phenolic hydroxyl substituents				
O-Methyl-DL-thyroxine		50	5	In myxedema patients
Altered ether linkage				
Thyroxine sulfur analog			>10	In myxedema patients
3,5-Diiodo-4-(3',5'-diiodo-4'-hydroxy-phenyl)-DL-phenylalanine			<0.3	Rat heart rate

[a] Abstracted from C. S. Pittman and J. A. Pittman, Relation of chemical structure to the action and metabolism of thyroactive substances. *In* "Handbook of Physiology" (M. A. Greer and D. H. Solomon, eds.), Sect. 7, Vol. III, p. 233. Am. Physiol. Soc., Washington, D.C., 1974.

is possible without major loss of biological activity. Methyl groups, bromine, fluorine, or nitrate are tolerated with decreasing activity in the 3,5,3' and 5' positions and the alanine side chain can be replaced by formate, acetate, propionate, or pyruvate groups with some decrease

---

one another and intersect at an angle of ~120°. Two conformations are possible for T_3 analogs that are monosubstituted in the ortho position relative to the 4'-OH group: (1) the proximal conformer with the single outer ring substituent oriented toward the inner ring; and (2) the distal conformer with the same substituent directed away from the inner ring. The distal conformation is believed to correspond to the active conformation of the molecule. (C) Structure of other thyroxine analogs.

but not loss of activity. Also, the ether link between the two phenolic rings can be replaced by a sulfur or methylene linkage. The biological properties of some thyroxine analogs are summarized in Table 6-1.

Thyroid-active compounds lacking a substitution in the 5' position have a higher biological activity than those retaining a group at this position. Thus, triiodothyronine (T_3) is some 5–8 times more active than tetraiodothyronine (T_4) (see Table 6-1). Compounds that are di- or tri-substituted but that lack two substituents in the first ring (e.g., 3,3',5'-triiodothyronine (reverse T_3), 3,3'-diiodothyronine, or 3',5'-diiodothy-ronine) usually have low or undetectable thyromimetic action.

Reverse T_3 or 3,3',5'-triiodothyronine is present in low concentrations in the thyroid and blood. It is largely produced by peripheral mono-deiodination of thyroxine (T_4). Reverse T_3 has only 10% of the thy-romimetic activity of T_4 and under some circumstances can antagonize the calorigenic effects of thyroxine.

Although D-thyroxine is not endogenously produced, the administra-tion of this analog will result in 5–20% of the calorigenic response of L-thyroxine. Surprisingly, D-T_3 and D-T_4 have been found to bind *in vitro* to the nuclear thyroid receptor protein with the same high affinity as the comparable L compounds. Thus, the differences in activity of the D compounds between *in vivo* and *in vitro* systems may relate to dif-ferences in blood transport or tissue metabolism.

The acetic acid analogs derived from T_3 and T_4, namely, tri- or tetraio-dothyroacetic acid (TRIAC or TETRAC) (see Fig. 6-3), are physiologically important since they are known to be endogenously produced by de-amination and decarboxylation of the parent compound.

IV. BIOCHEMISTRY

A. Iodide Metabolism

1. General Comments

The biosynthesis of thyroid hormone is dependent upon the continu-ous dietary availability of iodine. Approximately 90–95% of all iodide in the body is present in the thyroid. The dietary iodine is absorbed by the intestine after reduction to iodide. The inorganic iodide is then trans-ported in the blood by a variety of plasma proteins. The concentration of total iodide in the blood plasma is 8–15 μg/100 ml while the protein-bound concentration is normally 6–8 μg/100 ml. After arrival at the thyroid gland, the iodide is converted to the thyroid hormones in a series of metabolic steps which are summarized as follows:

1. Active transport of iodide into the thyroid gland follicular cells
2. Iodination of tyrosyl residues within the protein thyroglobulin
3. Transfer and coupling of iodotyrosines within thyroglobulin to form T_4 and T_3
4. Proteolysis of thyroglobulin with concomitant release of T_4 and T_3, as well as free iodotyrosines and iodothyronines
5. Scavenger deiodination of iodotyrosines within the thyroid follicular cells for reutilization of the liberated iodine

2. Iodide Transport

The transfer of iodide from the blood across the basal lateral membrane of the thyroid follicular cell is believed to proceed by an active transport process. Under normal conditions the relative amounts of the halide in the thyroid as compared with the serum or plasma (T:S or T:P ratio) are in the range of 20–30:1, but can be as high as 300:1 under circumstances of dietary iodine deprivation. The iodine is accumulated by the cell against both an electrical and a chemical gradient. The iodide transport is inhibited by ouabain, suggesting the involvement of an Na^+, K^+-ATPase. The K_m for iodide transport into the follicular cell is $\sim 3 \times 10^{-5} M$; the maximum concentration of iodide attainable by the rat thyroid is 1 mM. Certain anions such as ClO_4^-, SCN^-, and pertechnetate are able to effectively compete with I^+ for access to the transport process on the follicular cell. A similar transport system for iodide exists in the mammary gland, salivary glands, and parietal cells of the gastric mucosa, the placenta, and the ciliary body.

Thyrotropin or TSH is the most important physiologic factor affecting iodide uptake; however, cAMP also has been shown to stimulate follicular cell iodide uptake. The exact molecular details of the effect of cAMP on increasing the iodide accumulation by the follicles are not yet known. Once the iodide has entered the follicle cell, it is believed that a significant proportion moves across the cell and is stored in the lumen with the colloid. As yet no specific iodide binding protein has been identified in the colloid compartment.

The iodide transport system of the follicle is controlled in an autoregulatory fashion by the gland. Under conditions of chronic dietary excess of iodine the activity of the iodide transport system is downregulated. A small number of patients with familial goiter have been studied in which the disease is attributable to a defective thyroid gland iodide transport system.

3. Mechanism(s) of Iodination

After entry of iodide into the follicular cell, it must be first oxidized to

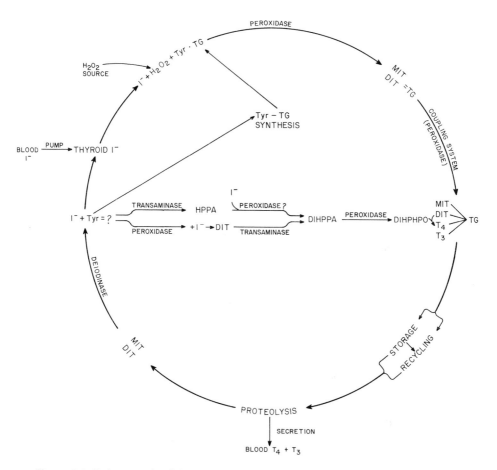

Figure 6-4. Pathways of iodide metabolism by the thyroid gland. Thyroidal iodide is oxidized by H_2O_2 in the presence of peroxidase to a higher valence state and bound enzymatically to tyrosyl residues of thyroglobulin. The coupling of iodotyrosines might be intramolecular or intermolecular. In the first case, peroxidase probably catalyzes the coupling reaction in the molecule of thyroglobulin. In the second instance, a series of steps producing free intermediates such as *p*-hydroxyphenylpyruvic acid (HPPA) and diiodo-*p*-hydroxyphenylpyruvic acid (DIHPPA) could lead to the formation of DIHPHPO (a hydroperoxide derivative of DIHPPA) that reacts with a DIT molecule of thyroglobulin to synthesize T_4 in an intermolecular coupling process. Modified from L. J. DeGroot and H. Niepomniszcze, *Metab., Clin. Exp.* **26,** 666 (1977).

a higher oxidation state before organification. The redox potential for the couple is

$$2I^- \rightarrow I_2 + 2e^- \qquad E^0 = +0.535 \text{ V}$$

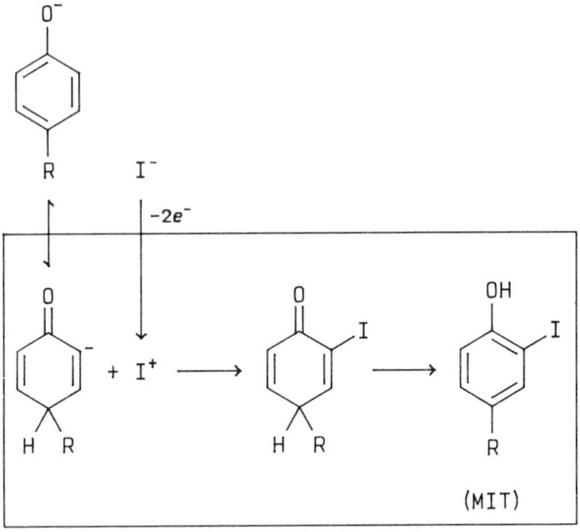

Figure 6-5. Iodination of tyrosine according to mechanism I. Iodide is oxidized by thyroid peroxidase in a two-electron oxidation step, forming I^+. The phenolate anion of tyrosine is in equilibrium with its quinoid form. Iodinium and tyrosine quinoid react to form an iodinated quinoid intermediate that forms MIT by electronic rearrangement. Modified from L. J. DeGroot and H. Niepomniszcze, *Metab., Clin. Exp.* **26,** 666 (1977).

This is relatively high in relation to the E^0 for most biological oxidants. Only O_2 and H_2O_2 are sufficiently good electron acceptors at pH 7 to be able to receive the electrons derived from the oxidation of iodide to iodine. Much evidence has been accumulated indicating that a thyroid follicular cell peroxidase is intimately involved with the oxidation of iodide to iodine. The peroxidase enzyme is a membrane-bound, heme-containing protein. It is likely that the peroxidase enzyme is oligomeric; molecular weight estimates range from 17,000 to 100,000 Da, depending upon the isolation conditions. Cytochemical studies have indicated that the peroxidase is present on the RER, Golgi vesicles, lateral and apical vesicles, as well as on the apical cell surface. The general pathways of iodide metabolism by the thyroid gland are given in Fig. 6-4.

Although the enzyme thyroid peroxidase has been closely implicated in the incorporation of iodide into the tyrosyl residues present in thyroglobulin, the exact pathway is not known. At least three possibilities, each involving a different oxidized form of I^-, have been put forth. (1) Enzyme-bound iodinium (E-I^+) as the iodinating species. This system involves the oxidation of iodide to iodinium by means of a two-electron loss catalyzed by the peroxidase and subsequent binding of I^+ to a tyrosine residue (in the quinoid form of the phenolate anion—see Fig. 6-5) present on thyroglobulin. In this mechanism the enzyme acts succes-

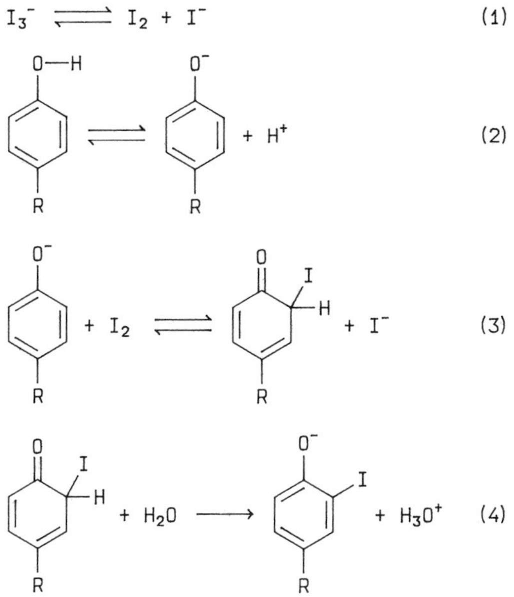

$$I_3^- \rightleftharpoons I_2 + I^- \tag{1}$$

(2)

(3)

(4)

Figure 6-6. Chemical iodination of tyrosine with I_2. In a solution containing iodide, iodine, and tyrosine, iodotyrosines are formed by a reaction between the phenolate anion and I_2 [Eqs. (3) and (4)]. I_2 is in equilibrium with iodide and I_3^- [Eq. (1)]. The phenolate anion is in equilibrium with undissociated tyrosine, according to Eq. (2). Modified from L. J. DeGroot and H. Niepomniszcze, *Metab., Clin. Exp.* **26,** 666 (1977).

sively as a peroxidase and then iodinase. This mechanism can readily explain the antithyroid activity of drugs such as thiouracil and thiourea (see below). (2) Formation of molecular iodine as the iodinating species. In this mechanism (see Fig. 6-6) the peroxidase generates iodine, which then effects chemical iodination of tyrosine residues on thyroglobulin. Some doubt has been expressed concerning this mechanism because the apparent K_m for iodide conversion to iodine is much higher than the K_m for iodide in the enzyme-mediated iodination of tyrosyl residues. However, this proposed mechanism cannot be totally excluded on the basis of the available data. (3) Enzyme-bound radical $E-I^0$ as the iodinating species. In this mechanism (see Fig. 6-7) the peroxidase enzyme is postulated to have two active sites; one site preferentially oxidizes I^- to the radical I^0, while the second site preferentially oxidizes tyrosyl to the tyrosyl radical. Iodotyrosine is then formed while both the iodine and tyrosyl free radicals are on the surface of the enzyme according to the reactions shown in Fig. 6-7.

In all three mechanisms the acceptor for the iodine is a tyrosine moiety which has already been incorporated into thyroglobulin. Experiments

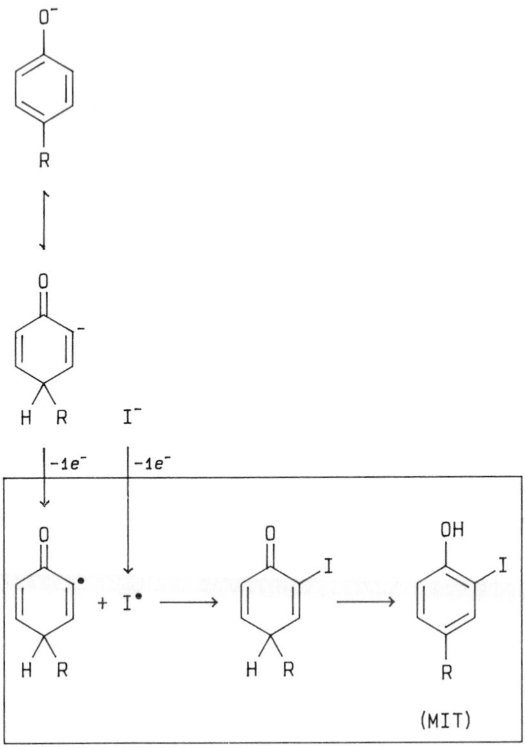

O⁻

R

O

H   R   I⁻

|-1e⁻ |-1e⁻

O   O   OH

+ I• ⟶   I   ⟶   I

H   R   H   R   R

(MIT)

Figure 6-7. Iodination of tyrosine according to mechanism II. Iodine is oxidized by thyroid peroxidase in a one-electron oxidation step forming a free radical (I^0). The quinoid anion of tyrosine is oxidized to a free radical by peroxidase or by another I^0. The quinoid free radical reacts with I^0 to form the iodinated quinoid intermediate that forms MIT by electronic rearrangement. Modified from L. J. DeGroot and H. Niepomniszcze, *Metab., Clin. Exp.* **26,** 666–681 (1977).

involving the protein synthesis inhibitors, puromycin or cycloheximide, have shown that tyrosine is not first iodinated and then incorporated into thyroglobulin. Also it should be noted that there is no genetic codon for monoiodotyrosine, thus the iodination can occur only after assembly of the polypeptide chain of thyroglobulin by a posttranslational mechanism.

The precise metabolic pathway employed in the thyroid follicular cell to generate the H_2O_2 is not known. Several factors are known to be capable of inhibiting the first iodination reaction which leads to the formation of monoiodotyrosine residues. Chronic TSH administration, as noted previously, stimulates the uptake of thyroid iodide. Although acute application of TSH will result in an increased availability of H_2O_2

without concomitant increased iodide transport, the acute effects are believed to occur without new protein synthesis, while the chronic effects require additional protein synthesis.

One of the major physiological controls on monoiodotyrosine formation is the dietary iodide supply. In the absence of ample dietary iodine, the iodotyrosine/iodothyronine and MIT/DIT ratios increase due to poor iodination of thyroglobulin.

It has also been observed that iodination of thyroglobulin is inhibited by excess iodide; this is known as the Wolff–Chaikoff effect. This inhibitory effect in intact animals is only transient, probably because the iodide transport system in the follicular cells undergoes some type of adaptation that results in a reduction in intracellular iodide levels. The adaptation to the circumstances of excess iodide appears to be due to a decrease in the unidirectional influx of iodide caused by an increase in the K_m for the pump.

B. Mechanisms of Iodothyronine Formation

Autoradiographic evidence indicates that iodination of the tyrosyl residues occurs very near the apical membrane of the thyroid follicular cell and the colloid interface. Although there is no clear evidence for the presence of the peroxidase in the colloid per se, it seems likely that iodination does occur near the cell–colloid interface, perhaps in the structure of cell pseudopods extending into the colloid (see Fig. 6-8). Because the origin of the peroxidase in the apical membrane appears due to the apparent fusion of apical vesicles containing peroxidase-positive granules, it is conceivable that exocytic thyroglobulin-containing granules fuse with the plasma membrane containing peroxidase, and then during the exocytotic process, which results in the passage of the peroxidase and thyroglobulin to the follicular lumen, the iodination takes place.

When thyroglobulin is iodinated by either enzymatic or chemical reactions, there is a progressive formation of MIT, DIT, T_3, and T_4. As the iodine content increases, the ratios DIT/MIT, T_4/T_3, and $(T_4 + T_3)/(DIT + MIT)$ all increase. Although thyroglobulin is obviously a successful substrate for the iodination process, it is not unique; bovine serum albumin, casein, fibrinogen, and lysozyme all have been employed as artificial substrates.

After the iodotyrosine is generated *in situ* on the thyroglobulin, a "secondary" coupling occurs which leads to the formation in the thyroglobulin molecule of both covalently bound thyroxine (T_4) and triiodothyronine (T_3). Associated with this coupling of one free iodinated tyrosine to a conjugated MIT or DIT is the obligatory release of the "lost

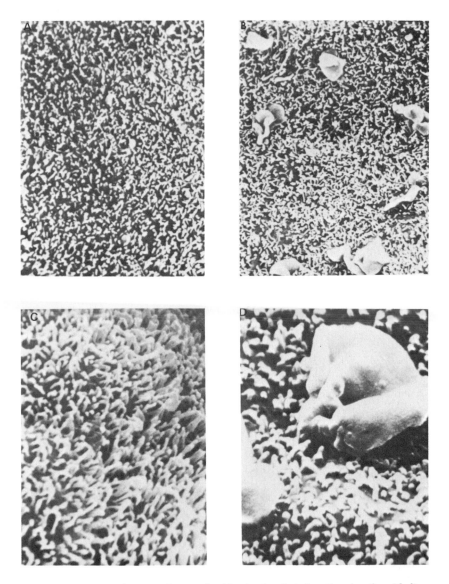

Figure 6-8. Scanning electron micrograph of *in vitro* incubated resting dog thyroid slices. (A) Apical surface of follicular cells. Digital microvilli are covering the cell surfaces (×7000). (B) Similar picture at higher magnification (×20,000). (C) Follicular cells after TSH stimulation. Pseudopods are emerging (×7000). (D) Similar picture at higher magnification (×20,000). (Courtesy of Dr. P. Ketelbant-Balasse.) Reproduced by permission of J. E. Dumont and G. Vassart, Thyroid gland metabolism and the action of TSH in endocrinology. *In* "Endocrinology" (L. J. DeGroot, G. F. Cahill, L. Martini, D. H. Nelson, W. D. Odell, J. T. Potts, E. Steinberger, and A. I. Winegrad, eds.), Vol. 1, p. 319. Grune & Stratton, New York, 1979.

side chain" either as dehydroalanine or pyruvate which is necessarily eliminated in the course of the reaction. Two general mechanisms have been proposed for the formation of these iodothyronines: They can occur either by (1) intramolecular coupling or (2) intermolecular coupling.

1. Intramolecular Coupling

Much evidence supports the concept that an intramolecular rearrangement is one pathway for formation of T_4 from DIT. A model for this mechanism is presented in Fig. 6-9A. This reaction can be catalyzed by peroxidase and iodide wherein an oxidation occurs leading to the formation of an iodotyrosyl free radical or positively charged ion which can be transferred within the thyroglobulin to an adjacent iodotyrosyl

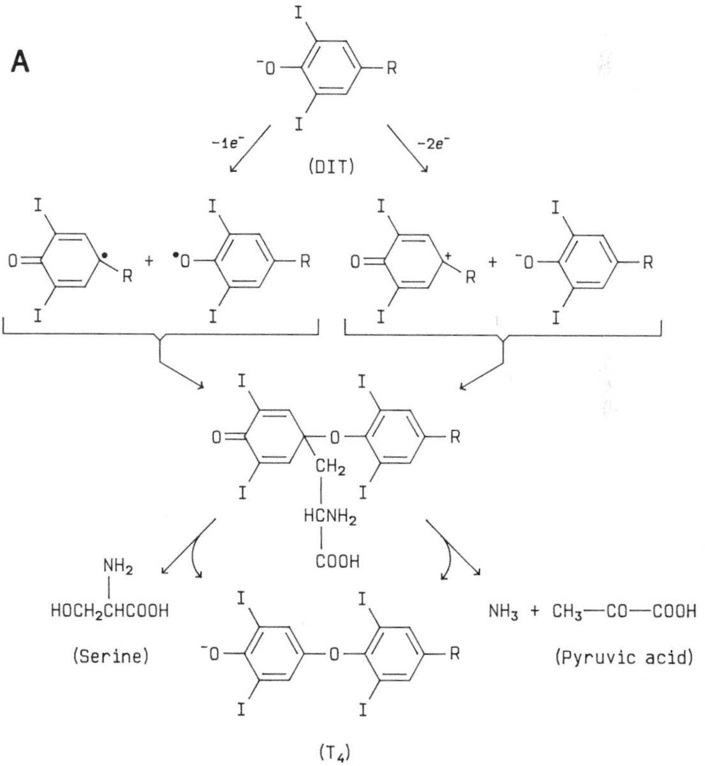

Figure 6-9. (A) Proposed intramolecular coupling mechanisms for formation of T_4 from DIT. (B) Hypothetical coupling scheme for intramolecular formation of T_4 in goiter thyroglobulin or other proteins iodinated with the TPO system. (A) is modified from L. J. DeGroot and H. Niepomniszcze, *Metab., Clin. Exp.* **26,** 694 (1977). (B) is modified from A. Taurog, Hormone synthesis. *In* "Endocrinology" (L. J. DeGroot, G. F. Cahill, L. Martini, D. H. Nelson, W. D. Odell, J. T. Potts, E. Steinberger, and A. I. Winegrad, eds.), Vol. 1, pp. 331–346. Grune & Stratton, New York, 1979.

238

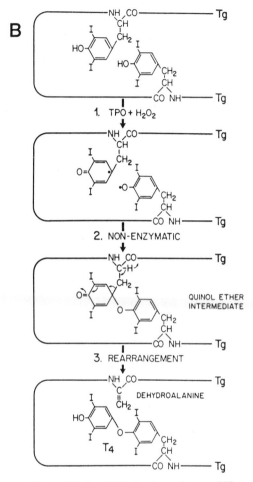

B

1. TPO + H₂O₂

2. NON-ENZYMATIC

QUINOL ETHER
INTERMEDIATE

3. REARRANGEMENT

DEHYDROALANINE

T₄

Figure 6-9. (cont'd.). See legend on p. 237.

See legend on p. 237.

group to form the iodothyronine. There are two basic concepts associated with this mechanism: (1) Free DIT radicals are generated inside the protein matrix through the action of the thyroid peroxidase; (2) then two DIT or one DIT and one MIT radicals couple to form a quinol ether intermediate, also within the thyroglobulin matrix. Next, the splitting of the quinol ether (in the instance of two DIT) could occur to yield either a serine or a dehydroalanine remaining in the position of the transferred DIT. The two DIT (yielding T_4) or DIT and MIT (yielding T_3) residues need not be on the same peptide chain of thyroglobulin. This mechanism does not involve the formation or breaking of peptide bonds. It is conceivable that this intramolecular rearrangement process might be facilitated by "maturation" of the thyroglobulin molecule through generation of a stabilized tertiary and quaternary structure or through the formation of new hydrogen, ionic, or disulfide bonds.

2. Intermolecular Coupling

This alternative mechanism postulates the intermolecular coupling of the pyruvic acid analog of DIT, namely, 3,5-diiodo-4-hydroxyphenylpyruvic acid (DIHPPA), to yield T_4 (see Fig. 6-3). Very low concentrations of free DIHPPA have been detected in the thyroid gland of rats following administration of radioactive iodide. The DIHPPA can be formed from free DIT in a reaction mediated by tyrosine aminotransferase. Next, a tautomerase present in the thyroid would convert the DIHPPA to its enol form which could then in turn be oxidized by H_2O_2 and the thyroid peroxidase to the hydroperoxide form, known to couple spontaneously with thyroglobulin-bound DIT to give T_4. At the present time the extent of this pathway in the thyroid is unknown.

C. Thyroglobulin

Thyroglobulin is a very large glycoprotein of molecular weight 660,000. It has a sedimentation coefficient, $s_{20,w}$, of 19 S. In some instances 12 S half molecules and 27 S dimers can be observed. Poorly iodinated 19 S thyroglobulin can readily dissociate into the 12 S subunits when exposed to denaturing conditions. Recent studies indicate that thyroglobulin is a dimer composed of two subunits of about 300,000 Da. As isolated from the mammalian thyroid, it represents at least 75% of the proteins present in the gland. The carbohydrate moieties of thyroglobulin are 10% by weight of the molecule; the principal sites of attachment are to aspargine, serine, and threonine.

The biosynthesis of thyroglobulin peptide chains takes place on very large membrane-bound polyribosomes. The messenger RNA for thyroglobulin sediments as a 33 S component. The 33 S mRNA is translated into a 300,000 Da peptide corresponding to the 12 S molecules which can dimerize spontaneously into the 19 S thyroglobulin. After the polypeptide chain has been discharged into the lumen of the RER, the polypeptide chain becomes glycosylated as it moves first to the Golgi and then to the exocytotic vesicles. Kinetic studies have indicated that the sugars mannose and galactose are inserted before the more distal sialic acids. The exocytosis of thyroglobulin is believed to precede its iodination (see previous section).

Purified thyroglobulin has been shown to have an iodine content proportionate to the dietary intake of iodide of the animal from which the protein was isolated. Normal human thyroglobulin has an iodine content varying from 0.1 to 1.1% by weight. Normal thyroglobulin, which contains 110 tyrosine residues, has the following iodoamino acid distribution (residues/molecule): MIT, 6.5; DIT, 4.8; T_4, 2.3; T_3, 0.29. These values correspond to 36% of the iodine being present as $T_4 + T_3$ and 58% present as iodotyrosines.

There are some clinical reports suggesting the existence of a familial goiter that has a "coupling defect." The implication is that there is a deficiency in this disease state of a specific enzyme involved in coupling; as yet there are no specific data to support this interesting possibility.

D. Secretion Mechanisms of Thyroid Hormones

1. Energy Metabolism of the Thyroid

The multistep process of iodide uptake and metabolism by the thyroid, the iodination reactions, and the biosynthesis, secretion, and proteolysis of thyroglobulin to yield the thyroid hormones T_4 and T_3, in response to the stimulatory actions of TSH, are complex and depend upon an integrated control process of cellular metabolism. Under normal circumstances there is a balance between oxidative phosphorylation (80%) and cytosol anaerobic metabolism (20%). TSH stimulates all facets of thyroid metabolism and can stimulate thyroid respiration by 10–50%. Extensive metabolic energy is required in the form of ATP to facilitate the iodide transport steps as well as the biosynthesis of thyroglobulin. Also, in view of the indispensible role of thyroid peroxidase in the oxidation of iodide as a prerequisite for the iodination reactions, it is essential that the thyroid cell have an efficient mechanism(s) to generate ample quantities of NADPH (see Fig. 6-10).

TSH is known to enhance glucose uptake into the dog thyroid and stimulate its cellular metabolism. The fraction of glucose converted to lactate is not changed, but the activity of the pentose phosphate pathway is markedly increased and the incorporation of the carbons of glucose into glycogen, proteins, and fatty acids decreases. Indeed, TSH activates hydrolysis and secretion of thyroglobulin and, possibly through the actions of its cellular mediator cAMP, may activate lipolysis and glycogenolysis. The activity of the pentose phosphate pathway is mainly dependent upon the rate of NADPH oxidation. TSH is known to stimulate not only an increase in the total cellular concentration of $NADP^+$ and NADPH, but to accelerate utilization of NADPH. Because it is not known with certainty whether the thyroid follicular peroxidase electron trans-

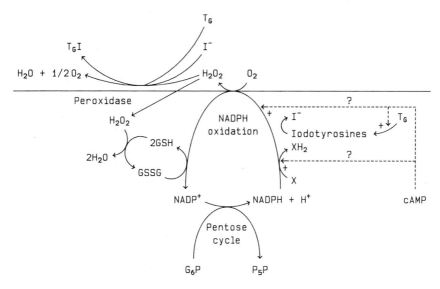

Figure 6-10. Postulated NADP oxidation–reduction cycle in thyroid. Four mechanisms of NADPH oxidation are outlined: the reduction of any intermediate X by an NADPH-linked dehydrogenase, the deiodination of iodotyrosines released by thyroglobulinolysis, the generation of H_2O_2, and the reduction of H_2O_2 through GSH peroxidase. T_G and T_GI: Uniodinated and iodinated thyroglobulin. - - -+, Activation. Modified from J. E. Dumont and G. Vassart, Thyroid gland metabolism and the actions of TSH in endocrinology. *In* "Endocrinology" (L. J. DeGroot, G. F. Cahill, L. Martini, D. H. Nelson, W. D. Odell, J. T. Potts, E. Steinberger, and A. I. Winegrad, eds.), Vol. 1, pp. 311–329. Grune & Stratton, New York, 1979.

port chain utilizes NADPH or NADH (there is a wide species variability), it seems reasonable to postulate the presence of transhydrogenases which can facilitate the ready availability of the correct reduced pyridine nucleotide.

2. Actions of TSH on Thyroid Hormone Release

a. Background. The chief intrathyroidal storage form of thyroid hormone is thyroglobulin. Under normal circumstances this protein is subjected to proteolysis by the thyroid, resulting in the release of thyroxine and T_3, probably in the ratio they are present in the protein. Small amounts of thyroglobulin can be detected in the blood of normal subjects. Proteolysis of thyroglobulin also results in the cellular production of free iodotyrosines; there is good evidence that most iodotyrosines do not leave the thyroid gland, but instead are rapidly deiodinated by a "scavenger" system (see below) that is specific for iodotyrosine but has no activity for the iodothyronines (e.g., T_3 and T_4).

The main control over T_4 and T_3 secretion is mediated in a complex manner by TSH. Basically TSH administration induces endocytosis of thyroglobulin from the colloid with concomitant thyroglobulin digestion and subsequent hormone release.

As detailed in Table 6-2, two major classes of TSH actions in the thyroid can be distinguished: (1) those that are rapid (occurring in seconds to minutes), such as activation of secretion, I^- binding to proteins, iodothyronine formation, and stimulation of cellular metabolism, including respiration and pentose phosphate metabolism; and (2) those that are delayed (hours to days), which include increased RNA and protein synthesis, and increased volume of the follicular cells. In general, the rapid effects of TSH action are not blocked by RNA or protein synthesis inhibitors, whereas the delayed responses (see Table 6-2) are inhibited by these agents. In terms of $T_4 + T_3$ homeostasis over a period of several days to weeks, it is apparent that there is a constant interplay and readjustment between the short-term and long-term actions of TSH.

A flow diagram for the regulation of thyroid follicular cell metabolism by TSH and iodide is given in Fig. 6-11. There are three interrelated regulator circuits: (1) the cAMP system; (2) the Ca^{2+}-cGMP system; and (3) the iodide feedback loop.

b. *The cAMP System.* It has been firmly established that most of the actions of TSH in the thyroid are secondary to the activation of the thyroid follicular cell adenylate cyclase. In some species there is also an activation of the adenylate cyclase by the β-adrenergic agents, catecholamines, or prostaglandins.

cAMP acts in cell metabolism through activation of cAMP-dependent protein kinases; phosphorylation of cellular proteins then may result in activation or inactivation which may produce specific hormonal effects. A prominent morphological change in the thyroid follicular cells after administration of TSH is the appearance of pseudopods on the apical membrane (see Fig. 6-8). These pseudopods are believed to be actively involved in the reabsorption of thyroglobulin from the colloid.

TSH is a protein with two peptide chains, designated alpha (α) and beta (β) (see Chapter 5). The α chain is believed to be the subunit activating the adenyl cyclase. The thyroid specificity of TSH is conferred on the molecule by the β subunit. The detailed sequence of molecular events and modulation of adenylate dose activity after activation by TSH is summarized in Fig. 6-11. Certainly the short-term actions of TSH are mediated through cAMP actions; what is not clear is whether the long-term actions of TSH on protein synthesis and cell growth (hypertrophy) are also exclusively the result of cAMP-mediated events.

Table 6–2. Multiple Effects of TSH on the Thyroid[a]

Time of appearance of response	Inhibition by[b] Actinomycin D	Puromycin	Site of action	Biochemical consequences	Biological consequence	Dependent effects of TSH
Seconds	0	0	Membranes	Permeability change	Stimulation	Uptake of glucose and amino acids
Minutes (few)	0	0	Membrane, cytoplasm	Formation of allosteric effectors (e.g., 3',5'-AMP)	Stimulation	Phagocytosis, energy metabolism
Minutes (many)	0	+	Cytoplasm	Translation (protein synthesis)	Stimulation	
Hours	+	+	Nucleus	Transcription (RNA synthesis)	Stimulation	Iodide uptake, weight, ribosomes, mitosis
Days	+	+	Nucleus	Transcription (RNA synthesis)	Differentiation	Appearance of Ig synthesis, I- uptake, I' oxidation, follicular structure

[a] Modified from J. E. Dumont and G. Vassart, Thyroid gland metabolism and the actions of TSH in endocrinology. *In* "Endocrinology" (L. J. DeGroot, G. F. Cahill, L. Martini, D. H. Nelson, W. D. Odell, J. T. Potts, E. Steinberger, and A. I. Winegrad, eds.), Vol. 1, pp. 311–329. Grune & Stratton, New York, 1979.

[b] Actinomycin D should inhibit DNA-directed RNA synthesis, while puromycin should block *de novo* protein synthesis.

244

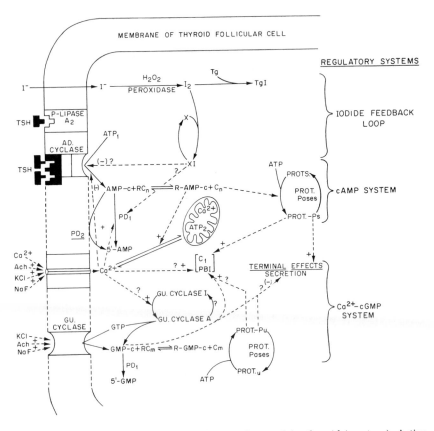

Figure 6-11. Postulated intracellular regulation scheme of the thyroid (- - -⁺ →), Activation; (- - - ⁻ →), inhibition. Tg and TgI, Uniodinated and iodinated thyroglobulin; P. lipase, phospholipase; Ad. cyclase, adenylate cyclase; X, postulated intermediate of iodide negative feedback; ATP_1, ATP_2, pools of ATP; PD_1, PD_2, cyclic nucleotide phosphodiesterases; RC_n, RC_m, cAMP(n)- and cGMP(m)-dependent protein kinase(s)—n or m indicates that the number of catalytic (C) and regulatory (R) subunits of the kinase need not be 1; Prot, protein substrates of the kinases; Prot Ps, Prot Pu, phosphorylated proteins of cAMP(s) and cGMP(u) protein kinases; AMPc, adenosine 3′,5′-cyclic monphosphate; GMPc, guanosine 3′,5′-cyclic monophosphate; Ach, acetylcholine; Gu. cyclase A,I, guanylate cyclase—A indicates active, I inactive. Modified from J. E. Dumont and G. Vassart, Thyroid gland metabolism and the actions of TSH in endocrinology. *In* "Endocrinology" (L. J. DeGroot, G. F. Cahill, L. Martini, D. H. Nelson, W. D. Odell, J. T. Potts, E. Steinberger, and A. I. Winegrad, eds.), Vol. 1, pp. 311–329. Grune & Stratton, New York, 1979.

c. The Ca^{2+}-Cyclic GMP System. The important role of Ca^{2+} as a signal in excitation secretion coupling and excitation–contraction coupling suggests the logical involvement of this divalent cation in regulation of thyroid follicular cell metabolism and $T_4 + T_3$ secretion. It has been proposed that changes in cellular Ca^{2+} concentration in conjunction with cholinergic (serotonin) activation of guanyl cyclase may have important regulatory actions in modulating the activity of the adenyl cyclase.

Extracellular Ca^{2+} is not necessary for the primary effect of TSH on the thyroid or the initial increase in cAMP levels and the subsequent immediate secretion of $T_4 + T_3$. However, calcium is essential for the activation of iodide binding to proteins and stimulation of glucose oxidation. The precise short-term effects of TSH on cellular Ca^{2+} concentrations remain to be elucidated.

All the agents increasing cGMP levels in the thyroid follicular cells also activate iodination of proteins, the pentose phosphate pathway, and probably inhibit cAMP accumulation and $T_4 + T_3$ accumulation. There is good evidence that these events are secondary to changes in cellular Ca^{2+} concentrations.

d. The Iodide Feedback Loop. Because the production of thyroid hormones is totally dependent upon the dietary availability of iodine, it is not surprising that regulatory mechanisms exist to shift the pattern of production of $T_3 + T_4$ under conditions of excess iodine intake. As mentioned earlier, high dietary levels of iodine via the Wolff–Chaikoff effect inhibit the iodination reactions of thryoglobulin and decrease the secretion of $T_3 + T_4$. Conversely iodine deficiency induces thyroid growth in hypophysectomized animals. As illustrated in Fig. 6-11, the cAMP system is negatively controlled by the iodide supply of the gland. This control is exerted by a postulated oxidized substance, termed XI. The site of action of factor XI (adenylate cyclase, cAMP efflux, phosphodiesterase, etc.) is not known.

e. Long-Acting Thyroid Stimulator. The blood of many hyperthyroid subjects contains a substance known as "long-acting thyroid stimulator" or LATS. A more recent terminology for LATS reclassifies them into mouse thyroid-stimulating autoantibodies (MTS) or human thyroid-stimulating autoantibodies (HTS). Physiologically, LATS is capable of mimicking over a somewhat slower time interval all the actions of TSH (10–12 hr instead of 2 hr for TSH) and the stimulation of thyroid follicular cell adenylate cyclase and consequent cascade of metabolic events, which lead to an increased secretion of $T_4 + T_3$.

Biochemically, LATS has been identified as a 7 S globulin of the IgG class of immunoglobulins; thus, it is an antibody. The formation of this antibody is believed to result from the inappropriate release of an antigen from the thyroid follicular cells and subsequent production of autoantibodies by the thymus-dependent lymphocytes. The molecular basis of the biological action(s) of LATS is that the antibody is postulated to be complementary to the TSH receptor protein in the basal membrane of the thyroid follicular cell.

An important difference between LATS and TSH is that the production of LATS is not suppressed by high blood levels of the thyroid hormones. Thus, LATS production is believed to be the pathophysiological mechanism leading to the generation of Graves' disease or hyperthyrodism.

f. Iodine Reutilization by the Thyroid. Normally the ratio of iodotyrosines to iodothyronines in the thyroid gland is approximately 4:1. Approximately 25% of the iodide derived from tyrosine is lost to the blood; thus, the secretion of iodothyronines and the loss of inorganic iodide by the thyroid gland are comparable. It is significant that the amount of iodide recaptured per day by the thyroid gland is two to three times the amount of "new" iodide captured by the gland from the blood.

The monoiodotyrosines released from the thyroglobulin that do not leave the gland are rapidly deiodinated inside the gland by an NADPH-dependent microsomal flavoprotein deiodinase. This enzyme has little affinity for iodothyronine compounds.

3. Feedback Actions of T_4/T_3 at the Pituitary/Hypothalamus

The physiological regulation of secretion of the thyroid hormone is a complex system that involves, in addition to the thyroid gland, participation by the hypothalamus, pituitary, and neural activity. In addition to the thyroid–pituitary–hypothalamus feedback control loop, a neural control of thyroid metabolism has been proposed. Recent work suggests that parasympathetic and sympathetic innervation may be capable of modulating thyroid metabolism and its response to TSH, as is the case for other endocrine glands. Certain distinct actions of acetylcholine, norepinephrine, and probably prostaglandins of the E series are capable of mimicking several of the cyclic AMP-dependent TSH effects.

The activity of the thyroid–pituitary loop is a balance between the peripheral consumption/catabolism of T_4/T_3 and the combined hypothalamic and feedback actions of $T_4 + T_3$ on the pituitary secretion of TSH.

Each day the body catabolizes ~100 μg of T_4 and 30 μg of T_3. These lost hormones are replenished by secretion of new $T_4 + T_3$ by the thyroid; as the blood levels of $T_4 + T_3$ fall, this is sensed by the hypothalamus with a resultant increase in secretion of TSH from the pituitary. The thyroid hormones, $T_4 + T_3$, appear not to have a negative feedback influence on the hypothalamus. The role of the hypothalamus is to stimulate the pituitary to biosynthesize and secrete TSH through the action of thyrotropin releasing hormone (TRH) (see Chapter 5).

The set point for the control of the system probably lies in the pituitary TSH secreting cells. The balance between the positive TRH signal and the negative feedback of thyroxine ultimately determines the actual amount of TSH secreted. In the pituicyte, thyroxine stimulates the synthesis of nucleic acids and proteins, which affect the secretion of TSH. Thus, it is a metabolic effect of T_4 rather than the actual blood level which determines the production of TSH by the pituicyte. In contrast, TRH, which travels to the pituitary via hypophyseal portal vessels, interacts with the pituicyte membrane at specific receptor sites, leading to an activation of adenyl cyclase and increase in intracellular cAMP (see Chapter 5). This causes increased synthesis and secretion of TSH which in its initial phases is not dependent upon protein synthesis. Thus, the influences of TRH and thyroid hormones operate in a delicate balance; however, excess of one may counteract the actions of the other regulator.

E. Systemic Transport of Thyroid Hormone

1. Plasma Concentrations of Thyroid Hormones

Table 6-3 lists the blood concentrations and kinetics in man of the principal iodine-containing compounds. The main secretory product of the thyroid is T_4. Thyroxine is present in the blood at a concentration of 40–100 times that of T_3. The concentrations of DIT and TETRAC are comparable to that of T_3 (i.e., ~110–140 ng/ml). The blood level of reverse T_3 is ~30–50% that of T_3 and 1% of T_4.

2. Thyroid Hormone Binding Proteins

In most vertebrates, the bulk of the thyroid hormone circulates in the blood bound to proteins. The three blood proteins responsible for systemic transport of the thyroid hormones are thyroxine binding globulin (TBG), thyroxine binding prealbumin (TBPA), and albumin (ALB) (see Table 6-4). The normal distribution of T_4 among these proteins is 70–75% bound to TBG, 15–20% bound to TBPA, and 5–10% bound to ALB. In contrast, T_3 is bound 70–75% to TBG and 25–30% to ALB, and T_3 has little or no affinity for TBPA. Several instances have been reported of

Table 6–3. Kinetics of T_4, T_3, and rT_3 Metabolism in Normal Human Subjects[a]

| | Hormone | | |
Parameter	T_4	T_3	rT_3
Serum concentration			
Total (μg/100 ml)	8.0	0.12	0.04
Free (ng/100 ml)	2.1	0.28	0.20
Body pool (μg)	810	46	40
Volume of distribution (liter)	10	38	98
Metabolic clearance rate (liter/day)	1.1	22	90
Disposal rate (μg/day)	82	28	28

[a] Modified from C. S. Pittman, Hormone metabolism in endocrinology. *In* "Endocrinology" (L. J. DeGroot, G. F. Cahill, L. Martini, D. H. Nelson, W. D. Odell, J. T. Potts, E. Steinberger, and A. I. Winegrad, eds.), Vol. 1, pp. 365–372. Grune & Stratton, New York, 1979.

Table 6–4. Some Properties and Metabolic Parameters of the Principal Thyroid Hormone-Binding Proteins in Serum[a]

Parameter	TBG	TBPA	Albumin
Molecular weight	63,000	55,000	69,000
Structure	Monomer	Tetramer	Predominantly monomeric
Carbohydrate content (%)	30	1	—
Number of binding sites for T_4 and T_3	1	1	1
Association constant, K_a (M^{-1})			
For T_4	2×10^{10}	1.5×10^8	1.5×10^6
For T_3	2×10^9	—	1×10^7
Concentration in serum (mean normal, mg/100 ml)	1.6	25	3500
Occupancy, or saturation (%)			
For T_4	30	0.5	0.0015
For T_3	0.6	0.001	0.001
Half-life	5	2	15
Degradation rate (mg/day)	15	650	17,000

[a] Modified from S. Refetoff, Thyroid hormone transport in endocrinology. *In* "Endocrinology" (L. J. DeGroot, G. F. Cahill, L. Martini, D. H. Nelson, W. D. Odell, J. T. Potts, E. Steinberger, and A. I. Winegrad, eds.), Vol. 1, pp. 347–356. Grune & Stratton, New York, 1979.

PUTATIVE DNA BINDING SITE

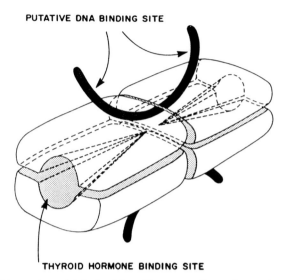

THYROID HORMONE BINDING SITE

Figure 6-12. Schematic model derived from X-ray crystallographic studies of prealbumin, illustrating the interaction of four identical subunits forming a channel through the interior of the molecule, thereby forming two identical thyroid hormone binding sites. The channel narrows at the center of the molecule. Although the binding sites are identical, T_4 binds cooperatively; occupation of T_4 at one site presumably alters the conformation of the second site, which results in a lower affinity for the second T_4 binding interaction. Depicted on the upper and lower side of the molecules is a symmetric β-pleated sheet structure that is relatively rich in amino acids with ionic side chains and that also contains tryptophan molecules. Based on computer graphic modeling studies, this site has been proposed to be a DNA binding site. Reproduced with permission from N. L. Eberhardt, J. W. Apriletti, and J. D. Baxter, The molecular biology of thyroid hormone action. *In* "Biochemical Actions of Hormones" (G. Litwack, ed.), Vol. 7, pp. 311–375. Academic Press, New York, 1980. © 1980 Macmillan Journals Limited.

inherited abnormalities in blood TBG levels. Absent or low TBG is more common than TBG excess; the incidence rate of abnormalities may approach 1 in 2000. No genetic abnormalities of TBPA have been found in man.

Gestation causes a marked increase in the thyroid physiological status of the mother. As estrogen secretion becomes elevated in the first weeks of pregnancy, there is a doubling of TBG concentration. This in turn stimulates T_4 secretion and shortly a new equilibrium is established wherein the blood levels of total T_4 are double that of the nonpregnant state. This occurs without any alteration of the "free" T_4 levels.

TBPA is composed of four identical polypeptide subunits, each containing 127 amino acids. It has a molecular weight of 55,000 and has two hormone binding sites. TBPA binds T_4 cooperatively with K_a values of 1.05×10^8/mol and 9.55×10^5/mol; TBPA binds T_3 only 1% as avidly as T_4. In plasma, TBPA binds 11% of the total T_4. Interestingly, TBPA also contains a separate specific binding site for the retinol binding protein. Retinol binding protein binds vitamin A precursors.

The crystallographic structure of TBPA is known. In fact, this is the only hormone binding protein for which such information is available (see Fig. 6-12). It has been proposed that TBPA may be structurally related to the thyroid hormone nuclear receptor because it was found to have a DNA binding site.

F. Thyroid Hormone Metabolism and Catabolism

1. Production of Thyroid Hormones

The blood concentration of the thyroid hormones for each substance is dependent upon not only the amount of hormone biosynthesized and eventually secreted, but also upon the hormone's affinity for carrier proteins, affinity for target tissues, its rate of catabolism, and finally its rate of clearance. It is apparent that the physiologically mediated changing relationships between the interconversions of $T_4 \to T_3$ and $T_4 \to rT_3$ provide insight into many aspects of disease states related to the thyroid hormones.

Figure 6-13 summarizes the daily production of T_4, T_3, and rT_3 in man. T_4 also is converted in the peripheral tissues to T_3 and rT_3 (see discussion, Section IV,G).

The conversion of T_4 to T_3 has clearly been shown to occur in many principal tissues of man, rats, and sheep. Because T_3 is 3 to 5 times more active than T_4 and because ~30% of the daily T_4 production is diverted to produce ~80% of the daily T_3 turnover, the key role of T_3 for meeting the energy requirements of man is obvious. The hormone T_4 is largely restricted to the vascular pool with a slow turnover, while T_3 has a small vascular pool, a high turnover rate, and is found in higher concentrations in the target tissues. From these considerations the view has emerged that T_4 may have little intrinsic biological activity.

In normal man ~40% of the T_4 is deiodinated by a pathway which yields reverse T_3 (rT_3). The biological role of rT_3 is not known. It has been suggested that a physiological concentration of rT_3 may regulate the conversion of $T_4 \to T_3$. The plasma concentration of rT_3 is known to vary from that of T_3 in a number of clinical conditions, including patients suffering from hepatic and renal disease, malnutrition, or after treatment with dexamethasone.

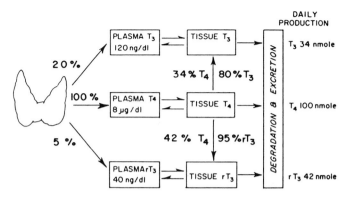

Figure 6-13. The daily production of T_3, T_4, and rT_3 in normal human subjects. Modified from C. S. Pittman, Hormone metabolism. *In* "Endocrinology" (L. J. DeGroot, G. F. Cahill, L. Martini, D. H. Nelson, W. D. Odell, J. T. Potts, E. Steinberger, and A. I. Winegrad, eds.), Vol. 1, p. 365. Grune & Stratton, New York, 1979.

2. Metabolic Transformations of Thyroid Hormones

Figure 6-14 depicts the metabolic pathways for the further metabolism of thyroxine. Only very small amounts of unaltered T_4 are excreted in the urine or feces. The liver and kidney are the major sites of metabo-

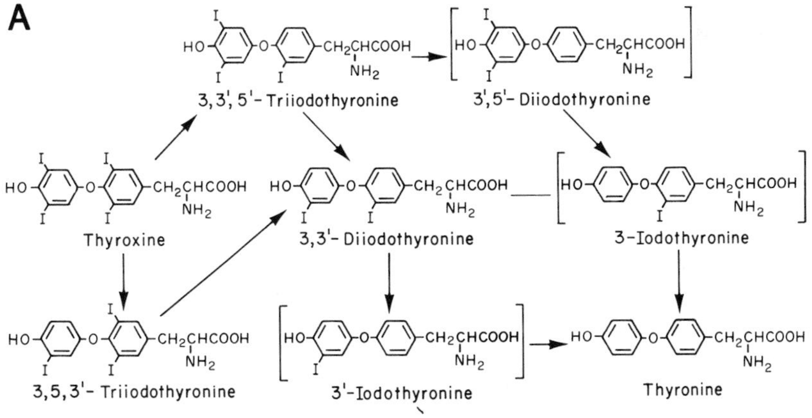

A

3,3',5'-Triiodothyronine

3',5'-Diiodothyronine

Thyroxine

3,3'-Diiodothyronine

3-Iodothyronine

3,5,3'-Triiodothyronine

3'-Iodothyronine

Thyronine

Figure 6-14. (A) Deiodination of thyroxine and its further metabolism (in brackets). (B) Metabolism of the thyroxine side chain. The metabolites have not been identified by *in vivo* studies. Modified from Figs. 28-2 and 28-3 in C.S. Pittman, *In* "Endocrinology" (L. J. DeGroot, G. F. Cahill, L. Martini, D. H. Nelson, W. D. Odell, J. T. Potts, E. Steinberger, and A. I. Winegrad, eds.), Vol. 1, p. 367. Grune & Stratton, New York, 1979.

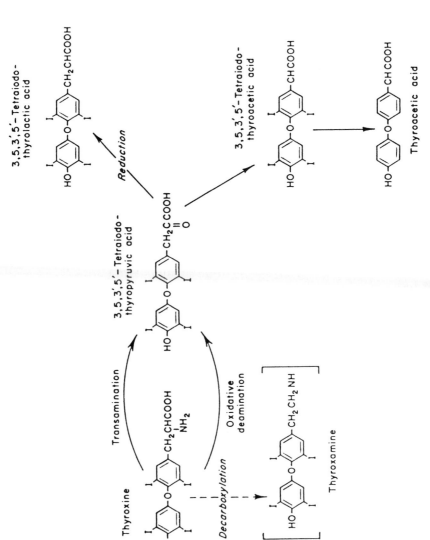

Figure 6-14 (cont'd). See legend on p. 251.

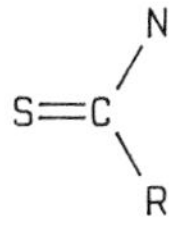

$$S=C \Big\langle {}^{N} _{R}$$

Figure 6-15. General structure of antithyroid compounds. The thionamide group R may be either an S, O, or N.

lism. In the liver stepwise deiodination is the prime pathway for inactivation (Fig. 6-14A). Other transformations that have been detected include β-glucuronide and sulfate conjugation with the phenol functionality, and transamination or deamination of the alanine side chain (Fig. 6-14B).

G. Antithyroid Drugs

Specific compounds that interfere with the thyroid follicular peroxidase are used both in research and certain clinical circumstances. In general, small doses of goitrogens preferentially block the coupling reactions in the thyroid, while large doses block the iodination of the tyrosyl residues in thyroglobulin. The most potent antithyroid compounds contain the thionamide group (see Fig. 6-15). The simplest member of the group is thiourea; the compounds thiouracil and 6-*n*-propylthiouracil are significantly more potent. The structures of several antithyroid drugs are given in Fig. 6-16.

V. BIOLOGICAL AND MOLECULAR ACTIONS

A. Interactions with Target Tissues— General Effects

In warm-blooded animals the principal biological effect mediated by thyroxine and T_3 is an increase in oxygen consumption and concomitant heat production. Associated with this is an increase in the metabolism of fats, proteins, and carbohydrates in the liver, kidney, heart, and muscle. Also, the cardiac output will be augmented and neural irritability increased. In poikilotherms adapted to low temperatures, T_3 has no calorigenic effects; this response will return if the animal is placed in an environment at 25–30°C. In amphibians, thyroid hormones are neces-

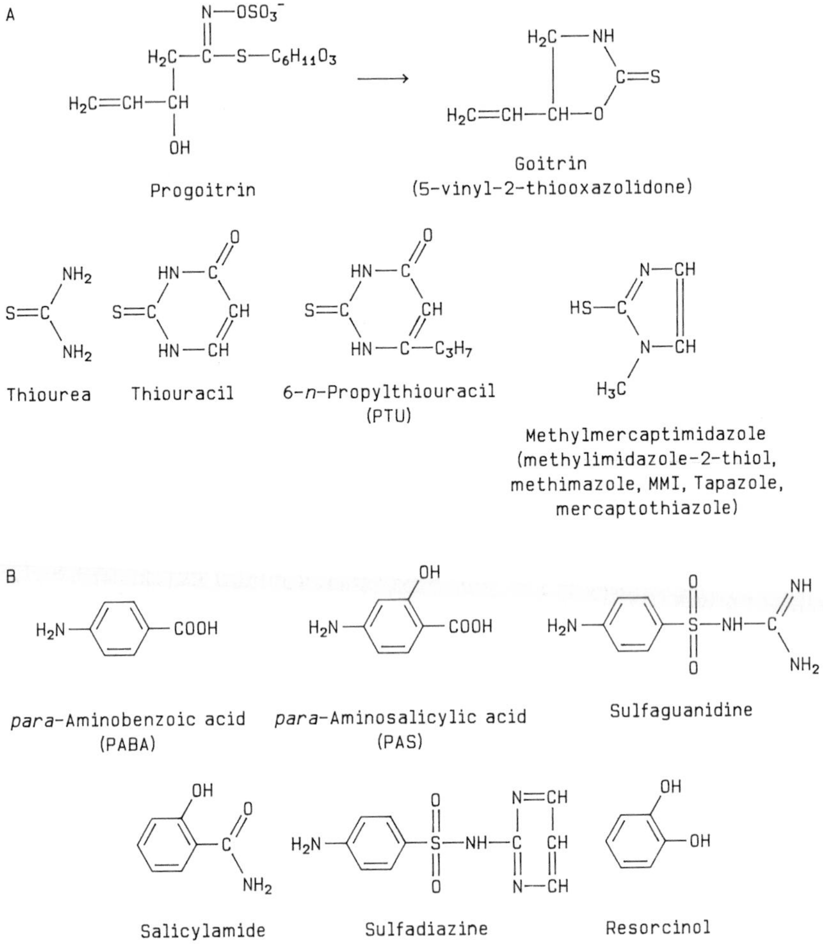

Figure 6-16. (A) Antithyroid compounds with the thionamide group. Progoitrin is present in a number of vegetables including cabbage, kale, and cauliflower. (B) Aromatic compounds with antithyroid activity.

sary for normal growth and cellular differentiation, and are directly responsible for the initiation of metamorphosis.

At the cellular level a myriad of effects of triiodothyronine can be detected from *in vitro* studies. These include stimulation of O_2 consumption, glycolysis, and succinate oxidation. Associated with these metabolic changes are increases in the activities of many enzymes including hexokinase, the respiratory enzymes NADPH—cytochrome-*c* reductase, and cytochrome oxidase. At the same time there is frequently an increase in RNA and protein synthesis. Thus, the biological consequences of the presence of thyroid hormones, particularly T_3, is that of a thermostat that synchronizes the metabolic activities in the responsive organs at "set points" or at a level of activity consistent with their feedback responses received under normal conditions. The precise biochemical mechanisms by which T_3 produces this wide spectrum of responses have involved three general models of action, described in the next section. No contemporary evidence as yet absolutely explains the general metabolic stimulation and growth response evoked by T_3.

B. Production of Biological Response

1. Actions in Oxidative Phosphorylation

An older theory of T_3 activation is related to observation of its dramatic effects on oxidative phosphorylation. The process of mitchondrial oxidation is normally quite tightly coupled to the production of adenosine triphosphate (ATP) (see Fig. 6-17). Compounds, such as 2,4-dinitrophenol or thyroxine given *in vivo* or *in vitro*, will "uncouple" the process of phosphorylation from the electron transfer oxidation steps, resulting in a lowering of the "P/O" ratio. Indeed, an increased oxygen consumption is characteristic of the thyrotoxic human or animal. Thus, an uncoupling of oxidative phosphorylation is a catabolic response.

The strongest arguments against the uncoupling hypothesis are that lowered P/O ratios have not been observed in preparations of muscle mitochondria obtained from thyrotoxic animals or humans. Such mitochondria are found to have an increased activity per milligram of protein with normal P/O ratios.

Alternative suggestions for mitochondrial actions of thyroid hormone include the possibility that T_3 causes effective uncoupling by stimulating extramitochondrial pathways which consume nutrients but generate fewer moles of ATP.

2. Stimulation of RNA and Protein Synthesis

Analogous to the general mechanism of action for steroid hormones (Chapters 10, 12, and 13) and 1,25-dihydroxyvitamin D_3 (Chapter 9), it has been proposed that triiodothyronine binds to specific receptor proteins in target tissues.

The generation of many biological responses by T_3 or T_4 is correlated with the presence of the hormone in the nucleus of the appropriate

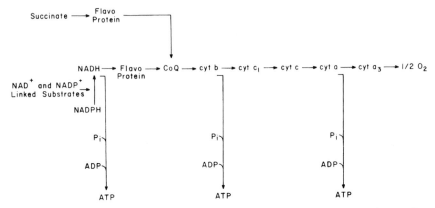

Figure 6-17. A scheme of mitochondrial oxidative phosphorylation showing the coupling of ATP synthesis to oxidative steps in the pathway leading from substrate pyridine nucleotide-linked oxidations to reduction of oxygen. Normally, as each equivalent of electrons flows along the pathway, three equivalents of ATP are generated.

target cells. Work in the laboratories of J. Oppenheimer, H. Samuels, and J. Baxter indicates that the cellular biological expression of response to T_3 and T_4 is mediated as a consequence of the nuclear localization and genomic activation by a ligand–receptor complex which results in the selective *de novo* synthesis of the new proteins required for the thyroid hormone's biological responses. Thus, the mode of action of many of the biological responses generated by thyroid hormones is analogous to that of steroid hormones. In this instance, T_3 (or T_4) binds to a high affinity, limited capacity, unoccupied receptor protein present in the nucleus of the target cell to form a hormone–receptor complex.

The evidence that the nuclear T_3 binding sites function as receptors in mediating the biological responses to T_3 and T_4 is largely correlative:

1. The relative binding affinities of several thyroid hormone-active compounds to the nuclear receptor parallel the biological activity of these compounds (see Table 6-5).

2. The nuclear receptors are only found in cells known to be responsive to thyroid hormones. These include the liver, brain, heart, lung, kidney, and anterior pituitary.

3. Changes in the cellular concentration of receptors for thyroid hormones are correlated with parallel changes in the cellular response to the hormone.

4. Thyroid hormones have been shown to stimulate the selective synthesis of RNA and protein.

Table 6–5. Biological Activity, Nuclear Binding, and Binding to Solubilized Nuclear Receptor of Thyroid Hormone Analogs[a]

Compound	Biological activity	In vivo nuclear binding	Cell-free nuclear binding	Binding to solubilized receptor
T_3	100	100	100	100
T_4	18	10	12.5	11
Isopropyl-T_2	142	100	104	89
TETRAC	9	5	16.3	—
Reverse T_3	0.1	0	0.1	.2
3,3'-T_2	1.5	1.8	—	0.7

[a] All data are expressed relative to L-T_3, which is arbitrarily equal to 100.

The unoccupied T_3/T_4 receptor is found in the nucleus of the cell bound to the chromatin. The molecular weight is estimated to be ~54,000; the protein has a frictional coefficient of 1.4 and is slightly asymmetric in shape. The partial purification of the thyroid receptor has been accomplished by ion-exchange molecular sieve and affinity chromatography. It is estimated that a 50,000-fold purification would be required for complete purification. The K_d of T_3 binding to the holoreceptor is $2–5 \times 10^{-10}$ M. The T_3 receptor, when extracted from the nucleus, migrates on a sucrose gradient with a 3.8 S mobility; however, when the T_3 receptor is released from the nucleus by DNase I digestion, it migrates with a mobility of 6.55. H. Samuels and co-workers suggest that the 6.5 S form of the receptor is comprised of a protein(s) of total molecular weight of 127,000 and DNA of 22,000 (equivalent to 36 base pairs of nucleotides of DNA). Whether the receptor protein(s) represents abundant chromatin proteins or unknown proteins of low abundance will require purification of the receptor to homogeneity.

The possible structural relationship of the thyroid hormone nuclear receptor to the TBPA of the blood is not known; however, the presence of a "groove" on the TBPA which can accommodate a DNA double strand suggests the possibility of a structural homology.

Figure 6-18 presents a general model for the receptor-mediated actions of thyroid hormone receptors. Thyroid hormones enter the cell by as yet undefined mechanisms and may then be subsequently metabolized to T_3. After association of T_3 with the holoreceptor, there ensues a structural change in the chromatin that has the consequence of affecting the transcription of specific genes. The domain of genes regulated by T_3 is

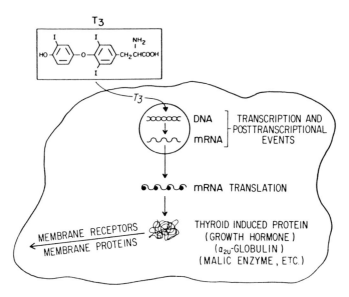

Figure 6-18. Working model for the mechanism of thyroid hormone action in a responsive cell. Thyroid hormones enter the cell by as yet unknown mechanisms and may be metabolized to the biologically active T_3. After association of T_3 with the "holoreceptor," there is a structural change in chromatin that influences the transcription of specific genes. Subsequent to transcription, processing of precursor forms of RNA may occur, yielding the mature mRNA. Translation of the mRNA results in the synthesis of proteins whose effects may be expressed intracellularly or extracellularly. Reproduced with permission from H. H. Samuels, Thyroid hormone receptors and action in cultured cells. *In* "Molecular Basis of Thyroid Hormone Action" (J. H. Oppenheimer and H. H. Samuels, eds.), pp. 33–65. Academic Press, New York, 1983.

not known precisely; it appears, though, that it overlaps in both a synergistic and antagonistic sense with gene domains that are regulated by glucocorticoids, insulin, and epidermal growth factor (EGF).

It is now clear that there is a structural homology, at the protein level, between the thyroid hormone receptor, steroid hormone receptors, and the *v*-erb-A oncogene (see Fig. 1-18). Thus, the thyroid hormone receptor and steroid hormone receptors all may have evolved from a common ancestral gene. Collectively, both thyroid receptors as well as steroid hormone receptors function to regulate gene transcription as cis-acting DNA-promoter elements in conjunction with other trans-acting proteins.

It remains to the future to learn whether all the biological effects of thyroid hormones are mediated through a nuclear receptor interaction or whether other pathways of action, such as direct effects on the mitochondria, are also significant.

3. Action of Thyroid Hormones on Cell Membrane Ion Transport

A third alternative model which describes the caloric effect of thyroxine and T_3 postulates a stimulation in target cells of a plasma membrane sodium transport process through the direct stimulation of the sodium pump. In this model, the Na^+, K^+-ATPase present in the basal membrane of many cells and which normally effects a coupled outward transport of Na^{2+} in exchange for an inward movement of K^+ is specifically stimulated by T_3.

VI. CLINICAL ASPECTS

A. Hormone Deficiency

Thyroid hormone deficiency may result in a wide variety of clinical and physiological disturbances in virtually every organ system. The classic disease state is myxedema; the accumulation of mucinous edema results in facial periorbital and peripheral edema involving both hands and feet. The periorbital edema contributes to the patient's haggard appearance and includes a "droop" of the upper eyelid.

Table 6-6 lists the major causes of hypothyroidism. Hashimoto's disease is an autoimmune thyroid disease in which the subject has circulating thyroid antibodies. (It is not known whether these antibodies functionally contribute to the state of hypothyroidism.) The typical patient with Hashimoto's disease is a middle-aged woman with an enlarged, but firm nodular goiter who is euthyroid or hypothyroid, that is, presenting an appearance of mild mxyedemas. (The thyroglobulin antibodies are usually of the IgG type. They are highly species specific.) Complexes of antibody and thyroglobulin are frequently deposited in the thyroid. Hypothyroidism in elderly patients is considered to be usually an inactive phase of Hashimoto's disease and the major cause of idiopathic hypothyrodism.

(Without question) in many sections of the world the prime cause of hypothyroidism is a dietary insufficiency of iodine. This results in the adaptive appearance of an endemic goiter. In large part the adaptive responses are triggered by an increased TSH secretion which attempts to stimulate the iodide trapping mechanisms and subsequent steps in the intrathyroidal metabolism of iodine. The morphological consequence of this sequelae is the development of a goiter.

Endemic cretinism is the most severe version of goiter. In countries such as Zaire, Ecuador, and regions of the Himalayas, 5–12% of whole

Table 6–6. Major Causes of Hypothyroidism

Loss of functional thyroid tissue
   Chronic autoimmune thyroiditis (Hashimoto's disease)
   Idiopathic hypothyroidism
   Postradioactive iodine treatment
   Postthyroidectomy
Biosynthetic defects in thyroid hormonogenesis
   Inherited defects
   Iodine deficiency
   Antithyroid agents
Hypothyrotropic hypothyroidism
   TSH deficiency
   TRH deficiency
Peripheral resistance to thyroid hormones

communities can be affected. Goiter is quite common, hypothyroidism frequent, but cretinism rare. The dominant characteristics of the disease are mental retardation, with an associated impairment of the central nervous system.

There are a variety of hereditary diseases in which there are defects in one or more of the many steps required for the biosynthesis of thyroid hormone. These include defects in (1) iodide concentration, (2) iodide organification, (3) thyroglobulin biosynthesis, (4) iodotyrosine dehalogenase, and (5) thyroid gland insensitivity to TSH. Another cause of hypothyroidism relates to perturbation in the thyroid–pituitary axis such that there may be a deficiency or total lack of pituitary-derived TSH or thyrotropin releasing hormone (TRF) (see Chapter 5).

B. Hormone Excess

There are two principal types of hyperthyroidism which result in thyrotoxicosis. These are Graves' disease and toxic adenoma. Clinically, Graves' disease is characterized by a distinct bulging of the eyeball (exophthalmos). This results from an accumulation of fluid and a connective tissue ground substance. Also characteristic is a goiter and pretibial myxedema.

Graves' disease is also an autoimmune disease that results from the presence in plasma of an IgG globulin—a long-acting thyroid stimulator (LATS) which causes responses on the thyroid gland qualitatively similar to TSH, but with a more persistent effect. LATS is believed to be produced by thymus-dependent lymphocytes in individuals with a genetic predisposition. It has been suggested that the disorder is inherited by a simple autosomal recessive mechanism with relative sex limitation to the female and with a reduced penetrance in homozygotes. The incidence of Graves' disease in England and probably the United States is estimated to be 23/100,000 overall population, with an established sex ratio of 4–5:1 for females over males.)

The presence of an adenoma in the thyroid gland (toxic adenoma) can lead to the overproduction of thyroid hormones. An understanding of toxic adenoma is best found by approaching the pathology of the disease as being due to a benign hyperplasia. There is a gradual transition from inordinate sensitivity to TSH, to autonomous function. Although the hyperthyroidism of toxic adenoma can be controlled by antithyroid drugs, the definitive resolution is normally achieved by ablation of the neoplasm(s).

There are also a variety of other minor types of hyperthyroidism. They include (1) a pituitary tumor secreting excess TSH, (2) thyrotoxicosis factitia wherein a patient chronically ingests an excess of T_4 or T_3, usually in an effort to lose weight, (3) a functioning metastatic carcinoma, and (4) multinodular goiter.

C. Measurement of Thyroid Function

Thyroid tests may be classified according to whether they provide insight into anatomical, etiological, or functional dysfunction of the gland. Given the complex cellular and molecular biology of the many steps associated with the production of thyroid hormones and the obvious multitude of thyroid-related diseases, there are now available to the clinician a wide battery of tests, assays, and manipulations which will assist in determination of the problem. A detailed discussion of these procedures is beyond the scope of this text.

References

A. Books

DeGroot, L. J., Cahill, G., O'Dell, W. D., Martini, L., Potts, J. T., Nelson, D. H., Steinberger, E., and Winegrad, A. I., eds. (1979). "Endocrinology," Vol. 1, pp. 305–547. Grune & Stratton, New York.

Oppenheimer, J. H., and Samuels, H. H., eds. (1983). "Molecular Basis of Thyroid Hormone." Academic Press, New York.

B. Review Articles

Burman, K. D. (1978). Recent developments in thyroid hormone metabolism: Interpretation and significance of measurements of reverse T_3, 3,3'T_2, and thyroglobulin. *Metab., Clin. Exp.* **27**, 615–630.

DeGroot, L. J., and Niepomniszcze, H. (1977). Biosynthesis of thyroid hormone and clinical aspects. *Metab., Clin. Exp.* **26**, 663–718.

Eberhardt, N. L., Apriletti, J. W., and Baxter, J. D. (1980). The molecular biology of thyroid hormone action. *In* "Biochemical Actions of Hormones" (G. L. Litwack, ed.), Vol. 7, Academic Press, New York.

Ganong, W. F. (1974). The role of catecholamines and acetylcholine in the regulation of endocrine function. *Life Sci.* **15**, 1401–1414.

Hearn, M. T. W. (1980). Graves' disease and the thyrotropin receptor. *Trends Biochem. Sci.* **5**, 75–78.

Sap, J., Munoz, A., Damm, K., Goldberg, Y., Ghysdael, J., Lentz, A., Beug, H., and Vennstrom, B. (1986). The c-*erb*-A protein is a high affinity receptor for thyroid hormone. *Nature (London)* **324**, 635–640.

Sterling, K. (1979). Thyroid hormone action at the cell level. *N. Engl. J. Med.* **300**, 117–123, 173–177.

Weinberger, C., Thompson, C. C., Ong, E. S., Lebo, R., Gruol, D. J., and Evans, R. M. (1986). The c-*erb*-A gene encodes a thyroid hormone receptor. *Nature (London)* **324**, 641–646.

C. Research Papers

DeGroot, L. J., Refetoff, S., Strausser, J., and Barsano, C. (1974). Nuclear triiodothyronine-binding protein: Partial characterization and binding to chromatin. *Proc. Natl. Acad. Sci. U.S.A.* **71**, 4042.

Field, J. B. (1975). Thyroid-stimulating hormone and cyclic adenosine 3′,5′ monophosphate in the regulation of thyroid gland function. *Metab., Clin. Exp.* **24**, 381–393.

Gavaret, J., Cahnmann, H. J., and Nuñez, J. (1981). Thyroid hormone synthesis in thyroglobulin: The mechanism of the coupling reaction. *J. Biol. Chem.* **256**, 9176–9173.

Heimann, P. (1966). Ultrastructure of human thyroid. *Acta Endocrinol. (Copenhagen)* **53**, Suppl. 110.

Ismail-Beigi, F., and Edelman, I. S. (1970). Mechanism of thyroid calorigenesis: Role of active sodium transport. *Proc. Natl. Acad. Sci. U.S.A.* **67**, 1071.

Kumara-Siri, M. H., Shapiro, L. E., and Surks, M. I. (1986). Association of the 3,5,3′-triiodo-L-thyronine nuclear receptor with the nuclear matrix of cultured growth hormone-producing rat pituitary tumor cells (GC cells). *J. Biol. Chem.* **261**, 2844–2852.

Kurtz, D. T., Sippel, A. E., and Feigelson, P. (1976). Effect of thyroid hormones on the level of the hepatic mRNA for globulin. *Biochemistry* **15**, 1031.

Pearlman, A. J., Stanley, F., and Samuels, H. H. (1982). Thyroid hormone nuclear receptor: Evidence for multimeric organization in chromatin. *J. Biol. Chem.* **257**, 930–938.

Williams, J. A. (1972). Effects of Ca^{2+} and Mg^{2+} on secretion *in vitro* by mouse thyroid glands. *Endocrinology (Baltimore)* **90**, 1459–1463.

Williams, J. A., and Wolff, J. (1970). Possible role of microtubules in thyroid secretion. *Proc. Natl. Acad. Sci. U.S.A.* **67**, 1901–1908.

Yamashita, K., and Field, J. B. (1972). Elevation of cyclic guanosine 3′,5′-monophosphate levels in dog thyroid slices caused by acetylcholine and sodium fluoride. *J. Biol. Chem.* **247**, 7062–7066.

Chapter **7**

Pancreatic Hormones: Insulin and Glucagon

263

I. INTRODUCTION

A. Background Information

A feature essential for life of higher vertebrates is their ability to maintain a relatively constant blood glucose concentration. In the higher animals, glucose is essential as an energy source for all cells. Although some cells can utilize alternate "fuel metabolites" such as amino acids or fatty acids, the brain and its neurons are dependent upon a continuous supply of blood-delivered glucose. Superimposed on the requirement for the maintenance of a constant blood glucose level are the perturbations in blood glucose that may naturally occur as a consequence of ongoing physiological and metabolic events. These can include (1) the intestinal absorption and concomitant systemic transport to storage depots (liver, muscle, and/or adipose tissue) of foodstuffs (e.g., carbohydrates, proteins, and fat); (2) muscular activity; (3) thermogenesis and the response to environmental extremes of heat and cold; (4) starvation; (5) pregnancy/lactation; or (6) disease or injury states. The endocrine system largely responsible for the maintenance of blood glucose levels and the proper cellular uptake and exchange of the "fuel metabolites" is the pancreas. The principal hormones secreted by the pancreas are insulin and glucagon. Additionally, somatostatin is secreted by the pancreas and gastrointestinal tract as well as by the hypothalamus (see Chapter 3 and this chapter). The pancreas is vital for the maintenance of homeostasis of glucose and other fuel metabolites.

Insulin is a potent hormone in that it has a wide sphere of influence; directly or indirectly it affects virtually every organ and tissue in the body. The main functions of insulin are to stimulate anabolic reactions for carbohydrates, proteins, and fats, all of which will have the metabolic consequences of producing a lowered blood glucose level. Glucagon can be thought of as an indirect antagonist of insulin. Glucagon stimulates catabolic reactions which lead ultimately to an elevation of blood glucose levels. Thus, the pancreas is continuously adjusting the relative amounts of glucagon and insulin secreted, in response to the continuous perturbations of blood glucose and other fuel metabolites occurring as a consequence of changes in anabolism and catabolism in the various tissues.

B. Regulation of Blood Glucose

The blood concentration of glucose normally lies within the range of 80–110 mg/100 ml (4.4–6.1 mM). Reduction in concentrations in blood glucose levels below 45–55 mg/100 ml for a continued interval of time will lead to an impairment of brain function, tremors, and convulsions due to activation of the sympathetic nervous system, and ultimately death. Conversely, prolonged hyperglycemia (a relative lack of insulin) leads to a devastating wasting of metabolic energy, osmotic diuresis, and metabolic acidosis. Because glucose is a "small molecule," all blood glucose is completely filtered by the glomerulus of the kidney. Under normal physiological circumstances virtually all of this filtered glucose is reabsorbed; since this reabsorptive process is saturable and can only accommodate a finite throughput of glucose in instances of excessive hyperglycemia, a significant fraction of the filtered blood glucose will be lost in the urine. If there is not a balanced increase in dietary intake of glucose there will be, of necessity, a compensatory breakdown or catabolism of the storage forms of glucose, namely, glycogen; over an extended interval of time this can result in a significant loss of "stored" metabolic energy.

Related to prolonged hyperglycemia and its concomitant glucosuria is an associated increase in loss of body water from the general circulatory system; this is due to the passive loss of water across the kidney tubule which occurs as a consequence of the high osmotic pressure of the sugar-rich urine. In extreme cases of chronic glucosuria there will be cellular dehydration leading to a loss of potassium and a reduction in blood volume, which can ultimately lead to a marked lowering of systemic blood pressure (see Chapter 15). In a normal (70 kg) man, the 24-hr urine volume ranges from 600 to 2500 ml, with a glucose concentration of 10–20 mg/100 ml. In a typical untreated diabetic (without renal complications), the 24-hr urine volume may exceed 3000–3500 ml, with a glucose concentration of 500–5000 mg/100 ml.

However, the adverse consequences of a relative lack of insulin (hyperglycemia) are not restricted to a derangement of carbohydrate metabolism. In the absence of insulin, triglycerides and fatty acids will be mobilized from adipose tissue and amino acids from muscle tissue (discussed in detail later). These substances then proceed to the liver where the fatty acids and branched chain amino acids are converted into ketone bodies. The ketone bodies include β-hydroxybutyrate, acetoacetate, and acetone. Eventually, this results in a progressive ketonemia and, when the renal threshold for acetoacetate and β-hydroxybutyrate are exceeded, both substances will appear in the urine. Because they are excreted as the sodium salt, this has the consequence, when extended over a period of time, of depleting the body of base. This in turn elevates the $[H_2CO_3]/[NaHCO_3]$ ratio and leads to the condition of metabolic acidosis. Ultimately this will trigger the rapid and deep respiratory rate which is diagnostic of diabetic acidosis. Tabulated in Table 7-1 is a re-

Table 7–1. Effects of Altered Blood Glucose Levels on Several Constituents of the Blood and Urine

Parameter	"Normal" state	Chronic elevated blood glucose (diabetes)	Chronic lowered blood glucose (starvation)
Blood			
Insulin (μU/ml)	50–100	8–16[a]	5–10
Glucagon (pg/ml)	<50	200–300	150
Glucose (mg/100 ml)	80–110	>130	50–60
Free fatty acids (mM)	0.4–0.7	2.0	4.0
Ketones (mM)	1–2	20	10–20
Urine			
Volume (ml/24 hr)	600–2500	3000–3500	600–1200
Glucose (mg/100 ml)	6–8	500–5000	5–10

[a] For type II or insulin-dependent diabetes.

sume of the changes of several blood and urine components which may result as a consequence of altered blood glucose levels.

In addition to the dominant partnership of insulin and glucagon in maintaining glucose homeostasis, there is an extensive contribution of other physiological factors and hormones to the regulation of blood glucose. These are summarized in Table 7-2.

Table 7–2. Factors Contributing to Glucose Homeostasis[a]

Factors resulting in a reduction in blood glucose	Factors resulting in an elevation in blood glucose
Insulin	Glucagon → liver
	Epinephrine → glycogenolysis
Glucose uptake by peripheral tissues	Cortisol (gluconeogenesis)
Glycosuria	Insulin antagonists; growth hormone; cortisol
Exercise	Dietary intake of carbohydrates and proteins; mobilization from storage sites (glycogenolysis)
Stimulation of glucagon catabolism	Stimulation of insulin catabolism

[a] This table was adapted with permission from J. Wahren, Metabolic adaptation to physical exercise in man. In "Endocrinology" (L. J. DeGroot, G. F. Cahill, L. Martini, D. H. Nelson, W. D. Odell, J. T. Potts, E. Steinberger, and A. I. Winegrad, eds.), Vol. 3, pp. 1911–1926. Grune & Stratton, New York, 1979.

C. Nutritional and Metabolic Interrelationships

1. Introduction

Any detailed understanding of the integrated actions of glucagon and insulin to effect blood glucose homeostasis cannot be achieved by limiting the assessment of their actions to those on carbohydrate metabolism alone. Due to the ready metabolic interchanges that occur between carbohydrate, protein, and fat constituents, it is essential to have a clear understanding of the intermediary metabolism of all these substances. In addition, some appreciation of the principles of dietary nutrition is required because many key enzymes of intermediary metabolism of higher animals are adaptively regulated to reflect the current dietary intake of carbohydrate, protein, and lipids. The general design is such that the ingested components are diverted to storage sites during periods of feeding and are later reutilized by the metabolic processes of glycogenolysis, gluconeogenesis, and ketogenesis during intervals of food deprivation.

2. Substrate Stores

Table 7-3 lists for normal man the body pools of carbohydrate, fat, and protein and their caloric equivalent.

Virtually the complete body pool of protein is in a continuous state of flux. In the steady state there is a balance between biosynthesis and degradation. The amino acid efflux from human muscle is 0.5–1.0 g/kg/day. Physiological amounts of insulin are known to markedly reduce amino acid efflux from muscle. The released amino acids are further catabolized principally by the liver. Although a normal 70-kg man has a total of 10 kg of protein, only ~60% of this is theoretically metabolically mobilizable; the remaining 40% represents structural proteins. In reality no more than 2 kg of body protein can be metabolically mobilized before there is a marked muscular hypertrophy and myopathy (weakness). In cases of extreme starvation, death ensues not from hypoglycemia, but from loss of respiratory muscle function, which usually leads to terminal pneumonia.

Fat is the body's principal form of stored energy; 77% of the calories derived from the substrate stores tabulated in Table 7-3 comes from metabolic oxidation of triglycerides and free fatty acids. Fat or adipose tissue represents the most efficient body storage form of energy. This results not only from the higher caloric yield per gram mass of adipose tissue, but also from the fact that the biological "packing" of triglycerides is more condensed than protein or glycogen due to the absence of water molecules in the triglyceride structures. It is the fat depots that

Table 7–3. Body Pools of Carbohydrate, Fat, and Protein in a Normal (70 kg) Man[a]

Class	Amount (g)	Caloric yield (kcal)
Carbohydrate		
Muscle glycogen	350	1450
Liver glycogen	85	350
Extracellular glucose	20	80
Fat		
Muscle triglycerides	300	2800
Adipose triglycerides	15,000	140,000
Plasma free fatty acids	0.4	4
Plasma triglycerides	4.0	40
Protein		
Muscle	10,000	41,000
	Total	185,600

[a] Adapted with permission of the authors and publisher from J. Wahren, Metabolic adaptation to physical exercise in man. *In* "Endocrinology" (L. J. DeGroot, G. F. Cahill, L. Martini, D. H. Nelson, W. D. Odell, J. T. Potts, E. Steinberger, and A. I. Winegrad, eds.), Vol. 3., p. 1912. Grune & Stratton, New York, 1979.

allow man to tolerate prolonged intervals of dietary calorie deprivation. The energy stored in the body fat depots is sufficient to permit the average individual to survive 2–3 months of total food deprivation. Lipolysis or hydrolysis of adipose tissue triglycerides leads to the release of glycerol and free fatty acids into the bloodstream. During intervals of exercise the sympathetic neurotransmitter, norepinephrine, is a potent stimulator of triglyceride mobilization. The free fatty acids are then further catabolized by both muscle and liver tissue.

Approximately 80% of the storage form of carbohydrate, namely, glycogen, is found in the muscle; the concentration is 9–16 g/kg wet muscle. The muscle glycogen levels are rapidly depleted during vigorous exercise, but reduced only slowly during prolonged fasting. Because muscle, in contrast to the liver, does not contain the enzyme glucose 6-phosphatase and because there is normally no hydrolysis of the phosphate esters of the various glycolytic pathway intermediates, it is not possible for significant amounts of glycogen (glucose) to leave the muscle. Thus, muscle glycogen can only serve as a metabolic fuel in the cell in which it is localized.

The liver glycogen pool plays a key role in facilitating the metabolic adjustment by the body to varying energy requirements. The concentration of hepatic glycogen is 50 g/kg wet tissue; it represents 20% of the total body glycogen pool. Liver glycogen may be depleted gradually during periods of fasting (within 10–12 hr of fasting, the hepatic glycogen is mobilized at a rate of 50 mg/min/kg liver) or very rapidly in response to exercise. During 40 min of severe exercise, the liver glycogen pool may be depleted by 18–20 g; that is, glycogen is mobilized at a rate of 330 mg/min/kg wet weight. Replenishment of the hepatic levels of glucose occurs relatively slowly; 12–36 hr are required, depending on the diet and extent of physical activity.

The body pool of extracellular glucose is quite modest by comparison with the muscle and liver stores; only ~20 g of free glucose is present in the extracellular water and the intracellular pool of the liver. The principal function of the blood pool of glucose is to provide a continuous supply of glucose to all the glucose-dependent tissues. In the basal state the brain is the chief glucose-consuming tissue. During a 24-hr interval the brain requires 125 g of glucose.

The exclusive source of replenishment of the blood glucose pool is the liver. Under usual circumstances, 70% of the hepatic output of glucose is derived from liver glycogenolysis and 30% from gluconeogenesis. During intervals of prolonged exercise (40 min), ~50% of the oxidative metabolism of skeletal muscle is derived from glucose uptake from blood.

The ketones or "ketone bodies" accumulate in the blood under normal circumstances where they function to assure survival of the organism and under pathological conditions where they can cause coma and death. The ketone bodies are produced almost exclusively by the liver from fatty acids and other carbon fragments derived from amino acids. The acetone is removed from the body through the lungs. The metabolic role of the ketones varies depending upon the nutritional state. Their principal function is to serve under conditions of fasting as a primary substrate for energy metabolism by the muscle, heart, and particularly the brain. Although muscle and heart have the capacity for cellular uptake and oxidation of free fatty acids (derived from lipolysis of adipose tissue), the brain does not have this capacity. Thus, under conditions of fasting when the liver glycogen and eventually blood glucose pools become depleted, the physiological significance of the ketone bodies assumes a far greater importance. Under conditions of adequate feeding, the blood levels of the ketones are relatively low (see Table 7-1).

Figure 7-1 summarizes the balance of glucose production and utilization in man that ensues over a 24-hr interval after dietary intake and in the absence of excessive exercise. Maintenance of a constant blood glucose level is governed by the liver and the regulatory actions of the pancreatic hormones. In the absence of hepatic glucose production, the blood level of glucose would fall by 50% in 40–60 min.

270

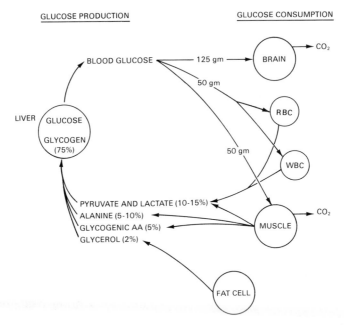

GLUCOSE PRODUCTION   GLUCOSE CONSUMPTION

Figure 7-1. Schematic diagram describing the utilization and production of glucose by normal man in a postabsorptive state (i.e., not actively ingesting a meal). The values for glucose uptake represent the amounts consumed per day; in the case 'of muscle this refers to the resting state. Glucose output from the liver derives from glycogenolysis (25%). As starvation extends beyond 12 hr, glycogen stores are depleted and the contribution from gluconeogenesis increases. RBC, Red blood cell; WBC, white blood cell. Reproduced with permission from P. Felig, Starvation. In "Endocrinology" (L. J. DeGroot, G. F. Cahill, L. Martini, D. H. Nelson, W. D. Odell, J. T. Potts, E. Steinberger, and A. I. Winegrad, eds.), Vol. 3, pp. 1927–1940. Grune & Stratton, New York, 1979.

3. Dietary Nutritional Requirements

The dietary caloric requirements necessary for normal bodily functions vary with age and sex; the recommended values are tabulated in Table 7-4A. Of course, the caloric intake must be increased appropriately during intervals of prolonged exercise.

The calorie referred to in nutritional or metabolic studies is the kilocalorie (1000 cal) and represents the energy required to raise the temperature of 1000 g of water from 15 to 16°C.* These caloric requirements can be met by adequate dietary intake of protein, carbohydrate, or fat. Each food substance has its own characteristic caloric yield (see Table

*The C of calorie, when it is used to denote a kilocalorie, must be capitalized; thus, 1000 cal = 1 kcal = 1 Cal.

Table 7–4A. Recommended Daily Dietary Allowances[a]

	Age (year)	Weight (kg)	Calories	Protein (g)
Men	18–35	70	2900	70
	35–55	70	2600	70
	55–77	70	2200	70
Women	18–35	58	2100	58
	35–55	58	1900	58
	55–75	58	1600	58
	Pregnant	—	+200	+20
	Lactating	—	+1000	+40
Children	1–3	13	1300	32
	3–6	18	1600	40
	6–9	24	2100	52
	9–12	33	2400	60
	12–15	46	2500–3000	—

[a] Recommended by the Food and Nutrition Board, *N.A.S.-N.R.C., Publ.* **1146** (1963).

7-4B) which reflects the relative extent of reduction of the carbon atoms of that food component.

In addition to calories, the diet must supply on a regular basis adequate amounts of the various essential dietary constituents; these include the water and fat-soluble vitamins, the essential unsaturated fatty acids, the essential amino acids, and both the bulk and trace minerals.

The basal metabolic rate (BMR) is defined as the energy expenditure required to maintain those cellular processes that are all essential for the continuing activities of the organism (e.g., the metabolic activity of the heart, lungs, kidneys, and other vital organs). The BMR of an adult 70-kg male is 35–40 Cal/m^2 body surface/hr. The comparable value for a woman of the same age is 29–36 Cal/m^2 body surface.

Table 7–4B. Caloric Yield of Food Substances

	Calories/gram	Respiratory quotient[a]
Carbohydrates	4.0	1.00
Proteins	4.1–4.2	0.8
Fat (triglycerides)	9.3	0.70

[a] Respiratory quotient is defined as the molar ratio of CO_2 released to O_2 consumed during the complete oxidation of a food substance to CO_2 and H_2O.

Not all of the caloric content of dietary constituents is available to support the daily calorie requirements. When food is eaten there is a rise in total body oxygen consumption; this is known as the specific dynamic action, or SDA, of foodstuffs. Although a detailed molecular explanation of the process of SDA has not been given, it in essence represents energy which is spent in the metabolic processing of food and which is therefore lost or not available to support other bodily energy requirements.

The specific dynamic action is ~30% for protein, 0% for carbohydrate, and 4% for lipid, each in terms of the theoretical energy value of the food component ingested.

The respiratory quotient (RQ) is defined as the molar ratio of carbon dioxide released to oxygen utilized during the complete oxidation of a substance to CO_2 and H_2O.

II. ANATOMICAL, MORPHOLOGICAL, AND PHYSIOLOGICAL RELATIONSHIPS

A. Introduction

The hepatopancreatic complex along with the gallbladder is responsible for the integrated digestion and subsequent processing of most dietary nutrients. The complex series of steps and the components of the digestive system are summarized in Table 8-1. The pancreas is both an exocrine and an endocrine gland. The exocrine pancreas biosynthesizes and secretes the major digestive enzymes, for example, the proteases (chymotrypsin and trypsin), amylase, and lipase, as well as bicarbonate, while the endocrine tissue of the pancreas produces the peptide hormones insulin, glucagon, pancreatic polypeptide, and also somatostatin (Table 7-5).

Table 7–5. Hormones Produced by the Pancreas

Hormone	Pancreatic cell of origin	Number of amino acid residues
Insulin	β or B	51
Glucagon	α or A	29
Somatostatin	δ or D	14
Pancreatic polypeptide	F	36

Figure 7-2A illustrates the gross anatomic features of the human pancreas. Anatomically, the pancreas has distinct dorsal and ventral lobes. The pancreas can be divided up into lobules which contain the exocrine acinar glands and the endocrine islets of Langerhans. The islet cells are separated from the surrounding acinar cells by a thin layer of reticular tissue. The endocrine protein of the pancreas is only 1–2% of the weight of the gland. Figure 7-2B schematically illustrates the relationship of the number and distribution of the insulin and glucagon secreting cells in an islet.

B. Development and Embryologic Origins

In invertebrates the functional cells of the exocrine pancreas and liver are combined and there is no clear-cut presence of the endocrine pancreas cells. In vertebrates there is increasing structural organization and differentiation of the exocrine and endocrine cells in relation to the liver as one proceeds from fish (endocrine pancreas is a separate organ; exocrine pancreas is partially incorporated into liver) up through amphibia (endocrine cells scattered in exocrine tissue or islets) to birds and mammals where the pancreas is a separate organ (endocrine pancreas found as vascularized islets imbedded in the exocrine tissue).

In mammals and birds the adult pancreas develops embryologically from two diverticula of the duodenum. It has been generally accepted that the endocrine cells of the pancreas develop from pancreatic ducts originally of endodermal origin. In the developing rat embryo, insulin biosynthesis can be detected by day 16.

C. Ultrastructure of Pancreatic Islets

In both man and the rat, pancreatic islets are composed of at least three major cell types: the α or glucagon-secreting cells, the β or insulin-secreting cells, and the δ cells which secrete somatostatin. By histological staining with Neutral Red it has been estimated that there are 13,500 or 890,000 islets, respectively, in the rat or human pancreas. The islets in the rat pancreas range in diameter from 50 to 400 μm. The distribution of cells in a typical rat islet is 15–18% α, 75–80% β, and 2–5% δ. The islets are surrounded by a basement membrane which encloses all three cell types.

The pancreas of a number of species is also known to secrete a substance known as pancreatic polypeptide (PP). Avian PP is a potent gastric secretagogue; it stimulates the release of both pepsin and HCl. In the chicken pancreas, immunofluorescent studies have indicated that PP is present in cells scattered throughout the exocrine pancreas. A homolo-

A

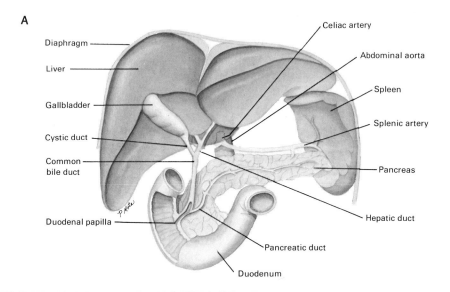

Diaphragm

Liver

Gallbladder

Cystic duct

Common bile duct

Duodenal papilla

Celiac artery

Abdominal aorta

Spleen

Splenic artery

Pancreas

Hepatic duct

Pancreatic duct

Duodenum

B

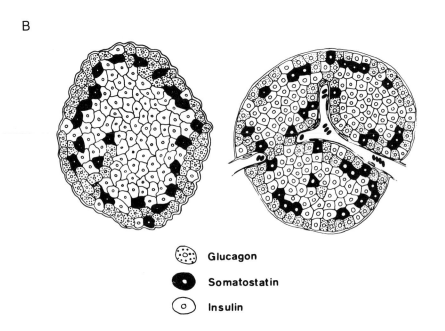

Glucagon

Somatostatin

Insulin

gous peptide to avian PP has been isolated from human pancreas; immunofluorescent studies have indicated human PP present in cells that are localized on the periphery of the human islet. There are also dispersed throughout the endocrine portions of the pancreas low concentrations of cells that secrete gastrin.

The α cells can be differentiated from other islet cells (see Fig. 7-3) on the basis of the ultrastructural appearance of their secretory granules. Usually the center of the granule is exceedingly electron dense. The β cells can be specifically identified histochemically by staining with aldehyde fuchsin or aldehyde thionin, which apparently react with sulfhydryl groups present in insulin. A remarkable feature of most β cells is the visible presence of a crystalline matrix or array; in the β cells of man, the bat, or dog, there is a repeating periodicity of ~50Å. This may be related to the property of insulin to form dimers and hexamers (see later).

It has been proposed by R. Unger, L. Orci, and others that the α and β and possibly δ cells function together as a hormonal secretory unit; this unit releases suitable proportions of glucagon and insulin necessary to regulate the minute-to-minute blood glucose levels and also modulates metabolism either toward anabolism or catabolism in accordance with physiological needs. The integrated secretion of glucagon and insulin by the α and β cells may well have a functional basis due to the close anatomic intimacy of these two cells. Orci has identified by electron microscopic, freeze-fracture methods a preponderance of both gap junctions and tight junctions between adjacent α and β cells. It is believed that the tight junctions may form dynamically to trap insulin released extracellularly from secretory granules, thus effectively compartmen-

---

Figure 7-2. (A) Gross anatomical features of the pancreas, liver, and biliary system. (B) Schematic diagram of a pancreatic islet. (Left) Schematic representation of the number and distribution of insulin-, glucagon-, and somatostatin-containing cells in the normal rat islet. Note the characteristic position of most glucagon- and somatostatin-containing cells at the periphery of the islet, surrounding the centrally located insulin-containing cells. Cell types in the islet for which a characteristic function and/or morphology is not defined are intentionally omitted. (Right) Schematic representation of the number and distribution of insulin-, glucagon-, and somatostatin-containing cells in the normal human islet. Large vascular channels penetrate the islet and are surrounded by glucagon- and somatostatin-containing cells. This pattern divides the total islet mass into small subunits, each of which contains a center formed mainly of insulin-containing cells and surrounded by glucagon- and somatostatin-containing cells. Cell types for which definite functions and/or morphologies have not yet been determined are intentionally omitted. Reproduced with permission from L. Orci, *in* "Insulin and Metabolism" (J. S. Bajaj, ed.), p. 262. Excerpta Medica, Amsterdam, 1977.

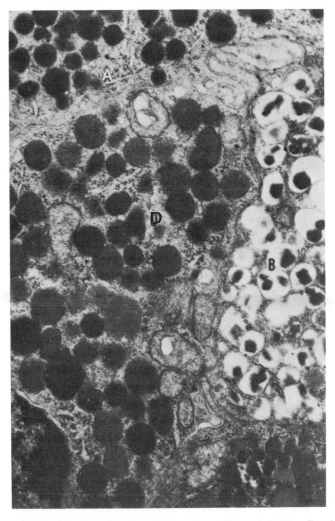

Figure 7-3. Electron micrograph of normal α (A), β (B), and δ (D) cells of a human pancreatic islet. Also present is part of a cell with small secretory granules (G) that may represent a gastrin cell (×32,000). Reproduced with permission from P. E. Lacy and M. H. Greider, Anatomy and ultrastructural organization of pancreatic islets. *In* "Endocrinology" (L. J. DeGroot, G. F. Cahill, L. Martini, D. H. Nelson, W. D. Odell, J. T. Potts, E. Steinberger, and A. I. Winegrad, eds.), Vol. 2, p. 909. Grune & Stratton, New York, 1979.

talizing the intercellular space between the islet cells and providing channels of access to the pancreatic capillary bed. The gap junctions could also well serve as pathways of intercellular communication between adjacent cells. In other systems, gap junctions have been shown to permit the interchange between cells of molecules of under 500 Da. The role of the δ cells and their secretory product, somatostatin, which can inhibit both insulin and glucagon secretion, is not yet known. Possibly somatostatin functions in the pancreas as a paracrine substance.

D. Vascularization and Innervation of Pancreatic Islets

Figure 7-2A illustrates the gross anatomic features of the pancreas in relation to the biliary system and liver.

The arterial supply of the pancreas arises from the splenic, hepatic, and mesenteric arteries and the venous drainage is into the splenic and mesenteric veins. As shown in Fig. 7-4, the individual islets of the pancreas are vascularized by an extensive labyrinth of capillaries. Each islet

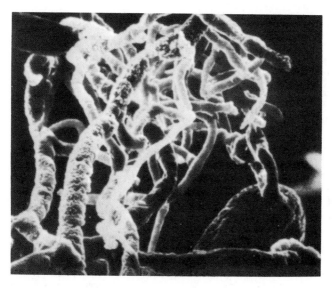

Figure 7-4. Scanning electron micrograph of capillary network in a pancreatic islet. Reproduced with permission from P. E. Lacy and M. H. Greider, Anatomy and ultrastructural organization of pancreatic islets. *In* "Endocrinology" (L. J. DeGroot, G. F. Cahill, L. Martini, D. H. Nelson, W. D. Odell, J. T. Potts, E. Steinberger, and A. I. Winegrad, eds.), Vol. 3, p. 911. Grune & Stratton, New York, 1979.

is normally vascularized by 1–3 arterioles which abruptly terminate into capillaries and 1–6 veinules, depending upon the size of the islet. Morphological studies of the islets indicate that their endocrine cells are arranged in cords or short bands of cells, with each islet cell being adjacent to a capillary. This permits the rapid transfer of the secreted hormones into the general vascular system.

The capillaries present in the pancreatic islets are comprised of endothelial cells which are fenestrated to permit the rapid uptake of the peptide hormones (see, e.g., Fig. 11-13). It has been estimated from infusion of horseradish peroxidase (40,000 Da) that the fenestrated islet capillary is 4–7 times more permeable than a nonfenestrated capillary. The hormonal products secreted by islet cells into the surrounding extracellular fluid must traverse the basement membrane of the endothelium before entering the bloodstream.

Figure 7-5 schematically illustrates the innervation of the pancreatic islets by both parasympathetic cholinergic neurons and sympathetic adrenergic neurons. There are no specialized morphologic membrane structures in the islet cells characteristic of neuromuscular synapses; the nerve terminals end abruptly within the islet underneath the basal lamina which surrounds the islet cell.

Both adrenergic and cholinergic nerve fibers are present in both the acinar as well as islet regions of the pancreas. Stimulation of the parasympathetic nervous system leads to insulin secretion and inhibition of glucagon secretion, irrespective of whether the stimuli occur at the lateral hypothalamic nuclei, the motor nuclei of the vagus, or the mixed pancreatic nerves. Stimulation of the sympathetic nervous system or application of epinephrine can likewise stimulate glucagon production and inhibit insulin secretion. The hypothalamus appears to play the major integrating role in the balance between the sympathetic and parasympathetic regulation of the islet.

III. CHEMISTRY

Table 7-5 lists the peptide hormones produced by the pancreas. The chemistry of each of these will be discussed separately.

A. Insulin

The history of insulin occupies a unique place in the evolution of our understanding of peptide hormones. Table 7-6 summarizes the notable

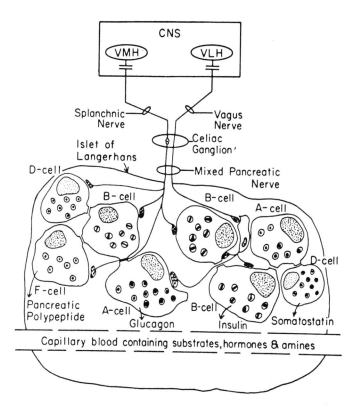

Figure 7-5. Schematic representation of the autonomic innervation of the pancreatic islets (VMH, ventromedial hypothalamus; VLH, ventrolateral hypothalamus; CNS, central nervous system). Reproduced with permission from S. C. Woods *et al.*, The role of the nervous system in metabolic regulation and its effect on diabetes and obesity. *In* "Handbook of Diabetes Mellitus" (M. Brownlee, ed), p. 213. Garland Publishing Co., New York, 1981.

series of "firsts" associated with the development of the chemistry and physiology of this important hormone. Due to its relatively modest size, insulin was an ideal molecule for the pioneering developments of peptide chemistry, amino acid sequencing techniques, and the recombinant DNA cloning of the insulin genome.

Insulin is a molecule of molecular weight 5700–6100 which falls on the borderline between large polypeptide and small protein. It is composed of two separate peptide chains, designated the A chain and the B chain. These two chains are joined together by two disulfide bridges. The A chain consists of 21 amino acid residues, and the B chain of 30 amino acid residues.

280

Table 7–6. History of Insulin

Year	Event	Investigator
1869	Discovery of pancreatic islets	P. Langerhans
1921	Discovery and isolation of insulin	F. G. Banting[a] and C. Best
1955	Determination of primary amino acid sequence	F. Sanger[a]
1967	Discovery and structure determination of proinsulin	D. F. Steiner and R. Chance
1969	Determination of three-dimensional structure of insulin	D. Crowfoot-Hodgkin[a]
1979	Cloning of the insulin gene	W. Rutter and H. Goodman

[a] Received Nobel Prize (see Appendix E).

To date the primary amino acid sequence of some 25 vertebrate insulins has been determined (see Fig. 7-6). Amino acid substitution can apparently occur at many positions without loss of biological activity; indeed, as many as 29 of the 51 positions can be replaced. It is at positions 8–10 (in the middle of the A chain internal disulfide bond) that the greatest biological variation occurs. These sequence differences are expected to exert important antigenic responses in heterologous species and accordingly determine the therapeutic effectiveness of a particular insulin preparation in the replacement therapy often associated with the management of diabetes.

From careful analysis of structure–function relationships of both naturally occurring and chemically modified insulins, it is apparent that certain structural features of insulin have been conserved throughout evolution. These include (1) the precise positions of the three disulfide bonds; (2) the N- and C-terminal regions of the A chain; and (3) the hydrophobic residues of the C-terminal region of the B chain. From biological studies, it has been shown that insulin binds to receptors from tissues of differing species in a way which supports the view that there has been little or no evolutionary drift of the binding site specificity of the insulin receptor. The insulin receptor specifically recognizes an extensive region of ~11 residues around residues A-21 and B-23–B-27 and is dependent upon an intact tertiary structure.

Since the amino acid sequence of the hagfish insulin differs from that

Figure 7-6. Primary amino acid sequence of insulin and related polypeptides. Modified from T. L. Blundell and R. E. Humbel, Hormone families and pancreatic hormones and homologous growth factors. *Nature (London)* **287**, 781–786 (1980). © 1980 Macmillan Journals Limited.

A Chains

	-2	-1	1	2	3	4	5	6	7	8	9	10	11	12	13	14	15	16	17	18	19	20	21	22	23	24	25	26	27	28	29	30
Insulin																																
Bovine	—	—	Gly	Ile	Val	Glu	Gln	Cys	Cys	Ala	Ser	Val	Cys	Ser	Leu	Tyr	Gln	Leu	Glu	Asn	Tyr	Cys	Asn	—	—	—	—	—	—	—	—	—
Human	—	—	Gly	Ile	Val	Glu	Gln	Cys	Cys	Thr	Ser	Ile	Cys	Ser	Leu	Tyr	Gln	Leu	Glu	Asn	Tyr	Cys	Asn	—	—	—	—	—	—	—	—	—
Rat 1	—	—	Gly	Ile	Val	Asp	Gln	Cys	Cys	Thr	Ser	Ile	Cys	Ser	Leu	Tyr	Gln	Leu	Glu	Asn	Tyr	Cys	Asn	—	—	—	—	—	—	—	—	—
Rat 2	—	—	Gly	Ile	Val	Asp	Gln	Cys	Cys	Thr	Ser	Ile	Cys	Ser	Leu	Tyr	Gln	Leu	Glu	Asn	Tyr	Cys	Asn	—	—	—	—	—	—	—	—	—
Guinea pig	—	—	Gly	Ile	Val	Asp	Gln	Cys	Cys	Thr	Gly	Thr	Cys	Thr	Arg	His	Gln	Leu	Gln	Ser	Tyr	Cys	Asn	—	—	—	—	—	—	—	—	—
Casiragua	—	—	Gly	Ile	Val	Asp	Gln	Cys	Cys	Thr	Asn	Ile	Cys	Ser	Leu	Tyr	Gln	Leu	Glu	Asn	Tyr	Cys	Asn	—	—	—	—	—	—	—	—	—
Coypu	—	—	Gly	Ile	Val	Glu	Gln	Cys	Cys	Thr	Asn	Ile	Cys	Ser	Leu	Met	Ser	Leu	Met	Ser	Tyr	Cys	Asn	Asp*	—	—	—	—	—	—	—	—
Hagfish	—	—	Gly	Ile	Val	Glu	Gln	Cys	Cys	His	Lys	Arg	Cys	Ser	Ile	Asn	Leu	Gln	Asn	Tyr	Cys	Asn	—	—	—	—	—	—	—	—	—	—
Insulin-like Growth factor																																
IGF 1	—	—	Gly	Ile	Val	Asp	Glu	Cys	Cys	Phe	Arg	Ser	Cys	Asp	Leu	Arg	Arg	Leu	Glu	Met	Tyr	Cys	Ala	Pro	Leu	Lys	Pro	Ala	Lys	Ser	Ala	
IGF 2	—	—	Gly	Ile	Val	Glu	Glu	Cys	Cys	Phe	Arg	Ser	Cys	Asp	Leu	Ala	Leu	Leu	Glu	Thr	Tyr	Cys	Ala	Thr	—	—	Pro	Ala	Lys	Ser	Glu	
Relaxin																																
Porcine	Arg	Met	Thr	Leu	Ser	Glu	Lys	Cys	Cys	Glu	Val	Gly	Cys	Ile	Arg	Lys	Asp	Ile	Ala	Arg	Leu	Cys	—	—	—	—	—	—	—	—	—	—

B Chains

	-2	-1	1	2	3	4	5	6	7	8	9	10	11	12	13	14	15	16	17	18	19	20	21	22	23	24	25	26	27	28	29	30	31
Insulin																																	
Bovine	—	—	Phe	Val	Asn	Gln	His	Leu	Cys	Gly	Ser	His	Leu	Val	Glu	Ala	Leu	Tyr	Leu	Val	Cys	Gly	Glu	Arg	Gly	Phe	Phe	Tyr	Thr	Pro	Lys	Ala	—
Human	—	—	Phe	Val	Asn	Gln	His	Leu	Cys	Gly	Ser	His	Leu	Val	Glu	Ala	Leu	Tyr	Leu	Val	Cys	Gly	Glu	Arg	Gly	Phe	Phe	Tyr	Thr	Pro	Lys	Thr	—
Rat 1	—	—	Phe	Val	Lys	Gln	His	Leu	Cys	Gly	Pro	His	Leu	Val	Glu	Ala	Leu	Tyr	Leu	Val	Cys	Gly	Glu	Arg	Gly	Phe	Phe	Tyr	Thr	Pro	Lys	Ser	—
Rat 2	—	—	Phe	Val	Lys	Gln	His	Leu	Cys	Gly	Pro	His	Leu	Val	Glu	Ala	Leu	Tyr	Leu	Val	Cys	Gly	Glu	Arg	Gly	Phe	Phe	Tyr	Thr	Pro	Lys	Ser	—
Guinea pig	—	—	Phe	Val	Ser	Arg	His	Leu	Cys	Gly	Ser	Asn	Leu	Val	Glu	Thr	Leu	Tyr	Ser	Val	Cys	Gln	Asp	Asp	Gly	Phe	Phe	Tyr	Ile	Pro	Lys	Asp	—
Casiragua	—	—	Tyr	Val	Gln	Arg	His	Leu	Cys	Gly	Ser	Gln	Leu	Val	Asp	Thr	Leu	Tyr	Leu	Val	Cys	Lys	His	Arg	Gly	Phe	Phe	Tyr	Arg	Pro	Ser	Glu	—
Coypu	—	—	Tyr	Val	Ser	Gln	His	Leu	Cys	Gly	Ser	Gln	Leu	Val	Asp	Ala	Leu	Tyr	Leu	Ala	Cys	Tyr	Arg	Arg	Gly	Phe	Phe	Tyr	Arg	Pro	Thr	Lys	Met
Hagfish	Arg	Thr	Thr	Gly	His	Leu	Cys	Gly	Lys	Asp	Leu	Val	Asn	Ala	Leu	Tyr	Ile	Ala	Cys	Gly	Val	Arg	Gly	Phe	Phe	Tyr	Asp	Pro	Thr	Lys	—	—	—
Insulin-like Growth factor																																	
IGF 1	—	—	Gly	—	Pro	Glu	Thr	Leu	Cys	Gly	Ala	Glu	Leu	Val	Asp	Ala	Leu	Gln	Phe	Val	Cys	Gly	Asp	Arg	Gly	Phe	Tyr	Phe	Asn	Lys	Pro	Thr	—
IGF 2	Ala	Tyr	Arg	Pro	Ser	Glu	Thr	Leu	Cys	Gly	Gly	Glu	Leu	Val	Asp	Thr	Leu	Gln	Phe	Val	Cys	Gly	Asp	Arg	Gly	Phe	Tyr	Phe	Ser	Arg	Pro	Ala	—
Relaxin																																	
Porcine	Ser	Thr	Asn	Asp	Phe	Ile	Lys	Ala	Cys	Gly	Arg	Glu	Leu	Val	Arg	Leu	Trp	Val	Glu	Ile	Cys	Gly	Ser	Val	Ser	Trp	Gly	Arg	—	—	—	Ser	

C-peptides / Connecting peptides

	1	2	3	4	5	6	7	8	9	10	11	12	13	14	15	16	17	18	19	20	21	22	23	24	25	26	27	28	29	30	31	32	33	34	35
Insulin																																			
Bovine	Arg	Arg	Glu	Val	Glu	Gly	Pro	Gln	Val	Gly	Ala	Leu	Glu	Leu	Ala	Gly	Gly	Pro	Gly	Ala	Gly	Gly	Leu	—	—	Glu	Gly	Pro	Pro	Gln	Lys	Arg			
Human	Arg	Arg	Glu	Ala	Glu	Asp	Leu	Gln	Val	Gly	Gln	Val	Glu	Leu	Gly	Gly	Gly	Pro	Gly	Ala	Gly	Ser	Leu	Gln	Pro	Leu	Ala	Leu	Glu	Gly	Ser	Leu	Gln	Lys	Arg
Rat 1	Arg	Arg	Glu	Val	Glu	Asp	Pro	Gln	Val	Pro	Gln	Leu	Glu	Leu	Gly	Gly	Gly	Pro	Glu	Ala	Gly	Asp	Leu	Gln	Thr	Leu	Ala	Leu	Glu	Val	Ala	Arg	Gln	Lys	Arg
Rat 2	Arg	Arg	Glu	Val	Glu	Asp	Pro	Gln	Val	Ala	Gln	Leu	Glu	Leu	Gly	Gly	Gly	Pro	Gly	Ala	Gly	Asp	Leu	Gln	Thr	Leu	Ala	Leu	Glu	Val	Ala	Arg	Gln	Lys	Arg
Guinea pig	X	X	Glu	Leu	Glu	Asp	Pro	Gln	Val	Glu	Gln	Thr	Glu	Leu	Gly	Met	Gly	Leu	Gly	Ala	Gly	Gly	Leu	Gln	Pro	Leu	Ala	Leu	Glu	Gly	Ala	Leu	Gln	X	X
Insulin-like Growth factor																																			
IGF 1	—	—	—	—	Gly	Tyr	Gly	Ser	Ser	Ser	Arg	Arg	Ala	Pro	Gln	Thr																			
IGF 2	—	—	—	—	Ser	Arg	Val	Ser	Arg	Arg	Ser	Arg																							

of man in only 38% of the residues, it can be calculated that amino acid substitutions (19 of 51 residues) have occurred in insulin at a rate of ~1 × 10⁻⁹ site/year; this is a typical figure for a highly conserved protein.

D. Crowfoot-Hodgkin and associates have determined via X-ray crystallographic techniques the three-dimensional structure of porcine insulin at a 1.9 Å resolution (see Fig. 7-7). Insulin can exist as a monomer, a dimer, or a hexamer. The insulin dimers in the crystalline state are held together by hydrogen bonds between the peptide groups of residues B-24 and B-26 which form an antiparallel pleated sheet structure (see Fig. 7-8). The hexameric structure of crystalline insulin consists of three dimers ordered around a major threefold axis containing two zinc atoms, each coordinated at the imidazole groups of three B-10 histidine residues (see Fig. 7-8). Indeed, the propensity for insulin to crystallize into hexamers may be related to the regular arrays seen in the electron microscopic evaluation of the storage granules of the β cell.

While for many years it was thought that insulin was not a member of

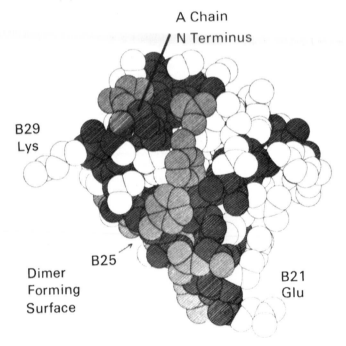

A Chain

N Terminus

B29
Lys

B25

Dimer
Forming
Surface

B21
Glu

Figure 7-7. Three-dimensional structure of the monomeric form of porcine insulin oriented perpendicular to the threefold axis. Only the side chains of known invariant residues are shown. Modified from T. L. Blundell, Chemistry and structure of insulin. *Adv. Protein Chem.* **26,** 279 (1972).

Monomer   Hexamer

Dimer   Tetramer

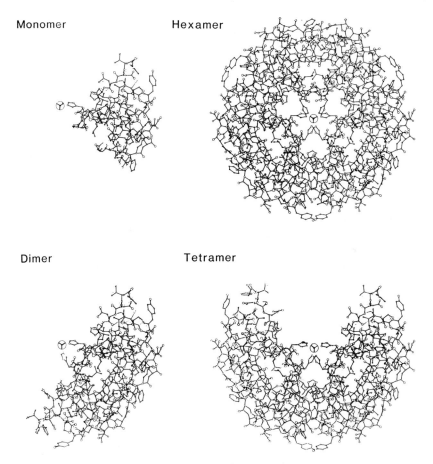

Figure 7-8. Hexameric, dimeric, and monomeric forms of insulin showing the development of dimers from monomers and their organization into the hexamer. The insulin structures were obtained courtesy of G. G. Dodson (York University) and redrawn by F. D. Coffman (University of California at Riverside).

any hormone family, either in a structural sense (e.g., oxytocin and vasopressin are structural analogs of one another) or in a protein-processing sense (proopiomelanocortin produces β-lipotropin, ACTH, endorphins, etc.), it now appears that there is a hormone family of homologous growth factors which includes proteins with regions of amino acid sequences identical to insulin. These include the following: (1) relaxin (a polypeptide hormone from the corpus luteum which is responsible for the dilation of the symphysis pubis prior to parturition); (2) insulin-like growth factors (IGFs) I or II (formerly known as NSILA or nonsuppressible insulin-like activity); (3) somatomedins (particularly somatomedin C); and possibly (4) nerve growth factor (NGF). Some of these factors are discussed in further detail in Chapter 19.

B. Glucagon

Glucagon, which is secreted by the α cells of the pancreas, has a molecular weight of 3450. It is the most potent hepatic glycogenolytic agent known. The amino acid sequence of glucagon is presented in Fig. 7-9. In contrast to insulin, glucagon is composed of a single amino acid chain of 29 residues and is devoid of disulfide linkages. To date the amino acid sequences of rat, rabbit, human, porcine, bovine, turkey, chicken, and duck glucagons have been determined. There is a high degree of structural conservation in all these peptides.

The secondary and tertiary structure of glucagon has been studied in solution by optical rotary dispersion/circular dichroism and in the crystalline state via X-ray crystallography (3 Å resolution). In dilute solutions, the glucagon peptide, due to its relatively short chain length, is flexible, with many different conformations and some indication of a stable interaction between valine-23 and tryptophan-25. In more concentrated solutions and in the crystalline state the molecules self-associated into α-helical trimers. The helical region extends from residues 6 to 27 and results in the formation of two hydrophobic "sticky" patches which are involved in the self-association process. Thus, the glucagon mole-

```
     1   2   3   4   5   6   7   8   9   10  11  12  13  14
NH₂-His-Ser-Gln-Gly-Thr-Phe-Thr-Ser-Asp-Tyr-Ser-Lys-Tyr-Leu-


    15  16  17  18  19  20  21  22  23  24  25  26  27  28  29
  -Asp-Ser-Arg-Arg-Ala-Gln-Asp-Phe-Val-Gln-Trp-Leu-Met-Asn-Thr-CO₂H
       Thr                                              Ser


    30  31  32  33  34  35  36  37
  -Lys-Arg-Asn-Asn-Lys-Asn-Ile-Ala-CO₂H
```

Figure 7-9. Primary amino acid sequence of glucagon (amino acid positions 1–29) and a fragment (amino acid positions 30–37) of the C-terminal proglucagon. This is the sequence for human, bovine, and porcine glucagon; the two amino acid substitutions for avian glucagon at positions 16 and 28 are shown beneath the sequence. Reproduced with permission from D. F. Steiner and H. S. Tager, Biosynthesis of insulin and glucagon. *In* "Endocrinology" (L. J. DeGroot, G. F. Cahill, L. Martini, D. H. Nelson, W. D. Odell, J. T. Potts, E. Steinberger, and A. I. Winegrad, eds.), Vol. 2, p. 929. Grune & Stratton, New York, 1979.

cule is unique among medium-sized polypeptides. Although it has a clearly definable secondary structure (α helix) and quaternary structure (self-association), it has no definable tertiary structure.

From biological studies it has been determined that virtually the entire glucagon peptide chain is required for optimal interaction with the glucagon-sensitive adenylate cyclase of hepatocyte membranes. The evidence suggests that glucagon binds to its receptor as a consequence of entropic considerations, resulting in the selection of the optimal solution helical conformer which has an available hydrophobic region for stereoselective interaction with the membrane receptor.

Glucagon also is structurally homologous with a family of peptide hormones found in the gastrointestinal tract. These include secretin, vasoactive intestinal polypeptide (VIP), and gastric inhibitory peptide (GIP), and glicentin (a 100 amino acid peptide isolated from the intestine). Interestingly, glicentin has many of the immunodeterminants of glucagon and can account for much of the glucagon-like activity of the intestine.

C. Pancreatic Polypeptide

Pancreatic polypeptide (PP) is a 36 amino acid peptide which appears to stimulate the gastric secretion of HCl and pepsin; it also may act as a satiety factor. PP is known to be released after a protein meal.

The amino acid sequence of several PP is given in Fig. 7-10. All sequenced PP have amidated carboxy termini. With the exception of the avian PP, which has 20 out of 36 residues different from human PP, there is strict conservation of sequences (only 2–3 amino acid differences) among the other four sequenced PP species.

Like insulin, PP molecules can self-associate to dimers; in addition, the avian PP, like insulin in the presence of zinc ions, can form higher oligomers. Because a homologous polypeptide has been isolated from pig intestine, it has been proposed that PP may be a member of a larger family of pancreatic-gastroenteric hormones.

D. Somatostatin

Somatostatin is the smallest of the pancreatic hormones; it contains 14 amino acids and one disulfide bridge (see Fig. 3-8). Although somatostatin was originally discovered in the hypothalamus, it is also known to be produced by the δ cells of the endocrine pancreas and dispersed cells in the gastrointestinal tract.

	1	2	3	4	5	6	7	8	9	10	11	12	13	14	15	16	17	18
Bovine	Ala	Pro	Leu	Glu	Pro	Gln	Tyr	Pro	Gly	Asp	Asp	Ala	Thr	Pro	Glu	Gln	Met	Ala
Human	Ala	Pro	Leu	Glu	Pro	Val	Tyr	Pro	Gly	Asp	Asp	Ala	Thr	Pro	Glu	Gln	Met	Ala
Ovine	Ala	Ser	Leu	Glu	Pro	Gln	Tyr	Pro	Gly	Asp	Asp	Ala	Thr	Pro	Glu	Gln	Met	Ala
Porcine	Ala	Pro	Leu	Glu	Pro	Val	Tyr	Pro	Gly	Asp	Asp	Ala	Thr	Pro	Glu	Gln	Met	Ala
Avian	Gly	Pro	Ser	Gln	Pro	Thr	Tyr	Pro	Gly	Asp	Asp	Ala	Pro	Val	Glu	Asp	Leu	Ile

	19	20	21	22	23	24	25	26	27	28	29	30	31	32	33	34	35	36
Bovine	Gln	Tyr	Ala	Ala	Gln	Leu	Arg	Arg	Tyr	Ile	Asn	Met	Leu	Thr	Arg	Pro	Arg	Tyr-NH$_2$
Human	Gln	Tyr	Ala	Ala	Asp	Leu	Arg	Arg	Tyr	Ile	Asn	Met	Leu	Thr	Arg	Pro	Arg	Tyr-NH$_2$
Ovine	Gln	Tyr	Ala	Ala	Glu	Leu	Arg	Arg	Tyr	Ile	Asn	Met	Leu	Thr	Arg	Pro	Arg	Tyr-NH$_2$
Porcine	Gln	Tyr	Ala	Ala	Glu	Leu	Arg	Arg	Tyr	Ile	Asn	Met	Leu	Thr	Arg	Pro	Arg	Tyr-NH$_2$
Avian	Arg	Phe	Tyr	Asp	Asn	Leu	Gln	Gln	Tyr	Leu	Asn	Val	Val	Thr	Arg	His	Arg	Tyr-NH$_2$

Figure 7-10. Primary amino acid sequence of bovine, human, ovine, porcine, and avian pancreatic polypeptides. Reproduced with permission from B. M. Jaffe, Hormones of the gastrointestinal tract. In "Endocrinology" (L. J. DeGroot, G. F. Cahill, L. Martini, D. H. Nelson, W. D. Odell, J. T. Potts, E. Steinberger, and A. I. Winegrad, eds.), Vol. 3, p. 1676. Grune & Stratton, New York, 1979.

IV. BIOCHEMISTRY

A. Biosynthesis of Hormones

1. Biosynthesis of Insulin

a. Identification of Proinsulin. For years one of the intriguing problems relating to insulin biosynthesis was that of describing the independent synthesis of the separate A and B chains followed by the correct formation of the three disulfide linkages. It was not at all clear whether these formed spontaneously based on peptide chain folding, conformation, and entropic considerations, or whether there were specialized "biological mechanisms" which mediated this precise process. The discovery by D. F. Steiner and colleagues in 1967 of proinsulin provided a resolution to this knotty problem.

Proinsulin is a precursor form of insulin which exists as a single-chain polypeptide of ~9000 Da; this chain contains within its sequence the 21 amino acid residues of the A chain and the 30 residues of the B chain of insulin. In addition, it contains a connecting sequence, known as the C peptide, which falls between the N terminus of the A chain and the C terminus of the B chain (see Fig. 7-11). It is now clear that proinsulin represents an intermediate species that appears on the biosynthetic pathway leading from the immediate polysomal translation product to the final β granule stored form of insulin. An extensive number of secreted proteins and hormonal peptides is now known to be synthesized in pro- or pre-pro- forms. These are all typically processed similar to proinsulin at an intracellular site [i.e., the rough endoplasmic reticulum (RER) for the peptide and the Golgi]. In the case of proinsulin, the excised C peptide is stored in the secretory granule with mature insulin.

Mammalian proinsulins contain from 78 (dog) to 86 (rat, man, horse) amino acid residues; these variations in amino acid units reflect only differences in the length of the connecting sequence between the A and B chains. Theoretically it is not necessary to have a connecting sequence of 28–36 amino acid residues; from model-building exercises related to the tertiary structure of insulin (Fig. 7-8) it appears that only 5–8 residues would be minimally required. The additional residues do not completely "mask" the biological activity of the molecule, since proinsulin contains 3–5% of the biological activity of native insulin.

Both the prospective N and C termini of the C peptide of all known mammalian proinsulins end in a pair of basic amino acid residues (either lysine or arginine). These represent the recognition signals for the pro-

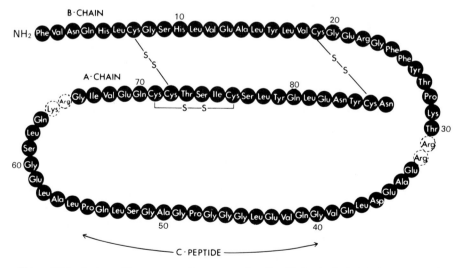

Figure 7-11. Amino acid sequence of human proinsulin. Circles in dashes indicate sites of cleavage. Modified from P. E. Oyer, S. Cha, J. D. Peterson, and D. F. Steiner, *J. Biol. Chem.* **246**, 1384 (1971).

288

teolytic cleavage that is necessary for conversion of proinsulin to insulin. To date the amino acid composition of the C peptide is known for nine mammalian and one avian species (see Fig. 7-12). It is apparent that there is a much higher rate of mutation in the C peptide than in the A or B chains of the related insulins; this is consistent with the hypothesis that the C peptide does not have any extrapancreatic hormonal function. The C peptide is secreted in equimolar amounts with insulin and is known to circulate in the blood; there are now available radioimmunoassays to measure this peptide.

   b. Biosynthetic Pathway for Insulin. There is now conclusive evidence that in the same species of animals (e.g., the laboratory rat, mouse, and spiny mouse, as well as the tuna and toadfish) two different insulins may be biosynthesized and secreted. In the rat, insulin I has three amino acid differences from insulin II. This implies that these different insulins in the same species are derived from two nonallelic insulin genes. Tumors deprived from single cells are known to produce both insulins simultaneously.

   H. Goodman and colleagues have determined the complete nucleotide sequence coding for rat insulin I and also for human insulin,

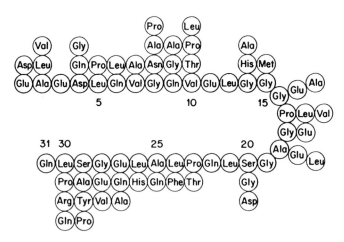

Figure 7-12. Amino acid sequence of human proinsulin C peptide combined with the known substitutions occurring in eight other mammalian species; one avian C peptide is also included. Deletions occur in the dog (residues 4–11), pig (residues 18 and 19), sheep and ox (residues 22–26), and guinea pig (residues 25 and 26). (These sequences do not include the basic residues at either end which link the C peptide to the insulin chains.) Reproduced with permission from D. F. Steiner and H. S. Tager, Biosynthesis of insulin and glucagon. *In* "Endocrinology" (L. J. DeGroot, G. F. Cahill, L. Martini, D. H. Nelson, W. D. Odell, J. T. Potts, E. Steinberger, and A. I. Winegrad, eds), Vol. 2, p. 928. Grune & Stratton, New York, 1979.

while D. Steiner and M. Efstradiates have determined the sequence coding for rat insulin II (Fig. 7-13). The rat insulins were found to contain an intervening sequence of 119 nucleotides in the untranslated 5' end of the mRNA. A major difference in the gene structure for rat insulins I and II was discovered; species II, but not species I, contains an additional 499 nucleotide intervening sequence in the middle of the region coding for the connecting C peptide. The gene for the human insulin also has an intervening sequence in this locus; however, it is 786 nucleotides long (see Fig. 7-14). The insulin genes of the chicken, dog, guinea pig, and hagfish all contain both introns, indicating that the canonical insulin gene in vertebrates has this structure. The gene for rat I insulin has lost the second intron during its duplication, which was a relatively recent evolutionary event.

As is the case with other secreted proteins (e.g., parathyroid hormone, honeybee mellitin, myeloma L chains, and serum albumin), in insulin-proinsulin the immediate translation product released from the polyribosomes has an N-terminal extension or "leader sequence" of ~ 23 amino acid residues (see Fig. 7-15). This product released from the polysomes is designated preproinsulin [by analogy, see preproparathyroid hormone (Fig. 9-4)]. The hydrophobic N terminus or leader sequence has been postulated to facilitate and direct the insertion and transfer of the nascent peptide across the membrane bilayer of the endoplasmic reticulum. This results in the "packaging" of the protein within a secretory granule which protects it from the environment of the cytoplasmic compartment of the cell and facilitates its export from the cell. As detailed in Fig. 7-15, preproinsulin is processed sequentially first to proinsulin and then to insulin. The formation of the three crucial insulin disulfide linkages is believed to occur spontaneously either while the almost complete nascent peptide is still attached to the polysome or immediately after insertion into the secretion granules.

The conversion of proinsulin to insulin is believed to occur in both the Golgi and the β granule. The proteolytic cleavages necessary for this transformation are detailed in Fig. 7-16; they require the sequential action of a trypsin-like protease and then a carboxypeptidase-like enzyme to remove the remaining basic amino acids which splice the C peptide between the A and B chains of insulin. As yet these specialized proteases have not been biochemically characterized in the pancreas. It is known that equimolar quantities of the C peptide are stored in the β granule and that C peptide is secreted at the time the β granule undergoes exocytosis. As the insulin is released from the proinsulin, it tends to crystallize with the relatively high levels of zinc ions which are present in the β granule. Morphological studies have shown that the re-

```
gH    156 ATCTGCCGACCCCCCCACCCCGCCCT:AATGGGCCAGGCGGCAGGGGTTGACAGGTAGGG
gRI     1 G CTA CTA    T :TAGA    T        AA  :TCAAA A T CATGG

                                                          *cap
      215 GAGATGGG::::CTCTGAGAC(TATAAAG)CCAGCGGGGGCCCAGCAGCCCTC AGCCCTCCA
       59 C   GA AGGTGCT TG        T  T AA T T AT C   A      AAG

                                   IVS1
      272 GGACAGGCTGCA:TCAGAAGAGGCCAT:::CAAGCAG (GTCTGTTCCAAGGGCCTTTGCGTCAG
      119 T   CA A  A   T:   ::   CAG        A   A TCTCCTGGG GAGCC G
      ------------------------------------------------------------

                                                  *cap
gH    221 GGGCTCTGAGAC[TATAAAG]CCAGCGGGGGCCCAGCAGCTCTC AGCCCTCCAGGACAGGCT
gRII    1 TGCT TG        T  T     ATT  T AT C      AAGT  CA

                             IVS1
      281 GCA:TCAGAAGAGGCCATCAAGCAG (GTCTGTTCCAAGGGCCTTTGCGTCAGGTGGGCTCA
       61 A G  G    ACCAT G        A   A :::::::::: CTCCA     CT

      340 TGGTTCCAGGGTGGCTGGACCCCAGGCCCCAGCTCTGCAGCAGGGAGGACGTGGCTGGGC
      111 CT C  CA :::::::::::::::::::::::::::::::::::::::::::::::::::::

      400 TCGTGAAGCATGTGGGGGTGAGCCCAGGGGCCCCAAGGCAGGGCACCTGGCCTTCAGCCT
      121   AA  CT CAAG ATTTGAG GA GCT TGGG TCTT TCTTACATGTA     TT  TA

                     IVS1                           fMet
      460 GCCTCAGCCCTGCCTGTCTCCCAG) ATCACTGTCCTTCTGCC ATGGCCCTGTGGATGCGCC
      181     A   A A  T       G  T   T :::CAA            C  T

      520 TCCTGCCCCTGCTGGCGCTGCTGGCCCTCTGGGGACCTGACCCAGCCGCAGCCTTTGTGA
      238           C    CAT      AG CCG   T  CAG T    C

      580 ACCAACACCTGTGCGGCTCACACCTGGTGGAAGCTCTCTACCTAGTGTGCGGGGAACGAG
      298 A G      T T T T  T              G    T    G T

                                            V IVS2
      640 GCTTCTTCTACACACCCAAGACCCGCCGGGAGGCAGAGGACCTGCAGG (GTGAGCCAACCG
      358 A          T T    C  A TG      CA A    A   ::::::

      700 CCCATTGCTGCCCCTGGCCGCCCCCAGCCACCCCCTGCTCCTGGCGCTCCCACCCAGCAT
      412 ::::::::::::::::::::::::::::::::T       :::::::::::::::::

      820 AAGTTCTCTTGGTCACGTCCTAAAAGTGACCAGCTCCCTGTGGCCCAGTCAGAATCTCAG
      422 ::::::::::::::::::::::::::::::::::::::::::::::::::::::::::::::

      880 CCTGAGGACGGTGTTGGCTTCGGCAGCCCCGAGATACATCAGAGGGTGGGCACGCTCCTC
      422 ::::::::::::::::::::::::::::::::::::::::::::::::::::::::::::::

      940 CCTCCACTCGCCCCCTCAAACAAATGCCCCGCAGCCCATTTCTCCACCCTCATTTGATGAC
      422 ::::::::::::::::::::::::::::::::::::::::::::::::::::AA TC AT

     1000 CGCAGATTCAAGTGTTTTGTTAACTAAAGTCCTGGGTGACCAGGGGTCACAGGGTGCCCT
      431 CA  TGCT  C ACCC      TGTCTTTCA  CTT A    TT TAAATTGT CCCTAGG

     1060 ACGCTGCCTGCCTCTGGGCGAACACCCCATCACGCCCGGAGGAGGGCGTGGCTGCCTGCC
      491 TGTGGAGGGT TCAC CTAACCAGTGGGGGGCACATTTCT TG  CA CTAGACATATGT

     1120 TGAGCGGGCCAGACCCCTGTCGCCAGCCTCACGGCAGCTCCATAGTCAGGAGATGGGGAA
      551 AA CAT  TAGCTG  AA AA GAGTGAGA TCCTTC  TA GTC  CTAG TG T ACG

     1180 GATGCTGGGGACAGGCCCTGGGGAGAAGTACTGGGATCACCTGTTCAGGCTCCCACTGTG
      611 G  GCTA  C CCAGGA A  T CCTA TTG    C  C A AGAGCACTG A TGAC

     1240 ACGCTGCCCCGGGGCGGGGGAAGGAGGTGGGACATGTGGGCGTTGGGGCCTGTAGGTCCA
      671 G GATGGTAACA GAT T  T   TTT   AGGCCCATATGTCCATTCATGACCA  GAC

     1300 CACCCAGTGTGGGTGACCCTCCCTCTAACCTGGGTCCAGCCCGGCTGGAGATGGGTGGGA
      731 TTGT TCACA CCATG AAC  T GCCT    T CTG CTTA CAG GATAAA   A

     1360 GTGCGACCTAGGGCTGGCGGGCAGGCGGGCACTGTGTCTCCCTGACTGTGTCCTCCTGTG
      791 AAA CTTGG CTAATCA   GGTCGCTCAG  CCTC AA   GA GTGTC TATG    C

                                               IVS2  a1
     1420 TCCCTCTGCCTCGCCGCTGTTCCGGAACCTGCTCTGCGCGGCACGTCCTGGCAG) TGGGGC
      851 TTGCT CTG GCTGCTGA G TCTGC    TC  ACAT AC TC         CA

     1480 AGGTGGAGCTGGGCGGGGGGCCCTGGTGCAGCGAGCCTGCAGCCCTTGGCCCTGGAGGGCT
      911 AC     T  A   G G C TGA T  A      A       T G

     1540 CCCTGCAGAAGCGTGGCATTGTGGAACAATGCTGTACCAGCATCTGCTCCCTCTACCAGC
      971 G       C   C    T G  C           T       A

                   AM
     1600 TGGAGAACTACTGCAACTAG ACGCAGCCTGCAGGCAGCCCCACACCCGCCGCCTCCTGCA
     1031              ::::::::::::::::::::::GC CA  A TA  CTG C

             poly(A)
     1660 CCGAGAGAGATGGAATAAAGCCCTTGAACCAGC CCTGCTGTGCCGTTCTGTGTCTGGGGG
     1071    CCTCTGC AT     A T      AG    A  A AAGTTGTG G ACA GC T CA

     1720 CCCTGGGCAAGCCCCA
     1131 TGTGCATATGTGGTGC
```

peating units characteristic of mature pancreatic β granules are quite similar to that found in the *in vitro* crystallized hexameric zinc insulin.

2. Biosynthesis of Glucagon

Much evidence has been accumulated to support the model that glucagon-like insulin is biosynthesized by way of a higher molecular weight precursor. These studies have been facilitated by the use of ^{3}H-labeled tryptophan because this amino acid occurs in glucagon but not insulin. Higher molecular weight biosynthetic species ($\sim$9,000–12,000) have been detected in the islet tissues of mammals, birds, and fish. In the angler fish a proglucagon of 78 amino acid residues has been isolated; it has been tentatively concluded that the 29 amino acids of glucagon reside in the amino-terminal protein of the pro species. Thus, the pro form of glucagon apparently represents a C-terminal extension of glucagon in marked contrast to the N-terminal extension of preproinsulin and the signal hypothesis for secreted proteins.

B. Secretion of Pancreatic Hormones

1. Background

The process of the regulated and integrated secretion of insulin and glucagon is very complex. Independently the α and β cells are ex-

---

Figure 7-13. Homology of the human insulin gene with the rat insulin I and II genes. The human insulin gene sequence (gH) is compared with the sequence of the rat genes for insulin I (gRI) and insulin II (gRII). "Maximum" homology was achieved by suitable additions, indicated in the sequence by colons, and by using a computer homology program. The program allows editing and moving of sequences while comparing one against the other. The upper, continuous sequence is that of the human gene. The lower, discontinuous sequence indicates the nature of the differences between the human and rat genes. The absence of a nucleotide in the lower sequence indicates that the human and rat sequences are the same; the presence of a colon in either sequence indicates a gap equal in length to the number of colons to be added to achieve maximum homology. The Hogness sequence, TATAAAG, is bracketed. The positions of the putative 5' end (capping site, *cap) and 3' end [poly(A) addition site; poly(A)] of the mRNA are indicated. The intervening sequences are indicated within parentheses and the left and right borders marked IVS1 or 2, respectively. The occurrence of IVS2 between the first and second base of the valine codon at proinsulin amino acid position 39 is indicated by a "V" at the left-hand boundary and "al" at the right. The initiation codon for preproinsulin is designated "fMet." The numbers in the left margin refer to the human sequence. The upper panel presents the homology of the human insulin gene with the rat insulin I gene in the region before the first intervening sequence (IVS1), and the lower panel the entire homology of the human insulin gene with that of rat insulin II. A schematic diagram of these three insulin genes is given in Fig. 7-14. Reproduced with permission from G. I. Bell, R. I. Pictet, W. J. Rutter, B. Cordell, E. Tischer, and H. M. Goodman, Sequence of the human insulin gene. *Nature (London)* **284,** 26–32 (1980). © 1980 Macmillan Journals Limited.

292

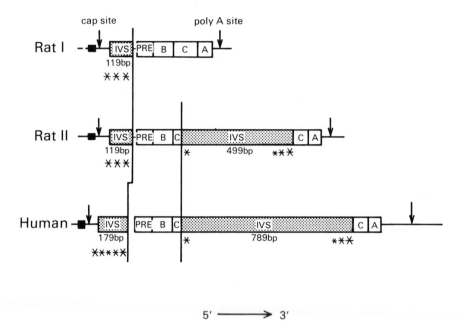

Figure 7-14. Schematic comparison of human insulin gene to rat insulin I and rat insulin II genes (see also Fig. 7-13). The topology of the two rat insulin genes (I and II) and the single human insulin gene is displayed. The coding sequences for the peptide chains (pre-, B, C, and A) of preproinsulin are represented by the clear boxes. Intervening sequences (IVS) are distinguished by the shaded areas, with the length of each intervening sequence indicated below. The extent and position of nucleotide homology between intervening sequences of the two species are represented by the size of the asterisks—the larger the asterisk, the greater the homology. Vertical lines describe the positions at which intervening sequences occur. The internal intervening sequence in the rat II and the human gene occurs in exactly the same position (valine 39 of the C-peptide region), whereas the position of the intervening sequence located in the 5'FT untranslated region is displaced by three nucleotides in the human gene as compared with both rat genes. Also indicated are the sites for polyadenylation and capping (shown by arrows) as well as the Hogness box, a potential site for the initiation of transcription (indicated by the small black box). The arrow indicates the direction of transcription. Reproduced with permission from G. I. Bell, R. I. Pictet, W. J. Rutter, B. Cordell, E. Tischer, and H. M. Goodman, Sequence of the human insulin gene. *Nature (London)* **284,** 26–32 (1980). © 1980 Macmillan Journals Limited.

quisitely sensitive glucose detectors; the output of glucagon is stimulated by a falling blood glucose while the output of insulin is stimulated by a rising blood glucose. Together the pancreatic cells function as a "fuel molecule" homeostat for the organism. The β cell can be envisioned as a fuel receptor which is responsible for the minute-to-minute monitoring of the changes in the organism's supply of calorigenic mole-

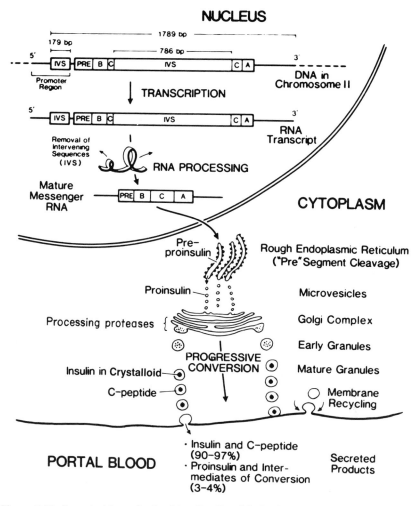

Figure 7-15. Steps in biosynthesis of insulin. Simplified scheme depicting molecular biological aspects of insulin formation. The proinsulin gene is represented schematically (upper panel). RNA polymerase is necessary for the transcription of preproinsulin messenger RNA (mRNA) from the gene and this then serves to guide the formation of preproinsulin chains on the polyribosomes. Preproinsulin is vectorially discharged and cleaved to proinsulin (center panel). The proinsulin is then transferred to the Golgi region where conversion to insulin and storage in secretion granules begin. Reproduced with permission from D. F. Steiner and H. S. Tager, Biosynthesis of insulin and glucagon. *In* "Endocrinology" (L. J. DeGroot, G. F. Cahill, L. Martini, D. H. Nelson, W. D. Odell, J. T. Potts, E. Steinberger, and A. I. Winegrad, eds.), Vol. 2, p. 926. Grune & Stratton, New York, 1979.

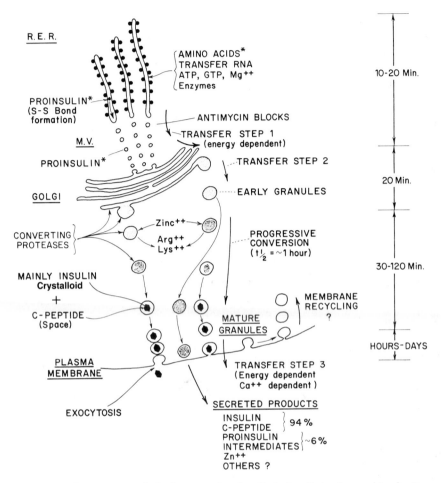

Figure 7-16. Steps in proteolytic cleavage of proinsulin to insulin by the combined action of trypsin-like and carboxypeptidase B-like proteases. Reproduced with permission from D. F. Steiner and H. S. Tager, Biosynthesis of insulin and glucagon. *In* "Endocrinology" (L. J. DeGroot, G. F. Cahill, L. Martini, D. H. Nelson, W. D. Odell, J. T. Potts, E. Steinberger, and A. I. Winegrad, eds.), Vol. 2, p. 927. Grune & Stratton, New York, 1979.

cules. The β cell secretes insulin in response to D-glucose, L-amino acids, fatty acids, and ketones. There are no known inhibitors of β cell function among the fuel molecules. However, insulin is only released by the β cell in response to the L-amino acids, fatty acids, and ketones in the presence of glucose. In contrast, α cells can be stimulated to secrete glucagon by L-amino acids and fatty acids in the absence of glucose; also, D-glucose is a potent inhibitor of glucagon release. These relationships are summarized in Table 7-7.

Table 7–7. Fuel Receptor Properties of Pancreatic α and β Cells

Stimulators of hormone secretion	Permissive agent	Inhibitors	Inert glycolytic metabolites
α Cells			
L-Amino acids	—	D-Glucose	⎰ Glycerol
Fatty acids	—		⎱ Pyruvate
β Cells			Lactate
D-Glucose	—		⎰ Glycerol
L-Amino acids ⎱			⎰ Pyruvate
Fatty acids ⎰	D-Glucose		⎱ Lactate
Ketones ⎱			

The typical response of both α and β cells to a maximal physiological signal for secretion is a biphasic output of their characteristic hormones (see Fig. 7-17). Thus, in the isolated pancreas, infusion of 20 m*M* D-glucose will elicit within 1 min a rapid burst of insulin secretion; this will be followed by a resting interval of 5–7 min and then a slowly rising "second phase" of insulin secretion which will last as long as the glucose is present. A similar biphasic release pattern is followed when the α cells sense the presence of 1–5 m*M* amino acids in the absence of glucose.

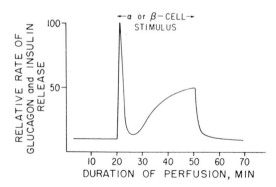

Figure 7-17. A typical biphasic hormone-releasing profile as seen with the isolated perfused pancreas from different species as a result of α or β cell stimulation. Reproduced with permission from F. M. Matschinsky, A. A. Pagliara, W. S. Zawalich, and M. D. Trus, Metabolism of pancreatic islets and regulation of insulin and glucagon secretion. *In* "Endocrinology" (L. J. DeGroot, G. F. Cahill, L. Martini, D. H. Nelson, W. D. Odell, J. T. Potts, E. Steinberger, and A. I. Winegrad, eds.), Vol. 2, p. 936. Grune & Stratton, New York, 1979.

2. Secretion of Insulin

Insulin is secreted from the β cells of the pancreatic islets by the process of emiocytosis (see Fig. 7-18). In this process the granules inside the cell are believed to migrate to the peripheral cell membrane down or along a microtubular network. In the region of the cell membrane the microtubules coalesce into a microfilamentous network that is immediately adjacent to the cell membrane. This microfilamentous system which contains actin has fibers that are 50–70 Å in diameter. Once the β granules encounter the cell membrane, there is a fusion of the cell and granule membranes (see Fig. 7-19) which results in the dissolution of the membrane at the point of contact, with concomitant extrusion of the granule contents out of the cell.

The most important physiological secretagogue for insulin release is glucose. It has been proposed that in the β cell specific glucoreceptors which are capable of recognizing D-glucose exist in the plasma membrane; in this regard, α-D-glucopyranose is known to be preferred over β-D-glucopyranose. Three general models of how the β cells respond to secretory stimuli are presented below.

a. Glucose Receptor/Amino Acid Receptor Model of Stimulus Recognition. The islet cells recognize and respond to "fuel molecules," including α-D-glucose and other hexoses, L-amino acids, fatty acids, and ketone bodies (see Table 7-8). This leads then to an activation of the stimulus-secretion process, resulting ultimately in the release of insulin.

b. Fuel Metabolism Model of Stimulus Recognition. The various fuel molecules are recognized as the consequence of their uptake into the β cell and subsequent metabolism via intermediary metabolism. Recognition might consist of the presence of a certain family of key metabolites or cofactors, such as NADH/NAD, ATP, and intracellular pH. This then could lead to activation of the stimulus-secretion mechanism, resulting in insulin secretion.

c. A Third Plausible Model Could Be a Combination of the Two Separate Models Described. Figure 7-20 presents a schematic working model proposed by F. Matschinsky to describe the coupling of the "fuel receptor" to the stimulus-secretion mechanism which results in insulin secretion. A key feature of this model is that it rationalizes two additional important facts relating to insulin secretion: (1) Physiological stimulation of the β cell is dependent upon an optimal concentration as well as intracellular calcium ions; (2) activation of the adenyl cyclase system (by glucagon or phosphodiesterase inhibitors) potentiates insulin release.

It is known that stimulation of the β cells by glucose or other fuel molecules transiently stimulates Ca^{2+} uptake, possibly by an increase in the "Ca^{2+} gate" membrane permeability. The precise role at the mo-

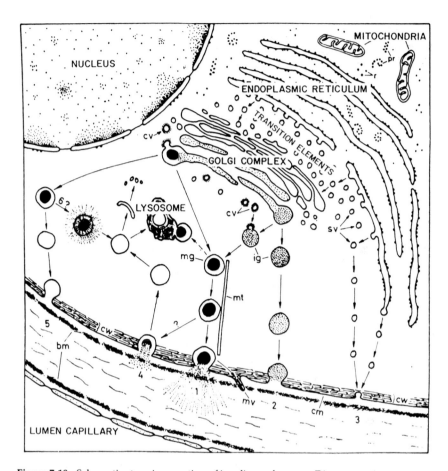

Figure 7-18. Schematic steps in secretion of insulin or glucagon. Diagrammatic representation of the morphological events of the secretory process in an insulin-producing cell. Proinsulin is synthesized on the membrane-associated ribosomes of the endoplasmic reticulum and transferred to the Golgi complex by way of transition elements where the granules are formed. Proinsulin-containing granules which bud from the Golgi cisternae can be hypothesized to be released by one or more of six possible processes: (1) conventional emiocytosis of mature secretory granules in conjunction with contractile microtubular elements; (2) emiocytosis of immature secretory granules; (3) release of microvesicles independent of the Golgi apparatus; (4) release of insulin from the granule as a result of increased permeability of the granular membrane, with retention of the membrane after evacuation of its contents; (5) emiocytosis of granules having previously undergone physical and chemical alteration of granule content; (6) physicochemical change in granule content followed by its passage into the cytoplasm. Although the majority of insulin is probably released by the first process, other methods have not been adequately explored. From A. E. Renold, *Diabetes* **21**, 622 (1971). Reproduced with permission from the American Diabetes Association, Inc.

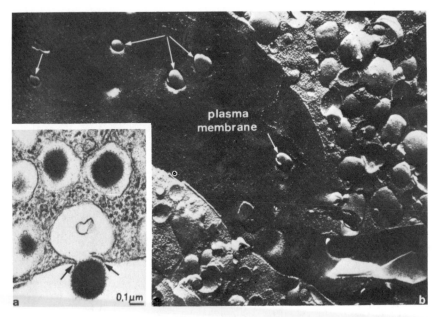

Figure 7-19. Electron micrograph and freeze-fracture study of insulin secretion. Isolated islets were exposed to a high (3.0 mg/ml) glucose concentration. (a) Thin section of part of a β cell. A granule core is being discharged into the extracellular space through the opening resulting from the coalescence of the membrane limiting the granule with the plasma membrane (arrows) (×56,000). (b) Freeze-fracture replica. On the exposed face of the plasma membrane there are several exocytotic (emiocytotic) stomata (thin arrows). The channel extending in the cytoplasm (large arrow) is possibly the result of the fusion of the membrane of several granules whose cores could be discharged through a single aperture in the plasma membrane (×31,000). Courtesy of Dr. Lelio Orci, Geneva. Reproduced with permission from P. E. Lacy and M. H. Greider, Anatomy and ultrastructural organization of pancreatic islets. *In* "Endocrinology" (L. J. DeGroot, G. F. Cahill, L. Martini, D. H. Nelson, W. D. Odell, J. T. Potts, E. Steinberger, and A. I. Winegrad, eds.), Vol. 2, p. 913. Grune & Stratton, New York, 1979.

lecular level of cAMP participation in the overall process is not clear. The altered ionic calcium concentration inside the cell, then in association with other as yet undefined factors, can be projected to initiate a contraction of the microtubule–microfilament system which initiates the emiocytosis process.

In terms of the biphasic secretion of insulin (Fig. 7-17) then, the first acute phase of insulin secretion represents release of insulin already stored in the granules of the β cell. The slower second phase of insulin release is likely supported by an initiation of *de novo* insulin biosynthesis.

Table 7–8. Modulators of Insulin and Glucagon Secretion

Modulator/secretagogue	Insulin secretion[a]	Glucagon secretion
Rising blood glucose	+	−
Falling serum calcium	−	+
Glucagon	+	−
Insulin	NE	−
Glucogenic amino acids		
Alanine, arginine	NE	+
Lysine	+	+
Leucine	+	NE
Growth hormone	+	NE
Nervous stimulation		
Sympathetic (norepinephrine)	−	+
Parasympathetic (epinephrine)	+	−
Stimulators of adenyl cyclase		
Glucagon	+	NE
ACTH	+	NE
TSH	+	NE
Isoproterenol	+	NE
cAMP	+	NE
Oral hypoglycemic agents		
Tolbutamide	+	NE
Chloropromamide	+	NE
Gastrointestinal peptides		
Enteroglucagon	+	NE
Secretin (*in vivo*—but not *in vitro*)	+	−
Cholecystokinin/pancreozymin	+	+
Somatostatin	−	−

[a] A + indicates stimulation of secretion; a − indicates inhibiton of secretion; NE indicates no effect.

3. Secretion of Glucagon

The principal physiological function of the pancreatic α cell is to prevent hypoglycemia by appropriately regulating secretion of glucagon. As documented in Table 7-8, there are an array of substances which are potent modulators of glucagon secretion. In addition, there is evidence of both adrenergic and cholinergic control of glucagon secretion which comes into play during insulin-induced hypoglycemia; this redundant neural mechanism apparently exists to combat the life-threatening situation of hypoglycemia. Glucagon release is clearly stimulated by epinephrine and blocked by the β-adrenergic blocking agent propanolol, which indicates the presence of a β-adrenergic receptor on the D cell membrane. Also, somatostatin can block glucagon release from the D

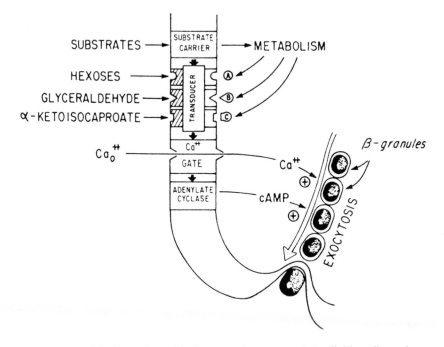

SUBSTRATES ⟶ SUBSTRATE CARRIER ⟶ METABOLISM

HEXOSES ⟶

GLYCERALDEHYDE ⟶

α-KETOISOCAPROATE ⟶

TRANSDUCER

Ⓐ

Ⓑ

Ⓒ

Ca_o^{++}

Ca^{++}

GATE

Ca^{++}

⊕

ADENYLATE CYCLASE

cAMP

⊕

β-granules

EXOCYTOSIS

Figure 7-20. Model of hypothetical fuel receptor in a pancreatic β cell. The cell membrane of the islet cell is postulated to contain five coupled systems: (1) the substrate carriers, which may or may not function as fuel receptors; (2) a receptor–transducer complex with fuel receptors (e.g., for hexoses, glyceraldehyde, and α-ketoisocaproate) on the outside and sites for various fuel-derived metabolites and cofactors (e.g., A, B, C) on the inside of the membrane; (3) a Ca^{2+} gate that controls Ca^{2+} entry; (4) the adenylate cyclase system; and (5) the secretory complex comprised of microtubule and secretory granules involved in the process of exocytosis driven by Ca^{2+} and cAMP. Modified from F. M. Matschinsky, A. A. Pagliara, W. S. Zawalich, and M. D. Trus, Metabolism of pancreatic islets and regulation of insulin and glucagon secretion. *In* "Endocrinology" (L. J. DeGroot, G. F. Cahill, L. Martini, D. H. Nelson, W. D. Odell, J. T. Potts, E. Steinberger, and A. I. Winegrad, eds.), Vol. 2, p. 946. Grune & Stratton, New York, 1979.

cell. Electron micrographic studies suggest that the basic mechanism for release of the glucagon-containing granules is emiocytosis. At the present time it is not clear whether there is an involvement of a microtubule–microfilament system or whether there is a glucose receptor in the plasma membrane.

4. Integrated Secretion of Insulin and Glucagon

The overriding responsibility of insulin and glucagon is to maintain blood glucose within normal limits. Shown in Fig. 7-21 is the dose–

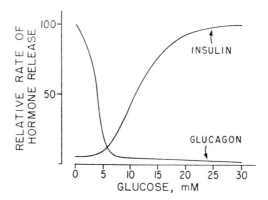

Figure 7-21. Dose–response of glucose suppression of glucagon release stimulated by amino acids and of glucose stimulation of insulin secretion as obtained by studies *in vitro* with the isolated perfused pancreas of the rat. Modified from F. M. Matschinsky, A. A. Pagliara, W. S. Zawalich, and M. D. Trus, Metabolism of pancreatic islets and regulation of insulin and glucagon. *In* "Endocrinology" (L. J. DeGroot, G. F. Cahill, L. Martini, D. H. Nelson, W. D. Odell, J. T. Potts, E. Steinberger, and A. I. Winegrad, eds.), Vol. 2, p. 937. Grune & Stratton, New York, 1979.

response curve of glucose suppression of glucagon release stimulated by amino acids and of glucose stimulation of insulin secretion. The chemistatic properties of the α and β cells to the prevailing blood glucose concentration are nicely interdependent. The β cell threshold for glucose is ~5 mM, while the threshold for an amino acid mixture is 10 mM, provided that glucose is already present. The steep portions of the insulin release curve occur at blood concentrations of amino acids and glucose that occur postprandially. Conversely, the half-maximal glucose-mediated suppression of glucagon secretion occurs at a glucose concentration of 3 mM. These two dose–response curves describe the responses of the α and β cells as they work to effect a stable blood glucose concentration.

Given the possibility of metabolic interconversion of amino acids, fatty acids, and glycogen into glucose in liver, muscle, or adipose tissue and the reality of a changing dietary intake of these same nutrients, it is to be anticipated that these fuel metabolites themselves would coordinately modulate glucagon and insulin secretion. These relationships are incorporated into the model of a fuel receptor in a pancreatic β cell receptor illustrated in Fig. 7-20 and are further illustrated schematically in Fig. 7-22.

Figure 7-22 schematically describes the secretion of insulin and glucagon under the condition of (1) a normal basal metabolic state, (2)

302

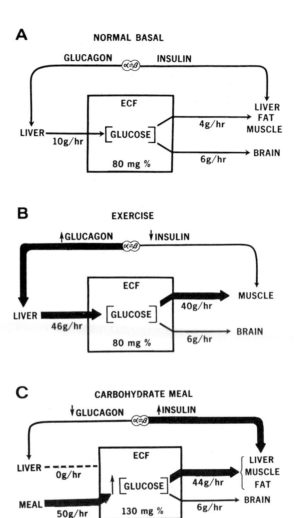

Figure 7-22. Comparison of the relative contributions of insulin and glucagon to maintenance of blood glucose homeostasis in (A) normal basal state; (B) an instance of exercise; and (C) after ingestion of a carbohydrate-rich meal. (A) The role of glucagon in maintaining glucose influx at a rate equal to glucose efflux into insulin-independent tissues so as to maintain extracellular fluid (ECF) glucose concentration above a hypoglycemic range is emphasized. (B) The role of glucagon in maintaining glucose influx equal to markedly increased glucose efflux into exercising muscle so as to maintain ECF glucose concentration above a hypoglycemic range and maintain cerebral glucose delivery is emphasized. (C) The role of insulin in increasing glucose efflux during the rapid influx of ingested glucose so as to prevent an abnormal rise in ECF glucose is emphasized. Reduced glucagon secretion may facilitate this by helping to diminish hepatic glucose production. Reproduced with permission from R. H. Unger and L. Orci, Glucagon and diabetes. *In* "Endocrinology" (L. J. DeGroot, G. F. Cahill, L. Martini, D. H. Nelson, W. D. Odell, J. T. Potts, E. Steinberger, and A. I. Winegrad, eds.), Vol. 2, p. 962. Grune & Stratton, New York, 1979.

exercise, and (3) after ingestion of a carbohydrate meal. A crucial function of the integrated operation of the α–β cell unit is to permit the appropriate regulation of the homeostasis of nutrients such as amino acids by allowing increases in the secretion of insulin secretion without danger of concomitant hypoglycemia. Thus, the aminogenic actions of insulin, which are manifest after ingestion of a "protein-rich" meal, do not lead to hypoglycemia because there is a coupled stimulation of glucagon release; the glucagon then initiates hepatic glycogenolysis and increased release by the liver of as much glucose as leaves the extracellular space as a consequence of the insulin-mediated cellular uptake of glucose. Similarly, this same coupling of α and β cells makes possible the inhibition of lipolysis without an associated fall in glucose. A key unresolved issue concerns the detailed role of somatostatin in pancreatic islet functioning. Although somatostatin is known to inhibit the secretion of both insulin and glucagon, the molecular basis and physiological rationale for this effect is not clear.

C. Pharmacological Agents Related to the Pancreas

Diabetes can be induced chemically by the acute administration of the drug alloxan (Fig. 7-23) or the antibiotic streptozotocin. Each of these agents will selectively destroy the pancreatic β cells, leaving the glucagon-secreting α cells relatively functional. The biological actions of alloxan apparently relate to its affinity for zinc; hence, it is selectively accumulated by the zinc-rich β cells. The 7-carbon sugar mannoheptulose also is known to disrupt the secretory response of the β cells. These agents are frequently used to produce diabetes in experimental animal systems.

There are two groups of drugs which, when given orally, are capable of effecting a sharp drop in the elevated blood glucose levels associated with diabetes (see Fig. 7-23). These are the sulfonyl urea derivatives (tolbutamide, chlorpropamide, glibenclamide, and glipizide) and the biguanide derivative (phenformin). When these oral drugs were first introduced in the early 1960s, there was much hope that they would provide a long-term solution to the management of diabetes. However, their general use has fallen off since the report in 1971 that persons treated with tolbutamide for 8 years had a higher death rate from cardiovascular disease than did control subjects.

The biological mechanism of action of the sulfonyl urea agents is believed to be dependent upon their ability to acutely stimulate the secretion of insulin by functionally responsive islets. Alternatively, there is some evidence to support a peripheral mode of action wherein the

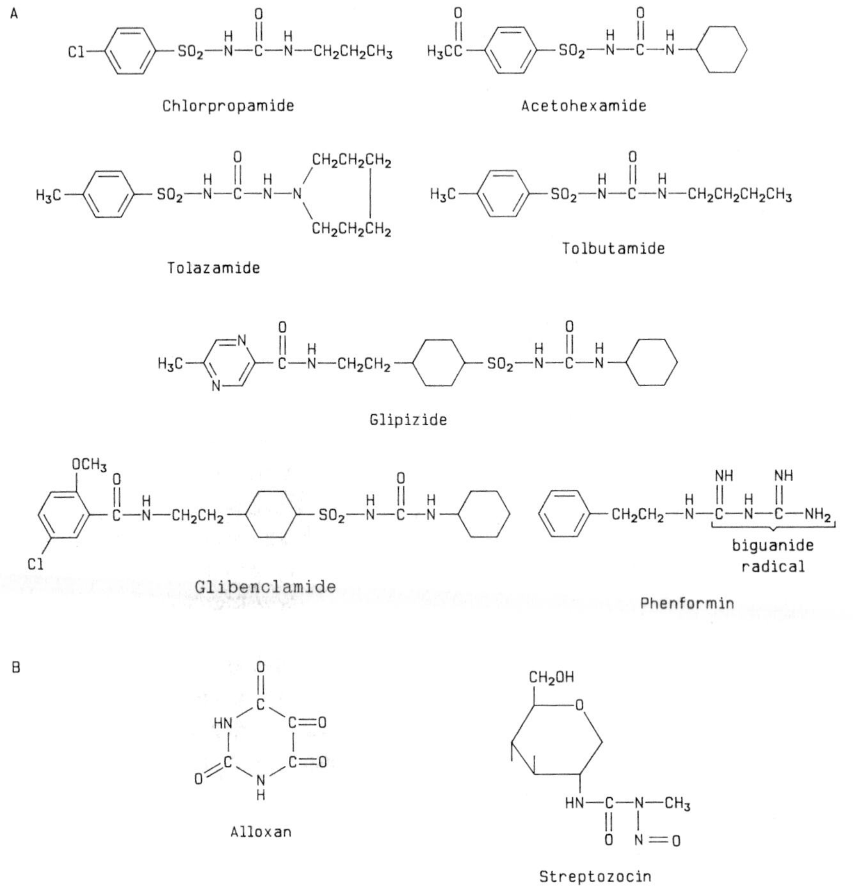

A

Chlorpropamide

Acetohexamide

Tolazamide

Tolbutamide

Glipizide

Glibenclamide

Phenformin

B

Alloxan

Streptozocin

Figure 7-23. (A) Structures of the most frequently employed oral antidiabetic compounds; the "active" portion of the molecule is the sulfonyl urea radical. (B) Structures of alloxan and streptozocin, 2-substituted D-glucose derivatives which are employed to selectively destroy pancreatic B cells.

sulfonyl urea agents increase the sensitivity of tissues such as the liver to the prevailing levels of insulin.

The biguanides have long been known to be potent hypoglycemic agents; regrettably they are also very toxic to many tissues. Although a detailed mode of action is not available, from *in vivo* studies it appears that these agents decrease the rate of intestinal absorption of glucose and increase the peripheral tissue uptake of blood glucose.

Thus, the principal agents now employed for the treatment of the some 6–10 million diabetic individuals in the United States who require drug-assisted management of their blood glucose levels are various preparations of insulin. These preparations have all been purified from extracts of either bovine or porcine pancreases. Because both bovine and porcine insulins have a significantly different amino acid sequence than human insulin, a complicating problem has been the generation of anti-bodies by the patient to the heterologous insulin drug. A major goal of the new recombinant DNA technology has been to clone the gene for human insulin and then to mass-produce it in quantities that would make it possible to provide human insulin as a drug for the diabetic population.

D. Metabolism of Insulin and Glucagon

The plasma half-life of insulin is 3–5 min. The principal pathway for lowering of plasma insulin levels is the receptor-mediated endocytosis of the insulin–receptor complex; a major site of this activity is in the liver, with the kidney as the second most important site. Mutant insulins that bind weakly to the insulin receptor are degraded 6–10 times more slowly.

The plasma half-life of glucagon is 6–7 min. Glucagon is largely inactivated by the liver and kidney. A glucagon-degrading enzyme has been purified from the liver; it specifically cleaves off the N-terminal tripeptide of H_2N-His–Ser–Gln-COOH.

V. BIOLOGICAL AND MOLECULAR ACTIONS

A. Interactions with Target Tissues

1. Glucagon

Glucagon secretion is stimulated by a fall in blood glucose level or a rise in the blood levels of free fatty acids or certain amino acids (see Table 7-8). Most of the biological consequences of glucagon lead to an increase in the blood level of glucose. Virtually all the glycagon secreted by the pancreatic α cell is sequestered by the hepatocyte cells of the liver; thus, the extrahepatic blood levels of glucagon are quite low.

Glucagon elicits its plasmic biological responses through activation of a membrane-bound adenylate cyclase. The second messenger, cyclic AMP, then is the intracellular initiator of specific responses. Glucagon has a high affinity for its liver cell membrane receptor; the K_d is 4×10^{-9} M. As yet there has not been complete isolation and purification of the glucagon receptor. However, molecular weight estimates have been made of the glucagon receptor *in situ* in membrane fractions prepared from liver cells using the technique of high-energy neutron irradiation or "target size analysis." In this technique, the membrane sample is bombarded with a defined intensity of neutrons for varying intervals of time and then the biological activity or functionality of the membrane receptor is determined by appropriate assay (e.g., glucagon-mediated stimulation of adenyl cyclase). The minimal size of the intact receptor was estimated to be 350,000 Da; evidence was obtained indicating the oligomeric nature of the receptor.

M. Rodbell has proposed a theoretical model for hormones that activate membrane-bound adenyl cyclase; this includes glucagon, ACTH, and the β-adrenergic stimulators such as epinephrine (see Fig. 1-26). The model is discussed in detail in Chapter 1.

2. Insulin

There is clear evidence that insulin interacts with stereospecific receptors present in the external membrane of a wide number of cell types. The highest concentration of insulin receptors is present in the cell membranes of liver, muscle, and adipose tissue, and also of lymphocytes, which is in accordance with the significant biological effects on cellular processes that occur in these tissues in the extremes of insulin excess or deficiency.

J. Roth and P. DeMeyts have found that insulin binding to its cultured lymphocyte receptor exhibits negative cooperativity. This implies that there are possible biologically important interactions between insulin receptor molecules in the membrane. In this instance the changing affinity provides a receptor that is sensitive at low hormone concentrations, but that may act as a buffer against very high insulin concentrations.

The insulin receptor retains both insulin binding and immunologic cross-reactivity to insulin receptor antibodies when it is solubilized in neutral detergents. The estimated molecular radius of the insulin receptor is 68–72 Å, which corresponds to a molecular weight of 300,000. Evidence has also been obtained for the existence of major subunits of 125,000 and 90,000 Da and some additional minor subunits. However, when the size of the insulin receptor is estimated *in situ* in the membrane (i.e., not solubilized) by the technique of neutron beam radiation inactivation, it is found that the functional receptor unit is ~1,000,000 molecular weight. This larger estimate may indicate the presence of accessory regulatory proteins around the receptor. R. Kahn and co-workers as well as M. Czech and colleagues have proposed a model for the insulin receptor (see Fig. 7-24) which postulates that its structure is analogous to that of immunoglobulin. The insulin binding component may exist in the membrane either free (90–130,000 Da), in which case it would have a high affinity for insulin, or associated with an inhibitor (40–50,000 Da), causing the affinity for insulin to be reduced. Further, it is proposed that the receptor is oligomeric. Thus, the insulin receptor is proposed to be composed of at least four subunits that are disulfide linked into a large receptor complex of apparent molecular weight of 350,000. Two of the subunits, referred to as α subunits (molecular weight 125,000), are thought to be linked by one or more disulfide bonds. The other two subunits, denoted β (molecular weight 90,000), are disulfide linked.

There is extensive homology in the organization and structure of the insulin receptor in all vertebrates (bony fish, birds, and mammals). In addition, it appears that the insulin receptor has been functionally well conserved over a period of evolution of 400 million years.

Although it is well established that many peptide hormones after interaction with their specific external membrane receptors stimulate adenylate cyclase to produce cyclic AMP, such is not universally the case with insulin. In fact, under certain circumstances, insulin can increase and under other circumstances can decrease the intracellular concentrations of cyclic AMP in liver and adipose tissue, and at the same time increase the levels of cyclic GMP; these changes have been shown to

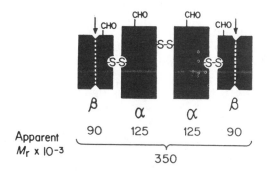

Figure 7-24. Model for the insulin receptor. The key features are two copies each of two glycoprotein subunits designated α and β; disulfide bonds link all the subunits. The high sensitivity of the β subunit to proteolytic cleavage near the center of the subunit is indicated by arrows. Modified from M. P. Czech, J. Massagne, and P. F. Pilch, The insulin receptor: Structural features. *Trends Biochem. Sci.* **6**, 222–225 (1981).

correlate with at least some of the biological effects of insulin in these tissues.

Two general models of receptor-mediated insulin action have been proposed (see Fig. 7-25). The first model (Fig. 7-25A) assumes that insulin itself, after entry into the cell, functions as its own second messenger. It has been clearly shown from electron micrographic studies using ferritin-labeled insulin or radioactively labeled insulin that after insulin is bound to the external membrane-receptor of its target cell, it is rapidly internalized. Exactly where the internalized insulin then goes remains a matter of some controversy. However, a significant proportion of the internalized insulin is degraded by lysozymes. This has led to the suggestion that either insulin or a fragment of insulin interacts with other intracellular proteins to initiate insulin-dependent biological responses.

In a second model, insulin binding to its receptor activates some membrane-associated enzyme or glucose transport protein which concomitantly generates an intracellular "second messenger" responsible for the mediation of the typical metabolic responses produced by insulin. As yet, the chemical nature of this second messenger is not known, although it may be a peptide. It has been demonstrated that treatment of cells with anti-insulin receptor antibodies produces a second messenger which is indistinguishable from that occurring after insulin treatment. This second messenger concept may be explainable in part by the recent considerable evidence supporting the view that the binding of insulin to its membrane-bound receptor results in a phosphorylation on the 90K β subunit of specific tyrosine and serine residues. Phosphorylation of receptors has also been shown to occur for the epidermal growth factor (EGF) and acetylcholine receptors. For the insulin receptor system, it has been determined that the β subunit itself possesses tyrosine kinase activity. The implications of this discovery may be far reaching; although the natural substrates for the insulin receptor kinase are not known, these findings suggest that a portion, if not all, of the insulin biological actions could be mediated through activation of insulin receptor–kinase activity which triggers a cascade of phosphorylation–dephosphorylation events elsewhere in the interior of the target cell (see Fig. 7-25B).

Any complete study of the interaction of insulin with its various target tissue receptors would have to include the resolution of the following biological responses: (1) transformation of glycogen synthetase of the liver from the D to the I form; (2) stimulation of the membrane translocation and cellular uptake by muscle and liver of selected sugars and amino acids as well as K^+; (3) stimulation in the absence of glucose of protein synthesis in liver, muscle, and adipose tissues; (4) suppression

A

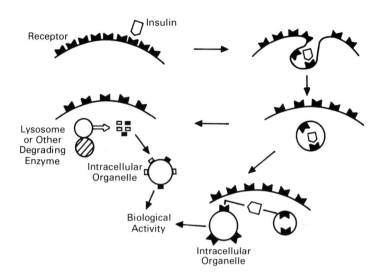

B

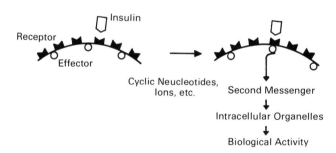

Figure 7-25. Two models of insulin receptor-mediated biological response. (A) A receptor-mediated internalization hypothesis and (B) a second messenger hypothesis. Modified from C. R. Kahn, K. L. Basird, J. S. Flier, C. Grunfeld, J. T. Harmon, L. C. Harrison, F. A. Karlson, M. Kasuga, G. L. King, U. Lang, J. Podskalny, and E. van Obberghen, Insulin receptors, receptor antibodies and the mechanism of insulin action. *Recent Prog. Horm. Res.* **37,** 521 (1981).

of hormone (glucagon or epinephrine) -stimulated lipolysis; and (5) in some instances stimulation of RNA and DNA synthesis [a growth-promoting effect (see also Chapter 19)].

B. Biological Actions

1. Introduction

The principal biological actions of insulin and glucose are complex and interdependent upon the presence or absence of the partner hormone and the delicate balancing of anabolism and catabolism that is occurring throughout the body to reflect changes in caloric intake, caloric composition, and the degree of physical activity. In most situations the roles of insulin and glucagon are antagonistic. Tables 7-9 and 7-10, respectively, summarize the actions of insulin and glucagon in their principal target tissues, the liver, muscle, and adipose tissue. Also, it should be appreciated that the fundamental intermediary metabolism capabilities of these three tissues and their "normal" oxidative substrates vary depending upon the prevailing metabolic condition. The actions of insulin and glucagon in the liver, muscle, and adipose tissue will be discussed sepa-

Table 7–9. Summary of Actions of Insulin on Several Tissues

Tissue	Insulin-sufficient state	Insulin-deficient state
Liver	No effect on glucose uptake Stimulates biosynthesis of hexokinase IV and activates glycogen synthetase I Promotes glycolysis and formation of ATP	Uptake of FFA and conversion to ketones
Muscle	Stimulation of glucose uptake Stimulates biosynthesis of hexokinase II and pyruvate kinase Stimulates glycolysis and formation of ATP Increases muscle glycogen levels and creatine phosphate	Impaired blood glucose
Adipose	Stimulation of glucose uptake Enhances glycolysis which makes available glycerol phosphate which, in turn, enhances triglyceride synthesis Inhibits lipase activity	Decreases triglyceride synthesis due to a lack of glycerol phosphate Stimulation of lipolysis and release of FFA into blood stream
Brain	No direct actions of insulin; brain dependent upon blood glucose	None

Table 7–10. Summary of Actions of Glucagon on Several Tissues
in the Glucagon-Sufficient State

Tissue	Effect
Liver	Inactivates glycogen synthetase and activates phosphorylase *a*, which leads to an activation of glycogenolysis
	Increases the activity of glucose 6-phosphatase
	Enhances synthesis of glucose from pyruvate and lactate as well as amino acids, especially arginine and alanine (i.e., activates gluconeogenesis)
Muscle	Muscle does not contain receptors for glucagon and accordingly it has no effect
	Major effects on muscle metabolism are mediated by epinephrine (see Chapter 11)
Adipose	In large doses can stimulate lipolysis—but under normal circumstances it has little or no effects
Pancreas	Stimulates insulin secretion, particularly after intestinal absorption of amino acids
Brain	None

rately. Figure 7-26 compares for liver, muscle, and adipose tissue the major metabolic effects that are found in the absence and presence of insulin.

2. Liver

The liver performs an indispensable role in maintaining an adequate blood level of glucose. It possesses the enzymatic capability either to generate glucose from stored glycogen or to store excess glucose as glycogen. In addition, the liver contains an active gluconeogenesis capability which will permit the production of glucose from 3- and 4-carbon fragments derived from amino acids. Also, the liver can oxidatively metabolize glucose and other smaller metabolites to H_2O and CO_2, which generates ATP, or convert 2-carbon fragments to larger free fatty acids which then are incorporated into triglycerides and phospholipids.

Figure 7-27 diagrams the enzyme reactions involved in storage of glucose and mobilization of glycogen. Several key enzymes in this scheme are markedly affected by the presence or absence of glucagon or insulin. Activation of the glycogenolytic system involves phosphorylation of key enzymes while inactivation necessitates dephosphorylation. On the one hand glycogen is phosphorylzed (broken down) by the cascade of cAMP-governed reactions which convert the relatively inactive phosphorylase *b* into the more active phosphorylase *a*. On the other hand, under conditions where it is appropriate to convert glucose into

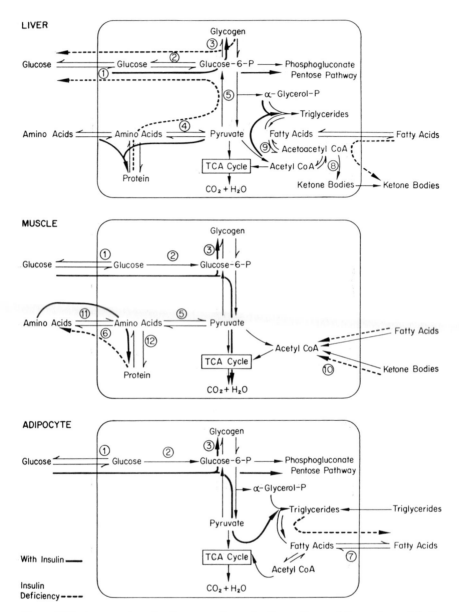

Figure 7-26. A comparison for liver, muscle, and adipose tissue of the major metabolic effects that occur in the absence and presence of insulin. Thick solid arrows ($\rightarrow$) show the pathways that are favored in the presence of insulin, while thick broken arrows ($\dashrightarrow$) depict those that predominate when the action of the hormone is insufficient. (For explanation, see the text.) Modified from A. G. Gilman, L. S. Goodman, and A. Gilman, "The Pharmacological Basis of Therapeutics," 6th ed. Macmillan, New York, 1980.

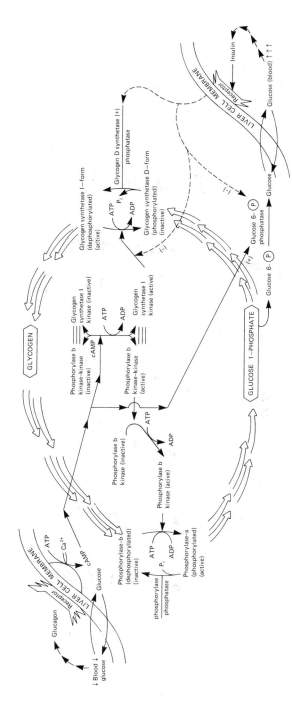

Figure 7-27. Summary of biochemical consequences of insulin and/or glucagon actions in the storage of glucose or the mobilization of glycogen in a liver cell. Events depicted occur in the cell cytoplasm after binding of insulin or glucagon to their respective membrane receptors.

glycogen, there is activation of a phosphatase which converts the phosphorylated D or dependent form of glycogen synthetase into the dephosphorylated I or independent form. It will be noted that a key feature of this system is the unique role played by the protein phosphorylase *b* kinase-kinase which has two distinct catalytic activities. When it is phosphorylated (as a consequence of the presence of glucagon), it initiates the cascade which ultimately leads to conversion of phosphorylase *b* into phosphorylase *a* and the production of glucose-1-P. Alternatively, when the phosphorylase-*b*-kinase-kinase is not phosphorylated, it acquires the activity of glycogen-I-synthetase-kinase. Thus, the presence of glucagon favors generation of an active phosphorylase-*b*-kinase-kinase while the presence of insulin activates a phosphatase which leads to glycogen formation.

In addition to the glucagon–insulin modulation of glycogen storage and mobilization in the liver, these two peptide hormones also modulate the balance between gluconeogenesis and lipogenesis. Under circumstances of glucose demand, gluconeogenesis will predominate to convert into glucose those carbon skeletons derived from amino acids or glycolytic intermediates produced prior to pyruvate. Under conditions of glucose excess, glycolytic intermediates and free fatty acids can be directed either to storage as triglycerides or to oxidation by the TCA cycle or to production of ketone bodies. It is not yet clear what detailed cellular or hormonal signals determine whether a given free fatty acid is dedicated to storage as triglyceride or conversion to CO_2 and/or ketones. These relationships are diagrammed in Fig. 7-28. Reversal of the glycolytic pathway requires access to NADH whereas lipogenesis is dependent upon access to NADPH for fatty acid biosynthesis.

In summary, glucagon has been shown to stimulate the conversion of pyruvate, lactate, alanine, and glycerol into glucose. This is accomplished largely by modulating key enzymes of the gluconeogenic pathway. There appear to be no effects of glucagon on stimulating substrate supply or in increasing amino acid uptake by the liver. Insulin appears to exert its inhibitory effects on liver gluconeogenesis by (1) inhibiting or slowing the enzymes of gluconeogenesis, and (2) diminishing the flow of amino acids from peripheral tissues, principally muscle, to the liver (see later).

Phosphorylated glycolytic intermediates are not capable of traversing the cell membrane of the liver. However, the liver contains an active glucose 6-phosphatase. The activity of this enzyme is increased in the absence of insulin or by the presence of cortisol; this ensures the ready conversion of glucose 6-phosphate to free glucose which may then be exported from the liver cell. By contrast, muscle cells do not have mea-

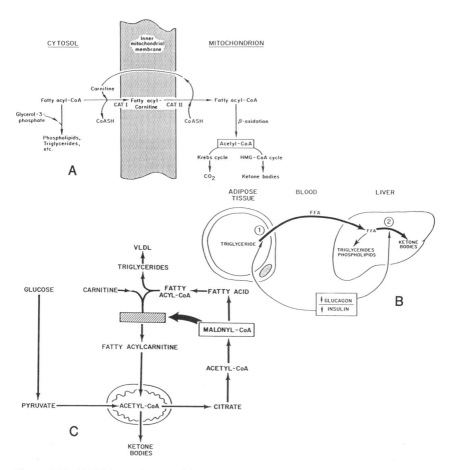

Figure 7-28. (A) Major pathways of fatty acid metabolism in the liver where CAT I and CAT II refer to carnitine acyltransferases located on the outer and inner surfaces of the inner mitochondrial membrane. (B) Summary of the effects of insulin and/or glucagon on hepatic ketone production. (C) Interrelationships between the pathways of fatty acid synthesis and oxidation in the liver. Modified from J. D. McGarry, New perspectives in the regulation of ketogenesis. *Diabetes* **28,** 517–523 (1979). Reproduced wih permission from the American Diabetes Association, Inc.

surable glucose-6-phosphatase activity and thus the muscle glycogen stores cannot be mobilized for maintenance of blood glucose levels.

3. Muscle

In the absence of insulin there is a stimulation of net protein catabolism in muscle. The resulting free amino acids are released into the bloodstream and delivered to the liver where they are oxidatively deaminated. The resulting carbon fragments are then committed to gluconeo-genesis or to catabolism to yield ketone bodies and/or CO_2. The resulting increase in nitrogen is converted to urea and excreted in the urine.

Muscle tissue is known to contain insulin but not glucagon receptors. Insulin occupancy of this receptor leads to an increased uptake of both glucose and amino aids; there is also an associated stimulation of protein synthesis. The biochemical bases for these effects are not yet clearly understood in that they cannot be explained by changes in cellular cyclic AMP levels. Also, actinomycin D does not block insulin-mediated stimulation of protein synthesis. It has been proposed that the 40 S large subunit of ribosomes obtained from the muscle of diabetic animals is defective.

After an overnight fast and in the absence of physical activity, muscle tissue is largely dependent upon the oxidation of free fatty acids to meet its energy demands. Under these conditions there would be a significant pool of muscle glycogen. With the initiation of mild to moderate exercise, the muscle tissue successively oxidizes its own glycogen, then blood glucose, and finally, blood-delivered free fatty acids derived from adipose and hepatic stores.

4. Adipose Tissue

Adipose tissue is one of the principal target organs for insulin action. The extensive amount of triglycerides stored in adipocytes serves as an important fuel source under conditions of dietary caloric restriction or prolonged exercise. The mobilized free fatty acids are systematically delivered to a number of key organs (heart and kidney) which can directly utilize them as substrate for oxidative metabolism. If the free fatty acids were taken up by the liver, they can be esterified into triglycerides or phospholipids, oxidized to CO_2, or more likely converted into ketones, particularly β-hydroxybutyrate and acetoacetate. These ketones in turn can also serve as fuels for most extrahepatic tissues, particularly the brain, under conditions of very low blood glucose levels.

Insulin can suppress ketogenesis via two general mechanisms: (1) In the adipocyte insulin inhibits lipolysis which generates free fatty acids, and (2) in the liver, insulin also blocks or reduces the extent of liver oxidation and enhances the storage of the free fatty acids as triglycerides.

The rate-limiting step in the biosynthesis of triglycerides by both the liver and adipose tissue is the availability of glycerol phosphate. This 3-carbon sugar is not transported systematically, hence it must be generated *in situ* in the cell where the triglyceride synthesis is occurring. This in turn implies that there should be adequate supplies of substrates to the glycolytic pathway to ensure the availability of the glycerol phosphate in sufficient amounts.

VI. CLINICAL ASPECTS

A. Insulin

Diabetes mellitus, or more usually diabetes, is the most common disease associated with the pancreatic islets; it may affect 1–5% of the total population. In the United States it is estimated that more than 12 million people have some form of diabetes; annually some 200,000 individuals are newly diagnosed as diabetic. Diabetes is the eighth leading health-related cause of death in the United States. More than 50% of diabetics die because of coronary disease; individuals with juvenile-onset diabetes usually succumb because of renal failure. Diabetes is the second highest causative factor of blindness.

The term diabetes means "running through"; characteristic features are polydipsia and polyuria. Mellitus is Latin for honey (i.e., sweet). In a classic sense diabetes mellitus is not a single disease because it has no single definable and distinct etiology.

The major pathophysiological abnormalities generated by diabetes mellitus include the following: (1) glucose intolerance or inappropriately high blood glucose levels in the presence of elevated or normal insulin concentrations; (2) acidosis and ketosis; (3) reduction of the enzymes for gluconeogenesis; (4) reduced growth; (5) a microangiopathy including a thickened basement membrane of capillaries in muscle, retinal blood vessels, and the capillaries of the renal glomerulus; and (6) a neuropathy, including peripheral sensory and motor defects.

Clinically there are two general classifications of diabetes: type I, or insulin-dependent diabetes mellitus, formally designated juvenile-onset diabetes, and type II, or insulin-independent mellitus, formally designated as maturity-onset diabetes. It is not yet clear for either form of diabetes what in molecular terms are the specific defects that likely are present in the complex biosynthetic and secretory steps required for normal insulin secretion by the β cell. What is clear is that in type I diabetes the β cells in the islet are partially or totally destroyed and consequently there is no endogenous insulin secretion. This is determined by the absence of plasma levels of C peptide and an absolute requirement of insulin for maintenance of life.

Individuals with type I diabetes are highly prone to develop metabolic ketosis and in the untreated state there are the acute symptoms of polyuria, polydipsia, weight loss, and fatigue, all of which are secondary to the absence of insulin. Patients with juvenile-onset diabetes require mandatory daily treatment with some form of drug insulin preparation.

Diabetic ketoacidosis is a clinical condition characterized by hyperglycemia, hyperketonemia, and a concomitant metabolic acidosis that results largely from elevated blood levels of β-hydroxybutyrate and acetoacetate. A propensity to diabetic ketoacidosis is the primary basis for clinical classification of a subject with juvenile-onset diabetes. The clinical symptoms arise from a low to undetectable blood level of insulin and result in the adverse consequences of persistent hyperglycemia. In the extreme, an afflicted subject will become unconscious due to "diabetic coma." Diabetic ketoacidosis is an acute life-threatening emergency and if left untreated leads to hypokalemia and cardiovascular failure. Diabetic ketoacidosis accounts for ~65% of all diabetic hospital admissions in the age group 1–20 years and 40% in the 21–34 age group.

Type II or maturity-onset diabetes is a form of diabetes mellitus in which there is only a relative lack of insulin, but the secretion is not correctly "geared" for glucose signals (i.e., the β cells are still functioning). It is frequently not diagnosed until the individual is middle-aged. In this form of the disease the diabetes is stated to be insulin independent, since the patient will not develop ketosis without insulin therapy. Type II diabetes may require only intermittent adjunctive insulin therapy, usually to manage fasting hyperglycemia. In many subjects adequate glucose and fuel metabolite homeostasis can be achieved by careful dietary management of nutritional and caloric intake.

The most commonly associated physical finding with maturity-onset diabetes is obesity. Obesity can be defined as an enlargement of the adipose depot and is usually associated with some kind of pancreatic dysfunction. For the population of hyperglycemic subjects older than 20 years, at least 90% are more than 10% overweight. Frequently after weight loss these individuals may regain a normal state of carbohydrate metabolism. A significant fact related to insulin-independent diabetes associated with or without obesity is that there is an apparent decrease in the sensitivity of the peripheral tissues to insulin. As a result, obese individuals have an elevated level of insulin secretion.

From the perspective of the insulin receptor present in the various target tissues, it should be emphasized that in the obese form of diabetes, characterized by glucose intolerance, hyperinsulemia, and resistance to both endogenous and exogenous insulin, there is no evidence for a "nonfunctional form" of the insulin. The circulating ratio of proinsulin to insulin is normal; both cross-react normally in radioimmunoassays for insulin. The defect appears to be both in the number of receptors present in the target cells and in postreceptor events.

The pathogenesis of diabetes mellitus, besides being related to environmental and dietary factors, also clearly contains a genetic or familial component. Although the precise statistics supporting this statement vary with their source, it is estimated that between 25 and 50% of diabetic patients have "family histories" consistent with a genetic component. The reported incidence of diabetes is much higher in children derived from parents who both have diabetes; also monozygotic twins (identical twins) have a significantly higher incidence of diabetes than dizygotic twins (fraternal twins). Current evidence favors the position that the inheritance is polygenic or multifactorial; in some specific instance there is clear evidence of a recessive gene for diabetes. The Puma Indians have an incidence rate of diabetes which approaches 50% or higher. Also, there are animal models of diabetes (the *ob/ob* and *db/db* diabetic mouse and the Zucker rat) which clearly reflect genetic transmission. It has also been suggested that type I or juvenile-onset diabetes may be the result of an acute viral infection of the pancreatic islets or an autoimmune reaction due to an abnormality in the immune system.

B. Glucagon

In contrast to the situation relating to insulin, there are relatively few disease states that can be ascribed specifically to dysfunctions of glucagon. Only in 1966 was the syndrome of hyperglucagonemia first described. This condition arises as a consequence of the presence of a glucagon-secreting tumor of the pancreatic α cell.

There is also mounting evidence that diabetes mellitus in its extreme form is a double disorder of pancreatic islet cell dysfunction. Thus, insulin deficiency by itself may not be solely responsible for the broad spectrum of intermediary metabolic changes associated with diabetes. Because insulin is a known inhibitor of liver glucose production and secretion, it may be that in diabetes there is an inappropriately high level of blood glucagon for the prevailing blood glucose levels (i.e., a "relative" excess of glucagon). If indeed future research clearly documents that there is an α cell dysfunction associated with diabetes mellitus, then a substantial revision of the pathophysiological concepts and treatment modalities for this disease will be necessary.

References

A. Books

Fritz, I. B., ed. (1972). "Insulin Action." Academic Press, New York.
Steiner, D. F., and Freinkel, N., eds. (1972). "Handbook of Physiology," Sec. 7, Vol. 1. Am. Physiol. Soc., Washington, D.C.

B. Review Articles

Bennett, P. H. (1984). The diagnosis of diabetes; new international classification and diagnostic criteria. *Annu. Rev. Med.* **34,** 295–310.

Blundell, T. L., and Humbel, R. E. (1980). Hormone families: Pancreatic hormones and homologous growth factors. *Nature (London)* **287,** 781–786.

Blundell, T. L., Dodson, G. G., Hodgkin, D. C., and Mercola, D. A. (1972). Chemistry and structure of insulin. *Adv. Protein Chem.* **26,** 279–402.

Cuatrecases, P., Hollenberg, M. D., Chang, K., and Bennett, V. (1979). Hormone receptor complexes and their modulation of membrane function. *Recent Prog. Horm. Res.* **31,** 37–84.

Czech, M. P., Massague, J., and Rich, P. F. (1981). The insulin receptor: Structural features. *Trends Biochem. Sci.* **6,** 222–225.

Kahn, C. R., Basird, K. L., Flier, J. S., Grunfeld, C., Harmon, J. T., Harrison, L. C., Karlsson, F. A., Kasuga, M., King, G. L., Lang, U. C., Podskalny, J., and van Obberghen, E. (1981). Insulin receptors, receptor antibodies, and the mechanism of insulin action. *Recent Prog. Horm. Res.* **37,** 477–532.

C. Research Papers

Bell, G. I., Picket, R. L., Rutter, W. J., Cordell, B., Tischer, E., and Goodman, H. M. (1980). Sequence of the human insulin gene. *Nature (London)* **284,** 26–32.

Cahill, G. (1971). Physiology of insulin in man. *Diabetes* **20,** 785–799.

Cordell, B., Bell, G., Tischer, E., DeNoto, F. M., Ullrich, A., Picket, R., Rutter, W. J., and Goodman, H. M. (1979). Isolation and characterization of a cloned rat insulin gene. *Cell* **18,** 533–543.

CreHaz, M., Jialal, I., Kasuga, M., and Kahn, C. R. (1984). Insulin receptor regulation and desensitization in rat hepatoma cells: The loss of the oligomeric forms of the receptor correlates with the change in receptor affinity. *J. Biol. Chem.* **259,** 11543–11549.

Czech, M. P. (1984). New perspectives on the mechanism of insulin action. *Recent Prog. Horm. Res.* **40,** 347–373.

Honeda, M., Chan, S. J., Kwok, S. C. M., Rubenstein, A. H., and Steiner, D. F. (1983). Studies on mutant human insulin genes: Identification and sequence analysis of a gene encoding [Ser^{B24}] insulin. *Proc. Natl. Acad. Sci. U.S.A.* **80,** 6366–6370.

Kwok, S. C. M., Steiner, D. F., Rubenstein, A. H., and Tager, H. S. (1983). Identification of a point mutation in the human insulin gene giving use to a structurally abnormal insulin (insulin Chicago). *Diabetes* **32,** 872–875.

McGarry, J. D., and Foster, D. W. (1977). Hormonal control of ketogenesis. *Arch. Intern. Med.* **137,** 495–501.

Rodbell, M. (1980). The role of hormone receptors and GTP regulatory proteins in membrane transduction. *Nature (London)* **284,** 17–22.

Roth, R. A., Morgan, D. D., Beaudoin, J., and Sara, V. (1986). Purification and characterization of the human brain insulin receptor. *J. Biol. Chem.* **261,** 3753–3757.

Unger, R. H., and Orci, L. (1977). Role of glucagon in diabetes. *Arch. Intern. Med.* **137,** 482–491.

Gastrointestinal Hormones

I. INTRODUCTION

A. Background

The stomach, intestine (small and large), liver, gallbladder, and pancreas operate as a physiological unit to effect digestion and absorption of the bodily nutrients. A discussion of the principal pancreatic hormones, insulin and glucagon, is presented in Chapter 7. This chapter will focus only on the gastrointestinal hormones.

The gastrointestinal hormones are a family of polypeptides produced by specialized endocrine cells present in the stomach and small and large intestine. These hormones mediate a variety of specific biological responses by the stomach, small intestine, endocrine and the exocrine pancreas, liver, and gallbladder which, when integrated, optimize the physiological conditions necessary to permit the efficient digestion and absorption of protein, carbohydrates, and fat from the lumen of the intestine.

Gastrointestinal function is modulated by a complex series of hormonal and neural interrelationships. There is also increasing evidence of neuroendocrine communication between the brain and gut which provides an additional level of integration and complexity to these digestive processes.

B. Problems of Food Processing and Digestion

All animals require a continued and regular intake of food so that they can meet their bodily nutrient requirements. Briefly, these include (1) an adequate caloric intake of carbohydrates and proteins providing the spectrum of substrates required for the generation of metabolic energy which is indispensable for the biosynthesis, modification, and repair of tissue components and the generation of mechanical energy (muscle contraction) and electrical energy (nerve impulse); (2) an adequate intake of essential substances not capable of being biosynthesized by the animal in question (i.e., essential amino acids, fatty acids, and vitamins); and (3) an adequate intake of macro and trace minerals. Thus, the term food is a general label to include the variety of chemical substances including proteins, carbohydrates, fats, minerals, and vitamins required to provide nourishment (i.e., maintenance of life).

However, the simple process of swallowing food does not mean that these food substances are available to sustain life. It is only after they have left the lumen of the intestine and appeared in the blood or lymph that they can be said to be "in the body." Although some food substances, such as minerals and free amino acids, can be absorbed with little or no change in the chemical form in which they are ingested, other food components must be subjected to extensive physical and chemical modification prior to their entry into the lymph or bloodstream. Thus, proteins, polysaccharides (both macromolecules), fats (triglycerides), and phospholipids all must be degraded to their constituent components—amino acids, mono- and disaccharides, fatty acids, and glycerol, respectively—before they can be efficiently absorbed.

The overall physical and chemical properties of the various foodstuffs (e.g., water solubility, net charge) as well as the nature of their structural units and bonding (amide, glycoside, ester) pose a diversity of biochemical problems to be resolved by the digestive system. The system of digestion, then, is the processing of the ingested bulk food into molecular forms capable of entering the intestinal absorptive process.

The digestive process involves the complex integration of voluntary and involuntary muscle contractions, parasympathetic and sympathetic neural actions, release of the gastrointestinal and other hormones, biosynthesis and release of a host of digestive enzymes (e.g., pepsin, trypsin, chymotrypsin, amylase) and digestive reagents (e.g., HCl and HCO_3^-), along with digestive detergents (e.g., bile acids). These all collectively work together to process the food and present it to the intestinal absorptive machinery in an optimal form for absorption. These include the integrated functioning of the mouth, stomach, small and large intestine, pancreas, liver, and gallbladder; the steps of the digestive process are outlined in Table 8-1.

As a consequence of evolutionary pressures, a number of hormonal systems have emerged to participate in the regulation of the digestion and absorption of the key dietary nutrients. These include the gastrointestinal hormones (this chapter), insulin and glucagon (see Chapter 7), and vitamin D + metabolites (one of the calcium-regulating hormones— see Chapter 9). In addition, many other hormones are known to exert "effects" on either the digestion process or the gastrointestinal tract to modulate the absorption of various nutrients.

C. Resume of the Gastrointestinal Hormones

As reviewed in Table 8-1, the gastrointestinal hormones play key roles in many of the steps and processes associated with the digestion and absorption of food. The three major gastrointestinal hormones are gastrin, secretin, and cholecystokinin–pancreozymin (CCK–PZ). The actions of these peptide hormones in the digestive process are summarized in Table 8-2. In addition, there are several other peptide hormones

Table 8–1. Steps and Components of the Digestive Process

Process	Anatomical location	Purpose
Food entry		
Consumption of food/mastication	Mouth	Support bodily nutrient requirements
Salivary secretion (stimulated by the nervous system): 1200 ml is secreted per day	Salivary glands	Conversion of starches into dextrins and maltose
Voluntary swallowing of food	Tongue/pharynx/esophagus	Entry of food into digestive tract
Involuntary peristaltic muscular contraction	Esophagus	To move food along the digestive tract
Digestion in the stomach		
Secretion of gastric juice (HCl + pepsin) as a consequence of neural, mechanical, and hormonal (gastrin) stimuli (2000 ml secreted/day)	Stomach	Conversion of proteins to polypeptides
Involuntary mechanical contractions	Stomach	Mixing of intestinal contents and when pylorus opens—transfer of stomach contents (chyme) to the small intestine
Digestion in the small intestine		
Neural and hormonal (secretion of pancreozymes) -mediated secretion of pancreatic juice (1200 ml secreted/day)	Exocine or acinar pancreas secretions are ducted into the duodenum	
Bicarbonate secretion		HCO_3^- neutralizes HCl from stomach and creates favorable duodenal pH (6.0–7.0) so that pancreatic enzymes may operate efficiently
Amylase, trypsinogen, chymotrypsinogen secretion and conversion to "active" enzymes		Hydrolysis of amide, glycoside, and ester bonds of peptides, carbohydrates, and lipids
Neural stimulation and duodenal muscular	Duodenum	

Table 8–1. (*Continued*)

Process	Anatomical location	Purpose
distension stimulation of intestinal juice (4000–5000 ml secreted/day)		
Enterokinase (activates trypsinogen into trypsin)		Further processing of proteins/peptides
Proteases (chymotrypsinogens, trypsinogen, lipases, amylases)		Further processing of proteins/peptides
Sucrase, maltase, lactase; specific transport systems (all bound to brush border membranes)		Further processing of dextrins and other partially hydrolyzed substances
Synthesis and secretion of bile acids (by the liver) followed by storage in the gallbladder; hormonally stimulated secretion (by cholecystokinin and secretin) of the gallbladder to release bile acids (600–800 ml secreted/day)	Liver (site of production), gallbladder (storage), transport (through bile duct) into duodenum	Emulsify fats to facilitate absorption of fatty acids
Involuntary mechanical activity		
Segmentation	Duodenum, jejunum, and ileum	Squeezing and mixing of intestinal contents (8–10 contractions/min in duodenum
Peristalsis	Duodenum, jejunum, and ileum	Onward movement of intestinal contents
Chemical activity	Duodenum, jejunum, and ileum	Continued saponification of fat and hydrolysis of proteins/peptides to amino acids and carbohydrates/dextrins to mono- and disaccharides followed by cellular absorption and transport to the blood or lymph compartments

(*continued*)

Table 8–1. (*Continued*)

Process	Anatomical location	Purpose
Digestion in the large intestine		
Involuntary mechanical activity	Large intestine	Mixing movements which promote reabsorption of H_2O and compaction of intestinal contents (7000–8000 ml H_2O reabsorbed/day)
Bacterial action	Large intestine	Acts on undigested residues to effect fermentation of carbohydrate and further degradation of proteins as well as biosynthesis of vitamin K

produced within the gastrointestinal tract which have significant biological actions related to the digestive processes.

II. ANATOMICAL, MORPHOLOGICAL, AND PHYSIOLOGICAL RELATIONSHIPS

A. The Gastro-Entero-Pancreatic System

The gross anatomical organization of the digestive tract, the stomach, the small intestine, and the large intestine of man is shown in Fig. 8-1. The anatomical relationships of the liver, pancreas, and gallbladder are given in Fig. 7-2A.

The digestive tube or alimentary canal in man is a 9-m-long muscular tube extending from the lips to the anus. Indicated in Fig. 8-1 are the individual components of the alimentary canal; each part makes an essential contribution to the process of making food available to the cells of the body. The operations within the digestive tube are supplemented by several accessory organs including the teeth, tongue, salivary glands, pancreas, and liver.

B. The Stomach

Figure 8-2 presents a cross-sectional view of the stomach. The gastric secretions of hydrochloric acid and pepsin are dependent upon the functional capacity and mass of the various secretory elements in the gastric

Table 8–2. Gastrointestinal Hormones

Hormone	Stimulatory agent(s)	Site of production	Actions on the digestive process
Major			
Gastrin	Distension of stomach	Gastric mucosa in the region of the pylorus	Stimulates acid secretion and, to a lesser extent, pepsin secretion; stimulates bile flow; inhibition of H_2O and electrolyte absorption in the intestine; contraction of gastroesophageal sphincter; relaxation of sphincter of Oddi α, the ileal–cecal sphincter
Secretin	Acidity of duodenal contents	Duodenal mucosa	Stimulates acinar pancreas and bile ducts to secrete H_2O and HCO_3^-; inhibits gastric secretion of gastrin and peristalsis; stimulates pepsin secretion; stimulates insulin secretion
Cholecystokinin– pancreozymin	Chyme, fats, fatty acids	Duodenal mucosa	Stimulates release of enzymes from the acinar pancreas (e.g., amylase, trypsinogen, lipase); stimulates contraction and evacuation of the gallbladder; inhibits gastric secretion
Other hormones			
Gastric inhibitory polypeptide (GIP)	Oral glucose and amino acids	Duodenal mucosa	Inhibits acid and pepsin secretion; stimulation of insulin secretion
Vasoactive intestinal polypeptide (VIP)	Vagal stimulation	Duodenal mucosa	Arterial vasodilation and hypotension; increased splanic blood flow; suppression of gastric acid secretion
Motilin	Alkaline conditions	Duodenal mucosa	Stimulation of gastric motor activity
Neurotensin	—	Ileum	Inhibition of gastric motor activity
Somatostatin	Electrical stimulation of the vagus; gastrin	Nerve cells in intestine	Exerts inhibitory actions on release of CCK, VIP, GIP, secretion; decreases intestinal contractions, gallbladder contractions and bile flow
Enteroglucagon	—	Ileum and colon	Tropic effects on enterocytes

mucosa as well as a consequence of the action of the several hormonal and neural stimulants and inhibitors.

The gastric mucosa is divided into three anatomical regions: the cardiac, oxyntic, and pyloric. The total surface area of the gastric mucosa is ~800 cm². Anatomically the cardiac portion encompasses the first few millimeters below the gastroesophageal junction and includes the cardiac mucus glands; it secretes alkaline mucus and a small amount of electrolytes.

The oxyntic or fundic portion comprises 75–80% of the entire stom-

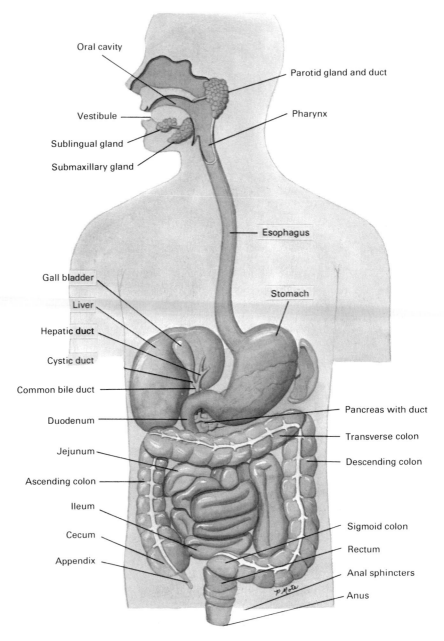

Figure 8-1. Diagram of the human digestive system.

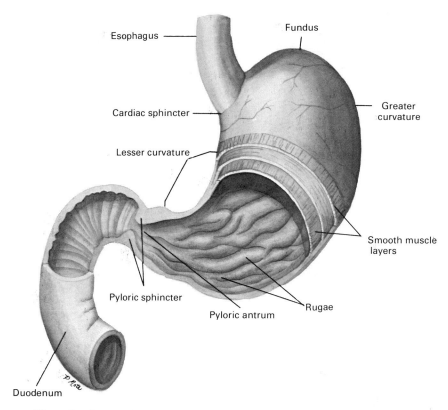

Esophagus

Fundus

Cardiac sphincter

Greater curvature

Lesser curvature

Smooth muscle layers

Pyloric sphincter

Rugae

Pyloric antrum

Duodenum

Figure 8-2. Longitudinal section of the human stomach and upper duodenum.

ach. The oxyntic glands, which number ~35 million in the stomach of man, are straight or slightly coiled tubules and are comprised largely of parietal cells and mucus-secreting cells (see Fig. 8-3A and B). The parietal cells, constituting 75% of the mucosal volume, have large numbers of mitochondria which are required for the metabolic energy demands involved in the production of concentrated hydrochloric acid. The parietal or oxyntic cells undergo a dramatic morphological transformation during stimulation so that the internal tubulovesicles coalesce and become transformed into microvillar membranes. The chief cells (see Fig. 8-3C) are the primary site of secretion of pepsin.

The pyloric gland area constitutes the lower 20% of the gastric mucosa and contains pyloric glands which are comprised largely of mucus-secreting cells.

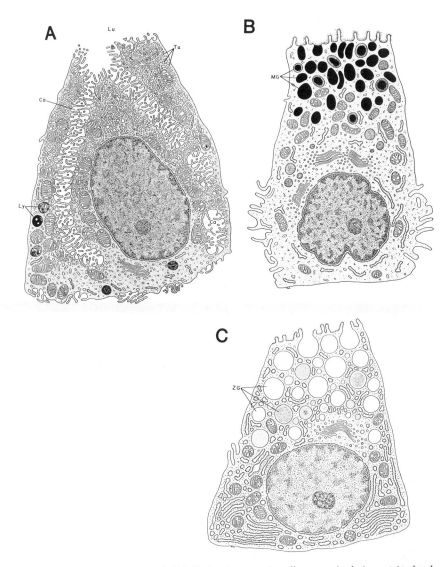

Figure 8-3. Cells of the stomach (A). Parietal or oxyntic cells occur singly in gastric glands and are the site of secretion of hydrochloric acid. Ca, Secretory caniculi that extend from the apex of the cell, pass lateral to the nucleus, and extend almost to the base of the cell; the caniculi open into a common outlet that is continuous with the lumen (Lu) of the gland. Tu, Cytoplasmic tubules. Ly, Lysozyme. (B) Surface mucous cells. The lumen of the stomach and the gastric pits are lined by the surface mucus-secreting cells. The mucous granules (MG) are concentrated in the upper portion of the cell. (C) Chief or zymogenic cells occupy the greater portion of the bases of gastric glands in the fundus. Chief cells secrete pepsin and the gastric intrinsic factor which facilitates the absorption of vitamin

C. Small and Large Intestine

The small intestine of man is divided anatomically into the duodenum (~20 cm), which is connected to the stomach via the pylorus, the jejunum (~275 cm), and the ileum (~425 cm), which connects to the large intestine. The large intestine (~180 cm) is sequentially divided into the colon, appendix, rectum, and anal canal.

The morphology and cellular organization of the intestine are superbly adapted to efficiently effect the absorption of dietary constituents. The lumen of the small intestine is composed of a multitude of finger-like projections which are termed villi (see Fig. 8-4A). Typically these villi range from 0.5 to 1.5 mm in length. They are composed principally of two types of cells: the columnar epithelial cell and the goblet or mucus-secreting cell. The cells on the villus are rapidly renewed. The mucosal cells originate in a progenitor population existent at the base of the villus in the crypt of Lieberkuhn, and ultimately after migration up the villus the cells are sloughed off into the lumen of the intestine. Only after epithelial cells enter the villus do they differentiate into fully functional absorptive cells. This differentiation process is characterized by a change in the RNA/protein ratio and a change in the activity of various enzymes as a function of the position of the epithelial cell on the villus. Intestinal epithelial cell turnover times of 70–100 hr have been reported in mice, rats, and human beings. The rate of epithelial cell renewal increases when there is an increased demand for new cells, as in recovery from radiation injury, response to parasite infestation, or adaptation to partial intestinal resection.

The apical surface of these cells, which is exposed to the lumen, is referred to as the brush border of the microvillar membrane (see Fig. 8-4B). These microvilli are ~1 μm long and 0.1 μm wide. As a consequence, the surface area of the mucosa is increased 600-fold as compared to the total area of a hypothetical cell without microvilli. A variety of carbohydrate hydrolases and an alkaline phosphatase are specifically associated with this brush border region of the intestinal mucosal cell. This is believed to be the site of localization of permeases that are postulated as being involved in the absorption of materials into the cell. Beneath the columnar epithelial cells lie the lymphatic and blood vascular systems which project into each villus and thus provide an efficient mechanism for the translocation of the various substrates once they exit from the epithelial cells.

B_{12}. The supranuclear region contains numerous zymogen (ZG) granules. Reproduced with permission from T. L. Lentz, "Cell Fine Structure." Saunders, Philadelphia, Pennsylvania, 1971.

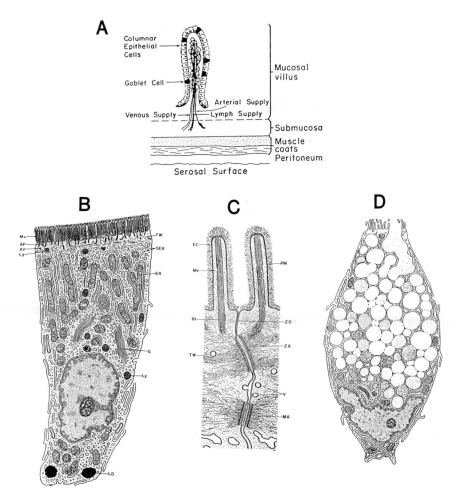

Figure 8-4. Organization of the intestinal mucosa. (A) Diagrammatic representation of the intestinal villus. (B) Intestinal columnar epithelial cell which lines the intestinal mucosa. Microvilli (Mv) extend from the free surface and form the striated edge. The surfaces of the microvilli are coated by a filamentous mucopolysaccharide material termed the glycocalyx. The terminal web (TW) lies immediately under the microvilli. G, Golgi; SER, smooth endoplasmic reticulum. (C) The junctional complex of an intestinal epithelial cell. The junction is comprised of three elements: the zonula occludens (ZO or tight junction), zonula adherens (ZA or intermediate junction), and macula adherens (MA or desmosome). PM, Plasma membrane; MA, macula adhesions; Rt, filamentous rootlets; EC, glycocalyx or filamentous coat. All three elements appear to be involved in cell-to-cell attachment. (D) Goblet cells occur singly in the intestinal epithelium and large intestine. The mucous secretion of the goblet cells lubricates the lumen of the gastrointestinal tract. Reproduced with permission from T. L. Lentz, "Cell Fine Structure," pp. 179, 181, 183. Saunders, Philadelphia, Pennsylvania, 1971.

The outermost surface of the columnar epithelial cell, that is, the microvilli or brush border region, is covered with a filamentous, muco-polysaccharide coat termed the glycocalyx or "fuzzy coat." The function of the glycocalyx is not specifically known.

D. Hormone-Secreting Cells: Their Distribution in the Gastro-Entero-Pancreatic Complex

A variety of endocrine cells are dispersed throughout the gastric mucosa, the small intestine, and colon. Two basic kinds of cells are identifiable by the classical histological procedures of staining with silver and chrome: (1) enterochromaffin cells, and (b) argophyl cells. The enterochromaffin cells are sparsely present in the gastric mucosa, but are fairly prevalent in the small and large intestine. Both cell types are located either between the bases of other gastrointestinal gland cells or they extend from the basal lamina to the lumen of the intestine. In man there are approximately twice as many argophyl cells as enterochromaffin cells in the intestine. However, as documented in Table 8-3 it is apparent that the endocrine properties of these cells are considerably more complex. Using immunofluorescent techniques it has been shown that in the gastro-entero-pancreatic complex there may be as many as 14 different hormone-secreting cells. It has been documented that these cells are capable of secreting gastrin, motilin, secretin, cholecystokinin/pancreozymin, somatostatin, GIP, VIP, enkephalins, insulin, and pancreatic polypeptide.

In many cases these cells have microvillous borders facing the lumen of the stomach or intestine so that they can respond to chemicals in the stomach or intestinal contents. Most of the cells appear to produce a single peptide hormone, but in some instances they also produce biogenic amines such as histamine or 5-OH-tryptamine. The peptide hormones produced by these cells can be delivered to their appropriate target cells by one of three paths: (1) an endocrine path by way of the blood; (2) a paracrine path by diffusion through the intercellular fluid to adjacent cells; and (3) an exocrine path via discharge of hormone contents into an adjacent lumen (as in the stomach of intestine). Thus, as illustrated in Fig. 8-5, gastroentero endocrine cells may either be "open" with luminal exposure or "closed." Closed cells do not have the potential for luminal discharge of their hormonal contents. But, some of these same gastro-entero-hormone-secreting cells have been shown histologically to be present in the nerves and ganglia of the gastric and intestinal wall. This then permits them to release their hormones as a consequence of nervous stimulation.

Table 8–3. Classification and Anatomical Distribution of the Hormone-Secreting Cells in the Gastro-Entero-Hepatic Tissues[a]

Hormone product	Cell designation	Pancreas	Stomach		Small intestine		Large intestine
			Oxyntic, cardial	Antral	Upper	Lower	
5-Hydroxytryptamine	EC	+	+	+	+	+	+
Somatostatin	D	+	+	+	+		
Pancreatic polypeptide	PP	+				+	+
Glucagon	A	+	+				
Insulin	B	+					
Unknown	X		+				
Gastrin	G			+			
Secretin	S				+		
Cholecystokinin	CCK				+		
GIP	K				+		
Neurotensin	N					+	
GLI	L					+	+

[a] Abstracted from E. Solcia, C. Capella, R. Buffa, B. Frigerio, L. Usellini, and R. Fiocca, Morphological and functional classification of endocrine cells and related growths in the gastrointestinal tract. In "Gastrointestinal Hormones" (G. B. Jerzy-Glass, ed.). Raven Press, New York, 1980.

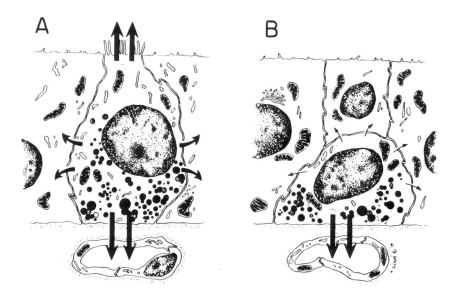

Figure 8-5. Diagram of (A) open and (B) closed endocrine cells. The open gastro-entero-endocrine cells have a membrane surface with luminal exposure, whereas closed cells, such as found in the pancreas, do not have a portion of their extracellular membrane bordering on a lumen. Modified from C. Creutzfeldt and W. Creutzfeldt, Cellular synthesis and release of gastro-entero-pancreatic hormones. *In* "Gastrointestinal Hormones" (G. B. Jerzy-Glass, ed.), p. 75. Raven Press, New York, 1980.

A. Pearse and colleagues have proposed that all the gastro-entero-pancreatic endocrine cells are derived from a common embryological ancestor—the APUD cell. The acronym APUD stands for "amine precursor uptake and decarboxylation," which reflects the common biochemical properties of all these cells to produce and metabolize amines. Pearce noted that both endocrine cells and neurons which produce peptide hormones share similar ultrastructural, cytochemical, and biochemical properties. He postulated that all hormonal peptide-producing cells are originally derived from the neural ectoderm.

E. Coordination of Gastro-Entero-Pancreatic Hormone Release

A number of gastrointestinal hormones can only be secreted by their cells of origin (see Table 8-3) as a consequence of the active digestion/absorption of nutrients in the stomach and duodenum. Thus, the stomach has been recognized to be a major control center to coordinate digestion. The ingestion of nutrients is postulated to be the initiating signal for gastro-entero-pancreatic hormone release. Carbohydrate ingestion leads to the secretion of GIP and enteroglucagon, while fat ingestion stimulates CCK, GIP, neurotensin, and possibly motilin release. Because these responses occur within 15 min of ingestion, it seems probable that cellular absorption cannot have played a significant role. This finding suggested to the Creutzfeldts that gastric hormones or releasing factors may function as control signals for hormone release from jejunal and ileal cells as well as the pancreas (see Fig. 8-6). Recently, a gastrin-releasing protein has been isolated from the fundic portion of the stomach.

It is also possible that the gastro-entero-pancreatic releasing hormones may be involved in an interchange of signals between the brain and intestine. The brain peptides somatostatin (14 amino acids) and neurotensin (13 amino acids) are known to be secreted by cells in the stomach and intestine. Also, cholecystokinin has been shown to be localized in the brain, and it has been suggested by R. Yalow to be involved in satiety and body weight control.

III. CHEMISTRY AND BIOCHEMISTRY

A. General Relationships

All of the gastrointestinal hormones are polypeptides and they are each produced in special endocrine cells which are dispersed throughout the stomach and small and large intestine. The gastrointestinal hormones were originally discovered during the search for physiological agents that regulated and stimulated the exocrine secretions and activities of the gut.

To date, there are three well-characterized gastrointestinal hormones: gastrin, secretin, and cholecystokinin–pancreozymin. In addition, there are a host of other peptide substances which have been isolated from the gastrointestinal tract (see Table 8-3) as well as the skin of certain amphibians (bombesin and cerulein). Advances in protein/peptide techniques have facilitated the isolation of many pure substances which in turn have permitted assessment of their biological actions and subsequent development of specific radioimmunoassay procedures. It has become apparent from a comparison of biological activities and the amino acid sequence homologies among the pure peptides that there are extensive areas of both functional as well as chemical overlap among the gastrointestinal hormones.

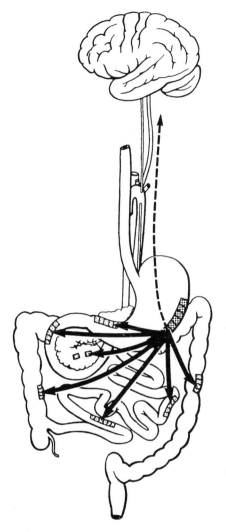

Figure 8-6. Schematic diagram illustrating how gastric hormones may regulate the release of various gastro-entero-pancreatic hormones. Modified from C. Creutzfeldt and W. Creutzfeldt, Cellular synthesis and release of gastro-entero-pancreatic hormones. *In* "Gastrointestinal Hormones" (G. B. Jerzy-Glass, ed.), pp. 71–84. Raven Press, New York, 1980.

B. Gastrin

1. Chemistry

In 1964 Gregory and Tracey isolated and purified gastrins I and II from the antrum of frog gastric mucosa (molecular weight 2100). Both gastrins I and II are identical heptadecapeptides in a single, linear polypeptide chain. Gastrin II differs from I in that the hydroxyl of tyrosine at position 12 is in a sulfate-ester linkage (see Fig. 8-7). Subsequently, gastrin has been isolated and sequenced as a heptadecapeptide from the dog, cow, sheep, cat, and man and found to differ by only 1–2 conservative amino acid substitutions in the middle (positions 5, 8, and 10) of the peptide chain. The substitutions require only a single base change of the codon triplet per substitution.

As is the case with many peptide hormones, multiple molecular species of gastrin have been detected in the blood by application of a radioimmunoassay to samples of serum which have been separated on the basis of "size" via chromatography over columns of Sephadex (see Table 8-4). These include "mini-gastrin" (molecular weight 1700; amino acid positions 4–17 of gastrin), "little gastrin" (the intact 17 amino acid native gastrin), "big gastrin" (molecular weight 3900; 34 amino acid residues), and "big big gastrin" (molecular weight 10,000). The physiological significance of the various gastrin peptides has not yet been clearly assessed. Although big gastrin is the predominant species present in the blood, the 17 amino acid gastrin is the predominant species in the pyloric mucosa and is believed to be the agent responsible for stimulation of parietal cells to produce HCl.

The smallest fragment capable of producing most of the biological responses of gastrin is the C-terminal tetrapeptide: H_2N-Trp–Met–Asp–Phe-$CONH_2$. Removal of the C terminal of this tetrapeptide abolishes its biological activity. The C-terminal pentapeptide of gastrin is also known to be identical with that of cholecystokinin–pancreozymin (see later).

The gastric peptide most frequently used both in research and clinically is pentagastrin. This peptide consists of an N-t-butyloxocarbonyl-β-alanine coupled to the N-terminal amino group of the four C-terminal amino acids of gastrin.

2. Biochemistry

Recently, the gene sequence of gastrin has been reported. It seems likely that big gastrin represents some form of progastrin reminiscent of the general mechanism for biosynthesis and secretion of other peptide hormones [e.g., proinsulin and proglucagon (Chapter 7), proopiomelanocortin (Chapter 5), or proparathyroid hormone (Chapter 9)]. Big

Gastrin-34 Man (MW 3839)

1	2	3	4	5	6	7	8	9	10	11	12	13	14	15	16
Pyroglu	Leu	Gly	Pro	Gln	Gly	His	Pro	Ser	Leu	Val	Ala	Asp	Pro	Ser	Lys

17	18	19	20	21	22	23	24	25	26	27	28	29	30	31	32	33	34
Lys	Gln	Gly	Pro	Trp	Leu	Glu	Glu	Glu	Glu	Glu	Ala	Tyr	Gly	Trp	Met	Asp	Phe-NH_2

Gastrin-17-I Man (MW 2096)

1	2	3	4	5	6	7	8	9	10	11	12	13	14	15	16	17
Pyroglu	Gly	Pro	Trp	Leu	Glu	Glu	Glu	Glu	Glu	Ala	Tyr	Gly	Trp	Met	Asp	Phe-NH_2

Gastrin-17-II Man (MW 2176)

Pyroglu Gly Pro Trp Leu Glu Glu Glu Glu Glu Ala Tyr(SO_3H) Gly Trp Met Asp Phe-NH_2

Gastrin-17 Hog

Pyroglu Gly Pro Trp Met Glu Glu Glu Glu Glu Ala Tyr(SO_3H) Gly Trp Met Asp Phe-NH_2

Gastrin-17 Dog

Pyroglu Gly Pro Trp Met Glu Glu Ala Glu Glu Ala Tyr Gly Trp Met Asp Phe-NH_2

Gastrin-17 Cow and sheep

Pyroglu Gly Pro Trp Val Glu Glu Glu Glu Ala Ala Tyr Gly Trp Met Asp Phe-NH_2

Gastrin-17 Cat

Pyroglu Gly Pro Trp Leu Glu Glu Glu Glu Glu Ala Tyr Gly Trp Met Asp Phe-NH_2

Gastrin-13-I Man

Trp Leu Glu Glu Glu Glu Glu Ala Tyr Gly Trp Met Asp Phe-NH_2

Pentapeptide

t-Boc-B Ala Trp Met Asp Phe-NH_2

Figure 8-7. Primary amino acid sequences of gastrin isolated from various species. Modified from G. Nilson, Gastrin; Isolation, characterization and functions. *In* "Gastrointestinal Hormones" (G. B. Jerzy-Glass, ed.), pp. 127–222. Raven Press, New York, 1980.

Table 8–4. Biochemical Characteristics of the Molecular Species of Gastrin[a]

Molecular species	Molecular weight	Number of amino acids	Percentage in fasting plasma	Antrum tissue	Potency of endogenous (relative)	Half-life (min)
Big big	>10,000	83	75	—	0	90
Big	3,900	34	15	10–20	0.17	16
Little	2,100	17	10	80–90	1.0	3
Mini	1,700	14	1	—	0.8	2

[a] This information was abstracted from B. M. Jaffe, Hormones of the gastrointestinal tract. In "Endocrinology" (L. J. DeGroot, G. F. Cahill, L. Martini, D. H. Nelson, W. D. Odell, J. T. Potts, E. Steinberger, and A. I. Winegrad, eds.), Vol. 3, p. 1684. Grune & Stratton, New York, 1979.

gastrin contains a Lys–Lys sequence at positions 18 and 19; this doublet of basic amino acids has been found to be the signal for cleavage of pro species at the time they undergo the secretion coupling process.

The secretion of gastrin from the antrum of the stomach is a complex process that involves the integrated actions of two systems: (1) direct stimulation of G cells by peptides and amino acids (especially aromatic amino acids) in the gastric lumen, which may be counteracted by lowering of the intragastric pH; and (2) neural stimulation by vagal, noncholinergic mechanisms that may involve either β-adrenergic or bombesin transmission. The latter actions can be inhibited by somatostatin released from adjacent cells. These tentative relationships are summarized in Table 8-5.

The gastrin-releasing peptide (GRP) has been isolated from porcine nonantral stomach and the amino acid sequence determined. GRP contains 27 amino acids; as a linear peptide, GRP shows structural homology to bombesin such that 9 of the 10 carboxyamino acid residues are identical (see Fig. 8-13). A detailed physiological role for GRP is not yet available. The half-lives and relative potencies of the gastrin species are summarized in Table 8-4.

C. Secretin

1. Chemistry

Secretin was the first hormone to be discovered. W. Bayliss and E. Starling, in 1902, reported the existence in acid extracts of the duodenum of a substance that when injected into the bloodstream led to the secretion by the pancreas of HCO_3^- and water. J. Jorpes and V. Mutt have isolated and sequenced secretin from the porcine duodenum. Se-

Table 8–5. Factors Affecting Gastrin Secretion[a]

Mode of delivery	Stimulating factors	Inhibitory factors
Gastric lumen	PEPTIDES	ACIDITY
	Amino acids	(pH below 3)
	Calcium	
Paracrine	BOMBESIN	SOMATOSTATIN
Nervous	β-adrenergic agents,	
	cholinergic agents	
Circulation	Epinephrine	GIP
		Secretin
		Somatostatin
		Glucagon
		Calcitonin

[a] Major factors affecting gastrin release are indicated by capital letters; possible factors are indicated by lowercased letters.

cretin is a linear heptacosapeptide (27 amino acids) with a C-terminal amide (see Fig. 8-8). It is of interest that 14 of the 27 amino acid residues are identical with those of pancreatic glucagon (compare with Fig. 7-9). Unlike cholecystokinin–pancreozymin and gastrin, it has been established that the entire 27 amino acid sequence is required for biological activity.

2. Biochemistry

Few biochemical details are yet available to describe the various steps which result in the release of secretin by the endocrine S cells present in the duodenal mucosa. The only known stimulant for the release of secretin from the S cells is the hydrogen ion. The threshold for release of secretin is pH 4.5. However, since acidification of the duodenal lumen rarely falls below 4.5, it is difficult to identify at the present time either the stimulatory agents for secretin release or to develop a clear understanding of its physiological significance.

The biological half-life of secretin in the plasma is ~3–4 min. The kidney is believed to play a major role in secretin inactivation.

D. Cholecystokinin–Pancreozymin

1. Chemistry

Cholecystokinin–pancreozymin (CCK–PZ) is a single molecular species with dual major physiological properties. CCK was discovered in 1928 by Ivy and Goldberg as a substance which, when released into the bloodstream, would stimulate gallbladder contraction. Then in 1944

His-Ser-Asp-Gly-Thr-Phe-Thr-Ser-Glu-Leu-Ser-Arg-Leu-Arg-
Asp-Ser-Ala-Arg-Leu-Gln-Arg-Leu-Leu-Gln-Gly-Leu-Val

Figure 8-8. Primary amino acid sequence of porcine secretin. Modified from V. Mutt, Secretin: Isolation, structure and function. *In* "Gastrointestinal Hormones" (G. B. Jerzy-Glass, ed.), pp. 85–126. Raven Press, New York, 1980.

Harper and Roper reported that extracts of porcine intestinal tissue contained a substance distinct from secretin which stimulated the acinar pancreas to secrete a spectrum of proteases. Later work by Jorpes and Mutt in 1966 established that the same molecular species contained both CCK and PZ properties. Because cholecystokinin was discovered earlier than pancreozymin, it has now been proposed that CCK–PZ be named CCK for short, it being understood that the designation CCK includes both pancreozymin and cholecystokinin activities.

Porcine CCK has been isolated from duodenal and jejunal tissue; it is a single-chain polypeptide of 33 amino acids (see Fig. 8-9). As is the case with gastrin II, the phenolic hydroxyl of the tyrosine in position 7 of CCK is esterified by sulfate. Also, the carboxy-terminal pentapeptide is identical to that of gastrin II (compare with Fig. 8-8).

One important structural variant of CCK-33 is the addition of an N-terminal hexapeptide to yield CCK-39. Again, as with big gastrin, CCK-39 contains the basic amino acid dimer, Arg–Lys, in positions 34 and 35, suggesting that CCK-39 may represent a "proform" of CCK-33 that is produced during biosynthetic events. Also, an even larger form of CCK (i.e., a CCK-58 species) has been shown to be present under some circumstances.

All known biological activities of CCK can be produced by the heptapeptide at the C terminal; the heptapeptide (C-terminal residues 1–7) has been reported to be 2–3 times more active on a molar basis than CCK-33 or CCK-39.

2. Biochemistry

The physiological release of CCK from the endocrine cells of the duodenum is stimulated by free fatty acids, but not triglycerides, and by

Tyr-Ile-Gln-Gln-Ala-Arg-Lys-Ala-Pro-Ser-Gly-Arg-Val-
Ser-Met-Ile-Lys-Asn-Leu-Gln-Ser-Leu-Asp-Pro-Ser-His-
Arg-Ile-Ser-Asp-Arg-Asp-Tyr*-Met-Gly-Trp-Met-Asp-Phe-NH₂

Figure 8-9. Primary amino acid sequence of cholecystokinin. Modified from V. Mutt, Secretin: Isolation, structure and function. *In* "Gastrointestinal Hormones" (G. B. Jerzy-Glass, ed.), pp. 85–126. Raven Press, New York, 1980.

certain free amino acids and hydrogen ions. However, no detailed models of secretion coupling for CCK have been put forth.

The metabolism and inactivation of plasma CCK have been studied. Both CCK-39 and CCK-33 are cleaved to yield CCK-12, which is then slowly converted into CCK-8. The plasma half-life of CCK biological activity is less than 3–4 min.

An intriguing observation was the discovery of the existence of CCK in cerebral tissue. Possibly brain CCK acts as a neurotransmitter. Also, there is structural similarity of the N-terminal pentapeptide of CCK-7 to that of methionine enkephalin.

E. Other Gastrointestinal Hormones

1. Gastrointestinal Inhibitory Polypeptide (GIP)

A substance termed the gastrointestinal inhibitory polypeptide, or GIP, has been isolated from porcine duodenum–jejunum. GIP is a linear peptide of 43 amino acids; the primary amino acid sequence is given in Fig. 8-10.

GIP was first identified as a substance capable of inhibiting the gastric secretion of HCl and pepsin as well as the motor activity of the stomach. However, the role of GIP as a physiologically relevant inhibitor of gastric secretion has been questioned because these effects could only be achieved by the infusion of supraphysiological levels of GIP. It has been shown that GIP is insulinotropic in the rat, dog, and man. The secretion of GIP is stimulated by ingestion of a meal or glucose. Conversely, GIP secretion is apparently inhibited by both insulin and glucagon.

2. Vasoactive Intestinal Peptide (VIP)

A polypeptide substance termed vasoactive intestinal peptide, or VIP, was first identified in 1970 on the basis of its vasodilator action. The peptide is a linear sequence of 29 amino acids (see Fig. 8-11). It has been

```
 1                                                              14
Tyr Ala Glu Gly Thr Phe Ile Ser Asp Tyr Ser Ile Ala Met

15                                                             28
Asp Lys Ile Arg Gln Gln Asp Phe Val Asn Trp Leu Leu Ala

29                                                             43
Gln Gln Lys Gly Lys Lys Ser Asp Trp Lys His Asn Ile Thr Gln
```

Figure 8-10. Primary amino acid sequence of gastrointestinal peptide (GIP). Modified from J. C. Grown, S. Kwank, S. C. Otte, and C. H. S. McIntosh, Gastric inhibitory polypeptide: Structure and basic function. *In* "Gastrointestinal Hormones" (G. B. Jerzy-Glass, ed.), pp. 245–274. Raven Press, New York, 1980.

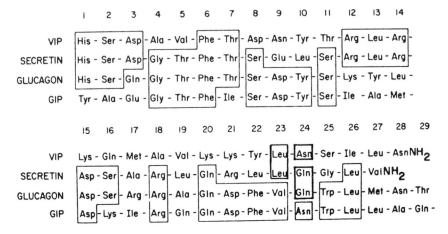

Figure 8-11. Primary amino acid sequence of porcine, vasoactive intestinal peptide (VIP), glucagon, and gastrointestinal peptide (GIP). Regions of identical sequences are outlined. Modified from S. I. Said, Vasoactive intestinal peptide (VIP): Isolation, distribution, biological actions, structure–function relationships and possible functions. *In* "Gastrointestinal Hormones" (G. B. Jerzy-Glass, ed.), pp. 245–274. Raven Press, New York, 1980.

shown to have extensive structural homology with both glucagon and secretin as well as some homology with GIP.

VIP occurs widely in both the intestinal and nervous systems of many mammals and lower animals. The biological actions of VIP include (1) suppression of gastric acid secretion; (2) stimulation of intestinal H_2O and ion secretion; (3) promotion of splanchnic blood flow; and (4) stimulation of cyclic AMP production in a wide variety of tissues. It has been suggested that VIP functions as a paracrine substance (i.e., a local hormone). The further biological actions of VIP are summarized in Table 8-6.

VIP secretion is stimulated by vagal nerve stimulation, by depolarizing concentrations of K^+, and by cholinergic agonists. Receptors for VIP have been identified in selected regions of the gastrointestinal tract as well as the brain.

3. Motilin

A 22 amino acid, linear polypeptide, termed motilin (see Fig. 8-12), was isolated in 1973 by J. Brown and co-workers. The amino acid sequence is entirely different from all the other known gastrointestinal hormones. Motilin is believed to play a role in the regulation of the small intestine motility during fasting. Its release from the endocrine EC cells of the duodenum is cyclical, occurring approximately every 2 hr. Signifi-

Table 8–6. Biological Actions of Vasoactive Intestinal Peptide (VIP)[a]

Cardiovascular system	Vasodilation (including peripheral, splanchnic, coronary, extracranial, and cerebral vessels), hypotension, moderate inotropic effect
Respiratory system	Bronchodilation, augmented ventilation, stimulation of adenylate cyclase activity
Digestive system	
Esophagus	Relaxation of lower sphincter
Stomach	Relaxation of fundic smooth muscle, suppression of acid, and pepsin secretion
Pancreas, liver	Stimulation of water and bicarbonate secretion (secretin-like action), increased bile flow
Gallbladder	Relaxation of isolated smooth muscle, inhibition of contractile effect of CCK–PZ
Small and large intestine	Inhibition of absorption, stimulation of water and ion secretion, stimulation of adenylate cyclase activity, relaxation of smooth muscle of colon
Metabolism	Stimulation of glycogenolysis, lipolysis, and adenylate cyclase activity (in liver, pancreatic acini, and adipocytes), hyperglycemia
Endocrine function	
Pancreas	Release of insulin, glucagon, and somatostatin
Pituitary-hypothalamus	Stimulation of release of prolactin, GH, and LH
Adrenal	ACTH-like action (stimulation of steroidogenesis and adenylate cyclase activity)
Central nervous system	Arousal, excitation of cerebral cortical and spinal cord neurons, hyperthermia, regional stimulation of adenylate cyclase activity

[a] Abstracted from S. I. Said, Vasoactive intestinal peptide (VIP): Isolation, distribution, biological actions, structure–function relationship, and possible functions. *In* "Gastrointestinal Hormones" (G. B. Jerzy-Glass, ed.). Raven Press, New York, 1980.

cantly, most of motilin's actions do not coincide with dietary intake, but with fasting. It has been suggested that it enhances movement of digested food particles in preparation for the next meal. The physiological role of motilin remains to be clarified.

4. *Pancreatic Polypeptide (PP)*

Pancreatic polypeptide or PP is a 36 amino acid peptide which appears to stimulate the gastric secretion of HCl and pepsin; it also may act as a satiety factor. PP is known to be released after ingestion of a protein meal. Cells secreting PP are scattered at a low concentration throughout the duodenum and in the pancreatic islets. The amino acid sequence of PP is given in Fig. 7-10. Despite the large number of factors known to

PHE-VAL-PRO-ILE-PHE-THR-TYR-GLY-GLU-LEU-GLN
  1   2   3   4   5   6   7   8   9   10   11

-ARG-MET-GLU-GLU-LYS-GLU-ARG-ASN-LYS-GLY-GLN
  12   13   14   15   16   17   18   19   20   21   22

Figure 8-12. Primary amino acid sequence of porcine motilin. Modified from C. H. S. McIntosh and J. C. Brown, Motilin: Isolation, structure and basic functions. *In* "Gastrointestinal Hormones" (G. B. Jerzy-Glass, ed.), pp. 233–244. Raven Press, New York, 1980.

stimulate the release of PP and the relatively high plasma concentration that is maintained following food intake, little is known concerning its precise physiological function.

5. Enteroglucagon

A protein substance can be extracted from the gastrointestinal tract which exhibits immuno-cross-reactivity to antibodies prepared against pure pancreatic glucagon (see Chapter 7). Intestinal glucagon appears to have a higher molecular weight than pancreatic glucagon. Its physiological role remains to be clarified.

F. Peptides from Amphibian Skin with Gastrointestinal Hormone Actions

The skin of amphibians is known to contain four classes of biologically active peptides: the bombesin-like, the physaelamin-like, the caevulein-like, and the bradykinin-like peptides.

The family of bombesin-like peptides has been extensively studied since the discovery that they have potent actions on the gastrointestinal tract. Bombesin is a tetradecapeptide present in the skin of two species of frogs, *Bombina bombina* and *Bombina variegata*, at a concentration of 200–700 µg/g wet weight. Their amino acid sequence is given in Fig. 8-13. The C-terminal nonapeptide is as biologically active as the intact bombesin. Alytesin, ranatensin, and litorin are structural analogs of bombesin also present in frog skin.

The principal biological effect of bombesin is stimulation of gastrin release and gastric acid secretion. Also, bombesin can stimulate the contraction of the gallbladder. In addition, bombesin has extragastrointestinal effects which include hypertension due to contraction of vascular muscle, contraction of smooth muscle, and antidiuretic effects on the kidney.

Another class of frog skin-derived peptides is caerulein (a decapep-

	1	2	3	4	5	6	7	8	9	10	11	12	13	14
Bombesin	Pyroglu	Glu	Arg	Leu	Gly	Asn	Gln	Trp	Ala	Val	Gly	His	Leu	Met-NH$_2$
Alytesin	Pyroglu	Gly	Arg	Leu	Gly	Thr	Gln	Trp	Ala	Val	Gly	His	Leu	Met-NH$_2$
Ranatensin			Pyroglu	Val	Pro	Gln	Trp	Ala	Val	Gly	His	Phe	Met-NH$_2$	
Litorin				Pyroglu	Gln	Trp	Ala	Val	Gly	His	Phe	Met-NH$_2$		

Figure 8-13. Primary amino acid sequence of peptides isolated from amphibian skin which can exert biological actions on the gastrointestinal tract. Modified from B. M. Jaffe, Hormones of the gastrointestinal tract. *In* "Endocrinology" (L. J. DeGroot, G. F. Cahill, L. Martini, D. H. Nelson, W. D. Odell, J. T. Potts, E. Steinberger, and A. I. Winegard, eds.) Vol. 3, p. 1676. Grune & Stratton, New York, 1979.

tide) and phyllcaerulein (a nonapeptide); both are isolated from the skin of the Australian tree frog, *Hyla caerulea*. There is a high sequence homology between the caeruleins and the C-terminal octapeptide of porcine cholecystokinin. The caeruleins also mimic the biological effects of CCK in that they are potent stimulators of the contraction of the gallbladder.

G. Brain–Gut Peptides

1. Neurotensin

Over 95% of the neurotensin in the body is in the gut and brain. Neurotensin has been isolated and sequenced from bovine hypothalamus and bovine and human intestine; all three sources gave a peptide with an identical tridecapeptide structure (see Fig. 8-14).

The biological actions mediated by neurotensins are diverse and include vascular effects (vasodilation, hypotension), gastrointestinal effects (contraction of fundus and ileum, relaxation of duodenum, increased gastrin secretion), pancreatic islet effects (increased insulin and glucagon secretion), and neuroendocrine effects (hypothermia, increased release of ACTH, LH, FSH, GH, and prolactin). The mode of action of neurotensin is not known. The plasma half-life of neurotensin is ~1 min.

2. Somatostatin

The amino acid sequence of the tetradecapeptide somatostatin is given in Fig. 3-8. The endocrine cells in the gastrointestinal system which secrete somatostatin are widely scattered. Also, somatostatin is

$$\text{H}_2\text{N-Glu-Leu-Tyr-Glu-Asn-Lys-Pro-Arg-Arg-}$$
$$\text{-Pro-Tyr-Ile-Leu-COOH}$$

Figure 8-14. Amino acid sequence of neurotensin.

released by nerve endings throughout the stomach and gastrointestinal tract. A large proportion of the actions of somatostatin appear to occur in very close proximity to its site of release. It has been shown to inhibit the release of CCK, VIP, GIP, and secretin and to decrease intestinal contractions. The half-life of somatostatin is 1–3 min.

IV. BIOLOGICAL AND MOLECULAR ACTIONS

A. Gastric Secretion

The parietal cells of the stomach secrete a solution of 0.10 M HCl and 7 mM KCl, with only a trace of other electrolytes. The concentration of hydrogen ions is 1 million times higher than that of plasma. The secretion of hydrochloric acid by the parietal cells of the stomach is effected by endocrine (gastrin), neuroendocrine (acetylcholine), and paracrine (histamine) pathways. In addition, an increase in the cytosolic concentration of calcium can trigger the release of HCl. The actions of acetylcholine can be blocked by anticholinergic agents, such as atropine. Cimetidine (an H_2 receptor antagonist) can specifically block the actions of histamine.

Pepsin is the principal proteolytic enzyme present in the gastric secretions. Pepsin is stored in an inactive form as pepsinogen in secretory granules of the chief cells of the oxyntic mucosa of the stomach. Smaller amounts of pepsinogen are also found in the cardiac and pyloric cells of the stomach and upper duodenal mucosa. As yet no detailed model has been proposed to describe the molecular steps of secretion of pepsinogen. The process is probably analogous to that of secretion of the proenzymes trypsinogen and chymotrypsinogen from the exocrine portion of the pancreas.

Pepsinogen secretion is strongly stimulated by gastrin and related peptides as well as by a vagal cholinergic stimulation which may be induced by feeding. Also, secretin is a strong stimulator of pepsinogen secretion. The enzymatically inactive pepsinogen (40,400 Da) is, in the presence of acid, autocatalytically converted to the active form, pepsin, by the cleavage of a 42 amino acid residue from the N-terminal portion of the peptide chain. Pepsins are active at acid pH (below 3.5) and are irreversibly inactivated at neutral or slightly alkaline pH. The active form of pepsin is 32,000 Da and has a proetolytic specificity for Trp, Phe, Tyr, Met, and Leu amino acid residues in a protein substrate. A model for secretagogue stimulation of the parietal cell is given in Fig. 8-15.

The parietal cell is known to have separate receptors for gastrin, histamine, and acetylcholine. The actions of histamine, but not gastrin or cholinergic agents, are coupled to the generation of the second messenger cyclic AMP, whereas the effects of acetylcholine, but not gastrin and histamine, are related to an enhanced influx of calcium across the epithelial cell membrane.

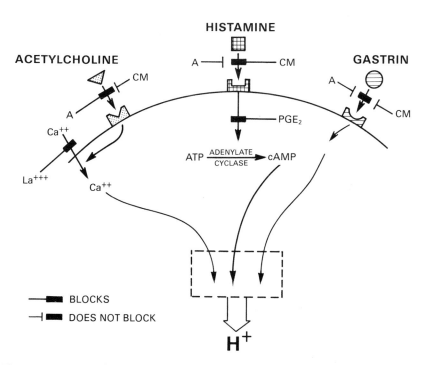

Figure 8-15. Proposed model to describe the actions of secretagogues on stomach parietal cells. Receptors for gastrin, acetylcholine, and histamine are indicated, as well as the proposed sites of the inhibitors cimetidine (CM) and atropine (A). Modified from A. H. Soll, Isolated canine parietal cells: Receptors and effectors regulating function. *In* "Physiology of the Gastrointestinal Tract" (L. R. Johnson, ed.), p. 686. Raven Press, New York, 1981.

B. Pancreatic, Biliary, and Intestinal Secretions

1. Exocrine Pancreas Secretion

After ingestion of a meal and associated with the appearance of the acidified chyme from the stomach in the duodenum, there is a coupled secretion by the exocrine pancreas of H_2O, bicarbonate, and the digestive enzymes, amylase, trypsinogen, chymotrypsinogen, and lipase. This pancreatic secretion is dependent upon the release of gut hormones from the antrum and small intestine (see Table 8-2). In addition, stimulation of appropriate cholinergic or peptidergic nerves leading to the pancreas can stimulate exocrine pancreatic secretions (see Fig. 8-16).

Pancreatic secretions of electrolytes and H_2O from the ductular and centroacinar cells are primarily under the influence of secretin. Secretin is believed to generate intracellular cyclic AMP in these cells which activates unknown factors necessary to alter the secretory cell membrane permeability to sodium and hydrogen ions. Thus, there is an increased exchange of external Na^+ ions for internal H^+ ions. The increased concentration of extracellular H^+ lowers the local pH, which then increases the production of CO_2 from circulating bicarbonate. This CO_2 then diffuses into the cells where it combines with water to form

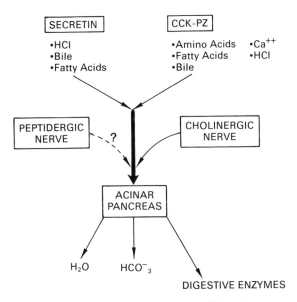

Figure 8-16. Schematic diagram of secretin stimulation of the acinar pancreas illustrating the roles of secretin, CCK, cholinergic, and peptidergic nerves. Modified from W. Y. Chey, Gastrointestinal hormones and pancreatic, biliary and intestinal secretions. *In* "Gastrointestinal Hormones" (G. B. Jerzy-Glass, ed.), pp. 565–584. Raven Press, New York, 1980.

carbonic acid (mediated by carbonic anhydrase) and results in the secretion of bicarbonate.

The pancreatic secretion of the digestive enzymes occurs in the acinar cells of the exocrine pancreas under the influence of CCK and VIP. Two pathways of hormone-mediated stimulus secretion are envisaged: (1) acetylcholine and CCK-mediated changes in phosphatidylinositol turnover, with an associated elevation of intracellular free Ca^{2+} and activation of a guanylate cyclase which, in turn, leads to a phosphorylation of membrane proteins; and (2) a VIP-mediated stimulation of an adenylate cyclase and subsequent membrane phosphorylation. The increased membrane phosphorylation is envisioned to stimulate emiocytosis and secretion of amylase, lipase, chymotrypsinogen, and trypsinogen stored in secretory granules.

2. Biliary Secretion

Hormonal regulation of bile secretion primarily by CCK and secretin occurs by action on the ductules and ducts of the gallbladder. Table 8-7 presents the major components of human bile. These constituents are secreted into the intestinal lumen in response to dietary fat and act as detergents to disrupt and disperse the oil droplets. Secretin increases the volume and bicarbonate concentration of the bile probably by a mechanism analogous to its actions on the exocrine pancreas. Also, the canalicular secretion of bile is known to be stimulated by thyroxine, insulin, glucagon, vasopressin, and cortisol and inhibited by estradiol; the physiological significance of these observations is not yet clear.

Table 8–7. Major Organic Components of Human Bile[a]

Component	Concentration (mg/ml bile)
Dihydroxycholanic acids	49
Cholic acid	32
Phospholipid (mostly lecithin)	27
Protein	5
Cholesterol	3
Bilirubin	3
Hexose and hexosamine	1

[a] Abstracted from F. Nakayma and H. Miyake, Species differences in cholesterol-complexing macromolecular fractions in bile in relation to gallstone formation. *J. Lab. Clin. Med.* **67,** 78–86 (1966).

3. Intestinal Secretion

Several gut hormones, including VIP, GIP, secretin, CCK, and glucagon, and prostaglandins E_1, E_2, and $F_{2\alpha}$, have been shown to affect the small intestine and colon by either inhibiting the active absorption of electrolytes and H_2O or by stimulating the secretion of H_2O and electrolytes. Both VIP and the prostaglandins are potent stimulators of the adenylate cyclase–cAMP system, and it is probable that this is the basis of their actions on the intestinal secretion of H_2O and electrolytes. The cellular mechanisms of the other gut hormones in this system are not known at present.

C. Motor Functions of the Intestinal Tract

The gastrointestinal hormones play an important physiological role in the regulation of the motor activity of the gastrointestinal tract. This includes effects on the stomach, small intestine, colon, gallbladder, and bile ducts. The hormones may have indirect effects (neurally mediated) or direct actions (muscular) on smooth muscle motor activity. The peptides which primarily stimulate motor activity are gastrin, CCK, and motilin, while the peptides which inhibit motor activity are secretin, VIP, and glucagon and enteroglucagon.

Gastrin exerts its effects partly via direct interaction with intestinal or stomach muscle cell receptors and partly via postganglionic cholinergic fibers; it is effective at very low concentrations (e.g., $1–100 \times 10^{-12}$ M).

The actions of CCK on gall bladder contraction are believed to be largely receptor mediated. Emptying of the bile is the result of a number of successive events: (1) First, there is a progressive increase in the tension of the gallbladder wall; (2) then an intermittent opening of the sphincter-like cholecystocystic junction occurs; (3) next, there are phasic contractions along the common axis of the bile duct; and (4) finally, sequential opening and closing of the choledochoduodenal sphincter occurs, resulting in periodic discharge of bile into the duodenum.

As yet no molecular mechanisms of hormone action are available to describe these complex and critical physiological processes.

V. CLINICAL ASPECTS

A. Peptic Ulcer Disease

The term peptic ulcer refers to an open sore on the esophagus, stomach, or duodenum. It is generally believed that excessive secretions of gastric acid and pepsin are necessary for development and persistence of an ulcer. Peptic ulcer disease can account for as many as 4,000,000 hospital days per year in the United States. Although individuals with duodenal ulcer disease have clearly increased rates of gastric acid secretion and although gastrin is a potent secretagogue of HCl secretion, it has not been directly possible to implicate gastrin in the etiology of duodenal ulcer disease. Patients with duodenal ulcer disease have fasting gastrin levels indistinguishable from control subjects. It has been suggested that these "normal" gastrin levels are inappropriately high for the degree of hypersecretion of HCl that occurs, which might indicate some failure of feedback inhibition in these ulcer patients.

The drug cimetidine has a proven value in the treatment of duodenal ulcer disease through its capacity to inhibit the secretion of gastric acid in hypersecretory states, particularly those involving peptic ulceration.

B. Zollinger–Ellison Syndrome

Zollinger–Ellison syndrome is characterized by an advanced ulcer disease of the upper gastrointestinal tract, hypersecretion of gastric acid, and tumors of the pancreas islets. It is estimated that ~1% of operative cases of peptic ulcer disease are individuals with Zollinger–Ellison syndrome.

The syndrome results from the release of large quantities of gastrin by the pancreatic islet tumors, probably D cells. This then results in an increased secretion of HCl by the parietal cells of the stomach.

C. Carcinoid Syndrome

The term carcinoid or argentaffinosis is employed to describe a group of intestinal tumors that grow more slowly than the more common intestinal carcinoma. The carcinoid tumor is derived from the enterochromaffin cells, which are cytochemically indistinguishable from many of the gastrointestinal hormone-secreting cells of the intestinal tract. The most frequent site of their location is the ileum and appendix. The chief clinical signs of carcinoid syndrome are flushing and diarrhea.

The chief biochemical lesion is an elevated production of 5-hydroxytryptamine which results from the conversion of tryptophan to 5-hydroxytryptophan followed by decarboxylation to yield 5-hydroxytryptamine. Elevated blood levels of 5-hydroxytryptamine and an increased urinary excretion of 5-hydroxyindole acetic acid are often diagnostic of the carcinoid syndrome. Also, the tumor contains the enzyme kallikrein (see Chapter 15), which leads to increased plasma levels of bradykinin.

354

Both pharmacological as well as surgical treatments are employed to treat the carcinoid syndrome.

References

A. Books

Bloom, S. R., and Polak, J. M., ed. (1981). "Gut Hormones," 2nd ed., Churchill-Livingstone, Edinburgh and London.
Jerzy-Glass, G. B., ed. (1980). "Gastrointestinal Hormones." Raven Press, New York.

B. Review Articles

Anderson, S. (1983). Secretion of gastrointestinal hormones. *Annu. Rev. Physiol.* **35,** 431–452.
Gugita, T., and Kobayashi, Y. (1977). Structures and function of gut endocrine cells. *Int. Rev. Cytology Suppl.* **6,** 187–229.
Pearse, A. G. E., and Takor, T. (1976). Neuroendocrine embryology and the APUD concept. *Clin. Endocrinol. (Oxford)* **5,** Suppl., 2295–2445.
Rayford, P. L., Miller, T. A., and Thompson, J. C. (1976). Secretin, cholecystokinin, and newer gastrointestinal hormones. *N. Engl. J. Med.* **294,** 1093–1101, 1157–1164.
Walsh, J. H. (1981). Gastrointestinal hormones and peptides in physiology of the gastrointestinal tract. *In* "Gastrointestinal Physiology" (L. R. Johnston, ed.), pp. 59–144. Raven Press, New York.
Walsh, J. H., and Grossman, M. I. (1975). Gastrin (parts I and II). *N. Engl. J. Med.* **292,** 1324–1334, 1377–1384.

C. Research Papers

Bayliss, W. M., and Starling, E. H. (1902). Mechanism of pancreatic secretion. *J. Physiol. (London)* **28,** 325–334. (Note: This paper describes the first hormone to be discovered.)
Gregory, R. A., and Tracy, H. J. (1964). The constitution and properties of two gastrins extracted from hog antral mucosa. *Gut* **5,** 103–111.
Hanks, J. B., Andersen, D. K., Wise, J. E., Putnam, W. S., Meyers, W. C., and Jones, R. S. (1984). The hepatic extraction of gastric inhibitory peptide. *Endocrinology (Baltimore)* **115,** 1011–1018.
Huang, C. G., Eng, J., and Yalow, R. S. (1986). Ontogeny of immunoreactive cholecystokinin, vasoactive intestinal peptide, and secretin in guinea pig brain and gut. *Endocrinology* **118,** 1096–1101.
Jorpes, J. E., and Mutt, V. (1961). Biological activity and amino acid sequence of porcine secretin. *Acta Chem. Scand.* **15,** 790–799.
Jorpes, J. E., and Mutt, V. (1966). Cholecystokinin and pancreozymin: One single hormone. *Acta Physiol. Scand.* **66,** 196–202.
Mutt, V., and Jorpes, J. E. (1968). Structure of porcine CCK–PZ. *Eur. J. Biochem.* **6,** 156–162.
Richter, K., Egger, R., and Kreil, G. (1986). Sequence of preprocaerulein cDNAs cloned from skin of *Xenopus laevis.* A small family of precursors containing one, three, or four copies of the final product. *J. Biol. Chem.* **261,** 3676–3680.

Chapter **9**

The Calcium-Regulating Hormones: Vitamin D, Parathyroid Hormone, Calcitonin

I. INTRODUCTION

A. Background Information

Calcium and phosphorus are the most abundant of the inorganic elements in man; together they are the key structural minerals of the human body. A 70-kg man contains about 1200 g of calcium and 770 mg of phosphorus present as phosphate. Calcium and phosphorus are also essential to a great number of cellular processes (see Table 9-1).

For optimal growth and function, living organisms require an adequate supply of calcium and phosphate to meet their metabolic and structural needs. Higher organisms must be supplied with calcium and phosphorus on a continuous basis. The plasma concentrations of these substances are maintained within a surprisingly narrow limit by an endogenous control mechanism, often of great subtlety and elegant precision.

The three prime target tissues involved in calcium and phosphorus homeostasis in man and higher animals are the intestine, where these ions enter into the physiological milieu, the bone, where they are stored and made available for minute-by-minute regulation of the serum level of these ions, and the kidney, where their rate of excretion can be monitored and regulated. The maintenance of calcium and phosphorus

Table 9-1. Biological Calcium and Phosphorus

Calcium	Phosphorus
Utilization	
Body content: 70-kg man has 1200 g Ca^{2+}	Body content: 70-kg man has 770 g P
Structural: Bone has 95% of body Ca	Structural: Bone has 90% of body P_i
Plasma [Ca^{2+}] is 2.5 mM, 10 mg%	Plasma [P_i] is 2.3 mM, 2.5–4.3 mg%
Muscle contraction	Intermediary metabolism
Nerve pulse transmission	(phosphorylated intermediates)
Blood clotting	Genetic information (DNA and RNA)
Membrane structure	Phospholipids
Enzyme cofactors	Enzyme/protein components
(amylase, trypsinogen, lipases, ATPases)	(phosphohistidine, phosphoserine)
Eggshell (birds)	Membrane structure
Daily requirements (70-kg man)	
Dietary intake: 700[a]	Dietary intake: 1200[a]
Fecal excretion: 300–600[a,b]	Fecal excretion: 350–370[a,b]
Urinary excretion: 100–400[a,b]	Urinary excretion: 200–600[a,b]

[a] Values in milligrams per day.
[b] Based on the indicated level of dietary intake.

homeostasis thus involves the delicate and coordinated interrelationships of absorption by the intestine, accretion and reabsorption by bone tissue, and urinary excretion by the kidney.

The three principal endocrine regulators of calcium and phosphorus metabolism are the two peptide hormones, parathyroid hormone and calcitonin, and vitamin D and its metabolites. The interdependent actions of these three hormones of calcium and phosphorus homeostasis reflect the crucial roles of both calcium and phosphate in the biological processes of higher animals. It is vital that the extracellular calcium ion concentration is maintained within narrow limits; accordingly, the higher the phylogenetic order, the greater the complexity of endocrinological interrelationships and mechanisms developed to ensure ion homeostatis.

Calcium in the plasma exists in three forms; free (ionized), complexed (chelated) by organic ions such as citrate, and protein bound (see Table 9-2). The total concentration of calcium in plasma is normally 2.5 mM or 10 mg/100 ml. Under usual circumstances ~45% of the total plasma

Table 9–2. Distribution of Calcium and Phosphate in Normal Human Plasma[a]

State		Plasma concentration		Percentage of total
		(mmol/liter)	(mg/100 ml)[b]	
Phosphorus				
Free HPO$_4^{2-}$		0.50	1.55	44
Free H$_2$PO$_4^-$		0.11	0.34	10
Protein-bound		0.14	0.43	12
NaHPO$_4$		0.33	1.02	28
CaHPO$_4$		0.04	0.12	3
MgHPO$_4$		0.03	0.10	3
	Total	1.15	3.56	
Calcium				
Free Ca^{2+}		1.18	4.72	48
Protein-bound		1.14	4.56	46
Complexed		0.08	0.32	3
Unidentified		0.08	0.32	3
	Total	2.48	9.92	

[a] Adapted from M. Walser, Ion association VI. Interaction between calcium, magnesium, inorganic phosphate, citrate and protein in normal human plasma. *J. Clin. Invest.* **40,** 723 (1961).

[b] For plasma inorganic phosphate (H$_2$PO$_4^-$, HPO$_4^{2-}$, and PO$_4^{3-}$) the values are expressed as milligrams of elemental phosphorus or P per 100 ml of plasma in accordance with long-standing clinical practice.

calcium is bound to protein, primarily to serum albumin; the remaining 55% is ultrafilterable. The normal physiological range of the blood concentration of Ca^{2+} is 9.0–10.5 mg/100 ml; deviations outside this narrow "range" of concentrations are reflective of significant perturbations of the calcium-regulating hormones. There are two basic mechanisms for generating free or ionized calcium in the plasma: that which can be mediated by endocrine mechanisms, and that which can occur by changing the concentration of plasma protein. All evidence indicates that the biologically functional and therefore regulated form of calcium is the ionized species.

The plasma concentrations of the several ionic species of phosphate are not so stringently regulated. Under normal circumstances phosphate is present in the plasma at a level of 1.2 mM or in the range of 2.5–4.3 mg of P per 100 ml of phosphorus. (In the United States, plasma concentrations of P are formally expressed as phosphorus, not phosphate.) Approximately 10% of the plasma phosphate is protein bound, and the remainder exists as free phosphate, either as HPO_4^{2-} or $H_2PO_4^{-}$. The relative proportion of these two species is dependent upon plasma pH. There are many biological functions of phosphate extending from its role as an inorganic ion to multiple involvements as organic phosphates in various enzymatic and structural proteins and nucleic acids.

B. Calcium and Phosphorus Homeostasis

The principal organs of the body involved in maintenance of calcium and phosphate homeostasis are the intestine, kidney, and bone; it is here that the three calcium-regulating hormones perform an integrated set of biological actions which results in calcium and phosphorus homeostasis. Vitamin D is known to play a dominant role in increasing the intestinal absorption of calcium and phosphorus; this uptake process is regulated according to the nutritional or physiological needs of the animal and is dictated by certain physiological signals. Once calcium and phosphorus are made available in the plasma, a delicate balancing occurs in the bone between accretion and mobilization and in the kidney between excretion and reabsorption. In the event that the dietary availability of calcium and phosphorus is diminished or increased, the balance is tipped in favor of increased bone mobilization or increased urinary excretion to meet the stringent requisite of a constant serum calcium level. Thus, serum calcium may become elevated by stimulation of intestinal calcium absorption, bone calcium mobilization, or by parathyroid hormone stimulation of the tubular reabsorption of calcium at the kidney. It is clear that bone is the central organ in calcium metabolism, acting as a reservoir for calcium and phosphorus. There are a variety of endocrine-mediated events that govern this organ's involvement in calcium and phosphorus metabolism. These will be discussed later in this chapter.

Figure 9-1 is a schematic diagram illustrating the 24-hr "metabolic balance" of calcium and phosphorus metabolism in a normal adult male. Calcium and phosphorus are both absorbed into the body primarily in the duodenum and jejunum. In addition to the calcium ingested in the diet (for normal man the dietary requirements range from 400 to 1200 mg/day), ~600–700 mg is added to the intestinal contents by intestinal secretions. Of the approximate total of 1600–1700 mg of calcium present in the lumen of the intestine, ~700 mg is absorbed or reabsorbed into

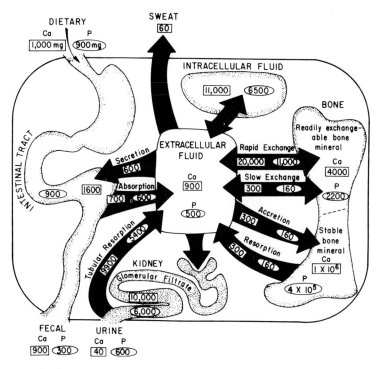

Figure 9-1. A schematic model of calcium and phosphorus metabolism in an adult man having a calcium intake of 1000 mg/day and a phosphorus intake of 800 mg/day. All numerical values are milligrams per day. All entries relating to phosphate are calculated as phosphorus and are enclosed in ovals. Entries related to calcium are enclosed in rectangles. Reproduced by permission from A. W. Norman, "Vitamin D: The Calcium Homeostatic Steroid Hormone," p. 278. Academic Press, New York, 1979.

the bloodstream, leaving the remaining 900–1000 mg to be excreted in the feces.

After calcium has entered the extracellular pool, it is in constant exchange with the calcium already present in the extra- and intracellular fluids of the body and in certain compartments of the bone and glomerular filtrate. The entire extracellular pool of calcium turns over between 40 and 50 times per day. The glomerulus of the kidney filters some 10,000 mg of calcium per day, but the renal tubular reabsorption of this ion is so efficient that under normal circumstances only between 100 and 150 mg of Ca appears in the urine. In the event of hypercalcemia, the urinary excretion of calcium rises in a compensatory fashion; however, it rarely exceeds a value of 400–600 mg/day. The renal tubular reabsorption of calcium is stimulated by parathyroid hormone and possibly by vitamin D or one of its metabolites. The increased urinary excretion of calcium is stimulated by phosphate deprivation, acidosis, adrenal steroids, and saline diuresis. Also, it should be noted that an additional 30–100 mg of calcium may be lost per day through the skin via sweating.

The dynamics of phosphate metabolism are not particularly different from that of calcium. Under normal circumstances ~70% of the phosphate in the diet is absorbed. Absorption of phosphate is interrelated in a complex fashion with the presence of calcium and can be stimulated by a low-calcium diet, and also by vitamin D or its metabolites. Intestinal absorption of phosphate is inhibited by high dietary calcium levels, aluminum hydroxide ingestion, and beryllium poisoning. Phosphate in the body is also partitioned among three major pools: the kidney ultrafiltrate, the readily exchangeable fraction of bone, and the intracellular compartments in the various soft tissues.

The major excretory route for phosphate (see Fig. 9-1) is through the kidney. The handling of phosphate by the kidney is determined by the rate of glomerular filtration, tubular reabsorption, and possibly tubular secretion. The kidney glomerulus filters every day some 6000–10,000 mg of phosphorus. A normal man, given a diet containing 900 mg of phosphorus, excretes ~600 mg/day in the urine.

II. ANATOMICAL, MORPHOLOGICAL, AND PHYSIOLOGICAL RELATIONSHIPS

A. Parathyroid Gland

Parathyroid glands have been identified in all vertebrate species higher than fishes. In humans there are normally four parathyroid glands. Anatomically they are localized on the surface of each side of the thyroid (see Fig. 6-1); in total there is ~120 mg of tissue. They are derived from the endoderm of the third and fourth pharyngeal pouches.

The two main classes of epithelial cells of the parathryoid gland are the more abundant chief cells (see Fig. 9-2A) and the less abundant oxyphil cells (see Fig. 9-2B). The chief cell is responsible for the biosynthesis of parathyroid hormone (PTH). This cell undergoes a series of cyclical changes which can be observed histologically and are associated with the synthesis, packaging, and secretion of PTH, then followed by cellular involution. Each individual chief cell appears to undergo its cycle independent of adjacent chief cells.

The oxyphil cell appears in the normal human parathyroid gland at the time of puberty. After puberty the number of oxyphil cells increases throughout life. The biological function of oxyphil cells is not known. Under some circumstances of pathological dysfunction of hyperparathyroidism (e.g., parathyroid adenomas and chief cell hyperplasia), the oxyphil cells are believed to secrete PTH.

B. Calcitonin-Secreting Cells

Calcitonin (CT) is secreted by the parafollicular or C cells, which are located in the thyroid glands of higher animals. The anatomical rela-

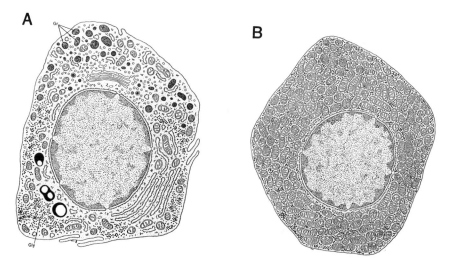

Figure 9-2. (A) Parathyroid principal or chief cells. They contain a prominent Golgi and many secretory granules and are the site of synthesis of PTH. (B) Parathyroid oxyphil cell. They occur singly or in small clumps and contain few or no secretory granules and are probably not engaged in the production of PTH. Gly, Glycogen granules; GR, granules. Reproduced by permission from T. L. Lentz, "Cell Fine Structure," pp. 329, 331. Saunders, Philadelphia, Pennsylvania, 1971.

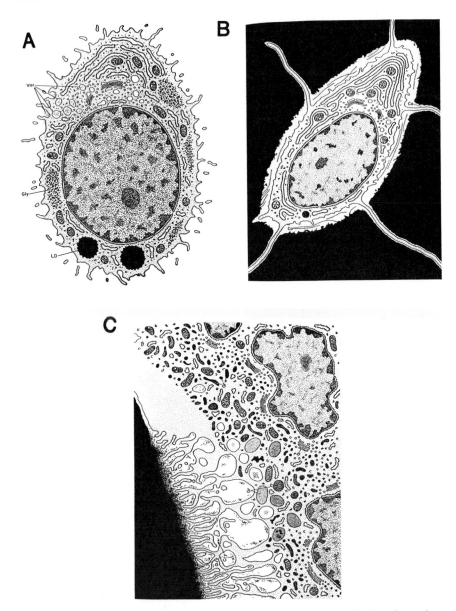

Figure 9-3. Typical cells of bone. (A) Chondrocytes or cartilage cells; they lie within lacunae in the matrix of the cartilage. Chondrocytes synthesize and release tropocollagen and a ground substance largely composed of chondroitin sulfate and a mucoprotein. (B) Osteoblasts or bone-forming cells lie within lacunae of fully formed bone. They actually secrete the bone matrix collagen and mucopolysaccharides. (C) Osteoclasts are large multi-nucleated cells involved with bone mineralization. The cell surface in contact with the

tionship of the C cells to the thyroid follicles varies with the species. The thyroid C cells have been established as being derived embryologically from the neural crest.

In lower vertebrates, including the teleost fish, elasmobranchs, anurans, urodeles, and aves, the calcitonin-secreting C cells are localized in the anatomically distinct ultimobranchial body. The ultimobranchial body persists as a separate gland in all jawed vertebrates except mammals.

C. Intestine

The morphology and cellular organization of the intestine is superbly adapted to efficiently effect the absorption of dietary constituents, including calcium and phosphorus. The anatomical organization of the intestinal mucosa which optimizes the surface/volume ratio of the cell and thereby facilitates the intestinal absorptive processes is discussed in Chapter 8 (see Fig. 8-4).

D. Bone

Bone is a complex tissue made up of cells and extracellular material; it is composed of organic and mineral components. The cells are of a wide variety of morphological and functional types, but all have a common origin in the mesenchymal tissue. The principal cell types are the (1) chondrocytes or cartilage cells which secrete the collagen matrix of the cartilage region; (2) osteoblasts or bone-forming cells; and (3) osteoclasts, which are multinucleated cells involved with bone resorption (see Fig. 9-3). On a dry weight basis, bone consists of ~65–70% inorganic crystals of the salt hydroxyapatite and 30–35% organic matrix known as osteoid. Of the osteoid, 40% is comprised of the protein collagen.

The formation of functional bone tissue can be divided into two phases: (1) that concerned with production and secretion of the extracellular collagen bone matrix, and (2) the deposition of the mineral calcium hydroxyapatite crystals in the matrix. It should be emphasized that bone is a dynamic tissue and that both these processes occur continuously throughout the life of the skeletal system.

Neither the collagen matrix, the extracellular mineral crystals, nor the several different cell types associated with bone exclusively determine

resorbing bone is specialized as a ruffled border. Inside are many granules or matrix vesicles which may be involved in the bone resorption process. Reproduced from T. L. Lentz, "Cell Fine Structure," pp. 74–79. Saunders, Philadelphia, Pennsylvania, 1971.

the behavior of the bone tissue. It is a unique combination of the organic and inorganic phases as well as the particular biochemical properties of these various cell types that confer on bone both its unusual mechanical properties (to support the weight of the soft tissues of the body) as well as its ability to serve as a dynamic reservoir for the calcium and phosphorus ions needed for mineral homeostasis in the whole organism. Table 9-3 is an outline of the elements of bone structure and metabolism.

Bone matrix is biosynthesized, secreted, organized, mineralized, and finally destroyed by reabsorption, all in accordance with the physiological and hormonal signals operative at any particular time. The production of organic matrix by osteoblast cells first involves the intracellular synthesis of protocollagen molecules by the ribosomal system through conventional protein biosynthetic pathways. The protocollagen is then polymerized to yield a three-stranded triple helix, each strand of which has a separate unique amino acid sequence. Next, approximately half of the proline residues and a small number of lysine residues of the protocollagen helix are enzymatically hydroxylated, and these new hydroxyamino acid residues are then glycosylated to yield the macromolecule known as procollagen. The procollagen is secreted into the extracellular space around the osteoblast cells, where it undergoes fur-

Table 9–3. Outline of the Elements of Bone Structure and Metabolism[a]

I. Structure of bone	
A. Macroscopic level	
1. Spongiosa or cancellous	Occurs in metaphyseal region of long bone and is composed of spicules known as trabeculae; is the most metabolically active region
2. Cortical bone	Occurs in cortex and diaphysis of long bone
B. Microscopic level	
1. Collagen fiber distribution	
a. Woven bone	Composed of loosely and randomly arranged collagen bundles; predominant in young bones
b. Lamellar bone	Composed of highly ordered bundles of collagen fibers arranged in layers interspersed between osteocytes; is characteristic of adult bone
2. Three dimensional collagen fiber network	Principally characteristic of adult bone
a. Trabecular	Synonymous with cancellous bone

Table 9–3. (*Continued*)

b. Haversian	Occurs as a consequence of remodeling of cortical bone
C. Types of bone cells	
1. Osteoprogenitor	Synonymous with mesenchymal cells
2. Osteoblasts	Cells that synthesize and secrete bone matrix
3. Osteoclasts	Cells that resorb bone; are multinucleate
4. Osteocytes	Precise function not known
II. Inorganic phase	On a dry-weight basis bone is 65–70% inorganic material
A. Components	
1. Crystalline calcium hydroxyapatite	Constitutes 55–60% of bone mineral; molecular formula $[(Ca^{2+})_{10-y}(H_3O)^{+}_{2y}\cdot(PO_4{}^{3-})_6(OH^-)_2]$
2. Amorphous calcium phosphate	Constitutes 40–45% of bone mineral; may be formed before crystalline Ca hydroxyapatite, which is then produced with time
B. Ionic composition	Other ions include K^+, Na^+, Mg^{2+}, Sr^{2+}, Cl^-, $CO_3{}^-$, F^-, citrate 3^-, and many trace constituents
III. Organic phase of bone	On a dry-weight basis bone is 30–35% organic material, often referred to as bone matrix or osteoid
A. Collagen	
1. Biosynthetic steps	
a. Intracellular phase	
i. Protocollagen biosynthesis	Occurs on ribosome; composed of 20% proline and 33% glycine
ii. Protocollagen hydroxylation	Specific hydroxylation of 50% of proline and a small number of lysines
iii. Glycosylation of protocollagen to yield procollagen	Procollagen molecular weight 360,000; is secreted into extracellular space
b. Extracellular phase	
i. Conversion of procollagen to tropocollagen	An N-terminal fragment of procollagen of 20,000 Da is removed; tropocollagen molecule is 3000 × 15 Å
ii. Tropocollagen polymerization into microfibrils	44 Å diameter × several centimeters length
iii. Polmerization of microfibrils into collagen fibrils	150–1300 Å diameter × several centimeters length
iv. Cross-linking of strands of collagen fibers	Formation of Schiff bases, followed by aldol condensation
B. Ground substance	5% bone matrix is ground substance
1. Mucopolysaccharide	
2. Mucoproteins	

[a] Reproduced with permission from A. W. Norman, "Vitamin D: The Calcium Homeostatic Hormone." Academic Press, New York, 1979.

ther conversion to yield tropocollagen via cleavage of an N-terminal fragment of 20,000 Da from each of the three individual peptide genes of the macromolecule. After proteolysis, the tropocollagen molecule is some 15 Å in diameter. It immediately undergoes polymerization to yield microfibrils several centimeters in length and consisting of five tropocollagen molecules across the diameter. These microfibril pentamers further polymerize to yield the final form of collagen fibers, which range in diameter from 150 to 1300 Å. The polymerization process, although spontaneous, is highly ordered and principally involves hydrophobic interactions between adjacent peptide chains. The final phase of formation of mature collagen molecules is the generation of covalent chemical bonds, either by an aldol condensation or by a Schiff base conjugation.

In the normal process of bone formation, there is usually a delay of 5–10 days between the synthesis of the extracellular organic matrix and its ultimate mineralization. It is believed that the normal coupling time between matrix formation and subsequent mineralization may depend on the presence of vitamin D and/or its metabolites. After final secretion of protocollagen by the osteoblasts and the ultimate formation of mature collagen, the osteoblasts differentiate and are incorporated into the bone matrix as osteocytes where they then subsequently further differentiate to become cells capable of secreting matrix calcification granules. These granules may facilitate the extracellular accumulation of calcium and phosphate, which ultimately results in the appearance of amorphous calcium phosphate. This in turn is crystallized into the formal hydroxyapatite structure of bone within the matrix of the mature collagen fibers. As yet a detailed molecular description of the total calcification process cannot be provided.

In understanding the hormonal regulation of calcium and phosphorus homeostasis, it is important to appreciate that bone tissue is dynamic, both in terms of the metabolic activity of the various cell populations present and the kinetics of mineral flux into and out of the various bone compartments. As summarized in Fig. 9-1, there are three "compartments" of bone mineral; they represent the various fractions of the total calcium present in bone that can be identified on the basis of radioactive tracer studies (utilizing either radioactive $^{45}Ca^{2+}$ or $^{47}Ca^{2+}$). These include the "readily exchangeable bone mineral compartment" which has both a "rapid" component (20,000 mg/day) as well as a "slow" (300 mg/day) component of calcium. The term rapid implies the capability of exchange on a minute-by-minute basis. The third compartment is "stable bone mineral," and it is that pool of calcium that participates in the bone remodeling processes associated with bone mineralization, accretion (as in growth), or resorption. Both the accretion and resorption processes are those that are affected by the hormonal regulators of calcium metabolism, whereas the rapid and slow exchange pools largely represent chemical equilibria between the bone and the bathing extracellular fluids.

E. Kidney

The kidney is responsible not only for indispensable homeostatic actions with regard to the electrolytes of the body and filtration and removal of nitrogenous wastes, but also as an endocrine gland for several classes of hormones, including the hormonally active forms of vitamin D. The anatomical organization of the kidney is presented in Chapter 15. Shown in Fig. 15-7 is the principal site of reabsorption of calcium and phosphorus as well as the putative sites of action of parathyroid hormone and of vitamin D and/or its metabolites. Figure 15-6 (A–C) illustrates the organization of several different kidney tubule epithelial cells.

The concentration of calcium in the blood, particularly its ionized form, is regulated stringently through complex interactions among (1) the movement of calcium in and out of the bone, (2) its absorption by the intestine, and (3) the renal tubular reabsorption of calcium lost into the renal tubule by glomerular filtration. The kidneys of a typical adult male transfer per day some 11,000 mg (275 mmol) of calcium from the plasma into the glomerular filtrate. However, only 0.5–1.0% of this large amount of filtered calcium is lost into the urine; this is a reflection of the remarkably effective tubular reabsorption mechanism(s) for calcium. Man normally loses 100–200 mg of calcium daily in the urine. It is known that several nonhormonal factors as well as parathyroid hormone, vitamin D, and its metabolites may alter the renal handling and excretory rate of calcium.

From consideration of the fluid dynamics of the kidney, it is possible to postulate that an increase in the urinary excretion of calcium may arise either from a decreased tubular reabsorption or from an increased filtered load of calcium, or both. An increase in the filtered load produced by an elevation in the rate of glomerular filtration normally has only a small effect on calcium excretion. However, an increase in the filtered load produced by hypercalcemia usually will result in a more marked reduction in the tubular reabsorption of this cation.

The concentration of phosphorus in the blood is not as stringently regulated as that of calcium. In the case of phosphate, 40–60% of that available in the diet is absorbed by the intestine. The inorganic phosphate in the blood also is very efficiently filtered at the glomerulus so that in a typical day ~6,000–10,000 mg are transferred from the blood to the glomerular filtrate. Of this amount, the renal tubule reabsorbs 80–90%. Man normally loses 700–1500 mg of phosphate daily in the urine. Thus, in comparison to calcium a significantly larger amount of phosphate is excreted on a daily basis (see Fig. 9-1). As will become evident later, both parathyroid hormone and vitamin D and its various metabolites play important roles in modulating the amount of phosphate actually excreted in the urine. Under circumstances of dietary phosphate restriction, the kidney becomes very efficient in its tubular reabsorption of phosphate from the glomerular filtrate, thus conserving this important anion for the body. In contrast, in situations of a dietary excess, the plasma phosphorus concentrations may become elevated, resulting ultimately in a significant increase in the amount of phosphorus excreted in the urine.

III. CHEMISTRY AND BIOCHEMISTRY

A. Parathyroid Hormone

Parathyroid hormone (PTH) is an 84 amino acid-containing protein that is secreted by the chief cells of the parathyroid gland (see Fig. 9-4A). PTH is a single-chain polypeptide of 84 amino acids (molecular weight 9300) with no cysteine residues and hence no disulfide bridges. There is a preponderance of basic residues (arginine + lysine) conferring an overall positive charge to the molecule. A distinctly hydrophobic region is found in the central portion of the sequence (residues 31–43), including the single tyrosine residue, which is the site of iodine-125 labeling for radioimmunoassay procedures. A fragment of the intact hormone

Figure 9-4. (A) Comparison of amino acid sequences of bovine, porcine, and human parathyroid hormone. The backbone sequence represents the human structure. Residues 22, 28, and 30 of the human have also been reported to be Gln, Lys, and Leu, respectively. (B) Complete amino acid sequence of bovine preproparathyroid hormone as determined by microsequencing technique. The radiolabeled prehormone was synthesized in the cell-free extract of wheat germ by addition of parathyroid messenger RNA and radioactive amino acids. The NH$_2$-terminal methionine (residue −31) is the initiator amino acid not removed in the wheat germ *in vitro* translation system. Reproduced by permission from J. F. Habener, Parathyroid hormone biosynthesis. *In* "Endocrinology" (L. J. DeGroot, G. F. Cahill, L. Martini, D. H. Nelson, W. D. Odell, J. T. Potts, E. Steinberger, and A. I. Winegard, ed.), Vol. 2, pp. 599–611. Grune & Stratton, New York, 1979.

A

		1								10										20
Human	Ser	Val	Ser	Glu	Ile	Gln	Leu	Met	His	Asn	Leu	Gly	Lys	His	Leu	Asn	Ser	Met	Glu	Arg
Bovine	Ala	Val	Ser	Glu	Ile	Gln	Phe	Met	His	Asn	Leu	Gly	Lys	His	Leu	Ser	Ser	Met	Glu	Arg
Porcine	Ser	Val	Ser	Glu	Ile	Gln	Leu	Met	His	Asn	Leu	Gly	Lys	His	Leu	Ser	Ser	Leu	Glu	Arg

										30										40
Human	Val	Glu	Trp	Leu	Arg	Lys	Lys	Leu	Gln	Asp	Val	His	Asn	Phe	Val	Ala	Leu	Gly	Ala	Pro
Bovine	Val	Glu	Trp	Leu	Arg	Lys	Lys	Leu	Gln	Asp	Val	His	Asn	Phe	Val	Ala	Leu	Gly	Ala	Ser
Porcine	Val	Glu	Trp	Leu	Arg	Lys	Lys	Leu	Gln	Asp	Val	His	Asn	Phe	Val	Ala	Leu	Gly	Ala	Ser

										50										60
Human	Leu	Ala	Pro	Arg	Asp	Ala	Gly	Ser	Gln	Arg	Pro	Arg	Lys	Lys	Glu	Asp	Asn	Val	Leu	Val
Bovine	Ile	Ala	Tyr	Arg	Asp	Gly	Ser	Ser	Gln	Arg	Pro	Arg	Lys	Lys	Glu	Asp	Asn	Val	Leu	Val
Porcine	Ile	Val	His	Arg	Asp	Gly	Gly	Ser	Gln	Arg	Pro	Arg	Lys	Lys	Glu	Asp	Asn	Val	Leu	Val

										70										80
Human	Glu	Ser	His	Glu	Lys	Ser	Leu	Gly	Glu	Ala	Asp	Lys	Ala	Asp	Val	Asp	Val	Leu	Thr	Lys
Bovine	Glu	Ser	His	Gln	Lys	Ser	Leu	Gly	Glu	Ala	Asp	Lys	Ala	Asp	Val	Asp	Val	Leu	Ile	Lys
Porcine	Glu	Ser	His	Gln	Lys	Ser	Leu	Gly	Glu	Ala	Asp	Lys	Ala	Asp	Val	Asp	Val	Leu	Ile	Lys

		84		
Human	Ala	Lys	Ser	Gln-COOH
Bovine	Ala	Lys	Pro	Gln-COOH
Porcine	Ala	Lys	Pro	Gln-COOH

B

```
     -31                                           -20                          -12
H2N  Met Met Ser Ala Lys Asp Met Val Lys Val Met Ile Val Met Leu Ala Ile Cys Phe Leu
     <----------------------------------------pre-hormone------------------------

     -11                                      -1  +1                            +9
     Ala Arg Ser Asp Gly Lys Ser Val Lys Lys Arg Ala Val Ser Glu Ile Gln Phe Met His
     ----------------->  <-----pro-hormone----->  <------------------PTH--------------

     +10                             +18    +84
     Asn Leu Gly Lys His Leu Ser Ser Met .... Gln-COOH
     ------------------------------------------>
```

consisting of the first 28–34 amino acids at the N-terminal region of the molecule is sufficient for the peptide to exert its entire spectrum of characteristic biological effects.

Because PTH represents a secreted protein, it is biosynthesized as a larger precursor by the parathyroid gland (see Fig. 9-4B). To date, two precursor species have been identified. This includes a prepro-PTH with 31 additional amino acids added onto the N-terminal region of PTH and represents the primary translation product of the mRNA in the ribosomal fraction of the parathyroid gland. This prepro-PTH then is secreted into the cisterna of the rough endoplasmic reticulum where it is processed within seconds into a form known as pro-PTH. This occurs by removal of the NH_2 terminal methionyl residue and the next 24 amino acids (e.g., residues -30 through -7) after biosynthesis. By 20 min after synthesis, pro-PTH reaches the Golgi region where it is stored in vesicles and is converted into PTH by removal of the NH_2 terminal hexapeptide. PTH is stored in the secretory granule until released into the circulation in response to a fall in the blood concentration of calcium. These steps are summarized schematically in Fig. 9-5. Through the application of recombinant DNA techniques by B. Kemperer and H. Kronenberg and associates, a cDNA probe to the prepro-PTH messenger RNA has been prepared and used to evaluate cloned genomic DNA sequences containing the gene for PTH.

The introduction of radioimmunoassay techniques has permitted the detection of circulating levels of PTH and its changing concentration in disease states. Three predominant peptide species have been identified in human plasma. The first appears identical to the intact or native form of the PTH hormone as isolated from the parathyroid tissue; this has 84 amino acids and a molecular weight of $\sim$9500. There are two other populations of PTH fragments, one with a molecular weight of $\sim$7000 and one which is smaller, having a molecular weight in the range of 4500. Conflicting views are held on the importance of these three peripheral forms of circulating PTH. One view is that only the 9500 molecular weight material is biologically active, with the smaller species representing degradation products. The other view is that one of the smaller species is the major biologically active form of the hormone. There is evidence that the liver Kupfer cells play an important role in the metabolism of the intact PTH molecule. The half-life of the intact PTH molecule in normal human plasma is only 20 min.

B. Calcitonin

Calcitonin (CT) is a small polypeptide hormone secreted by the ultimobranchial gland in fish, amphibians, reptiles, and birds; in mam-

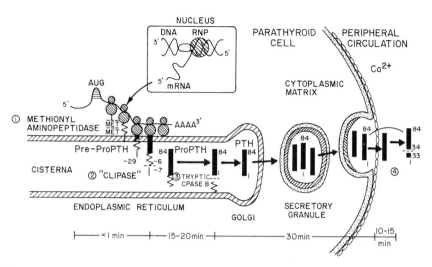

Figure 9-5. Schema depicting the proposed intracellular pathway of the biosynthesis of parathyroid hormone. Preproparathyroid hormone (Pre-ProPTH), an initial product of synthesis on the ribosomes, is converted into proparathyroid hormone (ProPTH) by removal of (1) the NH_2-terminal methionyl residues and (2) the NH_2-terminal sequence (-29 through -7) of 23 amino acids during or within seconds after synthesis, respectively. The conversion of Pre-ProPTH probably occurs during transport of the polypeptide into the cisterna of the rough endoplasmic reticulum. By 20 min after synthesis, ProPTH reaches the Golgi region and is converted into PTH by (3) removal of the NH_2-terminal hexapeptide. PTH is stored in the secondary granule until released into the circulation in response to a fall in the blood concentration of calcium. The time needed for these events is given below the schema. Modified from J. F. Habener, B. W. Kemper, A. Rich, and J. T. Potts, Biosynthesis of parathyroid hormone. *Recent Prog. Horm. Res.* **33**, 287 (1977).

mals it is secreted by the specialized C cells which are found primarily in the thyroid gland, but also at a small number of extrathyroidal sites. The amino acid sequences of nine calcitonins have now been determined; these include five mammalian species—porcine, bovine, ovine, human, and rat—as well as four nonmammalian species—salmon I, II, III, and eel. All have a similar structure consisting of a straight-chain peptide of 32 amino acids with a seven-membered disulfide ring at the N terminal and a prolinamide residue at the C terminal (see Fig. 9-6). Compared to the mammalian calcitonins, the nonmammalian hormones are much more stable and have a potency of 10–50 times greater in the standard hypocalcemic rat bioassay.

Studies of the molecular biology of the biosynthesis of calcitonin mRNA by M. G. Rosenfeld, R. Evans, and colleagues have demonstrated that the calcitonin gene can support the production of multiple protein products from a single transcription unit (see Fig. 9-7). Thus, the

Eel Cys-Ser-Asn-Leu-Ser-Thr-Cys-Val-Leu-Gly-Lys-Leu-Ser-Gln-Glu-
     1   5   10   15

     -Leu-His-Lys-Leu-Gln-Thr-Tyr-Pro-Arg-Thr-Asp-Val-Gly-Ala-Gly-
                      20   25   30

     -Thr-Pro-NH$_2$

Human Cys-Gly-Asn-Leu-Ser-Thr-Cys-Met-Leu-Gly-Thr-Tyr-Thr-Gln-Asp-
       1   5   10   15

       -Ph-Asn-Lys-Phe-His-Thr-Phe-Pro-Gln-Thr-Ala-Ile-Gly-Val-Gly-
                       20   25   30

       -Ala-Pro-NH$_2$

Salmon Cys-Ser-Asn-Leu-Ser-Thr-Cys-Val-Leu-Gly-Lys-Leu-Ser-Gln-Glu-
  I   1   5   10   15

        -Leu-His-Lys-Leu-Gln-Thr-Tyr-Pro-Arg-Thr-Asn-Thr-Gly-Ser-Gly-
                        20   25   30

        -Thr-Pro-NH$_2$

Figure 9-6. Amino acid sequences of eel, human, and salmon calcitonins. Reproduced through the courtesy of Excerpta Medica Foundation and the American Physiological Society.

Figure 9-7. Model to explain the alternative RNA processing pathways utilized in the expression of the calcitonin gene. The calcitonin gene supports the production of calcitonin (CT) in the thyroid and calcitonin gene-related peptide (CGRP) in the hypothalamus. The mature CT, which has 32 amino acid residues, and mature CGRP, which is postulated to have 37 amino acid residues, are derived from different precursor proteins. However, these two precursor proteins have an identical "common region" of 76 amino acid residues, which are derived from the C_1 and C_2 exons of the gene. Reproduced by permission of M. G. Rosenfeld, *Nature (London)* **304**, 129–135 (1983). © 1983 Macmillan Journals Limited.

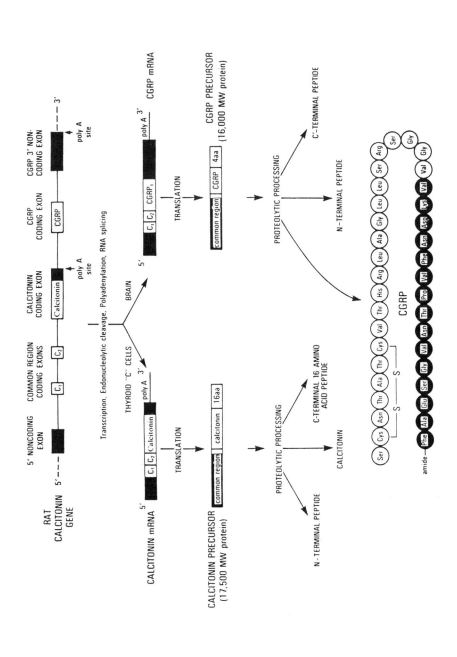

same gene produces as a consequence of alternative processing of RNA transcripts the hormone calcitonin in the thyroid and a protein termed calcitonin gene-related peptide (CGRP) in the hypothalamus. CGRP thus represents a putative hormone which was discovered through application of recombinant DNA methodology without prior knowledge of its structure or biological function. As yet the biological function of CGRP has not been clearly defined; it is distributed selectively in neural tissues and has been postulated to be involved with nociception (the ability to perceive noxious stimuli), ingestive behavior, and modulation of the autonomic and nervous systems.

The discovery that alternative mRNA processing can produce multiple protein products may provide insight into mechanisms by which endocrine genes increase the diversity and specificity of their biological responses.

The dominant biological action of calcitonin is to mediate a lowering of serum calcium. In addition to the onset of hypocalcemia, there is also normally an accompanying hypophosphatemia after administration of calcitonin. As yet no detailed mechanism of action of calcitonin is available. The hypocalcemic and hypophosphatemic effects of calcitonin are believed to be due to an inhibition of PTH-mediated calcium resorption from bone. These effects are believed to be mediated through cyclic AMP. In addition, calcitonin may have independent actions in the kidney where it can stimulate phosphate and calcium excretion.

Calcitonin may be measured via bioassay or radioimmunoassay. The bioassay of calcitonin is based on the hypocalcemic actions of the peptide or bone. Several radioimmunoassays for calcitonin have been developed; the radioimmunoassay for human calcitonin is important in the detection and treatment of medullary carcinoma of the thyroid.

C. Vitamin D

The molecular structure of vitamin D is closely allied to that of classical steroid hormones (see Fig. 9-8). Technically, vitamin D is a seco-steroid. Seco-steroids are those in which one of the rings of the cyclopentanoperhydrophenanthrene ring structure of classic steroids has undergone fission by breakage of a carbon–carbon bond; in the instance of vitamin D this is the 9,10 carbon bond of ring B. There are a family of vitamin D-related steroids, depending upon the precise structure of the side chain attached to carbon-17. The vitamin D_2 family is derived from 22,23-dihydroergosterol, while the vitamin D_3 family is derived from 7-dehydrocholesterol. The naturally occurring form of vitamin D is that which has the side chain structure identical to that of cholesterol; this is

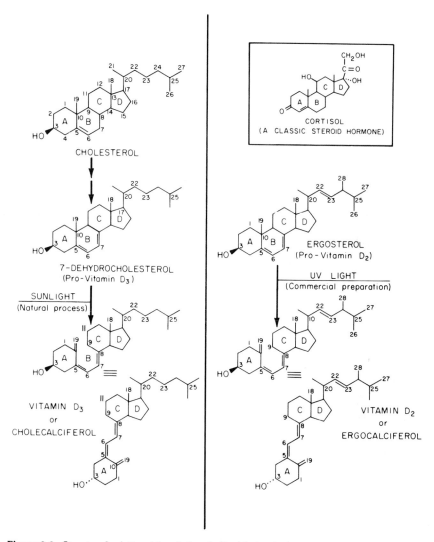

Figure 9-8. Structural relationship of vitamin D_3 (cholecalciferol) and vitamin D_2 (ergocalciferol) to their respective provitamins, to cholesterol, and to a classic steroid hormone, cortisol (see inset box). The two structural representations presented at the bottom for both vitamin D_3 and vitamin D_2 are equivalent; these are simply different ways of drawing the same molecule (see also Fig. 9-10). It is to be emphasized that vitamin D_3 is the naturally occurring form of the vitamin; it is produced from 7-dehydrocholesterol which is present in the skin by the action of sunlight. Vitamin D_2 (which is equivalently potent in man and many mammals, but not birds) is produced commercially by the irradiation of the plant sterol ergosterol with ultraviolet light.

known as vitamin D_3 or cholecalciferol. Vitamin D_2 or ergocalciferol, which has the side chain of ergosterol, is not a naturally occurring form of the vitamin. Collectively vitamin D_3 + vitamin D_2 can be termed calciferol.

Vitamin D_3 is normally derived by exposure to sunlight of the precursor, 7-dehydrocholesterol, present in the skin. Vitamin D_2 is produced synthetically via ultraviolet irradiation of the sterol ergosterol. In the United States this is the principal form of food supplementation for vitamin D. The minimum daily requirement of vitamin D (either D_2 or D_3) is 400 international units (IU); 1.0 IU is equivalent to 25 ng or 65 pmol.

A formal definition of a vitamin is that it is a trace dietary constituent required to effect normal functioning of a physiological process. Emphasis here is on *trace* and in the fact that the vitamin *must* be supplied in the diet; this implies that the body is unable to synthesize it. Thus, cholecalciferol is only a vitamin when the animal does not have access to sunlight or ultraviolet light. Under normal physiological circumstances, all mammals, including man, can generate via ultraviolet photolysis adequate quantities of vitamin D. It is largely through a historical accident that calciferol has been classified as a vitamin rather than as a steroid hormone. Chemists have certainly appreciated the strong structural similarity between vitamin D and other steroids, but this correlation had never been widely acknowledged in the biological/clinical or nutritional sciences until 1965–1970.

The chief structural prerequisite of a sterol to be classified as a provitamin D is its ability to be converted upon ultraviolet irradiation to a vitamin D; thus, it is mandatory that it have in its B ring a Δ^{5-7} conjugated double-bond system. Shown in Fig. 9-9 is a summary of the photochemical pathway involved in the production of calciferol. The molecular events associated with the photochemical reaction start with the orbital electrons in the molecule of 7-dehydrocholesterol existing in their ground state. After absorption of a discrete quantum of light, this "activated" molecule, which is no longer in thermodynamic equilibrium with its surroundings, ultimately loses energy to the environment either in the form of (1) fluorescence or phosphorescence, (2) chemical energy, or (3) thermal energy so that the molecule is again in a ground state. After return to the ground state, if the molecule has undergone a change in its chemical energy, it will be a new compound with a different structure (e.g., previtamin D, lumisterol, or tachysterol). In the skin, the principal ultraviolet irradiation product is previtamin D_3. The conversion of previtamin D to vitamin D involves an intermolecular hydrogen transfer from C-19 to C-9; this transformation can occur in the absence of further

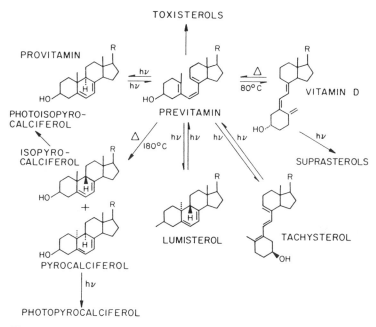

Figure 9-9. Photochemical pathway of production of vitamin D (calciferol).

ultraviolet exposure. Associated with the intramolecular hydrogen transfer is a rotation of the A ring around the 6-7 single bond, yielding the final structural species—vitamin D_3.

Although the chemical structure of vitamin D was determined in the 1930s, it was not until 1974 that the truly unique structural aspects of the molecule became apparent. Through the use of high-resolution NMR spectroscopy, it was possible to demonstrate the rapid interconversion of the A ring between two chair conformers (see Fig. 9-10, structures C and D). The existence of these A ring conformers is a direct consequence of the fact that vitamin D is a seco-steroid. Breakage of the 9,10 carbon bond of ring B "unlocks" the A ring which is rigidly fixed in other classic steroids, thus permitting a dynamic chair–chair interchange that occurs many thousands of times per second.

A totally new era in the field of vitamin D has opened since 1964 with the discovery of the metabolism of vitamin D into ~30 daughter metabolites (see Fig. 2-26). It is now recognized that there is an endocrine system for processing the prohormone, vitamin D, into its hormonally active daughter metabolite(s) (see Fig. 9-11). The biologically active form of vitamin D, particularly in the intestine, is the steroid 1,25-dihydroxy-

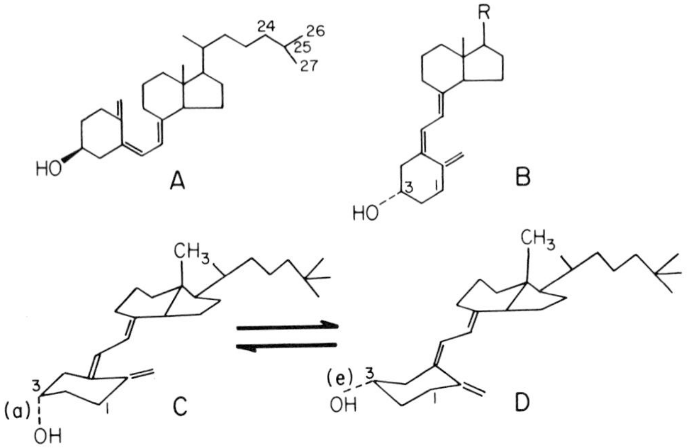

Figure 9-10. Evolution of conformational representations of vitamin D. Representation A resulted from the original chemical structure determination. The first X-ray crystallographic analysis by Nobel Laureate Dr. Dorothy Crowfoot-Hodgkin indicated the presence of a single A ring chair conformation as shown in C, but this was normally simplified to that shown in B. More recent studies emphasize that in solution there is a rapid equilibration between the two A ring chair conformations, as shown in C and D. In structures C and D, the (e) and (a) refer, respectively, to the equatorial and axial orientations of the 3-hydroxyl, which in both instances is geometrically β. Reproduced by permission from A. W. Norman, "Vitamin D: The Calcium Homeostatic Steroid Hormone," p. 54. Academic Press, New York, 1979.

vitamin D_3 [1,25$(OH)_2D_3$]. The endocrine gland producing the biologically active form(s) of vitamin D is the kidney. After metabolic conversion of vitamin D_3 into 25-hydroxyvitamin D_3 by a liver microsomal enzyme, this circulating form of the seco-steroid serves as a substrate for either the renal 25(OH)D-1-hydroxylase or the 25(OH)D-24-hydroxylase. Both enzymes are located in the mitochondrial fraction of the kidney cortex. The 1-hydroxylase is localized in the kidney of members of every vertebrate class from teleosts through amphibia, reptiles, and aves to mammals, including primates. It has been shown that the 25(OH)D-1-hydroxylase enzyme system is a classical mixed-function steroid hydroxylase similar to the steroid hormone hydroxylase that is located in the adrenal cortical mitochondria (see Fig. 2-30). The 1-hydroxylase is a cytochrome P-450-containing enzyme which involves an adrenodoxin component incorporating molecular oxygen into the 1-α-hydroxyl functionality of 25 $(OH)D_3$. The 1,25$(OH)_2D_3$ form of the vitamin is also known to induce the renal 24-hydroxylase to permit the coproduction of 24,25$(OH)_2D_3$. Emerging evidence suggests an important role for 24,25$(OH)_2D_3$ in mediating normal bone development and parathyroid function. Thus, 1,25$(OH)_2D_3$ and 24,25$(OH)_2D_3$ are the two

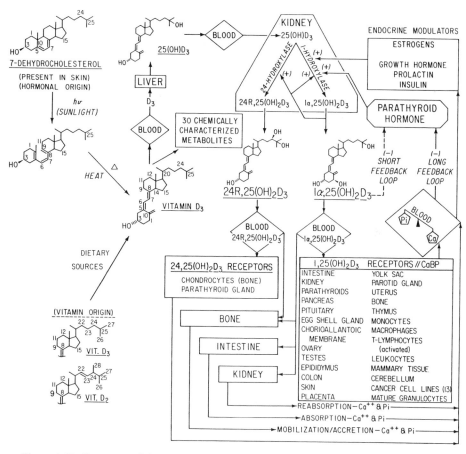

Figure 9-11. Summary of the vitamin D endocrine system. hv, Ultraviolet irradiation; P_i, inorganic phosphate.

principal forms of the parent vitamin D_3 which mediate the biological responses characteristic of this vitamin. The other metabolites shown in Fig. 2-26 are believed to represent pathways for inactivation of the pro forms and the biologically active metabolites of vitamin D.

IV. BIOLOGY AND PHYSIOLOGICAL SIGNIFICANCE

A. Parathyroid Hormone

The major target organs for PTH actions are kidney and bone. It also may act upon the intestine, but its effects here are probably indirect and are achieved by virtue of the tropic actions of PTH in stimulating the renal biosynthesis of $1,25(OH)_2D_3$.

The secretion of PTH is stimulated in response to a lowered blood concentration of calcium (see Fig. 9-12). In terms of the several forms of blood calcium summarized in Table 9-2, it is known that the biosynthesis and secretion of PTH is only responsive to the ionic and not to the protein-bound forms of calcium. The secretion of PTH can be (1) stimulated when hypocalcemia is induced by infusion of calcitonin or the divalent metal chelating agent, EDTA (ethylene diamine tetraacetic acid) or (2) decreased when hypercalcemia is induced by the infusion of calcium. Thus, there is an inverse correlation between serum calcium concentration and PTH concentration in the range of 4–10 mg calcium/100 ml (see Fig. 9-12). The most stringent control of serum calcium concentration is achieved in the range of 9–10.5 mg Ca^{2+}/100 ml serum, which is considered to be the normal physiological range of this divalent cation. Serum concentrations of calcium that fall above or below this range are likely to be due to the presence of disease states that perturb the integrated calcium–phosphorus homeostatic mechanisms.

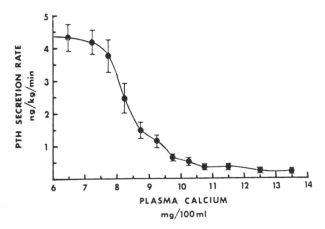

Figure 9-12. Secretory response of the parathyroid glands to changes in plasma calcium concentration. The secretion rate of a superior bovine parathyroid gland was measured by quantitative collection (flow rate measured) and radioimmunoassay of its venous effluent. The solid symbols indicate the mean secretion rate for either the 1.0 or 0.5 mg/100 ml range of plasma calcium concentration, and the vertical bars indicate the SE. Alterations in plasma calcium concentration were induced by intravenous infusion of solutions of either Na_2EDTA or calcium chloride. Reproduced by permission from G. P. Mayer, *in* "Calcium-Regulating Hormones" (R. V. Talmage, M. Owen, and J. A. Parsons, ed.), p. 123. Excerpta Medica, Amsterdam, 1975.

The most important biological actions of PTH are (1) to increase the plasma calcium concentrations; (2) to increase the urinary excretion of phosphate and hydroxyproline-containing peptides and to decrease the urinary excretion of calcium; (3) to increase the extent of osteoclastic and osteocytic osteolysis in bone (bone resorption and remodeling); and (4) to increase the rate of conversion of $25(OH)D_3$ to $1,25(OH)_2D_3$ in kidney tissue.

The actions of PTH on bone are complex and not yet fully understood. The response of bone to PTH is biphasic; the immediate action is largely that of bone mineral mobilization (i.e., an elevation of the blood levels of calcium and phosphorus). These effects may be seen within minutes following hormone administration and have in fact been used in parathyroidectomized animals as a bioassay for PTH. A second or slower action of PTH is its effect upon bone cell activity. PTH is believed to increase the size and number of the bone-resorbing cells, namely, the osetoclasts. This, then, upsets the balance between osteoblasts (bone-forming cells) and osteoclasts and can lead to an increased remodeling rate of bone. The net effect is normally that resorption is somewhat greater than accretion so that a net negative skeletal balance of Ca and P is observed. Also associated with prolonged bone resorption is an increased release of lysosomal enzymes so that there is a mobilization of the bone matrix which results in increased blood levels of the amino acid hydroxyproline.

The principal actions of PTH on the kidney are to stimulate the renal excretion of phosphate and to enhance the renal tubular reabsorption of calcium. The site of action of PTH in the kidney has been localized to be in the proximal tubule (see Fig. 15-7). Also, there are well-documented physiologically important effects of PTH which lead to increased excretion of potassium, bicarbonate, sodium, and amino acids and decreased excretion of ammonia and calcium.

The biochemical mode of action of PTH on bone cells or kidney cells is not clearly understood. Evidence has been presented in both organ systems that PTH is capable of stimulating adenylate cyclase and cyclic AMP production. Although specific membrane receptors for PTH have not yet been identified in bone, they have been characterized in the kidney. Decreasing the extracellular sodium concentration will prevent both PTH-stimulated bone and kidney calcium resorption. Accordingly, it has been proposed that PTH also acts to stimulate calcium release from bone and calcium reabsorption from the kidney tubule by means of a Na^+-Ca^{2+} exchange mechanism. Such agents as ouabain, veratridine, and monovalent cation ionophores will specifically block PTH-stimulated bone resorption *in vitro*. What is not clear is whether all of the biological actions of PTH in these tissues are mediated through the cAMP axis or whether there are other independent pathways for the elicitation of biological responses by this peptide hormone.

B. Calcitonin

Calcitonin is secreted in response to elevated blood levels of ionized calcium; the rate of calcitonin secretion is a direct function of the plasma calcium concentration. Extensive studies have demonstrated that one or more hormones of the digestive tract have the ability to elicit increased calcitonin secretion. The most widely tested hormone in this regard has been gastrin and its synthetic analog, pentagastrin. These results are consistent with the observation that the secretion of calcitonin is stimulated shortly after the ingestion of high dietary levels of calcium. Also, in experimental animals, blood levels of calcitonin are elevated during pregnancy and lactation.

At least three important biological functions for calcitonin have been proposed: (1) protection of the young animal or newborn against postprandial hypercalcemia; (2) blocking the actions of PTH in mobilizing bone calcium and phosphorus; and (3) stimulating the urinary excretion of both calcium and phosphate in the kidney. The net effect of these three actions is to mediate a reduction in serum calcium levels.

The mode of action of calcitonin is not well understood. It has been shown to stimulate adenylate cyclase activity in both skeletal and renal tissues. However, the specific consequences of the increased intracellular levels of cAMP is unclear at the present time.

C. Vitamin D and Its Metabolites

The molecule vitamin D itself has no intrinsic biological activity. All biological responses attributed to vitamin D are now known to arise only as a consequence of the metabolism of this seco-steroid into its biologically active daughter metabolites, namely, $1,25(OH)_2D_3$ and $24,25(OH)_2D_3$.

Figure 9-11 summarizes the scope of the vitamin D endocrine system. The steroid hormone $1,25(OH)_2D_3$ is produced only in accord with strict physiological signals dictated by the calcium "demand" of the organism; a bimodal mode of regulation has been suggested. On a time scale of minutes, changes in the ionic environment of the kidney mitochondria resulting from accumulation and release of calcium and/or inorganic phosphate may alter the enzymatic activity of the 1-hydroxylase. In addition, parathyroid hormone has been shown on a time scale of hours to be capable of stimulating the production of $1,25(OH)_2D_3$, possibly by stimulating the biosynthesis of the 1-hydroxylase. It is also relevant that $1,25(OH)_2D_3$ is a stimulant for the renal production of $24,25(OH)_2D_3$. Thus, under normal physiological circumstances, both renal dihydroxy-lated metabolites are secreted and are circulating in the plasma. There is evidence for a "short feedback loop" for both of these metabolites to modulate and/or reduce the secretion of PTH. There is also some evidence that other endocrine modulators such as estrogens, androgens, growth hormone, prolactin, and insulin may affect the renal production of $1,25(OH)_2D_3$. Thus, the kidney is clearly an endocrine gland, in the classic sense, which is capable of producing in a physiologically regulated manner appropriate amounts of $1,25(OH)_2D_3$ and $24,25(OH)_2D_3$.

The plasma compartment contains a specific protein termed the vitamin D binding protein (DBP), which is utilized to transport vitamin D seco-sterols. DBP is similar in function to the corticosteroid binding globulin (CBG), which carries glucocorticoids (see Chapter 10), and the steroid hormone binding globulin (SHBG), which transports estrogens or androgens (see Chapter 12). DBP is a slightly acidic (pI 5.2) monomeric glycoprotein of 53,000 D which is synthesized and secreted by the liver as a major plasma constituent. From analysis of the cloned cDNA, it has been determined that DBP is structurally homologous to albumin and α-fetoprotein; these three plasma proteins are members of the same multigene family which likely is derived from the duplication of a common ancestral gene. DBP, originally called group-specific component (Gc), was initially studied electrophoretically as a polymorphic marker in the α-globulin region of human serum.

DBP appears to be a multifunctional protein. It possesses one ligand binding site for seco-sterols of the vitamin D family; thus, it may carry the parent, D_3, or the daughter metabolites: $25(OH)D_3$, $1,25(OH)_2D_3$, and $24,25(OH)_2D_3$.

Since the total plasma concentration of D sterols is only ~0.2 μM, while DPP circulates at 9–13 μM, under normal circumstances only 1–2% of the sterol binding sites on DBP are occupied. DBP is also able to bind with high affinity to monomers of actin, thereby preventing their polymerization in the blood compartment. Also, DBP has been found to be associated with immunoglobulin on the surface of B lymphocytes; as yet its biological function in this locus has not been elucidated.

The principal mode of action of the vitamin D metabolites is believed to occur by a steroid hormone-like mechanism. Definitive biochemical evidence supports the existence of receptors for $1,25(OH)_2D_3$ in at least 28 different tissues (see Fig. 9-11). While it is not surprising to find $1,25(OH)_2D_3$ receptors in the classic target organs of intestine, kidney, and bone, the presence of these vitamin D "markers" in such diverse tissues as the pancreas, eggshell gland, parathyroid gland, pituitary, cells of the reticuloendothelial system, and cerebellum emphasizes the diversity of the vitamin D endocrine system and $1,25(OH)_2D_3$ in mediating calcium homeostasis.

The $1,25(OH)_2D_3$ receptor is a protein with a molecular weight of 67,000; it binds $1,25(OH)_2D_3$ tightly, $K_d = 1–5 \times 10^{-11}$ M, and with great ligand specificity. For optimal binding, the ligand should have 1α-, 3β-, and 25-hydroxy groups, an 8-carbon side chain, as well as a seco B ring. In contrast to the glucocorticoid receptor (Chapter 10) and the progesterone and estradiol receptors (Chapter 13), no formal temperature-dependent activation process for the $1,25(OH)_2D_3$ receptor system has yet been identified. Extensive evidence exists supporting the view that the unoccupied $1,25(OH)_2D_3$ receptor is largely associated with the nuclear chromatin fraction which is in accord with the new model of action of steroid hormones and their receptors (see Chapter 1). Thus, $1,25(OH)_2D_3$ receptors may be more similar to the thyroxine receptor (see Fig. 6-18), which is an intrinsic nonhistone nuclear protein. However, it is known that the occupied $1,25(OH)_2D_3$ receptor complex has a higher affinity for chromatin or DNA cellulose than the unoccupied receptor.

Preliminary evidence has suggested the existence of protein receptors for $24,25(OH)_2D_3$ in chondrocytes (bone cartilage cells) and the parathyroid gland. As yet no specific function for the $24,25(OH)_2D_3$ receptor has been identified, although there is a possibility of its involvement in proteoglycan biosynthesis.

Three distinct vitamin D-induced calcium binding proteins have been isolated and biochemically characterized. These proteins are all produced *de novo* in target tissues as a consequence of the $1,25(OH)_2D_3$ receptor complex selective genome activation. Their biochemical properties are summarized in Table 9-4. The two proteins with a K_d for Ca^{2+} of 10^{-6} M are termed calbindins and belong to a family of tight calcium binding proteins; other members of this family include the muscle proteins troponin C and parvalbumin and the widely distributed calmodulin. All of these proteins are believed to have a high degree of structural similarity in their calcium binding sites. The third vitamin D-induced calcium binding protein is an extracellular protein found associated with bone; it is termed osteocalcin or the bone gla protein (BGP), since it has many γ-carboxyglutamic acid residues.

A detailed biochemical function of the vitamin D-dependent calbindins (CaBP) has not yet been elucidated. Both the 11,000 and the 28,000 D CaBP species are soluble proteins found exclusively inside the intestinal and kidney cells, and they constitute 1–3% of the soluble cellular proteins. As yet there is no evidence to implicate these CaBPs in any of the

Table 9–4. Vitamin D-Induced Calcium-Binding Proteins

	Molecular weight	Number of Ca^{2+} bound per protein molecule	Dissociation (K_D) for Ca^2 binding
All avian vitamin D-responsive tissues	28,000	4	10^{-6}
Mammalian kidney and brain	~28,000	4	
Mammalian intestine	11,000	2	10^{-6}
Mammalian bone (BGP)[a]	6,000		10^{-3}

[a] BGP, Bone gla protein, i.e., a protein with several γ-carboxyl glutamyl residues.

steps involved in the translocation of calcium ions across the cell. Normally in all cells the intracellular concentration of "free" Ca^{2+} is maintained below $10^{-6} M$. It has been suggested that calbindin may function in the intestinal and kidney cells which are actively involved in calcium translocation as an intracellular calcium buffer to prevent the adverse effects of a high free Ca^{2+} concentration.

Intriguingly, the presence of the D-dependent CaBP or calbindins has been reported in a number of cells which were not previously known to possess responsivity to vitamin D_3 and its active hormone $1,25(OH)_2D_3$. These include the pancreas B cell (site of insulin secretion), placenta, eggshell gland (chicken), and cerebellum (Purkinje cells). It is to be anticipated that future research will define the actions of the calbindins in these new loci.

The principal biological effects of vitamin D (mediated by its daughter metabolites) are at the intestine to stimulate the absorption of dietary calcium and phosphorus, at the skeleton to promote both the mineralization of bone matrix as well as to stimulate bone resorption, and at the kidney to reduce the urinary excretion of phosphate and calcium (i.e., to stimulate the renal tubular reabsorption of these two ions). Of these three systems, the most thoroughly studied biochemically is the intestine.

The mode of action of $1,25(OH)_2D_3$ in the target organ, intestinal mucosa, in stimulating intestinal calcium and phosphorus absorption is analogous to that of other steroid hormones. As a consequence of the presence of the steroid–receptor complex in the nucleus, there ensues a stimulation of template activity, including the biosynthesis of a messenger RNA for the CaBP. The amount of intestinal CaBP in the intestine has been shown to be correlated with the amount of $1,25(OH)_2D_3$ localized in the intestinal mucosa and the level of vitamin D-mediated intestinal calcium absorption.

The process of intestinal calcium translocation and the effects of the vitamin D metabolites therein are complex. At least three steps are involved: (1) uptake of the Ca^{2+} ions across the brush border membrane; (2) translocation of the Ca^{2+} across the cell; and (3) efflux of the Ca^{2+} out of the cell across the basal lateral membrane.

A model for the action of $1,25(OH)_2D_3$ in the intestine is given in Fig. 9-13. Vitamin D and $1,25(OH)_2D_3$ increases the permeability of the brush border membrane to Ca^{2+} by altering the membrane protein composition and topology, which may include induction of a membrane-bound ATP-ase. It is believed that Ca^{2+} enters the cell passively via a selective Ca^{2+} gate. No molecular details on the path of movement of Ca^{2+} across the inside of the cell are known, although it is possible that the calbindin participates in this process. Next, Ca^{2+} ions are exported out of the cell via the involvement of an energy-dependent Na^+, Ca^{2+}-ATPase. The specific effects of vitamin D and its metabolites on this process have not been identified.

In addition to the role of $1,25(OH)_2D_3$ in mediating the synthesis of calcium binding proteins in selected cells, a new action(s) of this seco-steroid has recently been described within the hematopoietic system (see Fig. 9-14). Receptors for $1,25(OH)_2D_3$ exist in promonocytes, monocytes,

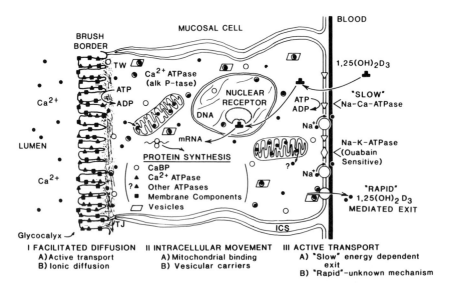

Figure 9-13. Schematic model to describe the action of $1,25(OH)_2D_3$ in the intestine in stimulating intestinal calcium transport. Reproduced with permission from I. Nemere and A. W. Norman, *Biochim. Biophys. Acta* **694,** 307–327 (1982).

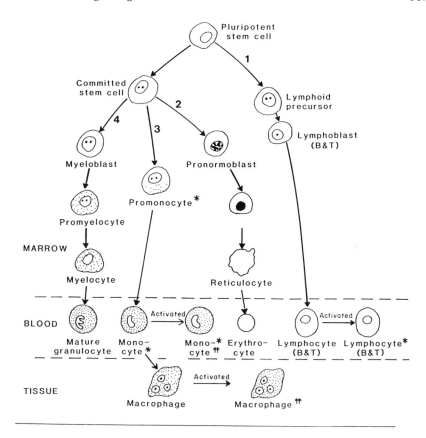

Figure 9-14. Flow chart of stem cell differentiation. A pluripotent stem cell can differentiate along one of four lineages toward (1) B and T lymphocytes, (2) erythrocytes, (3) monocytes and macrophages, and (4) granulocytes. *, Cells which possess 1,25(OH)$_2$D$_3$ receptors; #, cells which can produce small amounts of 1,25(OH)$_2$D$_3$.

and activated B and T lymphocytes. The principal biological effect of 1,25(OH)$_2$D$_3$ is to promote cell differentiation along the lineage from the committed stem cell to promonocyte→monocyte→macrophage. Macrophages are believed to be precursors of osteoclasts, the cells responsible for bone resorption. Further, γ-interferon from activated T lymphocytes will induce bone marrow macrophages to biosynthesize small amounts of 1,25(OH)$_2$D$_3$. Thus, there is the possibility of a paracrine system for 1,25(OH)$_2$D$_3$ such that "locally" produced 1,25(OH)$_2$D$_3$ could act on neighboring cells to promote differentiation toward macrophages and osteoclasts, thereby increasing the bone calcium resorption capability.

D. Integrated Actions of Parathyroid Hormone, Calcitonin, and Vitamin D Metabolites

The maintenance of calcium and phosphorus homeostasis involves the integration of absorption by the intestine, accretion and reabsorption by bone tissue, and urinary excretion of these two cations by the kidney. Table 9-5 summarizes the physiological effects of calcitonin, parathyroid hormone, and vitamin D metabolites in these three organs. The steroid $1,25(OH)_2D_3$ plays a dominant role in increasing the intestinal absorption of calcium and phosphorus; however, this uptake process is carefully regulated according to the needs of the animal and is dictated by certain physiological signals which are dependent in large part on the plasma levels of calcium and possibly phosphorus. Once calcium and phosphate enter into the plasma, a delicate balancing operation occurs between accretion and mobilization in the bone and excretion and reabsorption by the kidney. In the event that the dietary intake or availability of calcium and phosphorus is diminished or increased, it is possible to tip the balance in favor of increased bone mobilization or increased urinary excretion, respectively, to meet the stringent requirement of a constant serum calcium level. Thus, serum calcium may become ele-

Table 9–5. Physiological Effects of Calcitonin, Parathyroid Hormone, and Vitamin D (and Metabolites) Related to Mineral Metabolism

	Calcitonin	Parathyroid hormone	Vitamin D (+ metabolites)
Intestinal			
Calcium absorption	↓ ?	↑ (indirect)	↑
Phosphate absorption	?	?	↑
Renal			
Phosphate excretion	↑	↑	↓
Calcium excretion	↑	↓	↓
Hydrogen excretion	→	↓	?
Potassium excretion	Slight ↑	↑	?
Sodium excretion	↑	↑	?
Adenyl cyclase activity	↑	↑	?
Skeletal			
Calcium mobilization	↓	↑	↑
Mineralization of bone matrix	—	—	↑
Other			
Plasma levels of calcium	↓	↑	↑
Plasma levels of phosphate	↓	↓	—
Body weight	?	?	Increases

vated by a PTH/1,25(OH)$_2$D-mediated stimulation of bone calcium mobilization, or via parathyroid hormone stimulation of the tubular reabsorption of calcium at the kidney. Concomitantly, PTH also stimulates urinary phosphate excretion so that as the serum calcium concentration increases, there is usually an associated reduction in the plasma phosphate level. This then prevents the inappropriate precipitation of calcium phosphate in soft tissues which would be the logical consequence of exceeding the solubility product, K$_{sp}$, for [calcium] × [phosphate].

When serum calcium levels become too elevated, the action of calcitonin may come into play. Simply speaking, calcitonin is believed to block many of the actions of PTH at the skeletal level, thereby preventing further elevation of serum calcium levels. Secretion of calcitonin may be stimulated during intervals of gastrointestinal absorption of calcium to prevent short-term intervals of hypercalcemia. Also associated with the increased secretion of calcitonin is an increase in calcium excretion by the kidney which can contribute to a reduction in circulating levels of serum calcium and prevent soft tissue calcification.

Bone is a central organ in calcium and phosphorus metabolism, acting both as a source of and a reservoir for these two ions. It is apparent that bone remodeling processes may contribute to both short- and long-term events necessary for calcium and phosphorus homeostasis. The relative actions of bone formation and resorption are known to be modulated by various endocrine regulators during times of skeletal growth and lactation and in birds during the process of egg laying. Also, it is not surprising that bone is involved in a wide variety of disease states which reflect perturbations in calcium and phosphorus homeostasis.

V. CLINICAL ASPECTS

A. Parathyroid Hormone

The common disorders of the parathyroid gland fall into two main categories; (1) those associated with hypofunction (e.g., hypoparathyroidism), and (2) those associated with hyperfunction (e.g., hyperparathyroidism).

The most common cause of hypoparathyroidism is damage to or removal of the parathyroid glands in the course of an operation on the thyroid gland. A much less common cause of hypoparathyroidism is an idiopathic lack of function. Most cases are in children; approximately twice as many females as males are affected. The most prominent clinical feature of hypoparathyroidism is hypocalcemia and, in extreme instances, tetany.

Pseudohypoparathyroidism is a rare genetic disorder involving bone and mineral metabolism. It is probably inherited as an X-linked dominant trait with variable penetrance and is characterized by signs and symptoms similar to those of hypoparathyroidism. However, in this disease state there is a peripheral resistance to the biological actions of parathyroid hormone and an elevated secretion of PTH. Characteristic clinical features include a round face, short stature, brachydactylia—especially of the metacarpal and metatarsal bones as a result of early epiphyseal closure (see Fig. 9-15)—and in some instances ectopic soft tissue calcifications.

Primary hyperparathyroidism is a disorder of mineral metabolism characterized by a defect in the normal feedback control of PTH secretion by the plasma calcium concentration. Secondary hyperparathyroidism is a disorder characterized by primary disruption of mineral homeostasis such as impaired production of $1,25(OH)_2D_3$ or low dietary intake of calcium, which leads to a low blood calcium and a compensatory increase in parathyroid gland function, size, and secretion of PTH. Hyperparathyroidism is the most common disorder involving the parathyroid glands. It can result from single adenoma, multiple adenomas, hyperplasia, usually of the chief cells, and carcinoma. The principal clinical features of hyperparathyroidism are a markedly elevated plasma level of serum calcium (11–13 mg/100 ml) and, when present for prolonged intervals of time, extensive resorption of the skeleton. At the kidney level, the presence of renal kidney stones or calculi is a consequence. Deposition of calcium in the collecting tubules of the kidney produces nephrocalcinosis. The hyperactive gland may be removed surgically, resulting in the fall of serum calcium levels and often minimization of the urolithiasis, but the principal deleterious consequence of prolonged hyperparathyroidism is the greatly decreased mineral content of the bone. Also, calcitonin deficiency may be present in patients with surgically removed or congenitally absent thyroid glands, putting them at risk for bone disease.

B. Calcitonin

The only disease state known to be related to calcitonin is that resulting from a disorder of C cell function. This is medullary carcinoma of the thyroid, which results in hypersecretion of calcitonin. The etiology of this condition is unknown. Over 50% of the cases exhibit a familial

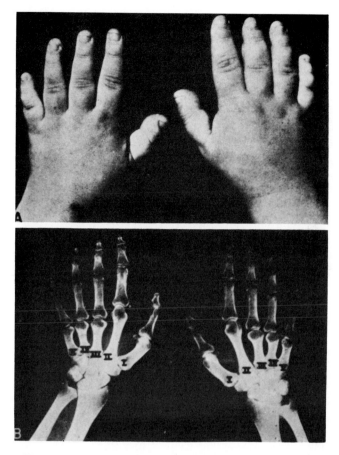

Figure 9-15. Photograph and X-ray film of hands of a patient with pseudohypopara-thyroidism. Note that all digits except the thumbs and index fingers are shorter than normal. The shortness results mainly from short metacarpals. Modified from F. Albright and E. C. Reifenstein, "The Parathyroid Glands and Metabolic Bone Disease." © 1948, Williams & Wilkins, Baltimore.

incidence, and the pattern of inheritance indicates an autosomal dominant mode of transmission. The disease is rare, occurring only in 1 of every several thousand patients seeking medical attention. It is one of the few forms of cancer that can be detected by radioimmunoassay of the plasma level of calcitonin. This is carried out by measurement of its concentration before and after a standard provocative infusion with either calcium or pentagastrin. Ectopic calcitonin production is commonly seen in some tissues, especially small-cell carcinoma of the lung.

392

C. Vitamin D

Conceptually, human clinical disorders related to vitamin D can be considered as those arising because of (1) altered availability of vitamin D; (2) altered conversion of vitamin D to its principal daughter metabolites $1,25(OH)_2D_3$ or $24,25(OH)_2D_3$; (3) conditions that may be due to variations in organ responsiveness to these dihydroxylated metabolites; and (4) perturbations in the integrated interactions of these metabolites with PTH and calcitonin. Figure 9-16 presents a schematic diagram of the relationship between human disease states related to vitamin D and the metabolic processing of vitamin D via its endocrine system. It is possible to identify diseases that are present in the intestine (e.g., malabsorption and tropical sprue) or diseases of the parathyroid gland (hyper- and hypoparathyroidism), of the bone (e.g., osteomalacia, osteoporosis, rickets), or the kidney, such as chronic renal failure. All of these in their own way reflect a disturbance in or a malfunctioning of the body's normal endocrine processing of vitamin D and its interaction with the other calcemic hormones.

The classic deficiency state resulting from a dietary absence of vitamin

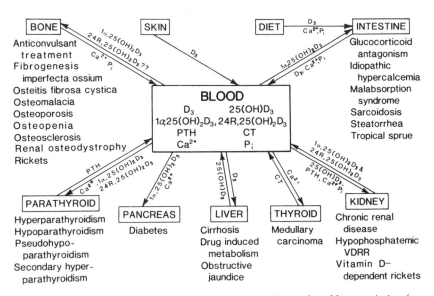

Figure 9-16. Human disease states related to vitamin D. Reproduced by permission from A. W. Norman, "Vitamin D: The Calcium Homeostatic Steroid Hormone," p. 411. Academic Press, New York, 1979.

D or lack of ultraviolet (sunlight) exposure is the bone disease called rickets in children or osteomalacia in adults. Historically the identification of rickets as a disease state allowed G. Mellanby in 1920 to induce rickets in puppies experimentally by nutritionally withholding vitamin D. This work demonstrated that in the absence of sunlight, vitamin D was truly a trace essential dietary constituent (e.g., a vitamin).

The clinical features of rickets and osteomalacia depend upon the age of onset. The classical skeletal disorders of rickets include deformity of the bones, especially in the knees, wrists, and ankles (see Fig. 9-17A), as well as associated changes in the costochondrial joint junctions, which have been termed by some as the rachitic rosary (see Fig. 9-17B). If rickets develops in the first 6 months of life, infants may suffer from convulsions or develop tetany due to a low blood calcium level (usually <7 mg/100 ml), but may have only minor skeletal changes. After 6 months, bone pain as well as tetany are likely to be present.

Since osteomalacia occurs after growth and development of the skeleton is complete (i.e., the adult stage of life), its main symptoms are muscular weakness and bone pain, with little bone deformity.

A characteristic feature of bone osteomalacia and rickets is the failure of the organic matrix of bone (osteoid) to calcify. This leads to the appearance of excessive quantities of uncalcified bone matrix, termed the osteoid. In addition, there is often a high serum level of alkaline phosphatase, a fact that is often used to assist in the clinical diagnosis of the presence of osteomalacia.

Osteoporosis is the most common generalized disorder of bone; it is estimated that over 3 million women in the United States may have osteoporosis. It is most simply characterized as a state of insufficiently calcified bone and is the end result of a number of metabolic abnormalities that affect the skeleton. Some of the causes of osteoporosis that have been recognized include (1) adrenal cortical hyperfunction, (2) acromegaly, (3) a prolonged calcium deficiency, (4) prolonged immobilization, and (5) a reduced level of estrogen, as in postmenopausal women.

The chief clinical sign of osteoporosis is a thinning of the bones with a concomitant increase in the number of fractures. Osteoporosis is often characterized by a crushed fracture of the vertebra with associated back pain or a hip fracture. In the 1980s, it is estimated that ~2 billion dollars is expended annually to provide health care for hip fractures attributable to postmenopausal osteoporosis. Two theories have been advanced to account for the development of osteoporosis: There may be either an increase of bone resorption or a decrease in the rate of new bone formation, or both.

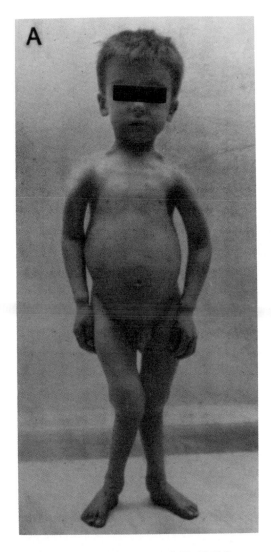

Figure 9-17. (A) Classic appearance of rickets in a child. (B) X-Ray appearance of rib cage and classic rachitic "rosary." The beaded appearance results from enlarged costochondrial regions of the bone. Reproduced by permission from A. W. Norman, "Vitamin D: The Calcium Homeostatic Steroid Hormone," p. 442. Academic Press, New York, 1979.

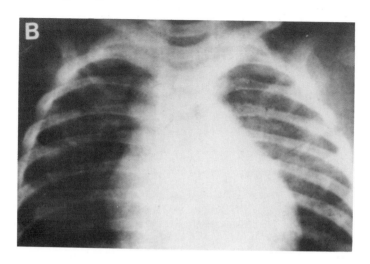

Figure 9-17B

References

A. Books

Kumar, R., ed. (1984). "Vitamin D: Basic and Clinical Aspects." Martinus Nijhoff, Amsterdam.

Norman, A. W. (1979). "Vitamin D: The Calcium Homeostatic Steroid Hormone." Academic Press, New York.

Rasmussen, H., and Bordier, P. (1974). "The Physiological and Cellular Basis of Metabolic Bone Disease." Williams & Wilkins, Baltimore, Maryland.

B. Review Articles

Cohn, D. V. (1981). Parathyroid hormone. *Endocr. Rev.* **2**, 1–26.

Copp, D. H. (1972). Evolution of calcium regulation in vertebrates. *Clin. Endocrinol. Metab.* **1**, 21–32.

Haussler, M. R., and McCain, T. A. (1977). Basic and clinical concepts related to vitamin D metabolism and action. *N. Engl. J. Med.* **297**, 974–983.

Henry, H. L., and Norman, A. W. (1984). Vitamin D: Metabolism and biological actions. *Annu. Rev. Nutr.* **4**, 493–520.

Norman, A. W., and Henry, H. L. (1979). Vitamin D to 1,25-dihydroxycholecalciferol: Evolution of a steroid hormone. *Trends Biochem. Sci.* **4**, 14–18.

Norman, A. W., Roth, J., and Orci, L. (1982). The vitamin D encodrine system: Steroid metabolism, hormone receptors and biological response (calcium binding proteins). *Endocr. Rev.* **3**, 331–366.

C. Research Papers

Cooke, N. E. (1986). Rat vitamin D binding protein. Determination of the full-length primary structure from cloned cDNA. *J. Biol. Chem.* **261**, 3441–3450.

Deftos, L. J., Weisman, M. H., Williams, G. W., Karf, D. B., Frumar, A. M., Davidson, B. J., Parihemore, J. G., and Judd, H. L. (1980). Influence of age and sex on plasma calcitonin in human beings. *N. Engl. J. Med.* **302**, 1351–1353.

Koeffler, H. P., Reichel, H., Munker, R., Barbers, R., and Norman, A. W. (1985). Interaction of 1,25-dihydroxyvitamin D$_3$ and the hematopoietic system. *In* "Leukemia: Recent Advances in Biology and Treatment" (R. P. Gale and D. W. Golde, eds.), pp. 399–413. Alan R. Liss, New York.

MacGregor, R. L., Jilka. R. L., and Hamilton, J. W. (1986). Formation and secretion of fragments of parathormone. Identification of cleavage sites. *J. Biol. Chem.* **261**, 1929–1934.

Riggs, B. L., Seeman, E., Hodgson, S. F., Taves, D. R., and O'Fallon, W. M. (1982). Effect of the fluoride/calcium regimen on vertebral fracture occurrence in postmenopausal osteoporosis. *N. Engl. J. Med.* **306**, 446–450.

Rosenfeld, M. G., Mermod, J. J., Amara, S. G., Swanson, L. W., Sawchenko, P. E., Rivier, J., Vale, W. W., and Evans, R. M. (1983). Production of a novel neuropeptide encoded by the calcitonin gene via tissue-specific RNA processing. *Nature (London)* **304**, 129–135.

Chapter 10

Adrenal Corticoids

HORMONES

I. INTRODUCTION

The hormones produced by the cells of the human adrenal cortex in response to appropriate stimuli are steroid hormones: cortisol, the major substance secreted in response to stress, and aldosterone, the steroid hormone acting on the kidney to conserve sodium ion from being excreted in the urine. Aldosterone, consequently, plays an important role in water balance and regulation of blood pressure. Secretion of these two hormones is controlled by different systems. A third major hormone, dehydroepiandrosterone (DHEA), and its sulfatide/sulfate derivative are secreted by the innermost layer of cells of the adrenal cortex in considerable amounts. Little is known about the physiological activities of this hormone except that it is a weak androgen and it can be converted in various cells by the aromatase enzyme system to an active estrogen.

Glucocorticoids are essential to life and they act on different cells in different ways. Often they induce proteins or repress the expression of certain proteins by transcriptional actions. A general result of glucocorticoid action is the direct effect of increasing glycogen, especially in liver, and of increasing the level of circulating glucose. The latter effect may occur through direct stimulation of certain rate-limiting enzymes in the gluconeogenesis pathway and through the negative effects of the hormone on peripheral cells which cause them to cease taking up nutrients (glucose) from the blood. Prolonged high levels of glucocorticoids can lead to cell death of susceptible cells, which accounts for muscle wasting and immunodeficiency. However, early effects of glucocorticoids probably do not include immunodeficiency and some recent information indicates that β-endorphin, which is secreted from the pituitary together with ACTH in the stress response, may actually stimulate the action of certain immune cells. Glucocorticoids are known to exert permissive effects on cells, without which many other hormones could not induce particular cellular proteins. The permissive action of glucocorticoids is not well understood, but may require mediation through the transcriptional level. In this regard some recent studies suggest that permissive actions of glucocorticoids are related to their ability to induce cyclic AMP-dependent protein kinase. As a powerful antiinflammatory agent, glucocorticoid acts on many cells through the normal receptor mechanism to induce a protein(s) known as "lipomodulin." Lipomodulin is an inhibitor of phospholipase A_2 and thus prevents the release of arachidonic acid (and other fatty acids) from phospholipids in the cell membrane. These fatty acids are precursors of prostaglandins, prostacyclin, thromboxanes, and leukotrienes, some of which mediate processes of inflammation and pain. Their production is depressed by the glucocorticoid-induced lipomodulin whose action may represent the principal pathway by which glucocorticoids exert their anti-inflammatory effects. Glucocorticoids have been shown to stimulate the uptake of Na^+ into tubular epithelial cells of the large intestine and kidney by a process (presumably involving the Na^+/H^+ antiporter) which is discrete from that regulated by mineralocorticoids (Na^+ conductance channel), so that Na^+ uptake into tissues appears to be a specific response to glucocorticoids. Water balance would also be effected by this activity. All of these effects, i.e., cell-specific metabolic changes, specific cell death in certain cases, permissive effects in a wide variety of cell types, profound antiinflammatory effects exerted through the induction of lipomodulin, and effects upon Na^+ retention, contribute to the systemic effects of this hormone.

Mineralocorticoids promote sodium and potassium transport, usually followed by changes in water balance. This function is essential to life, but in some cells can be produced by glucocorticoids. Glucocorticoids and mineralocorticoids generally act through their own specific receptors, but in certain situations can bind to the same hormone receptor. Thus, each can be expected to exert effects typical of the other, especially when large amounts are administered. In fact, both hormones seem to be involved in Na^+ ion uptake in tubular epithelial cells. Mineralocorticoids act on the kidney to maintain water balance through control of sodium ion uptake and mesh in function with the vasopressin system through control of water reabsorption. Potassium ion transport is also affected by mineralocorticoids. Because of the overlapping specificities of mineralocorticoids and glucocorticoids, much of the molecular interactions of these two hormones remain to be sorted out. A critical feature of aldosterone is that it is secreted in effective amounts only during stress.

Dehydroepiandrosterone circulates at very high levels in the bloodstream, mainly as the sulfate derivative. A receptor for this hormone has not been discovered. It is probably the main source for androgens (via testosterone) in the female. It is apparently important in fetal development, in supplying cells with a precursor for estrogen synthesis, and for certain tissue-protective functions which are as yet not understood.

II. ANATOMY, DEVELOPMENT, AND CELLULAR FINE STRUCTURE OF THE ADRENAL CORTEX

The adrenal glands are small organs embedded in fat and enclosed by coverings located above the kidneys. For this reason, they are often referred to as the suprarenal glands. The glands on each side of the body have different shapes; the right one is shaped like a pyramid, whereas the left one is crescent shaped. Nevertheless, they are easily recognized even in small experimental animals. In man, the glands weigh about 5 g each and their general locations are indicated in Fig. 10-1. These glands are well supplied with blood vessels, including a branch from the aorta and a branch from the renal artery (Fig. 10-2). The blood entering the adrenal cortex is drained out through the adrenal medulla. This is significant in view of the regulation of an important enzyme of the medulla by cortisol from the adrenal cortex. The adrenal blood supply empties into a major single central vein which merges with the renal vein (Fig. 10-2). The adrenal gland consists of two major parts, an outer cortex and a central medulla. The cortex is the part responsible for the formation of the steroid hormones, aldosterone, cortisol (hydrocortisone), and dehydroepiandrosterone (DHEA), as well as amounts of analogous hormones which are metabolites in the pathways of syntheses of these hormones.

The adrenal medulla is made up of nervous tissue and secretes the catecholamines, principally epinephrine (and norepinephrine) (see Chapter 11). The cortex is involved in short- and long-term stress reactions, whereas the medulla takes part in sudden or alarm reactions and it is under nervous system control. Catecholamines and enkephalins are released from the medulla instantaneously following a signal transmitted by the nervous system. This signal probably originates in the hypothalamus and arrives in the medulla by way of splanchnic nerves from the spinal cord.

As expected from their greatly differing functions, the cortex and medulla arise from different precursor tissues during development. The adrenal cortex is mesodermal in origin, formed by ingrowth of the peritoneum. The medulla arises from the neural crest and is ectodermal in origin. Essentially, the medulla may be thought of as a specialized nervous tissue designed for secretion.

By the fifth week of development a suprarenal groove appears above and on each side of the dorsal mesentary (Fig. 10-3A). The cells lining the groove (mesothelial cells) begin to proliferate (Fig. 10-3B) and a "primary cortex" is derived from this proliferation (Fig. 10-3C) by the seventh week of development. While this process has been going on, neural crest cells have moved downward toward the cortex. By 7 weeks the mesothelial layer becomes active again (Fig. 10-3C) and produces a new group of cells which are laid down upon the cells of the primary cortex and become the "secondary cortex" (Fig. 10-3D). Eventually this will be covered by a connective tissue capsule. In the meantime, the cells

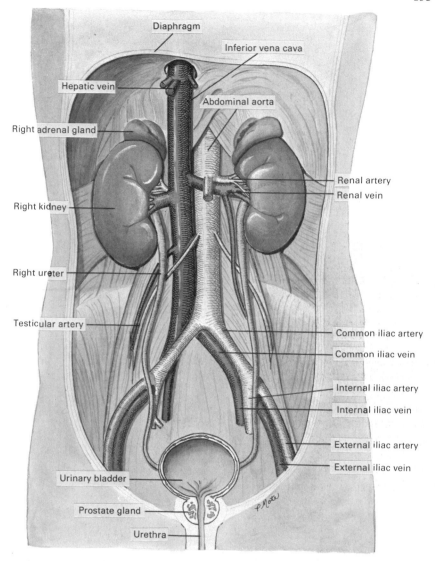

Figure 10-1. Summary of the major anatomical components of the urine-forming system. Reproduced with permission from E. E. Chaffee and I. M. Lytle, "Basic Physiology and Anatomy," 4th ed., p. 483. Lippincott, Philadelphia, Pennsylvania, 1980.

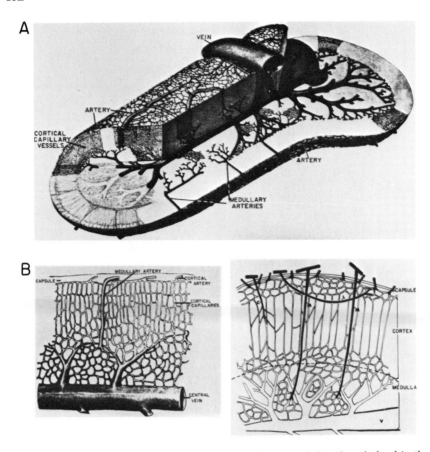

Figure 10-2. (A) Arterial blood supply and venous drainage of the adrenal gland in the dog. (B) Blood supply of the adrenal cortex and medulla in the dog. Reproduced from R. E. Coupland, *in* "Handbook of Physiology" (R. O. Greep and E. B. Astwood, eds.), Sect. 7, Vol. VI, pp. 282–294. Am. Physiol. Soc., Washington, D.C., 1975.

of the sympathetic ganglia (neural crest cells) have invaded the primary cortex to form the forerunner of the medulla (Fig. 10-3E and F).

In fetal life the human adrenal is large. At term and for the first postnatal year or longer the primary cortex begins to atrophy while the cells of the secondary cortex actively divide. The primary cortex is often referred to as the "fetal cortex" because of its transient life. It functions like the testis and is uncharacteristic of the mature adrenal (see Chapter 14). As the fetal cortex disappears, the *zona glomerulosa* appears immediately adjacent to the capsule. It is present at termination of pregnancy. With continued proliferation, the next inward zone, the *zona fasciculata*,

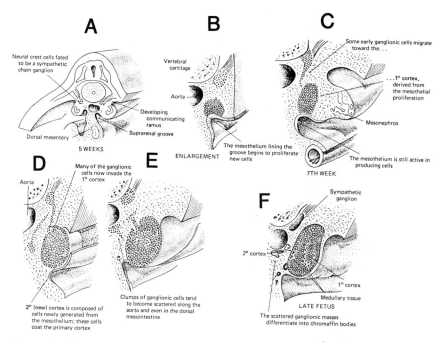

Figure 10-3. Development of the adrenal glands. (A) At 5 weeks development of the human fetus. (B) Enlargement of the mesothelium. (C) Seventh week of development. (D) Secondary cortex. (E) Appearance of ganglionic cells. (F) Differentiation into chromaffin bodies in the late fetus. Reproduced from D. A. Langebartel, "The Anatomical Primer," p. 443. University Park Press, Baltimore, Maryland, 1977.

arises and within a few months after birth the most inward layer of cells, the *zona reticularis,* is formed.

The zones of adrenal cortex cells are shown in Fig. 10-4. The *zona glomerulosa* is associated with the production of aldosterone, the salt-retaining hormone. Its cells are tall, rather unpigmented, and arranged in clusters. The *zona fasciculata,* the main producer of cortisol, the major glucocorticoid in man, is comprised by cells with many sides (poly-gonal). This is the largest of the three zones in the cortex. The *zona reticularis* is the innermost layer of cells adjacent to the medulla. The *fasciculata–reticularis zona* probably functions as a unit to produce cortisol and DHEA. ACTH converts *fasciculata* cells to *reticularis* cells that are responsible for most of the steroid production. Capillaries are found in this cellular network (Fig. 10-2). These cells are smaller and more pig-mented (golden brown) than *fasciculata* cells. The pigment is lipofuscin. Lipofuscin granules are derived from lysosomes and are called second-

404

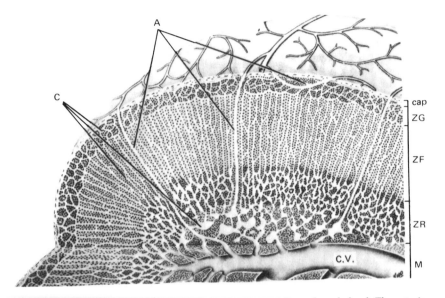

Figure 10-4. Schematic view of the circulation in a mammalian adrenal gland. The arteries and arterioles are shown in the capsule (cap) of which the outer layer has been removed. Other vessels shown are the radially arranged capillaries (C), a few arterioles (A) in the cortex, and "arterial" and "venous" capillaries in the medulla. The zones of the cortex are identified as *zona glomerulosa* (ZG), *zona fasciculata* (ZF), and *zona reticularis* (ZR). M denotes the medulla. CV, Central vein. Reproduced from R. G. Harrison, "A Textbook of Human Embryology," Vol. 1, p. 48. Blackwell Scientific, London, 1959.

ary lysosomes. Although cells of the *zona reticularis* are able to secrete glucocorticoids, primarily they produce and secrete the weak androgen, dehydroepiandrosterone (DHEA), in rather large quantities (15–25 mg/day). In addition to DHEA, a small amount of testosterone is formed in the reticularis layer.

The fine structure of each of the three cell types is shown in Fig. 10-5. The cells of the *zona glomerulosa* contain relatively long mitochondria with lamellar cristae, and these differ from the mitochondria in cells of the other adrenal cortical layers. The *zona fasciculata* is the largest of the three zones and is made up of columnar cells which are polygonal and form cords that radiate from the zone above. Mitochondria of these cells vary in size, but are usually larger than mitochondria in cells of the other zones. The *zona reticularis* contains networks of interconnecting cells. Mitochondria in these cells resemble those in cells of the *zona fasciculata*.

Glucocorticoid Targets

Although the glucocorticoids act on many cells of the body, the liver is an important target organ because of the relatively large concentration of glucocorticoid receptors in the hepatocyte. In Fig. 10-6 are shown various levels of organization of the liver. A basic subdivision is the liver lobule shown in the upper right. Cords of hepatocytes are clustered together with portal canals at each apex. The portal triad consists of bile duct, hepatic artery, and portal vein as shown in the upper center. From this drawing it is clear how the circulation efficiently bathes the hepatocytes. Clear also from this figure is the fact that the large majority of cells in the liver are hepatocytes, with bile duct cells and Kupffer (scavenging) cells in the minority. Probably at least 65% of the liver cells are hepatocytes. In Fig. 10-7 is a drawing of the idealized hepatocyte at the electron microscopic level and a discussion of salient features occurs in the figure legend.

Another major target of glucocorticoid hormones is the thymus. It is located above the upper end of the heart. The thymus has a relatively large size in the newborn and is invested with immunological functions. Its size decreases with age until adult proportions are attained largely due to the death of glucocorticoid-sensitive cells as the adrenal *zona fasciculata* becomes more active in secreting cortisol. The thymus cells killed off in this way during development probably contain large numbers of glucocorticoid receptors per cell. The histology of the thymus is shown in Chapter 17. Besides a capsule, there are two main layers of cells, the cortex and the medulla. Thymocytes are similar to the lymphocytes of other lymphoid organs and in the circulation. There are many free ribosomes and a large nucleus containing chromatin condensed in large masses in close proximity to the inside nuclear envelope.

III. CHEMISTRY AND BIOCHEMISTRY

The structures of principal steroid hormones of the adrenal cortex are shown in Fig. 10-8. The chemistry and structural relationships of the glucocorticoids compared to the other steroid hormones are reviewed in Chapter 2. The metabolic pathway for the production of glucocorticoids is presented in Fig. 2-22.

A

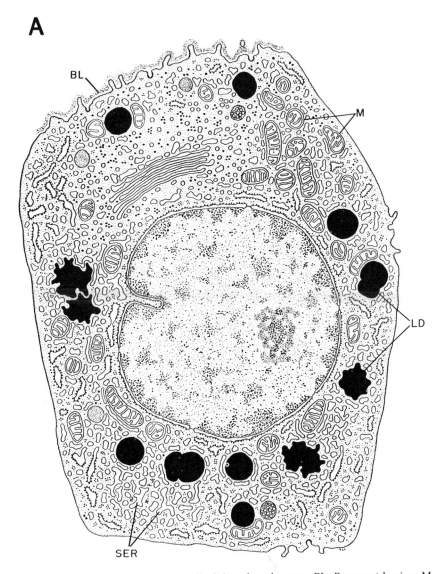

Figure 10-5. (A) A *zona glomerulosa* cell of the adrenal cortex. BL, Basement lamina; M, mitochondria; LD, lipid droplets; SER, smooth endoplasmic reticulum. This cell which secretes mineralocorticoids is columnar, with a spherical nucleus. The cell is smooth except on the surface(s) bordering a space where absorption or secretion may occur. Reproduced from T. L. Lentz, "Cell Fine Structure," p. 333. Saunders, Philadelphia, Pennsylvania, 1971. (B) Cell of the *zona fasciculata* of the adrenal gland. This glucocorticoid-secreting cell is a large polyhedral cell with a central nucleus. Ly, Lysosome; LPG, lipofuscin pigment granule; LD, lipid droplet; M, mitochondria; SER, smooth endoplasmic

B

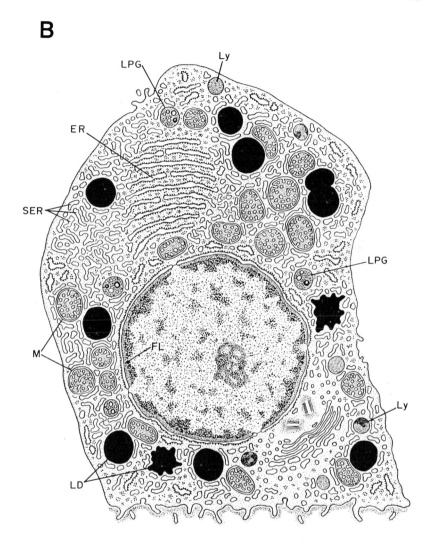

reticulum; ER, rough endoplasmic reticulum; FL, fibrous lamina. Lipid droplets are in close association with mitochondria. Reproduced from T. L. Lentz, "Cell Fine Structure," p. 335. Saunders, Philadelphia, Pennsylvania, 1971. (C, p. 408) Cell of the *zona reticularis* which secretes weak androgens (DHEA and DHEA sulfate). LPG, Lipofuscin granule. Mitochondria are elongated compared to the *zona fasciculata* and the number of lipofuscin granules is different. Otherwise the features of the cells of the two zones are rather similar. Reproduced from T. L. Lentz, "Cell Fine Structure," p. 337. Saunders, Philadelphia, Pennsylvania, 1971.

408

C

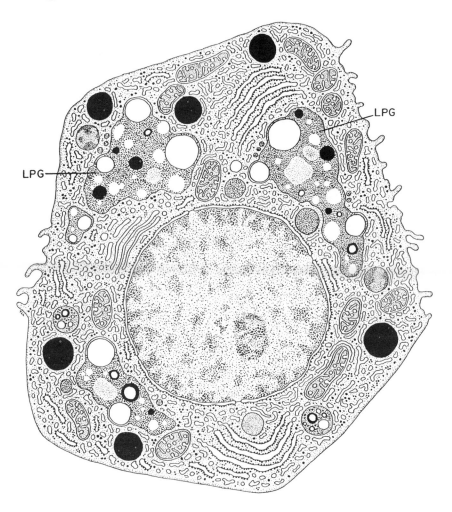

Figure 10-5C. See legend on p. 407.

A. Glucocorticoids and Stress

Glucocorticoids are secreted in large amounts in man, up to 25 mg or more per day, and represent a major chemical response of the body to stress. A person undergoing long-term stress will have higher amounts of cortisol circulating in the bloodstream than the unstressed person. The steroid acts on many of the tissues of the body to an extent undoubt-

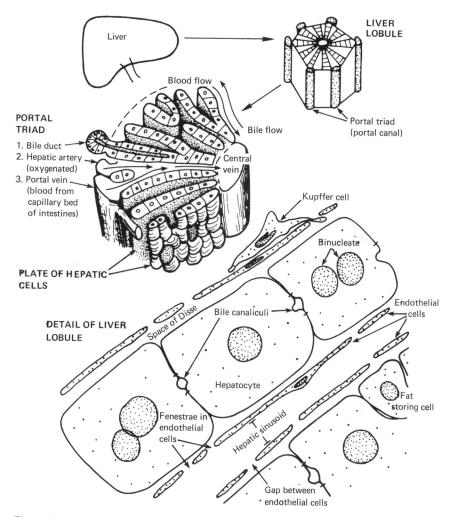

Figure 10-6. Anatomical components of the liver and hepatocyte, a major target cell for glucocorticoids. This drawing was made originally by Dr. Laurie Paavola, Department of Anatomy, Temple Medical School, and is redrawn here with her permission. Recent work with a polyclonal antibody to the glucocorticoid receptor indicates that the hepatocyte is the cell in the liver having a large number of receptor antigens, while the bile and Kupffer cells have little or no antigenic activity.

edly determined by the number of glucocorticoid receptors present in the cell of a particular tissue. The liver, which contains about 65,000 receptor molecules per cell in an experimental animal (rat), predominates as a major target of corticosterone (principal glucocorticoid in rat).

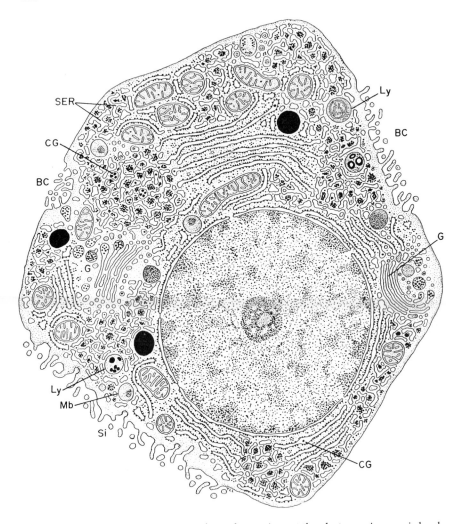

Figure 10-7. Drawing of a hepatocyte from observations at the electron microscopic level. SER, Smooth endoplasmic reticulum; CG, cisternae of endoplasmic reticulum; G, Golgi apparatus; Ly, lysosome; BC, bile canaliculi, Mb, microbody; Si, sinusoids. The hepatocyte is polygonal with a large round nucleus and nucleolus. Pores are present in the nuclear membrane and are a potential (but unproven) portal for nuclear translocation of steroid–receptor complexes. Free as well as membrane-bound ribosomes are evident in the cytoplasm, as is the smooth-surfaced endoplasmic reticulum. Glycogen granules in aggregates (α particles) are enclosed by networks of smooth endoplasmic reticulum. Single granules of glycogen (β particles) are present also. Some of the Golgi vacuoles contain dense granules of ~500 Å diameter. There are many mitochondria and a few lipid droplets (in contrast to adrenal cortical cells where steroid hormone synthesis takes place). Microbodies are evident. These are spherical structures containing urate oxidase, catalase, and D-

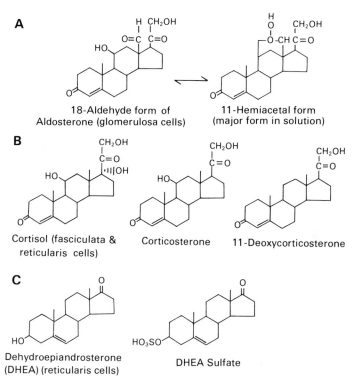

A

18-Aldehyde form of
Aldosterone (glomerulosa cells)

11-Hemiacetal form
(major form in solution)

B

Cortisol (fasciculata &
reticularis cells)

Corticosterone

11-Deoxycorticosterone

C

Dehydroepiandrosterone
(DHEA) (reticularis cells)

DHEA Sulfate

Figure 10-8. Structures of major hormones of the adrenal cortex. Aldosterone is secreted from the outer layer of the adrenal cortex, the *zona glomerulosa*. Two forms are in equilibrium, as shown in (A). (B) The structures of cortisol, the major human product of the *zona fasciculata*, together with corticosterone and deoxycorticosterone. (C) The structures of dehydroepiandrosterone (DHEA) and its sulfate derivative secreted from the inner layer of cells of the cortex, the *zona reticularis*.

Other important targets are the lymphoid cells, thymus gland, and kidney. Many other tissues seem to have enough receptor molecules to give a response to stress, especially if it is long-term. In fact, most tissues of animals or of cells in culture seem to contain measurable amounts of receptor, making it theoretically possible for nearly all tissues of the

amino acid oxidase, sometimes referred to as peroxisomes. In man, uricase is lacking. The SER near glycogen deposits may be associated with the secretion of glucose from the cell during glycogenolysis. Glucose 6-phosphatase present in these membranes may be active in outward glucose transport. The small dense granules in the Golgi region may be serum lipoproteins en route to cellular release. Reproduced from T. L. Lentz, "Cell Fine Structure," p. 189. Saunders, Philadelphia, Pennsylvania, 1971.

412

body to be affected by stress. Some recent studies using antibodies to the receptor indicate that rat biliary and Kupffer cells of the liver contain small amounts of receptor, and cells of the *pars intermedia* have small amounts or lack receptor altogether. Long-term stress may be distinguished from short-term stress, often referred to as "alarm" or "fright." In short-term stress, the minute-to-minute changes in metabolism are under control of catecholamine hormones, primarily epinephrine, secreted by the adrenal medulla. The secretion of epinephrine is in turn controlled by the autonomic nervous system. Both stresses, long- or short-term, lead to release of glucocorticoids. Figure 10-9 delineates the overall pathways by which the two types of stress call into play the secretion of glucocorticoid hormones or epinephrine. Glucocor-

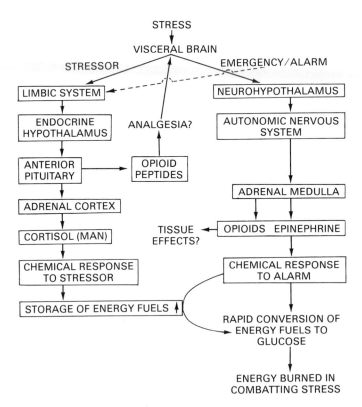

Figure 10-9. Overall pathways used in response to stressors. Note that cortisol can be produced either in classical long-term or alarm reactions.

ticoids are so named because they influence the storage of carbohydrate macromolecules in the form of energy supplies (glycogen) which can be tapped by conversion of glycogen to glucose on a minute-to-minute basis by epinephrine for instantly usable energy in "flight or fight" situations or for expenditure of "nervous energy." Many other hormones are involved in stress, and they include glucagon, growth hormone, prolactin, β-endorphin, vasopressin, angiotensin II, and prostaglandins.

Thus, we can classify two types of stressors: those that are relatively long-term and evoke glucocorticoids from the adrenal cortex, such as intensive cold, prolonged loud noise, serious injury, and burns, and changes in the environment necessitating adaptation by the organism, with serious consequences if adaptation does not occur. The alarm emergency or shorter term stressor would be an event of a surprise nature, such as fright induced by a specific happening. This type of stressor would evoke primarily the secretion of epinephrine (and norepinephrine) from the adrenal medulla as well as cortisol from the adrenal cortex. Both types usually occur simultaneously; one chain of events (Fig. 10-9) in operation does not preclude the utilization of the other pathway.

The reactions to stressors (Fig. 10-9) now can be defined in more detail (Fig. 10-10). The catecholamines, however, will be considered in depth in Chapter 11, but are presented in outline here because stress reactions involve both the glucocorticoids and catecholamines. The metabolic changes in the organism induced by elevated levels of glucocorticoids, such as cortisol, are mediated by the amount of available glucocorticoid receptor proteins located in the cytoplasm of target tissues. Very important organs are liver, lymphocytes including thymus cells, adipose cells, kidney, anterior pituitary, and various parts of the brain. The question of physiological subcellular location of unoccupied steroid receptors has been raised recently. Some work suggests that the estrogen receptor is located in the nucleus exclusively while cytoplasmic forms could be artifacts of cell breakage causing the nuclear form to leak in these preparations. The case for glucocorticoid receptors is not clear, and it seems possible that functional forms of the unoccupied receptor may occur in the cytoplasm. Continued research efforts are needed to resolve the question of whether cytoplasmic unoccupied receptors occur in the unbroken cell (see Chapter 1). Some of the effects of cortisol on tissues of normal or adrenalectomized rats are shown in Table 10-1.

Thus, as detailed later, the glucocorticoid hormone affects transcription and stimulates production of certain mRNAs which are translated

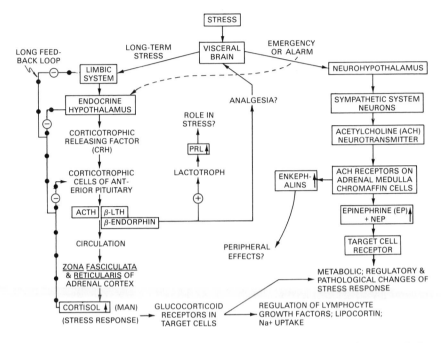

Figure 10-10. Summary of overall changes in stress. Circled plus signs refer to stimulation and upward arrows at the right of a name of a substance refer to an increase; circled minus signs refer to a negative effect or depression.

subsequently into proteins whose actions culminate in an anabolic (liver and kidney) or catabolic (lymphatic and other tissues) shift in cellular activity. This anabolic effect has been shown clearly for glucocorticoid action on tyrosine aminotransferase in hepatoma cells. The changes in metabolism in each cell containing the hormone receptor are the culmination of the hormonal effect at the level of the cell. The summation of metabolic changes in different tissues constitutes the adaptation of the organism to stress at this level. Antiinflammatory and antipain effects and Na^+ movements contribute as major alterations produced by glucocorticoids. Not all of these biochemical changes are understood. For example, the stress signals mediated by the brain and the feedback effects of cortisol on elements of the brain remain to be elucidated clearly. Behavioral modifications, if any, to stress may be clarified by future research in this direction. Elaboration of β-endorphin by the anterior

Table 10–1. Effects of Glucorticoids in Various Tissues[a]

Time after glucocorticoid administration	Sequence of responses
2 min	Liver uptake of hormone, accumulation of unmetabolized hormone in liver
<5 min	Binding to liver cytosol macromolecules
~15 min	Cortisol metabolized to anions in liver, conversion of rough endoplasmic reticulum to smooth endoplasmic reticulum
<30 min	Feedback inhibition of CRH and ACTH
<30 min	Steroid–receptor complex in liver nucleus
~90 min	Glycogen deposition
30–120 min	Nuclear RNA polymerase activity increased
2–4 hr	Increased RNA synthesis, increased fatty acid release from adipose, decreased glucose utilization in many sensitive tissues peripheral to liver
	Protein breakdown in peripheral tissues: decreased glucose utilization, nucleic acid synthesis and protein synthesis decreased; ornithine decarboxylase activity increased in liver, tyrosine aminotransferase activity peaks in liver, tryptophan oxygenase activity peaks in liver, polysome aggregation
8–20 hr	Increased general liver protein synthesis, decreased glucose utilization, increased hepatic gluconeogenesis, lympholysis
4 hr–days	Small increase in threonine dehydrase activity (liver), alanine aminotransferase activity increases (liver), many glycolytic enzyme activities increase (liver, kidney), urea cycle enzymes increase: arginine synthetase system; arginine succinase; arginase

[a] Some of the data of this table are reproduced from D. Shulster, S. Burstein, and B. A. Cooke, "Molecular Endocrinology of the Steroid Hormones," p. 275. Wiley, New York, 1976.

pituitary in response to stress is bound to have important stress adaptation effects, perhaps in the central nervous system.

B. Corticotropin Releasing Hormone (CRH)

The primary sequence of CRH peptide of 41 amino acid residues is given in Fig. 3-8. In Fig. 10-10, the response of the hypothalamus to signals from the limbic system is the secretion and subsequent resynthesis of the CRH. CRH is released from specific cells in the hypothalamus. CRH activity appears to be present in other tissues, such as cerebral cortex and liver.

C. Mode of Action of Releasing Hormones (e.g., CRH)

In Fig. 10-10 we see that following signals from the limbic system to the hypothalamus, CRH is released into a closed portal circulation intimately connected with the anterior pituitary (Fig. 3-2). Detailed information on anatomical considerations and mode of action of hypothalamic releasing hormones will be found in Chapters 3 and 5.

D. Mode of Action of ACTH

ACTH is the peptide hormone secreted from the anterior pituitary in response to CRH. ACTH is a 39 amino acid peptide; the structure is presented in Fig. 5-14. The common N-terminal sequence of residues 1–13 of ACTH and residues 1–13 of α-MSH constitutes an important homologous structure. Also, the sequence 11–17 of β-MSH and the residues 4–10 of ACTH are homologous. These homologies in amino acid sequence are suggestive of a close relationship or of a common precursor between ACTH and MSH. However, in man, only ACTH and β-endorphin appear to be secreted by corticotrophic cells of the anterior pituitary. In diseases characterized by altered secretion of ACTH, skin pigmentation (due to MSH action) can occur (see Section VII). It is not completely clear how MSH is secreted in this case; possibly in certain diseases ACTH is degraded to α-MSH.

It is now known that ACTH, MSH, and β-lipotropin are all coded for by a single gene. The gene gives rise to an mRNA which is translated to a preprotein called the "opiocortin precursor" or "proopiomelanocortin." This is represented diagrammatically in Fig. 5-13. Not all of the information in the preprotein sequence is known, as depicted by the blank spaces in the parent peptide chain.

Following the secretion of ACTH into the blood circulation after stimulation by CRH from the hypothalamus, ACTH molecules bind to a specific receptor on the outer cell membranes of the two inner layers of cells of the adrenal cortex, the *zona fasciculata* and the *zona reticularis* (ACTH probably also plays a role in stimulating aldosterone secretion). The results of many experiments appear in Fig. 10-11 in the form of a speculative mechanism of action.

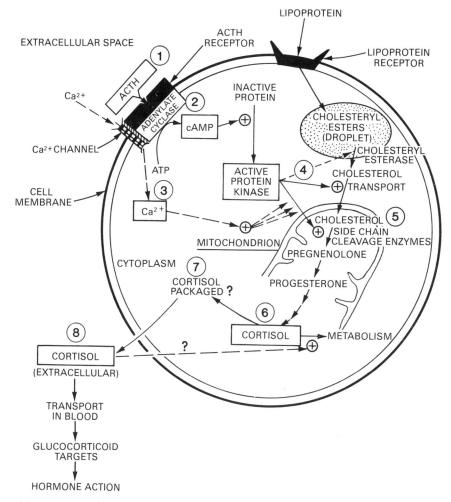

Figure 10-11. ACTH action on a cell of the *zona fasciculata* of the adrenal cortex. ACTH from the blood and the extracellular space binds to the ACTH receptor in the cell membrane (1). This results in the stimulation of adenylate cyclase and the formation of cyclic AMP from ATP (2). The calcium channel may be stimulated as well (3), allowing an increase of cytoplasmic Ca^{2+}. Elevated levels of cAMP activate protein kinase which phosphorylates certain proteins. This leads to increased hydrolysis of cholesteryl esters to form more cholesterol, increased transport of free cholesterol into the mitochondrion, and increased rates of synthesis of the side chain cleavage enzymes in the mitochondrion responsible for catalyzing the rate-limiting step of cortisol synthesis (4 and 5). Elevated cytoplasmic Ca^{2+} may also stimulate some of these reactions. Resulting cortisol (6) is probably packaged (7) and secreted to the extracellular space (8). High levels of cortisol in the extracellular space could have a negative feedback effect on the adrenal cell by increasing the rate of metabolism of intracellular cortisol to inactive forms, possibly by enhancing the activity (synthesis?) of cellular 5α-reductase. The hormone would be taken up by cells containing the glucocorticoid receptor where hormone action takes place (e.g., Fig. 10-14).

Molecules of ACTH bind to an outer cell membrane receptor. Formation of this complex activates adenylate cyclase of the inner membrane and increases the affinity of the enzyme for ATP. This could be accomplished by a mechanism described in Chapter 1. The cytoplasmic level of cyclic AMP is increased and inactive protein kinases are converted to active catalytic subunits and cyclic AMP-bound regulatory subunits (see Chapter 1). The active catalytic subunits phosphorylate proteins, as yet unidentified, which cause increased protein synthesis, possibly increased rates of hydrolysis of cholesteryl esters to free cholesterol, increased rate of transport of free cholesterol into the mitochondria (possibly by the sterol carrier protein), and, perhaps most importantly, a stimulation (by an unknown mechanism) of the cholesterol side chain cleavage reaction in the mitochondrion. This last effect may involve increased rate of synthesis of the enzymes of the side chain cleavage (Fig. 2-21). Recently, a novel adrenal peptide of low molecular weight, about 2000, has been shown to appear after ACTH stimulation. It could arise from a precursor protein or by synthesis *de novo*. Conversion of a precursor to the active peptide could be under the control of ACTH, operating perhaps by way of cyclic AMP, which would control some step in the system, for example, proteolytic processing. Generation of this peptide in cells of the adrenal cortex stimulates, in some way, the side chain cleavage system of enzymes in the mitochondrion, converting cholesterol to Δ^5-pregnenolone. This system is reminiscent of the hypothetical insulin mediator peptide which is claimed to regulate phosphoprotein phosphatases (see Chapter 7).

Since side chain cleavage of cholesterol appears to be the rate-limiting step in steroid hormone biosynthesis, the overall effect of ACTH is to increase the production and secretion of cortisol from cells of the *zona fasciculata* (and *zona reticularis*). This stimulation of cortisol production, however, depends on an increase in the concentration of Ca^{2+} in the cellular cytoplasm. This appears to occur through two processes: uptake from the extracellular space and mobilization of calcium phosphate stores from the mitochondrion (Fig. 10-11) and possibly from other subcellular locations. The precise role of Ca^{2+}, whose cytoplasmic levels are increased as a result of the increase in intracellular cyclic AMP or of an increase in cell membrane phospholipid metabolism, is unknown. It could involve activation of the contractile elements of the secretory process as well as an interaction of the outer membrane of the hormonal secretory components helping to bridge them to the inner cytoplasmic membrane. Ca^{2+} has been shown to stimulate activity of 11β-hydroxylase in adrenal mitochondria.

E. Sources of Cholesterol and Production of Glucocorticoids

The immediate substrate for steroid hormone biosynthesis is cholesterol (derived from circulating lipoproteins) from intracellular stores of cholesteryl esters or from free cholesterol (Fig. 10-11). For a discussion of cholesterol biosynthesis, see Chapter 2, Figs. 2-13–2-17.

Cholesterol is synthesized by the liver and intestine as major sources and to a smaller extent in other tissues. Cholesterol can be transported to peripheral cells as components of circulating lipoproteins. Lipoproteins are absorbed by many cells, such as the adrenal cortical cells (Fig. 10-11), and degraded within the cell to avail free cholesterol which is stored as fatty acid esters of cholesterol in the "lipid droplet." Activation of cholesteryl esterase may result from cellular stimulation by ACTH, which elevates levels of cyclic AMP, and the esterase may be activated by phosphorylation or by Ca^{2+} ions.

Cortisol is the main product in the *zona fasciculata* of human adrenal cortex. Aldosterone is the major steroid of the outer *zona glomerulosa*. Dehydroepiandrosterone and its sulfate are the principal products of the *zona reticularis*. These biochemical conversions are shown in Fig. 2-22. It is important to realize that the nature of the steroid hormone product is governed by the specificities of the converting enzymes produced in a given cell type. In essence, this specialization constitutes the cell's phenotypic function. For example, genes are expressed in the *fasciculata* cell encoding information for cytosolic 17α-hydroxylase, 21-hydroxylase, and mitochondrial 11β-hydroxylase whose reactions together with other cellular enzymes produce cortisol. A *zona glomerulosa* cell expresses genes for cytosolic 21-hydroxylase, but 17α-hydroxylase is not expressed. Mitochondrial 11β-hydroxylase and 18-hydroxylase are expressed also, resulting in the production of aldosterone rather than cortisol. Note that the side chain cleavage of cholesterol, the rate-limiting step in steroid hormone biosynthesis, occurs in the mitochondria. This is not a simple one-step reaction and the cleavage may involve as many as four enzymes, as shown in Fig. 2-21. Specific signals to the cells of the adrenal cortex determine which steroid hormone will be synthesized at an increased rate compared to the unstimulated state. Thus, ACTH stimulates *fasciculata* and *reticularis* cells to produce cortisol and dehydroepiandrosterone. The regulation of aldosterone synthesis will be discussed later.

F. Mechanism of Secretion of Glucocorticoids

Secretion can be said to occur at two levels in the process of synthesis and release of steroid hormones. Biosynthetic intermediates move between cytoplasmic and mitochondrial compartments and finally to the cytoplasm and to the cell exterior in the case of cortisol as the end product. Thus, the removal of Δ^5-pregnenolone from the mitochondria to the cytoplasm for action by the microsomal 3β-hydroxy-Δ^5-steroid dehydrogenase to produce progesterone is a transportation event. 17α-Hydroxylase is also located on the microsomes in the cytoplasm, as is 21-hydroxylase. The resulting 17α-hydroxydeoxycorticosterone must be transported back to the mitochondria, perhaps by way of a transporting protein, but 11β-hydroxylation to form cortisol occurs on the inner mitochondrial membrane (see Table 2-5). Cortisol comes out of the mitochondrion, presumably is packaged, and is secreted out of the cell into the extracellular space and into the bloodstream. Unfortunately, almost all of the foregoing scenario is lacking an understanding at the molecular level. Calcium is required for secretion and may help to attach secretory granules to the inner cell membrane.

Cholesterol and its ester are substrates for the mitochondrial synthesis of cortisol. Electron microscopy shows that lipid droplets reside near mitochondria (Fig. 10-5B). Cholesterol ester hydrolase and cholesterol transporting proteins could be activated by enhanced levels of cyclic AMP produced by ACTH action (if they are active as phosphorylated forms). Other lipid droplets may be depleted after ACTH, suggesting that cortisol may be stored in some droplets (Fig. 10-12), although evidence is weak on this point.

Values for the normal ranges of corticosteroids produced in a day, the plasma levels, protein binding, and urinary excretion are presented in Table 10-2.

G. Transport of Glucocorticoids in the Blood (CBG)

A corticosteroid binding globulin (CBG) is present in blood. This protein is also referred to as transcortin. It is synthesized in the liver and exported to the circulation. This protein binds cortisol with relatively high affinity (binding constant $\cong 10^8 \, M^{-1}$; the dissociation constant for the reaction: CBG + cortisol $\rightleftarrows$ CBG cortisol is about $10^{-8} \, M$ cortisol). Because of the affinity of the protein for cortisol, most of the hormone circulates in the bound form as reflected in the equilibrium which favors the complex: CBG + cortisol $\rightleftarrows$ CBG cortisol; there is only a small

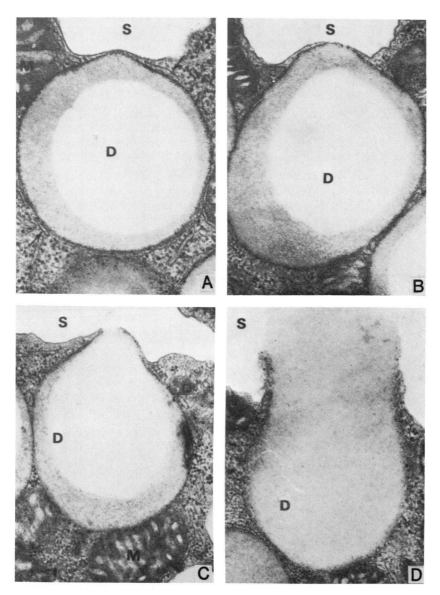

Figure 10-12. Sections of the rat *zona glomerulosa*. These pictures are arranged to show lipid droplets participating in a hypothetical mechanism of discharge (secretion?). D, Lipid droplet; S, extracellular space. (A), ×67,000; (B), ×52,000; (C), ×38,000; (D), ×39,500. Reproduced from J. A. G. Rhodin, *J. Ultrastruct. Res.* **34,** 23–71 (1971).

Table 10-2. Normal Values in Investigation of Adrenal Cortex[a]

Hormones and steroids	Normal range	Hormones and steroids	Normal range
Production rates of major hormones		Urine excretion	
Cortisol (mg/day)	10–20	Free cortisol	150 μg/day
Aldosterone (μg/day)	60–200	Cortisol in certain disease states	Several 100-thousand μg/day
Testosterone (mg/day)		Estrogens, total (μg/day)	
Males →	5–8	Males	4–25
Females →	0.3–0.8	Females	4–60
Dehydroepiandrosterone (mg/day)	25–30	Pregnanetriol (mg/day)	0–4
Plasma levels (μg/100 ml)		Pregnanediol (mg/day)	
Cortisol	5–20 (at 8:00 a.m.)	Males	0–1.5
Aldosterone	0.002–0.01	Females	
Testosterone		Follicular	0.5–1.5
Males	0.5–1.0	Postmenopausal	0.2–1.0
Females	0.03–0.06	Aldosterone (μg/day)	4–17
Protein binding (%)		Free cortisol (μg/day)	0–200
Cortisol	80		
Aldosterone	70		
Testosterone			
Males	90		
Females	95		

[a] Reproduced from C. Ezrin, J. O. Godden, R. Volpe, and R. Wilson, eds., "Systematic Endocrinology," p. 170. Harper & Row, New York, 1973.

amount of the free hormone. Nevertheless, at the target cell it is the free steroid which appears to enter the cell probably by a process of free diffusion. The driving force behind the movement of free hormone into the target cell appears to be proportionate to the number of specific hormone receptor molecules in the target cell cytoplasm which have unfilled ligand binding sites (unoccupied receptors). The affinity of this receptor for cortisol is similar (20 nM) to that of the circulating CBG–cortisol complex (10^8 M^{-1}). As the free hormone is taken up by target cells, more free hormone will be released from the CBG–cortisol complex.

H. Feedback Effects of Glucocorticoids

When cortisol is produced in response to ACTH, it has negative feedback effects on various elements of the hormonal cascade system (Fig. 10-10). Thus, the negative long feedback loop refers to the effect of elevated cortisol on the limbic system, the hypothalamus and the anterior pituitary. Feedback inhibition of ACTH is very fast. Feedback on the hippocampus may shut off further electrical activity responsible for the release of CRH and the subsequent release of ACTH. These actions are presumed to be mediated by glucocorticoid receptors located in these cells and which operate transcriptionally.

IV. BIOLOGICAL AND MOLECULAR ACTIONS

A. Molecular Actions of Glucocorticoids

1. *Immunosuppression by Glucocorticoids*

Among the cell types that involute and ultimately die under prolonged elevated levels of glucocorticoids are the cells involved in the production of immunoglobulin. Generally speaking, antibody production is only marginally affected by glucocorticoids in man. The effects of increased glucocorticoids in the circulation by stress are exemplified by *in vitro* experiments with immunoglobulin-producing plasma cells (derived from B cells).

Diminished immunoglobulin responses occur after treatment with relatively large amounts of glucocorticoid. Suppressor T cells seem to be very sensitive to steroid treatment, but helper T cells are relatively unaffected. B cell-derived plasma cells, the primary immunoglobulin producers, are depressed in their ability to produce all classes of immunoglobulins. Immunosuppression by glucocorticoids seems to result from the hormonal suppression of various lymphokines and monokines which are required for the function of antibody production. This is part of the catabolic response of certain cell types to glucocorticoids, as discussed below (see Fig. 10-13).

While clinical treatment with pharmacological doses of glucocorticoids represents one end of the spectrum, the physiological rise in circulating levels of cortisol following stress represents the other. Some workers believe there is a close link between stress, elevated glucocorticoids resulting from it, and injury to the immunological apparatus which may leave the individual vulnerable to the action of latent oncogenic viruses,

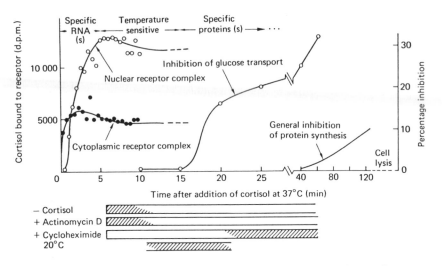

Figure 10-13. Time course in rat thymus cell suspensions at 37°C of cortisol–receptor complex formation, cortisol-induced inhibition of glucose transport, and inhibition of protein synthesis. Kinetics of receptor complex formation were determined with [³H]cortisol at about 0.1 μM. Inhibitory metabolic effects were produced with about 1 μM of cortisol. Glucose transport was measured with 2-min pulses of radioactive hexose initiated at the times indicated. Shaded segments of the horizontal bars in the lower part of the figure indicate roughly the time intervals during which emergence of the cortisol effect on glucose metabolism can be blocked by treatment with cortexolone (which displaces cortisol from the glucocorticoid receptors), actinomycin D, and cycloheximide, and delayed by lowering temperature. Open bars indicate periods during which these treatments have no effect. At the top of the figure is the sequence of steps by which it is hypothesized that the cortisol–receptor complex leads to synthesis of a specific protein that inhibits glucose transport. Reproduced from A. Munck and G. R. Crabtree, Glucocorticoid-induced lymphocyte death. *In* "Cell Death in Biology and Pathology" (I. D. Bower and R. A. Lockshin, eds.), pp. 329–357. Chapman and Hall, London and New York, 1981.

newly transformed cancer cells, or other disease processes that are normally held in control by the immunological apparatus. On the other hand, A. Munck and colleagues have proposed that in stress, elevated levels of glucocorticoids serve to suppress the body's normal defenses against stress, preventing them from overshooting and causing damage to the organism.

A more detailed discussion of the immune system and the effects of various factors on its function is found in Chapter 17 on thymus hormones. At issue under this subject is the mechanism involved in cell death produced by glucocorticoids. Although it has long been considered that the mechanism is a transcriptional one in which the expressed phenotypes are killer enzymes that might modify the cell membrane so that its uptake of essential nutrients (e.g., glucose) is seriously impaired, there has been little progress until recently in providing evidence to justify this model. Newer evidence shows that fragmentation of DNA is a rapid response in cell death. Glucocorticoids may induce, via a receptor, a nuclease activity to account for DNA breakdown.

2. Actions of Glucocorticoids on Hepatic Cells

The cellular mode of action of glucocorticoid hormone is summarized in Fig. 10-14 where the target gland is the liver cell representing the predominant tissue whose overall response is anabolic. Later, the actions of the hormone on the thymus cell, which responds to the hormone catabolically, will be described.

In this model (Fig. 10-14), the free hormone is shown permeating the liver cell membrane, as previously discussed. Once inside the cytoplasm of the cell, it can combine with the specific, high-affinity receptor to form a steroid–receptor complex. The possibility exists that the unoccupied receptor may actually reside in the nucleus (see Chapter 1). Probably the conformation (shape) of the receptor molecule changes upon combining with the steroid hormone. However, it is difficult to make the necessary physical measurements to describe this conformational change. Although the receptor has been highly purified, it so far cannot be isolated in the absence of steroid, required for these measurements, because of its lability.

The glucocorticoid receptor has been purified from rat liver, and polyclonal as well as monoclonal antibodies have been prepared to it. In rat liver the properties of the activated receptor include the following. It appears to be a single polypeptide chain of molecular weight about 94,000. It has one steroid binding site per molecule and a DNA binding site. The DNA binding site is unavailable at the surface of the unactivated form of the larger receptor complex. The properties listed here

426

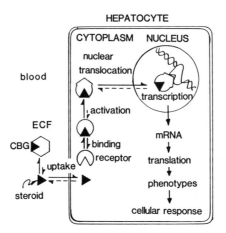

Figure 10-14. Molecular actions of the glucocorticoid hormone on the hepatocyte. ECF, Extracellular space; CBG, corticosteroid binding globulin of blood, also known as transcortin. Reproduced from G. Litwack, *In* "Altered Endocrine States During Aging" (V. J. Cristofalo, G. T. Baker, R. C. Adelman, and J. Roberts, eds.), p. 11. Alan R. Liss, Inc., New York, 1984.

pertain to the activated, or DNA binding (or nuclear binding) form of the steroid–receptor complex. The protein appears to be somewhat asymmetric, having a frictional coefficient (f/f_0) of about 1.4 and axial ratio (prolate ellipsoid) of about 5–6. The pI value of the activated form is still in the acidic range, although it is less acidic than the unactivated form. This shift in pI may derive from two sources: (1) a group of positive charges probably appears on the surface of the activated form, and (2) the unactivated form may be an aggregate of proteins, each component of which is the size of the activated form. The unactivated form is usually observed as an aggregate *in vitro*. The components of the activation process converting a non-DNA binding receptor to a DNA binding one are unknown. A Ca^{2+}-activated protease was considered early to be one of many possibilities for activation of the uterine estrogen receptor. Much current investigation is focused on this problem. Lysosomal proteases which act like trypsin can degrade the glucocorticoid–receptor complex. Whether proteolytic products so formed can be produced physiologically is not known. Although activation can be accomplished in the test tube by simply raising the temperature from 0–4°C to 12°C or above, there are experiments showing that this process may occur in a time-dependent manner in the whole cell or animal.

A large number of *in vitro* experiments describe the conditions under which the activation process occurs (see Fig. 10-14). One idea is that the steroid–receptor complex undergoes a further conformational change which enables it to translocate to the cell nucleus where it brings about an increase in the rate of synthesis of certain mRNAs coding for the translation of specific enzymes in the cytoplasm. The activated/ transformed state of the steroid–receptor complex can be determined by its ability to bind to DNA. Frequently, DNA cellulose is used to facilitate such studies. Another view of activation, which is not incompatible with the conformational change idea, is that a low-molecular-weight inhibitor is bound to the receptor in the unactivated form, thereby holding receptor subunits together in a way that obscures its DNA binding sites. Upon activation, this inhibitor dissociates from the surface of the receptor, exposing a group of putative positive charges. An RNA molecule may also be implicated in obscuring the DNA binding domain of the receptor, although its participation is debatable. Once in the nucleus, the exposed positive charges of the activated receptor complex permit electrostatic interaction with the negative charges of the phosphate groups on DNA. By itself, this interaction would not be specific. Further information suggests that a second site (or additional sites) on the steroid–receptor complex is responsible for specific binding to DNA.

With the use of cells in culture, several types of mouse lymphosarcoma cells have been isolated: cells with normal functioning of the receptor which respond to glucocorticoids, and cells which apparently have a defective receptor. Other types are cells which have a "receptor" that does not translocate to the nucleus [it probably has an altered DNA binding site (see below)], and cells which have a receptor and translocate to the nucleus, but are unresponsive to the hormone. In this last case, which resembles the condition of the late rat fetus, the receptor complex can bind to its acceptor on chromatin, but there is a block in steps of the receptor mechanism beyond the interaction of receptor and acceptor. It is also possible that the glucocorticoid receptor has a developmental program of its own and its expression in cells corresponds to the time during development when glucocorticoid responsiveness first appears. Another possibility in developing tissues is that receptor polymorphism exists and that different forms of receptor appear at different times during development with each form mediating the induction of different phenotypes. This remains to be substantiated. Thus, the mRNAs produced in the responsive cell might not be expressed in the unresponsive mutant cell. Among several possibilities there might be included the inability to process heterogeneous RNA precursors of mRNAs, and so on. Obviously a molecular analysis of these mutant cells, which have blocks at various points in the receptor mechanism, will help to explain receptor functions. In addition to the types described here, there are also mutations that lead to the rapid degradation of receptor once it has been activated.

In addition to the isolation and analysis of mutant cells with defects in glucocorticoid receptor functions, there are other genetic approaches. These include the possibility of mapping the chromosomal location of the gene encoding information for the synthesis of the receptor molecule. This can be done by hybridizing two cells of different species, for example, a mutant mouse cell which does not express the glucocorticoid receptor and a human cell which does express the glucocorticoid receptor or where both types are expressed, but can be distinguished experimentally. The fusion of cells can be accomplished by use of polyethylene glycol, with killed Sendai virus, or by electrofusion. The fusion agent essentially binds to the cell surface of neighboring cells.

In the synkaryon (hybrid), the chromosomes from the cell of the more recently evolved species usually begin to degrade (the opposite occurs, but rarely). Ultimately a connection would be established between expression of the receptor and a specific human chromosome. Then one or more gene products of the same chromosome would be measured along with the receptor. Clones that fail to express receptor would also fail to express the marker phenotype characteristic of that chromosome. If the expression of the human glucocorticoid receptor were linked to more than one chromosome, genes for receptor as well as a regulatory product might be expected. This kind of research is in progress at the present time. Some of the karyotypes of mutant lymphosarcomas from the mouse (Fig. 10-15) have been quantified by U. Francke and U. Gehring. Chromosome 18 was concluded to contain the gene for the mouse glucocorticoid receptor. Studies with human cells have also contributed to receptor genetics. The gene for the glucocorticoid receptor has been cloned in three laboratories and the primary sequence of the human receptor and a speculated map of its active groups are shown in Fig. 10-16.

The liver enzymes synthesized in response to glucocorticoid action are involved in the metabolism of amino acids or in the synthesis of glycogen and to a limited extent with the synthesis of glucose (Fig. 10-17). Many of these enzymes are listed in Table 10-1.

B. Glucocorticoids, Analogs, and Antiglucocorticoid Compounds

So far, we have discussed the actions of the major natural glucocorticoids: cortisol in the human and corticosterone in the rat. Other compounds have been synthesized in the laboratory and some of these have

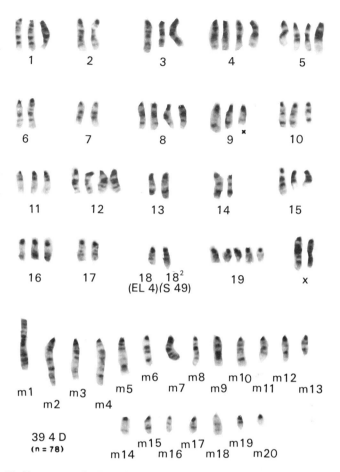

Figure 10-15. Karyotype of a hybrid cell crossed between S49.1 × EL4. Clone 39.4D, a dexamethasone-resistant derivative of 39.4N. Chromosome 18 derived from S49.1 is absent, while the remainder of the karyotype is identical to 39.4N. Reproduced from U. Francke and U. Gehring, *Cell* **22**, 657–664 (1980). © 1980 Massachusetts Institute of Technology.

greater potency than the natural hormones. Steroids may be divided into classes, depending on (1) ability to compete for binding to the ligand binding site of the glucocorticoid receptor and act like glucocorticoids (permit binding to DNA or the cell nucleus compared to the native hormone); (2) ability to bind to the ligand binding site and permit binding of the ligand–receptor complex to DNA, but to a considerably smaller extent than the natural glucocorticoids; and (3) ability to bind to the glucocorticoid receptor and prevent its binding to DNA in the cell

A

```
480                    490                    500                    510
ArgTyrArgLysCysLeuGlnAlaGlyMetAsnLeuGluAlaArgLysThrLysLysLysLysIleLeuLysLysLysIleLeuGlnGlnAlaThrThrGlyValSerGlnGluThrSerGlnAsnProGly
CGCTATCGAAAATGTCTTCAGGCTGGAATGAACCTGGAAGCAAGAAAAACAAAGAAAAATAAAAAAGAAAATTCTCAAGAAGCCACTACAGGAGTCTCAAGAGACCTCGAAAATCCTGGT   1,680

520                    530                    540                    550
AsnLysThrIleValProAlaThrLeuProGlnLeuThrProLeuSerLeuLeuValIleGluProGluValTyrAlaGlyTyrAspSerSerValProAspSerThr
AACAAAACAATAGTTCCTGCAACTTTACCACAACTCACCCCTACCCTGTCTCACTGTTGGAGTTATTGAGCCTGAAGTTTATGCAGGATATGATTCTAGTCCTGATTCCAGACTCAACT   1,800

560                    570                    580                    590
TrpArgIleMetThrThrLeuAsnMetLeuGlyGlyArgGlnValArgGlnValIleAlaIleAlaValAlaValLysTrpLysAlaValLeuAlaIleLeuProGlyPheArgAsnLeuHisLeuAspAspSerGlnMetThrLeuLeu
TGGAGGATCATGACTACGCTCAACATGTTAGGAGGCGGCAAGTGATTGCAGCAGTGAAATGGCAAAGGCAAGCAATACCAGTTTCAGGAACTTACACCTGGATACCAAAATGACCCTACTG   1,920

600                    610                    620                    630
GlnTyrSerTrpMetThrPheLeuMetAlaPheAlaLeuValGlyTyrTrpArgSerTyrArgGlnSerSerAlaAsnLeuAsnLeuCysPheAlaProLeuLeuIleIleLeuAsnGlnGlnAsnArgMetThrLeu
CAGTACTCCTGGATGACTTTCTTTATGGCATTTGCACTTGTAGGTTATTGGCGTAGCTACAGACAATCAAGTGCAAACCTGAATCTATGTTTTGCTCCTCTCTTAATAATAGAGCAGAAATGACCCTA   2,040

640                    650                    660                    670
ProCysMetThrTyrAspGlnCysLysSerHisCysLysHisArgLeuHisArgLeuGlnValSerGluGluHisArgLeuGlnValSerMetLysSerTyrGluGlyTyrLeuLysSerSerValPro
CCCTGCATGTACGACCAATGTAAAACCATGTAAACAGAGGCTTCATAGGCTGCAGGTATCTGAGGAACATAGGCTTCAGGTATCTATGAAAAGCTATGAAGGGTATCTGAAAAGCTCTGTTCCT   2,160

680                    690                    700                    710
LysAspGlyLeuLeuSerSerGlnGluLeuGluPheAspGluArgMetThrPheTyrIleLeuGluGlyLeuValValAsnLeuLeuAsnAsnTyrCysPheGlnIlePheGlyAlaIleAlaValAlaLysTyrArgGluGlyValAsnSerSerGlnAsnTrpGlnAsnPheTyr
AAGGACGGTCTGAAGAGCCAAGAGCTATTTGATGAAAGAATGACCTTCTATATCCTTGAGGGCTTAGTAGTGAATCTGCTGAACAAGCTCTATTGCTTTCAAATCAAAGACCTAGGGAGCAAAGCCATTGCAGTTGCAAAATACAGAGAAGGTGTTAATAGTTCTCAGAACTGGCAGAATTTCTAT   2,280

720                    730                    740                    750
GlnLeuThrLysLeuLeuAspSerSerMetHisGlyValValGlnAlaAsnLeuLeuAsnTyrCysPheGlnIlePhePheMetSerIleGlyLeuPheProGluMetLeuAlaGluIle
CAACTGACAAAACTCTTGGATTCTACGATGCATGGAGTGGTGCAAGCTAATTTACTCCTTAACTCCTCAAACATTTTGATAAGACCCATAGTATTGAATCCCGAGATGTTAGCTGAAATC   2,400

760                    770
IleThrAlaAsnGlnIleLeuProLeuTyrSerAsnGlyAsnIleLysLeuLysLeuPheHisGlnLysLysSTOP
ATCACCAATCAGATACCAATATTTCAGAATGGAAATATCAAAAACTTCTGTTTCATCAAAAGTGACTGCCTTAATAAGAAAGTGAATTAATAACTTTTATTG   2,520

TATAAACATATCAGTTTGTCCTGTAGAGGTTTGTTTTTGTTTTTCATCTGTGTTTTAAATAGCCACTACATGTGGTTATAGAGGGCCAAGACTTGCCAACAG   2,640
AAGCAGTTGAGTCGTCACATCCTTTGCAGTGAATGGTGCAAATTTATTAGTTAATATATCCCAGAAATTTAGAAAACCTAATATGGAGGTAATTCCAGTCAAAGAAG   2,880
GATNGCCACCTAAACCACCAGTGCCCCAAAGTCTGTGTGATGAAACTTTCCTTCACTACTTTTTTTCACAGTGGCCTGGATGAAATTTCTAGACTTTCTGTGTATCCCCCCTGTAT   3,120
AGTTAGGATAGCACATTTTTGATTTATGCATGGAAAAAAGTTTACAAGTGTATATCAGAAAAGGGAAGTTGTGCCCTTTTATAGCTATTACTGTCTGGTTTAAACAATTTCCTTT   
ATATTTAGTGAACTACGCTTGCTCCATTTTTCTTACATAAATTTTTATTTACAAGTTATTGTGCAAATTAACAGGTCGTTCCCAAATAAACTCTAAACATTAAT   3,360
CAATCATCTGTGTGAAAATGGGTTTGGTTCTTAACAGGTCGCAAATTAACCAGCTATGTTGCAATATTGACTATTTCCTTCGTGTCAAAAAAAAAAAAAAGCTCA   
TTGTATAACTTCTTAAAAGTTGTGATTCCAGATAAACAGCTTGCAAATAACCGTATACTGTATGGCTTCAGTCTGGCCTGGTAAACTGTGGATGAGTGTGCAA   3,600
AGACTAATTTAAAAAATAACTACCAGAGGCCCCATTTGCAAATGGTTAATCAGCCAGCTGAGCAGTAATTCCTCACTAAACTTTACCCAAAAACTAAATCTCTAATAT   
GGCAAAAATGGCTAGCACACCCATTTCACATTTCCCATGTGTCCATAGAGTTAACAACAGTTAATCTTTCCTGAATGTAAAATAATTATTGTAAAATTGTATGTCAGCA   3,840
TCCATGTTTGTAAAACTACACATCCCTAATGTGTCCCATAGAGTTCTGCATTTCCTTAAGTAAACAAATTTATTTGTGTAAATTATTTTGTAATTAGAACTGAAAAGTCAGAA   
TGTGCACCTTACACACTTCTCCCCAAAGTCTGTCTAAACTCAAAGCCACCAAGAAAATTTAGATATTTCAGGTGGCAAATTTATTTGCTAATCAAAATCTAATAAAAATACTAATA   4,080
TTAAAAAATATGCAGACTTCTAATATATTTAGTTAAGAAGTTATTTTAGATGAGTTTATTGTCTTTATTTTTGTAGGCTCAAAGAAATCGCTAGAATAAACCTAT   
ATGATTTATAGTTCTACATGCATTCATAAAAATGGGTTGCTCTTCTAACCATGCCACTACCCAGTTTACTATTACTTTTACTCAATCTCCCTTGCACTAAA   4,320
TCTCACCCGTGCAGTTACAGGAGAGCAGGGAGGTGTGCTTACATCCTTCACCTACCTTCACATCAGCCCCCCCCACAGCAGTTGAATGACAAGAAATCCTGAATAACCTAT   
GTATGTAAAGTATGTAAACAGGGAGCACCCTTTGCATAGGAAGTACCCAGCAAATCTCCAATAATGGAAATTATTTATAAGGTTCTTTCTATCTTACAACAAGAGTTTATTTCCAAA   4,560
TAAAATGAGGACAGTGTTTTGTTTCTTTAGTTTATTTGGGCAAGAATTATTTAATAAAAAAGAATCATTTGCTTTTGAAAAAAAAAAA                                   4,800
```

Figure 10-16A.   See legend on p. 432.

431

432

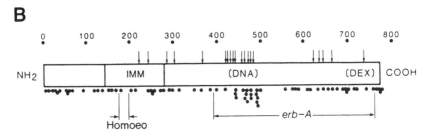

Figure 10-16. (A, pp. 430 and 431) Nucleotide sequence of the cDNA and the predicted protein sequence of the human glucocorticoid receptor. The complete coding sequence and the OB73′-untranslated region are shown, with the deduced amino acids given above the long open reading frame. An upstream in-frame stop codon at nucleotides 121–123 and putative additional polyadenylation signals in OB7 are underlined. Reproduced from S. M. Hollenberg, C. Weinberger, E. S. Ong, G. Cerelli, A. Oro, R. Lebo, E. B. Thompson, M. G. Rosenfeld, and R. M. Evans, Primary structure and expression of a functional human glucocorticoid receptor cDNA. *Nature (London)* **318**, 635–641 (1985). (B) Schematic representation of the primary amino acid structure of the human glucocorticoid receptor, with oncogene (*erb*-A) and homoeo box homologies indicated. Cysteine residues are represented by arrows above the boxed coding region and basic amino acids (arginine and lysine) are denoted by solid circles. The immunogenic domain (IMM), determined from overlapping expression cDNA clones, the putative steroid-binding region (DEX), and DNA-binding domain (DNA) are indicated within the boxed receptor coding region. Numbers indicate amino acid residues. Reproduced from C. Weinberger, S. M. Hollenberg, M. G. Rosenfeld, and R. M. Evans, Domain structure of human glucocorticoid receptor and its relationship to the v-*erb*-A oncogene product. *Nature (London)* **318**, 670–672 (1985). (A and B) © 1985 Macmillan Journals Limited.

nucleus under activating conditions. Steroids have been classified according to their potency in inducing specific enzymes in cell culture. The enzymatic activity which has been used is that of tyrosine aminotransferase (TAT) in hepatoma cells in culture. These cells are immortal in culture and have retained the property of TAT induction by glucocorticoids after transformation. The three groups of agents alluded to above reflect glucocorticoid potency in induction of this enzyme *in vitro*. The groups of compounds cluster into those described above for ligand binding to the glucocorticoid receptor and ability to induce TAT. They are called (1) agonists, (2) weak agonists, and (3) antagonists (Table 10-3).

C. Catabolism of Glucocorticoids

The major site of inactivation of glucocorticoids is the liver and to some extent the kidney. Enzymes are present which reduce the double bond at C-4 to C-5 of the unsaturated 3-ketosteroids. The product contains either a 5α or 5β proton and reduced steroids generally are much less active. The principal routes of metabolism of cortisol and cor-

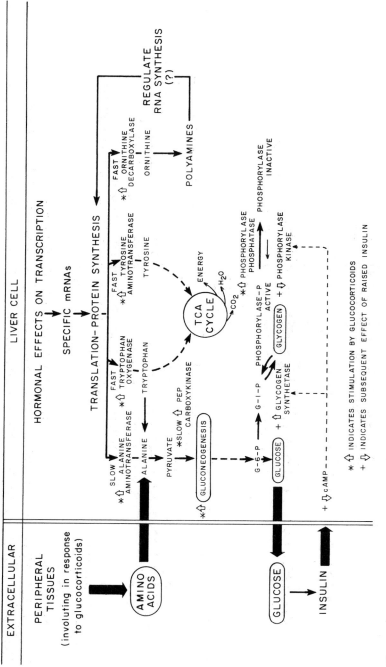

Figure 10-17. Overview of the actions of glucocorticoids on metabolism and on specific enzyme levels in the rat hepatocyte. Reproduced from M. H. Cake and G. Litwack, *In* "Biochemical Actions of Hormones" (G. Litwack, ed.), Vol. 3, pp. 317–190. Academic Press, New York, 1975.

Table 10–3. Potency of Natural and Synthetic Glucocorticoids

Steroid	Structure	Binding to ligand binding site of glucocorticoid receptor (affinity)	Ability to induce TAT in hepatoma cell culture	Classification (N, natural steroid; S, synthetic steroid)
Cortisol		(Strong binding)	+ + + +	(N) Optimal inducer
Corticosterone		(Strong binding)	+ + + +	(N) Optimal inducer
Dexamethasone		(Strong binding)	+ + + +	(S) Optimal inducer

434

Triamcinolone acetonide

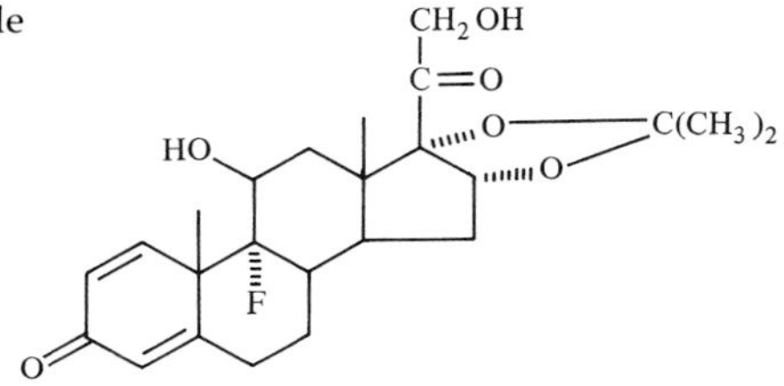

(Strong binding)

$+ + + +$

(S) Optimal inducer

11β-Hydroxyprogesterone

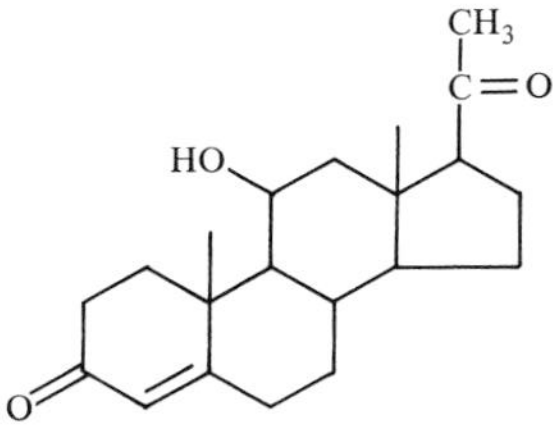

(Strong binding)

$+ +$

(N) Suboptimal inducer

5α-Dihydrocortisol

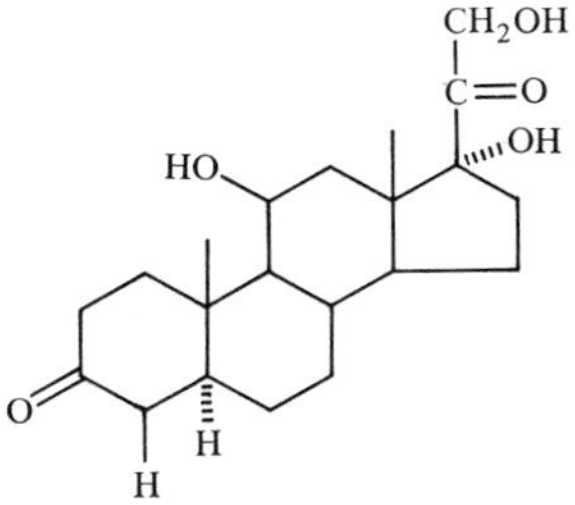

(Strong binding)

$+ +$

(N) Suboptimal inducer

(*continued*)

435

Table 10–3. (*Continued*)

Steroid	Structure	Binding to ligand binding site of glucocorticoid receptor (affinity)	Ability to induce TAT in hepatoma cell culture	Classification (N, natural steroid; S, synthetic steroid)
Dexamethasone mesylate	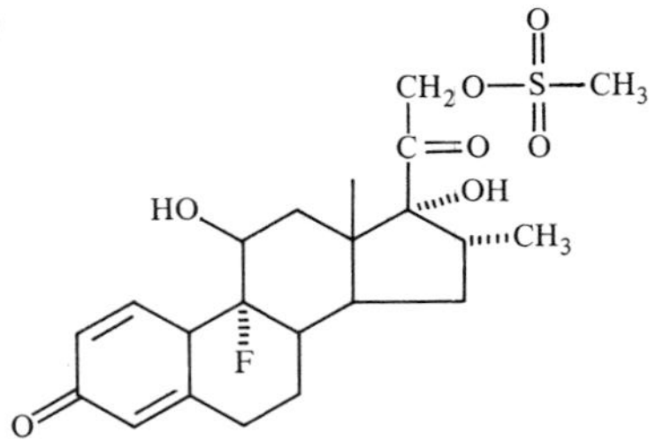 *(chemical structure)*	(Moderately strong binding)	++	(S) Optimal (?) inducer
Deacylcortivasol	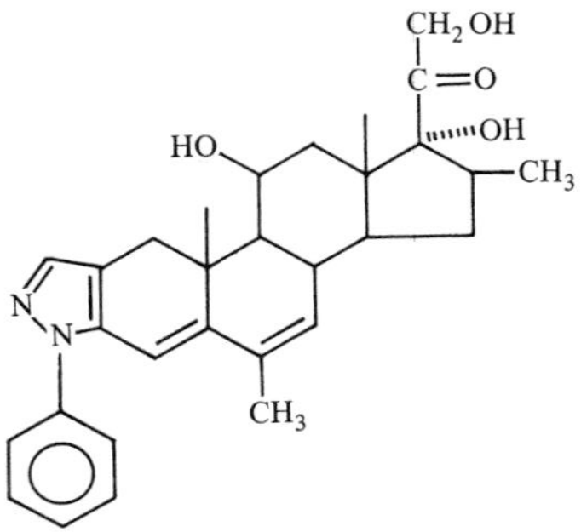 *(chemical structure)*	(Very strong binding)	++++	(S) Optimal inducer

436

Progesterone

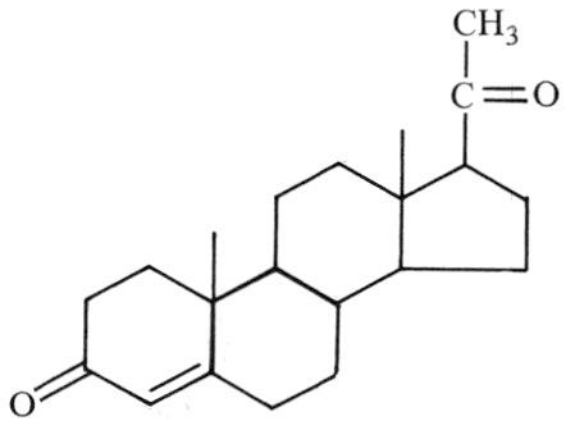

(Weak binding)

0

(N) Noninducer or antiinducer[a]

17α-Hydroxyprogesterone

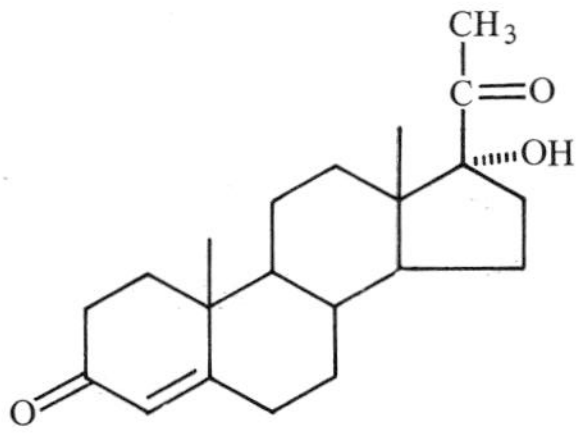

(Strong binding)

0+

(N) Antiinducer[a]

[a] An antiinducer binds to receptor, but will not induce TAT. Therefore it does not translocate to the nucleus, or if it does it cannot act productively in the nucleus.

ticosterone are shown in Fig. 10-17A. These are NADPH-requiring enzymes, one in the microsomal fraction which produces the 5α product and the other producing mainly the 5β isomer, while corticosterone is converted to a mixture of both products. As shown in Fig. 10-18, further reductions or oxidations occur on the 3-ketone, 11β-hydroxyl, and 20-ketone. Most of the urinary metabolites are glucuronides conjugated to hydroxyl groups. Sulfate derivates are formed also and these often occur in the bile as 3 or 21 monosulfates or 3,21 disulfates. Cortisone (Fig. 10-18) is relatively inactive as a glucocorticoid. When given in pharmacological amounts, it probably exerts glucocorticoid effects after its reduction to cortisol, an active hormone.

D. Drugs Antagonizing Glucocorticoids

The only means to remove the hormone nearly completely from the circulation of an experimental animal is to surgically remove the adrenal glands, the major source of the hormone. The rat is most depleted of corticosterone 3 days after adrenalectomy and can also be depleted by hypophysectomy. Such animals must be housed in well-controlled environments, since they will not survive stress. They must be given salt in drinking water because adrenalectomy removes steroid hormones from all three layers of the adrenal cortex, including aldosterone. There are no means to render an animal devoid of endogenous glucocorticoids by the use of drugs. Two agents are worth mentioning because they lower the amount of glucocorticoids in the circulation. Drugs of this type are *metyrapone* and *aminoglutethimide*, shown in Fig. 10-19. Metyrapone inhibits 11β-hydroxylation in adrenal cortex, leading to decreased cortisol production, and it may inhibit the side chain cleavage reaction. The 11β-hydroxylase is a mitochondrial enzyme and would be expected to cause accumulation of inactive precursors of cortisol, such as 11-deoxycorticosterone structure **95** or 11-deoxycortisol structure **94** in Fig. 2-22. As a consequence of decreased cortisol, the long-loop negative feedback by cortisol on the anterior pituitary, hypothalamus, and limbic system (Fig. 10-10) is much reduced, with the result that there is increased output of ACTH by the corticotrophic cells of the anterior pituitary. 11-Deoxycortisol can bind weakly to the glucocorticoid receptor and has minimal glucocorticoid activity. Measurement of elevated plasma concentrations of ACTH, usually by radioimmunoassay, is diagnostic of hypofunction of the adrenal cortex (Addison's disease).

E. Antiinflammatory Actions

Experiments, especially with cell culture systems and lung tissue, demonstrate that cortisol and other glucocorticoids inhibit the appearance of prostaglandins. The glucocorticoids via a receptor mechanism appear to cause the synthesis of a protein called "macrocortin" of about 40,000 molecular weight. This polypeptide is an inhibitor of cell membrane phospholipase A_2 responsible for the release of fatty acid precursors of prostaglandin synthetase, such as arachidonic acid (Fig. 10-20A; refer also to Chapter 16). This mechanism may represent the major part of the antiinflammatory action of the glucocorticoids. The 40,000-molecular weight lipocortin gene has now been cloned and its cDNA sequence is shown in Fig. 10-20B.

V. THE *ZONA RETICULARIS* AND DEHYDROEPIANDROSTERONE

Up to 30 mg of DHEA is secreted daily by the innermost zone of the adrenal cortex, and the blood levels of this hormone and its sulfate derivative are fairly high (Table 12-2). DHEA is considered to be a weak androgen. It can be converted to testosterone and androstenediol, as shown in Fig. 2-23. When the aromatase system of enzymes is present, DHEA can be converted to estrogens, as summarized in Fig. 14-11. Surprisingly, there is little known concerning direct actions of DHEA other than its serving as a substrate for production of the sex hormones.

VI. THE MINERALOCORTICOID HORMONE

A. Introduction

The mechanisms of response to stress involve the glucocorticoid hormone secretion activated by a cascade system consisting of the limbic system of the brain, the hypothalamus, the anterior pituitary (ACTH), and the *zona fasciculata* and *zona reticularis* of the adrenal cortex. The mineralocorticoid, aldosterone, is synthesized and secreted by cells of the outerlayer of the adrenal cortex, the *zona glomerulosa* (Fig. 10-4A). The secretion of this hormone involves a set of signals different from those we have introduced for cortisol. Aldosterone has salt-conserving actions, specifically Na^+, and therefore is a part of the system of water balance in the body. K^+ is pumped out of cells in response to aldosterone. However, the aldosterone-secreting system is not the only system controlling water balance. The topic of water homeostasis is covered in Chapter 15 where the mode of action of aldosterone is reviewed and in Chapter 4 where the actions of vasopressin are presented.

A

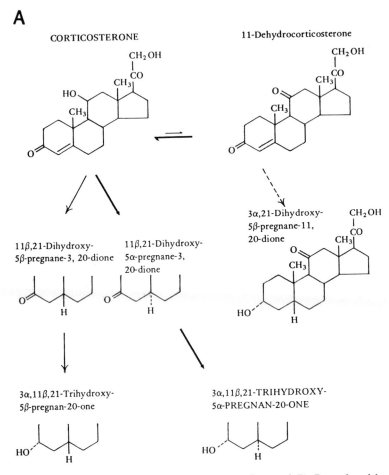

CORTICOSTERONE

11-Dehydrocorticosterone

11β,21-Dihydroxy-
5β-pregnane-3, 20-dione

11β,21-Dihydroxy-
5α-pregnane-3,
20-dione

3α,21-Dihydroxy-
5β-pregnane-11,
20-dione

3α,11β,21-Trihydroxy-
5β-pregnan-20-one

3α,11β,21-TRIHYDROXY-
5α-PREGNAN-20-ONE

Figure 10-18. Metabolic routes of corticosterone (A) and cortisol (B). Reproduced from D. Schulster, S. Burstein, and B. A. Cooke, "Molecular Endocrinology of the Steroid Hormones," pp. 156, 157. Wiley, New York, 1976, by copyright permission.

B. The Aldosterone-Producing System

This system is diagrammed in Fig. 15-8. The initial signal is a fall in blood volume, a decrease in Na$^+$ concentration in blood, a fall in blood pressure or release of catecholamines at the juxtaglomerular apparatus of the kidney, and the effect of angiotensin II. Any of these stimuli cause the release of *renin*, an enzyme with proteolytic activity from juxtaglomerular cells. Renin acts on a plasma α$_2$-globulin releasing an N-terminal decapeptide by hydrolyzing, at a hydrophobic sequence (ami-

B

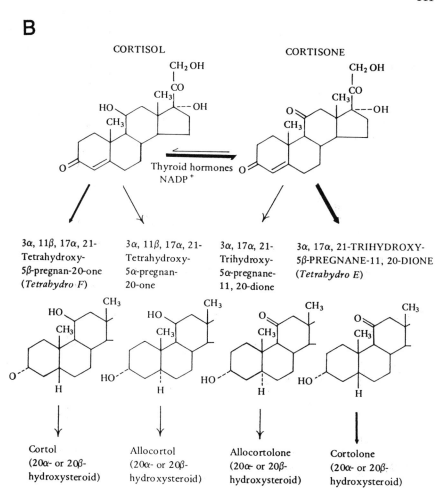

Figure 10-18B.

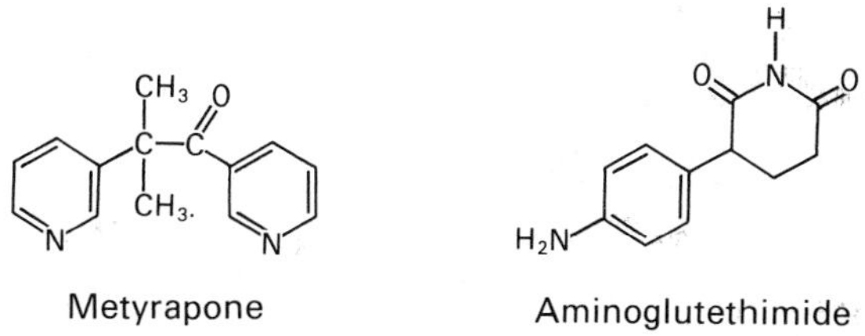

Metyrapone   Aminoglutethimide

Figure 10-19. Structures of metyrapone and aminoglutethimide.

442

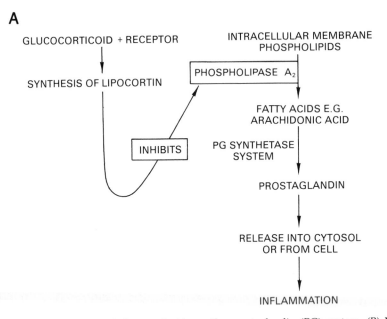

A

GLUCOCORTICOID + RECEPTOR

SYNTHESIS OF LIPOCORTIN

INHIBITS

INTRACELLULAR MEMBRANE
PHOSPHOLIPIDS

PHOSPHOLIPASE A₂

FATTY ACIDS E.G.
ARACHIDONIC ACID

PG SYNTHETASE
SYSTEM

PROSTAGLANDIN

RELEASE INTO CYTOSOL
OR FROM CELL

INFLAMMATION

Figure 10-20. (A) Action of glucocorticoids on the prostaglandin (PG) system. (B) Nucleotide and predicted amino acid sequence of human lipocortin. Nucleotides are numbered from the presumed initiator ATG. Rat data for comparison are derived from protein sequencing. Reproduced from B. P. Wallner, R. J. Mattaliano, C. Hession, R. L. Cate, R. Tizard, L. K. Sinclair, C. Foeller, E. P. Chow, J. L. Browning, K. L. Ramachandran, and R. B. Pepinsky, Cloning and expression of human lipocortin, a phospholipase A₂ inhibitor with potential antiinflammatory activity. *Nature (London)* **320,** 77–81 (1986). © 1986 Macmillan Journals Limited.

no acids 10–13), a leucyl-leucyl peptide bond. The resulting decapeptide is angiotensin I, an intermediate with no hormonal activity. Angiotensin I is then attacked by a *converting enzyme,* which has a broad distribution in the vascular epithelium, lung, liver, adrenal cortex, pancreas, kidney, spleen, and neurohypophysis. This enzyme is a carboxypeptidase which cleaves off the carboxy-terminal dipeptide, His–Leu, at a peptide bond connecting Phe and His. The resulting dipeptide is inactive and the octapeptide is angiotensin II, a hormone. This hormone has a short half-life of about 1 min because its activity is destroyed by angiotensinase, a Ca^{2+}-activated enzyme found in the peripheral vascular beds. This hormone, in addition to its effects on *zona glomerulosa* cells of the adrenal cortex, sensitizes vascular smooth muscles to the contractile effects of norepinephrine. There are specific outer cell membrane receptors for angiotensin II in the *zona glomerulosa* of the adrenal cortex. Binding of the hormone to the receptor causes an activation of the adenylate cyclase on the cytoplasmic side of the receptor–enzyme couple and stim-

B

```
Met Ala Met Val Ser Glu Phe Leu Lys Gln Ala Trp Phe Ile Glu Asn Glu
ATG GCA ATG GTA TCA GAA TTC CTC AAG CAG GCC TGG TTT ATT GAA AAT GAA
Glu Gln Glu Tyr Val Gln Thr Val Lys Ser Ser Lys Gly Gly Pro Gly Ser
GAG CAG GAA TAT GTT CAA ACT GTG AAG TCA TCC AAA GGT GGT CCC GGA TCA
Ala Val Ser Pro Tyr Pro Thr Phe Asn Pro Ser Ser Asp Val Ala Ala Leu
GCG GTG AGC CCC TAT CCT ACC TTC AAT CCA TCC TCG GAT GTC GCT GCC TTG
His Lys Ala Ile Met Val Lys Gly Val Asp Glu Ala Thr Ile Ile Asp Ile
CAT AAG GCC ATA ATG GTT AAA GGT GTG GAT GAA GCA ACC ATC ATT GAC ATT
Leu Thr Lys Arg Asn Asn Ala Gln Arg Gln Gln Ile Lys Ala Ala Tyr Leu
CTA ACT AAG CGA AAC AAT GCA CAG CGT CAA CAG ATC AAA GCA GCA TAT CTC
Gln Glu Thr Gly Lys Pro Leu Asp Glu Thr Leu Lys Lys Ala Leu Thr Gly
CAG GAA ACA GGA AAG CCC CTG GAT GAA ACA CTT AAG AAA GCC CTT ACA GGT
His Leu Glu Glu Val Val Leu Ala Leu Leu Lys Thr Pro Ala Gln Phe Asp
CAC CTT GAG GAG GTT GTT TTA GCT CTG CTA AAA ACT CCA GCG CAA TTT GAT
Ala Asp Glu Leu Arg Ala Ala Met Lys Gly Leu Gly Thr Asp Glu Asp Thr
GCT GAT GAA CTT CGT GCT GCC ATG AAG GGC CTT GGA ACT GAT GAA GAT ACT
Leu Ile Glu Ile Leu Ala Ser Arg Thr Asn Lys Glu Ile Arg Asp Ile Asn
CTA ATT GAG ATT TTG GCA TCA AGA ACT AAC AAA GAA ATC AGA GAC ATT AAC
Arg Val Tyr Arg Glu Glu Leu Lys Arg Asp Leu Ala Lys Asp Ile Thr Ser
AGG GTC TAC AGA GAG GAA CTG AAG AGA GAT CTG GCC AAA GAC ATA ACC TCA
Asp Thr Ser Gly Asp Phe Arg Asn Ala Leu Leu Ser Leu Ala Lys Gly Asp
GAC ACA TCT GGA GAT TTT CGG AAC GCT TTG CTT TCT CTT GCT AAG GGT GAC
Arg Ser Glu Asp Phe Gly Val Asn Glu Asp Leu Ala Asp Ser Asp Ala Arg
CGA TCT GAG GAC TTT GGT GTG AAT GAA GAC TTG GCT GAT TCA GAT GCC AGG
Ala Leu Tyr Glu Ala Gly Glu Arg Arg Lys Gly Thr Asp Val Asn Val Phe
GCC TTG TAT GAA GCA GGA GAA AGG ACA AAG GGG ACA GAC GTA AAC GTG TTC
Asn Thr Ile Leu Thr Thr Arg Ser Tyr Pro Gln Leu Arg Arg Val Phe Gln
AAT ACC ATC CTT ACC ACC AGA AGC TAT CCA CAA CTT CGC AGA GTG TTT CAG
Lys Tyr Thr Lys Tyr Ser Lys His Asp Met Asn Lys Val Leu Asp Leu Glu
AAA TAC ACC AAG TAC AGT AAG CAT GAC ATG AAC AAA GTT CTG GAC CTG GAG
Leu Lys Gly Asp Ile Glu Lys Cys Leu Thr Ala Ile Val Lys Cys Ala Thr
TTG AAA GGT GAC ATT GAG AAA TGC CTC ACA GCT ATC GTG AAG TGC GCC ACA
Ser Lys Pro Ala Phe Phe Ala Glu Lys Leu His Gln Ala Met Lys Gly Val
AGC AAA CCA GCT TTC TTT GCA GAA AAG CTT CAT CAA GCC ATG AAA GGT GTT
Gly Thr Arg His Lys Ala Leu Ile Arg Ile Met Val Ser Arg Ser Glu Ile
GGA ACT CGC CAT AAG GCA TTG ATC AGG ATT ATG GTT TCC CGT TCT GAA ATT
Asp Met Asn Asp Ile Lys Ala Phe Tyr Gln Lys Met Tyr Gly Ile Ser Leu
GAC ATG AAT GAT ATC AAA GCA TTC TAT CAG AAG ATG TAT GGT ATC TCC CTT
Cys Gln Ala Ile Leu Asp Glu Thr Lys Gly Asp Tyr Glu Lys Ile Leu Val
TGC CAA GCC ATC CTG GAT GAA ACC AAA GGA GAT TAT GAG AAA ATC CTG GTG
Ala Leu Cys Gly Gly Asn
GCT CTT TGT GGA GGA AAC.................................................
```

Figure 10-20B.

ulates the intracellular level of cyclic AMP by mechanisms we have already discussed in Chapter 1 (see also Chapter 15). This accounts for the enhanced synthesis of aldosterone. Appreciable levels of this hormone are generated only in stress.

C. Aldosterone Antagonists

Synthetic antagonists of aldosterone action are available and are known as spironolactones. The structure of spironolactone is given in Fig. 10-21. This substance has no Na$^+$-conserving action on its own and

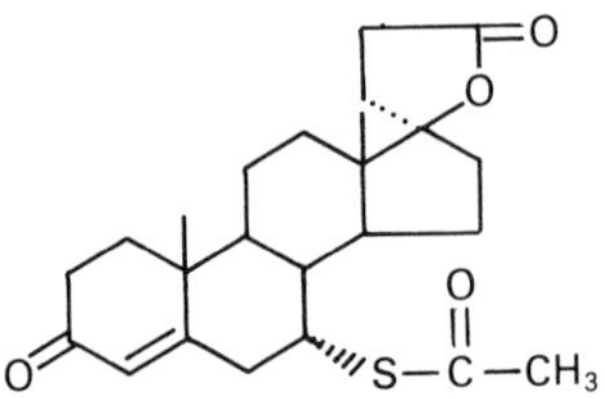

Figure 10-21. Structure of spironolactone.

its action appears to be through competition for aldosterone binding at the ligand binding site of the aldosterone receptor. Although some other compounds have indirect antimineralocorticoid effects, spironolactone is the compound most frequently used.

D. Aldosterone Metabolism

More than a dozen metabolites of radioactive aldosterone have been characterized in the urine. Nearly all of the hormone is metabolized within 48 hr. The major urinary form is a glucuronide derivative by substitution of the reduced C-3 position (Fig. 2-32). Conjugation occurs in liver and kidney.

VII. CLINICAL ASPECTS

A. Glucocorticoids

Major clinical problems associated with the adrenal cortex center around hyper- or hypoproduction of adrenal steroids. The causes of these conditions can be quite complicated, since there are several organs involved in the hormonal cascade. In the case of the glucocorticoids, the limbic system of the brain, the hypothalamus, the blood portal system connecting the hypothalamus with the anterior pituitary, and the adrenal gland are parts of the system. The normal values of steroidal hormones produced by the adrenal are presented in Table 10-2. When cortisol is overproduced, often by a pituitary tumor causing high levels of circulating ACTH, the resulting disease is known as Cushing's disease. When cortisol is underproduced, the resulting disease is known as Addison's disease, most frequently the result of adrenal destruction. The effects of Cushing's disease are summarized in Table 10-4. Hyperproduction of cortisol from the adrenal gland would be expected to occur if there is a tumor of the adrenal producing abnormal amounts of

Table 10–4. Effects of Overproduction of Cortisol (Cushing's Syndrome)[a,b]

Protein metabolism
   Thinning of skin
   Reddish striae
   Loss of bone matrix and demineralization
   Poor wound healing
   Muscle wasting and weakness
   Capillary fragility and bruising
   Impaired growth (children)
Carbohydrate metabolism
   Abnormal glucose tolerance curve
   Overt diabetes mellitus
Lipid metabolism
   Centripetal fat distribution
   Moon facies
Electrolyte balance
   Sodium retention, potassium loss
   Hypertension
   Hypervolemia
Hematopoietic effects
   Eosinopenia, lymphopenia
   Polymorphonuclear leukocytosis
   Erythrocytosis
General effects
   Hypercalciuria and renal calculi
   Gastric ulceration
   Psychosis
   Impaired immunological tolerance

---

[a] Cushing's syndrome is most often caused iatrogenically by administration of large amounts of glucocorticoids.
[b] Reproduced from C. Ezrin, J. O. Godden, R. Volpe, and R. Wilson, eds., "Systematic Endocrinology," p. 171. Harper & Row, New York, 1973.

the steroid, if there is a pituitary tumor producing high levels of ACTH (or if there is overproduction of CRH at the hypothalamic level which apparently has, so far, not been documented). Adrenalectomy is often a treatment of the primary disease, with maintenance levels of glucocorticoids taken orally. Adrenal tumors are more common in women. In Fig. 10-22 is shown a case of adrenocortical hyperplasia in a 5-year-old girl with congenital adrenogenital syndrome. The more malignant forms of adrenal tumors result in excess androgen production.

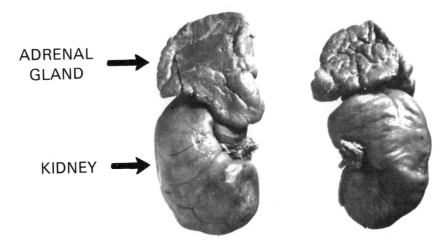

ADRENAL
GLAND

KIDNEY

Figure 10-22. Bilateral diffuse adrenocortical hyperplasia with moderate folding and segmentation of the surface in a 5-year-old girl with congenital adrenogenital syndrome. The bean-shaped organ below is the kidney and the arrow points to the hyperplastic adrenal glands. Reproduced from A. Labhart, ed., "Clinical Endocrinology," p. 362. Springer-Verlag, Berlin and New York, 1976.

Addison's disease or hypoproduction of cortisol is usually the result of atrophy of the adrenal cortex by unexplained causes (idiopathic). This can be the result of failure at other levels of the cascade from the limbic system downward. The results of Addison's disease are sodium loss (since aldosterone is usually also deficient), excess potassium in the blood, low blood pressure, hypoglycemia, high levels of ACTH and MSH (loss of negative feedback), with pigmentation of the skin due to the high levels of MSH (Fig. 10-23). The acute onset of Addison's disease, referred to as Addisonian shock, is shock associated with adrenal insufficiency and most commonly occurs when an individual with long-standing adrenal insufficiency is exposed to a stressful stimulus. It is treated with large intravenous doses of cortisol, fluid replacement, and antibiotics.

B. Mineralocorticoids and Androgens

Mineralocorticoid excess can be a feature of Cushing's syndrome, mentioned earlier. It can be the cause of reduced potassium levels in blood, resulting in weakness, sodium retention, and hypertension.

An inborn error of metabolism can result in a deficiency of the adrenal cortical enzyme, C-21 hydroxylase, whose function is required for the

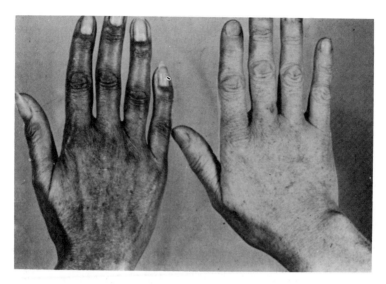

Figure 10-23. Idiopathic Addison's disease. The pigmentation of the hand at the left is contrasted with that of a normal hand. Reproduced from C. Ezrin, J. O. Godden, R. Volpe, and R. Wilson, eds., "Systematic Endocrinology," p. 178. Harper & Row, New York, 1973.

synthesis of cortisol. This deficiency results in lowered cortisol levels and enlarged output of ACTH by the anterior pituitary owing to reduced negative feedback. High ACTH results in adrenal hyperplasia and hypersecretion, especially in the products of the *zona reticularis* (DHEA) which, together with adrenal testosterone, can lead to masculinization of the female baby. Precocious puberty in the male can also result from this condition. Treatment is centered on cortisol replacement therapy which restores the negative feedback mechanism.

References

A. Books

Baxter, J. D., and Rousseau, G. G., eds. (1979). "Glucocorticoid Hormone Action." Springer-Verlag, Berlin and New York.

Chrousos, G. P., Loriaux, D. L., and Lipsett, M. B., eds. (1986). "Steroid Hormone Resistance." Plenum, New York and London.

Krieger, D. T., and Hughes, J. C., eds. (1980). "Neuroendocrinology." Sinauer Associates, Sunderland, Massachusetts.

B. Review Articles

Cake, M. H., and Litwack, G. (1975). The glucocorticoid receptor. *In* "Biochemical Actions of Hormones" (G. Litwack, ed.), Vol. 3, pp. 317–390, Academic Press, New York.

Flower, R. J. (1986). The mediators of steroid action. *Nature (London)* **320,** 20.

Gehring, U. (1980). Cell genetics of glucocorticoid responsiveness. *In* "Biochemical Actions of Hormones" (G. Litwack, ed.), Vol. 7, pp. 205–243. Academic Press, New York.

Munck, A., and Crabtree, G. R. (1981). Glucocorticoid-induced lymphocyte death. *In* "Cell Death in Biology and Pathology" (I. D. Bowen and R. A. Lockshin, eds.), pp. 329–357. Chapman and Hall, London and New York.

Munck, A., Guyre, P. M., and Holbrook, N. J. (1984). Physiological functions of glucocorticoids in stress and their relation to pharmacological actions. *Endocr. Rev.* **5,** 25–44.

Schmidt, T. J., and Litwack, G. (1982). Activation of the glucocorticoid receptor complex. *Physiol. Rev.* **62,** 1131–1192.

C. Research Papers

Compton, M. M., and Cidlowski, J. A. (1986) Rapid *in vivo* effects of glucocorticoids on the integrity of rat lymphocyte genomic deoxyribonucleic acid. *Endocrinology (Baltimore)* **118,** 38–45.

Harmon, J. M., Schmidt, T. J., and Thompson, E. B. (1984). Molybdate-sensitive and molybdate-resistant activation-labile glucocorticoid receptor mutants of the human lymphoid cell line CEM-C7. *J. Steroid Biochem.* **21,** 227–236.

Hollenberg, S. M., Weinberger, C., Ong, E. S., Cerelli, G., Oro, A., Lebo, R., Thompson, E. B., Rosenfeld, M. G., and Evans, R. M. (1985). Primary structure and expression of a functional human glucocorticoid receptor cDNA. *Nature (London)* **318,** 635–641.

Keller, S. E., Weiss, J. M., Schleifer, S. J., Miller, N. E., and Stein, M. (1981). Suppression of immunity by stress: Effect of a graded series of stressors on lymphocyte stimulation in the rat. *Science* **213,** 1397–1400.

Meisfeld, R., Okret, S., Wikstrom, A.-C., Wrange, O., Gustafson, J.-A., and Yamamoto, K. R. (1984). Characterization of a steroid hormone receptor gene and mRNA in wild-type and mutant cells. *Nature (London)* **312,** 779–781.

Munck, A., and Holbrook, N. J. (1981). Glucocorticoid receptor complexes in rat thymus cells. Rapid kinetic behavior and a cyclic model. *J. Biol. Chem.* **259,** 820–831.

Chapter **11**

Hormones of the Adrenal Medulla

I. INTRODUCTION

Catecholamines are synthesized and released from adrenergic neurons of the nervous system and together with cholinergic neurons represent two of the major vehicles for chemical neural communication. The adrenergic neurons of the nervous system synthesize and secrete norepinephrine (noradrenaline) and the cholinergic neurons synthesize and secrete acetylcholine. There are a variety of other neurons which synthesize additional neurotransmitters: serotonergic neurons, dopaminergic neurons, melatonergic neurons, enkephalinergic neurons, etc. Even some polypeptides such as insulin, now known to be present in the brain as well as in the pancreas, may act as neurotransmitters. Consequently, the demarcation between the central nervous system and the endocrine system is less well defined.

For the moment, however, the emphasis on catecholamines as hormones is a subject focusing on the adrenal medulla rather than upon the central nervous system. Whereas in the nervous system the adrenergic neurotransmitter is invariably norepinephrine (noradrenaline), the product of the adrenal medulla is uniquely epinephrine (adrenaline) in most species but not all, in addition to some norepinephrine. In this case epinephrine, released as a result of sudden environmental stress (e.g., fright), is a hormone.

The adrenal medulla is made up of modified neurons no longer possessing axons or nerve endings and are essentially cell bodies that have been adapted to secretory function. Thus, in the endocrine sense, the trigger to the adrenal medulla is a unique environmental signal. This is transmitted by way of a single cholinergic neuron from the sympathetic nervous system terminating in a synapse with the chromaffin cell of the adrenal medulla.

The catecholamine hormone binds to a receptor on the hepatocyte and elsewhere, generating the breakdown of glycogen to glucose which is passed into the circulation for use as a ready fuel during stress. Other physiological changes attributable to the adrenal catecholamines include changes in blood pressure and heart functions, which also occur through adrenergic receptors.

The overall system is not essential to life in the same sense as the requirement for the adrenal cortex. The adrenal medulla can be removed (sympathectomy) and, clinically, this is done sometimes without endangering survival in cases of oversecretion of catecholamines. However, when the adrenal cortex is removed, life can be sustained only in a totally nonstressful environment, with salt provided to the experimental animal unless glucocorticoid therapy is given.

II. ANATOMICAL, MORPHOLOGICAL, AND PHYSIOLOGICAL RELATIONSHIPS

A. Introduction

The adrenal glands are embedded and enclosed by coverings located (Fig. 10-1) in fat above the kidneys. The blood circulation of the adrenal is described in Fig. 10-2. The important detail to remember is that blood drains the adrenal cortex, carrying its secretions (e.g., cortisol, aldosterone) into the medulla, and then joins larger vessels which ultimately merge with the bloodstream. Thus, the intimacy of the cortical steroids with the medulla is apparent. Since the glucocorticoids induce the enzyme converting norepinephrine to epinephrine in the chromaffin cell and glucocorticoids as well as epinephrine are increased by stress, the capacity for the response of the specific secretion of the adrenal medulla is guaranteed by the events occurring in the cortex.

B. Development of the Adrenal Medulla

The adrenal medulla arises from the neural crest and is ectodermal in origin. As described in Chapter 10, the development of the primary cortex is signaled by the appearance of a suprarenal groove above the dorsal mesentary on each side (Fig. 10-3). The cells lining the groove proliferate into the primary cortex. Neural crest cells, which give rise to sympathetic neuroblasts, move down toward the cortex and invade it to form the precursor of the medulla. The cells of the medulla, postnatally, display a segmental arrangement which may relate to the structures of the nerve fibers from the sixth thoracic to the first lumbar segments, probably representing the sources of the migrating nerve cells forming the medulla. Ultimately, the medulla becomes invested with cells that secrete norepinephrine in addition to those secreting epinephrine. The persistence of the former suggests their relationship with the postganglionic sympathetic neurons.

C. Autonomic Nervous System and the Adrenal Medulla

It is becoming clear that the same structures are involved, at the central nervous system level, for triggering the adrenal cortex and the medulla. Thus, the limbic system is a candidate for the early stimulation followed by the hypothalamus. It has been shown experimentally that electrical stimulation of the dorsomedial nuclei and posterior hypothala-

452

mic areas lead to increased secretion of epinephrine and norepinephrine from the adrenal medulla. One possibility is that there exist separate hypothalamic centers which control secretion of norepinephrine and epinephrine, since there are situations when one type of medullary catecholamine is secreted predominantly. Signals are transmitted from the hypothalamus to the sympathetic nervous system, specifically a neuron located in the lateral horn gray matter of the thoracolumbar spinal cord (Fig. 11-1). This neuron sends out a long axon which travels in splanchnic nerves, passing through the celiac ganglion, and continues to the adrenal medulla. This first neuron releases acetylcholine from its nerve ending.

The acetylcholine-containing secretory vesicles are about 40–65 nm in

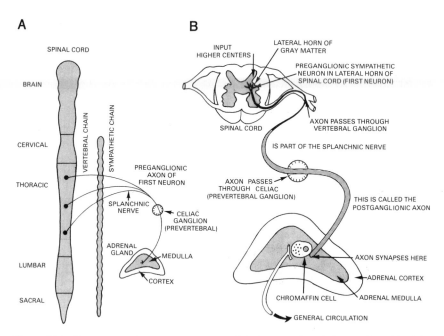

Figure 11-1. The autonomic nervous system and the innervation of chromaffin cells of the adrenal medulla. (A) The connections between the central nervous system and the adrenal medulla. Signals emanate from the hypothalamus down the spinal cord by way of descending autonomic pathways to the appropriate level in the spinal cord (segment 7 of the thoracic spinal cord). The signal is transported further from segment 7 over the long preganglionic axon which passes through the celiac ganglion and innervates the adrenal medulla by releasing acetylcholine at the level of the chromaffin cell. (B) Details of the pathway from the spinal column described in (A). Redrawn from notes compiled by Dr. Laurie Paavola, Department of Anatomy, Temple University School of Medicine, with permission.

diameter. The acetylcholine released binds to a receptor in the synaptic junction to the cell body of a second neuron in this chain, which contains the acetylcholine receptor. In this case, the second neuron of the sympathetic autonomic nervous system is the specialized chromaffin cell.

The chromaffin cell itself may be considered to be a modified postganglionic sympathetic neuron. It is analogous to the second neuron of the sympathetic nervous system and releases catecholamines. Whereas the catecholamines of the usual postganglionic second neuron synapse with an effector organ or tissue, chromaffin cells release catecholamines directly into the blood circulation. The nature of the precise signals at the beginning of the overall network is unclear. It would not be surprising to learn that the limbic system stimulates the hypothalamus electrically by alteration in the firing rate of the electrical signal. Presumably, further transmission from the hypothalamus to the sympathetic system is neuronal.

D. Histology of the Adrenal Medulla

The cells of the medulla are polyhedral, epithelioid, and arranged in connnecting cords. Many capillaries and venules are present (Fig. 11-1). As previously described, the neuron of the autonomic sympathetic nervous system delivers acetylcholine to the chromaffin cell and makes terminal contact with it. In most mammals, the epinephrine-containing chromaffin cell is more abundant than the norepinephrine chromaffin cell.

Idealized chromaffin cells of both types are shown in Fig. 11-2. The two different types of cells share many common features. The cell is polyhedral, with a large round nucleus containing one or more nucleoli. A large number of catecholamine-containing granules 1000–3000 Å in diameter are obvious in the cytoplasm. Chromaffin cells are also found in the kidney, ovary, testis, liver, heart, and gastrointestinal tract. Similar cell types are found in the carotid and aortic bodies which function as chemoreceptors (see Chapter 4).

A target tissue of interest with respect to epinephrine is the hepatocyte. A discussion of the cell biology of this cell and the liver has been presented in Chapter 10. Important target cells for the action of epinephrine are pericytes and vascular smooth muscle cells. The membranes of these cells contain α receptors which, when occupied by ligand, lead to movements of ions in and out of the cell and activation of contractile elements of the cell. Figure 11-3 shows an idealized pericyte, a cell occurring outside the endothelial lining of arterioles, capillaries, and sinuses. Although the function of these cells is not clearly understood, they have been suggested to regulate the size of the vessel lumen in that they possess contractile elements. There are tight junctions between pericytes and endothelial cells suggestive of ion transfer. An idealized smooth muscle cell is shown in Fig. 11-4. Smooth muscle cells are elongated with a contractile apparatus probably similar to the myosin system. Actin is undoubtedly present in these cells but the scarcity of thick filaments characteristic of myosin makes it difficult to explain contractile behavior on a basis similar to that occurring in striated muscle.

III. CHEMISTRY

The structures of norepinephrine, epinephrine, and a number of other compounds are shown in Fig. 11-5. Various epinephrine-like compounds are compared for their ability to elevate blood pressure or ability to cause contraction of an aortal strip *in vitro*. The phenylethylamine structure is basic to this activity. Hydroxylation of the ring amplifies pressor activity. Some substituted imidazolines, such as benzylimidazoline (see Fig. 11-6), have adrenergic activity. This type of structure can be

---

Figure 11-2. (A) Line drawing from electron micrographic data of an epinephrine-storing chromaffin cell of the adrenal medulla. These cells are similar in structure to the cells storing and secreting norepinephrine and differ only from those cells in the structure of the granules. Epinephrine-containing granules are moderately dense and finely granular with a thin halo between the granule and the enclosing membrane. Chromaffin cells similar to those in the adrenal medulla occur elsewhere and constitute the chromaffin system. Chromaffin cells are also found in the kidney, ovary, testis, liver, heart, and gastrointestinal tract. The carotid and aortic bodies, which function as chemoreceptors, contain similar types of cells. Reproduced with permission from T. L. Lentz, "Cell Fine Structure." Saunders, Philadelphia, Pennsylvania, 1971. (B, p. 456) Chromaffin cell storing norepinephrine. The adrenal medulla, in addition to containing a few sympathetic ganglion cells, contains two types of chromaffin cells, those which store epinephrine (A), and those which store norepinephrine. The cells of the adrenal medulla arise from neural crest tissue and are innervated by preganglionic sympathetic fibers which control the secretion of catecholamines into the bloodstream. Chromaffin cells contain cytoplasmic granules bounded by membranes of 1000–3000 Å in diameter. While granules of epinephrine-storing cells are moderately dense, those containing norepinephrine are opaque after fixation and osmium staining. Mitochondria, lysosomes, multivesicular bodies, vacuoles, and cisternae of rough-surfaced endoplasmic reticulum are distributed in the cytoplasm among the granules. Reproduced with permission from T. L. Lentz, "Cell Fine Structure." Saunders, Philadelphia, Pennsylvania, 1971.

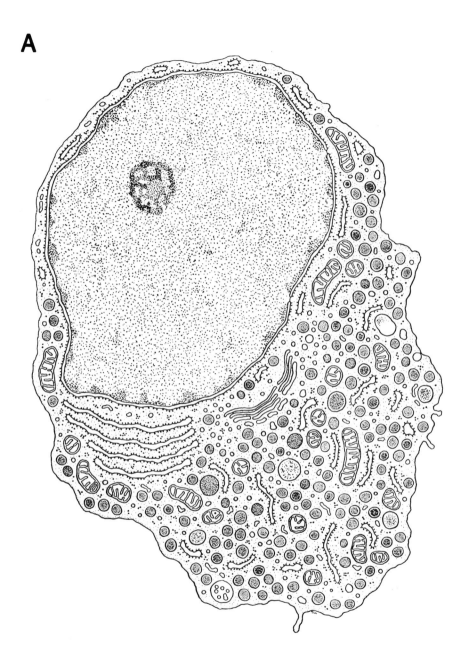

B

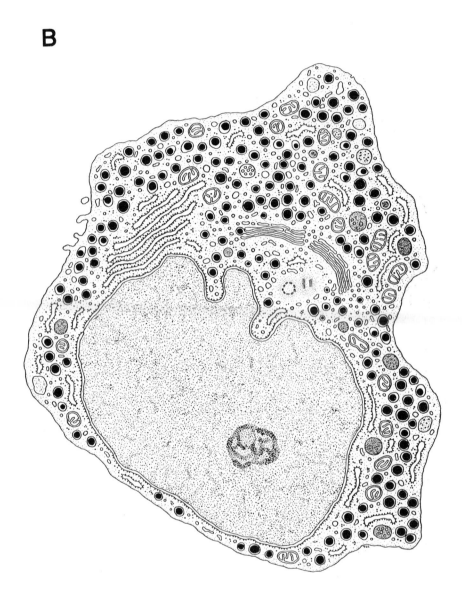

Figure 11-2B. See legend on p. 454.

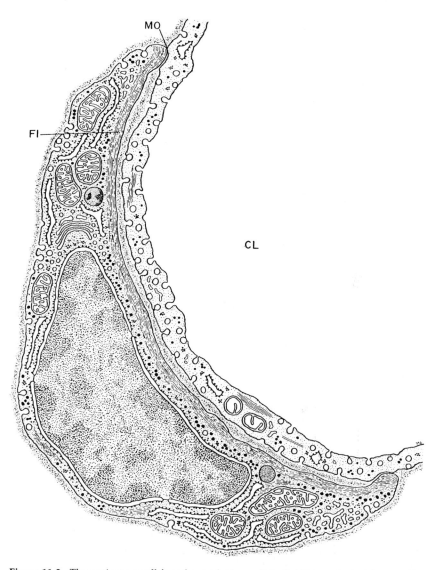

Figure 11-3. The pericyte, a cell found outside the endothelial lining of arterioles, capillaries, and sinuses. These cells may regulate the size of the vessel lumen in that they contain contractile elements. α Receptors in cell membranes could respond to epinephrine from the adrenal medulla to aid in the vascular contraction connected with epinephrine action. In capillaries (CL, capillary lumen), pericytes are located between leaflets of the basal lamina. The cells are polymorphous, some of which have long cytoplasmic processes which may encircle the vessel or extend along it. Mitochondria are large and numerous. Filaments (Fl) are abundant and often occur in bundles. A bundle of fibrillar material extends between small foot processes which penetrate the basement membrane and makes contact with the endothelium. A small area of membrane fusion, *macula occludens* (MO), may occur in these areas. Tight junctions between pericytes and endothelial cells are indicative of low-resistance coupling or ion transfer. Reproduced with permission from T. L. Lentz, "Cell Fine Structure." Saunders, Philadelphia, Pennsylvania, 1971.

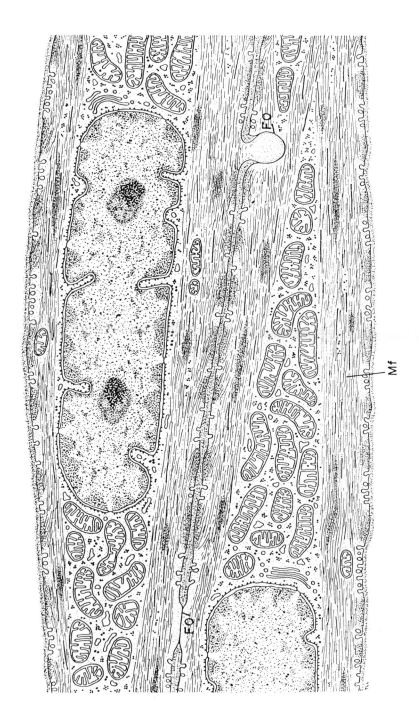

viewed as a phenylethylamine in which the ethylamine portion has been cyclized. A further development of structure–function and antagonism occurs with the later discussion of specific receptors of catecholamines.

IV. HORMONE ACTION AND BIOCHEMISTRY

A. Biochemistry of the Chromaffin Cell of the Adrenal Medulla

The relationship of the adrenal cortex to the medulla is shown in Fig. 11-7. In Fig. 11-7A, the vascular relationships are evident. The secretions from the cortex bathe the medulla on their way to the general circulation. Since similar unique environmental signals which cause epinephrine secretion from the medulla also stimulate glucocorticoid synthesis in the cortex, a ready supply of cortisol is available to the medulla for enhancement in the rate of conversion of norepinephrine to epinephrine. The availability of glucocorticoid is demonstrated in Fig. 11-7B. Here it is shown that the initial signals resulting in ACTH stimulation of the *zona fasciculata* of the cortex also stimulate the release of neurosecretory granules by way of the limbic system, hypothalamus, and autonomic nervous system via a cholinergic neuron which is shown to release acetylcholine synapsing with a receptor on the membrane of a chromaffin cell. Some rearrangement of macromolecules in the cell membrane occurs, probably involving phospholipids, and a "calcium channel" is constituted permitting influx of this ion from the extra-

---

Figure 11-4. Diagram of a smooth muscle cell from electron micrographic observations. These cells which are associated with the vasculature may play a role in elevated blood pressure through the action of epinephrine from the adrenal medulla. Epinephrine could bind to α receptors on the surface of these cells, generating increases in cytosolic calcium levels and bringing about contraction. These cells are elongated with a cytoplasm filled with myofilaments (Mf) arranged in the long axis of the cell. The two types of filaments are numerous thin filaments and fewer thicker filaments which are randomly distributed and seem unrelated to the thin filaments. Myofilaments terminate in the subsarcolemmal densities which oppose densities in neighboring cells. Pinocytotic vesicles occur between the densities. Some regions of the plasma membranes form tight junctions (*facia occludeus*, FO) where one cell contacts another. A major problem in explaining the mechanism of contraction of smooth muscle is that the structural counterpart of myosin has not been identified. The thin myofilaments may correspond to actin. The few thicker filaments probably correspond to myosin and are too scarce to explain the contraction mechanism. Reproduced with permission from T. L. Lentz, "Cell Fine Structure." Saunders, Philadelphia, Pennsylvania, 1971.

A

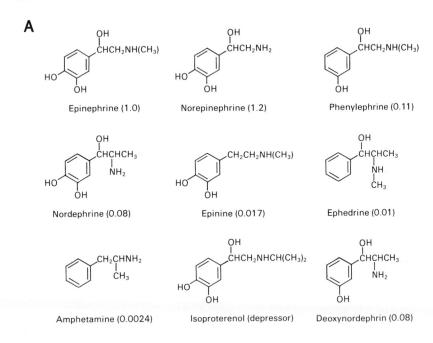

Epinephrine (1.0) Norepinephrine (1.2) Phenylephrine (0.11)

Nordephrine (0.08) Epinine (0.017) Ephedrine (0.01)

Amphetamine (0.0024) Isoproterenol (depressor) Deoxynordephrin (0.08)

B

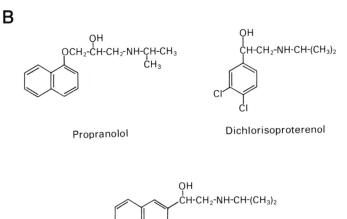

Propranolol Dichlorisoproterenol

Pronethalol

Figure 11-5. (A) Compounds with epinephrine-like (pressor) activity. The numbers in brackets represent the relative pressor activity (epinephrine = 1.0). Reproduced from E. H. Frieden, "Chemical Endocrinology," p. 46. Academic Press, New York, 1976. (B) Specific antagonists of β-adrenergic receptors. (C) Specific antagonists of α-adrenergic receptors.

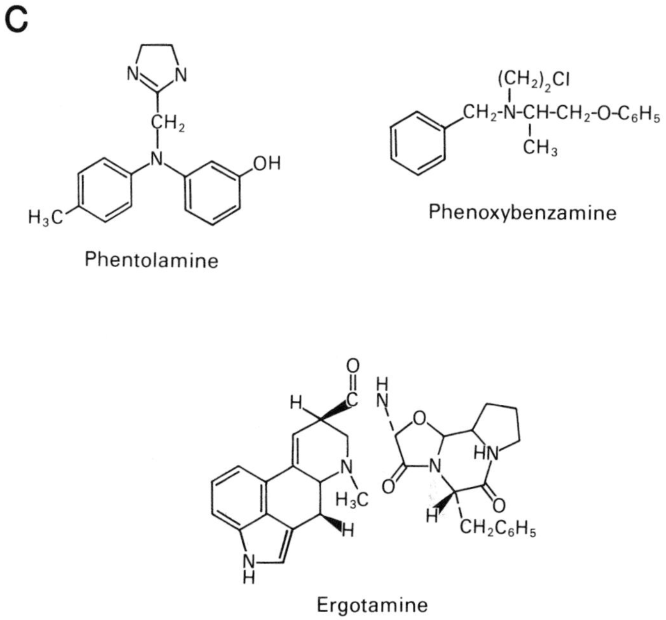

C

Phentolamine

Phenoxybenzamine

Ergotamine

Figure 11-5C.

cellular space. In some way the Ca^{2+} facilitates secretion of the neurosecretory granules. This may occur by the binding of Ca^{2+} to the granules and also to the inner plasma membrane, acting as a bridge and facilitating the process of exocytosis, pouring the contents of the granule into the venous sinus and then into local arterioles through fenestrations.

In the chromaffin cell the process of catecholamine synthesis is ongoing, as shown in Fig. 11-8. Tyrosine (or phenylalanine) enters the cell via the blood circulation and the extracellular fluid. In the cytosol, tyrosine is converted by tyrosine hydroxylase to dihydroxyphenylalanine (dopa) (Fig. 11-9). Tyrosine hydroxylase is the rate-limiting enzyme in the synthesis of catecholamines in all adrenergic neurons. L-Dopa is converted to dopamine by an L-amino acid decarboxylase located in the

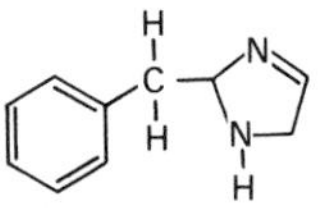

Figure 11-6. Structure of 2-benzylimidazoline.

462

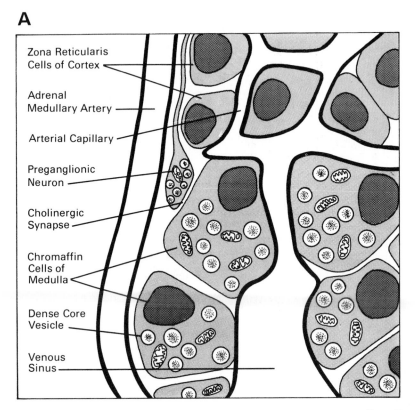

A

Zona Reticularis
Cells of Cortex

Adrenal
Medullary Artery

Arterial Capillary

Preganglionic
Neuron

Cholinergic
Synapse

Chromaffin
Cells of
Medulla

Dense Core
Vesicle

Venous
Sinus

Figure 11-7. Diagrams showing the relationship of adrenal medulla chromaffin cells to preganglionic neuron innervation and the structural elements involved in the synthesis of epinephrine and the discharge of catecholamines in response to acetylcholine. (A) Functional relationship between cortex and medulla for the control of synthesis of adrenal catecholamines. Glucocorticoids that stimulate enzymes catalyzing the conversion of nor-

cytosol. Dopamine must then enter the neurosecretory granule, since the enzyme catalyzing the subsequent catalytic biosynthetic pathway is localized there. Norepinephrine formed within the granule must perfuse out in order to be converted to epinephrine by the final enzyme of the pathway, phenylethanolamine N-methyltransferase (PNMT), which is located in the cytosol. Obviously, the epinephrine in the cytosol must move back into the neurosecretory granule and is stored there awaiting secretion. The reuptake process is linked to an ATPase of the granule membrane. The scenario of movement of intermediates in a biosynthetic pathway between intracellular compartments is not new, and we have seen similar movements during the synthesis of the steroid hormones.

B

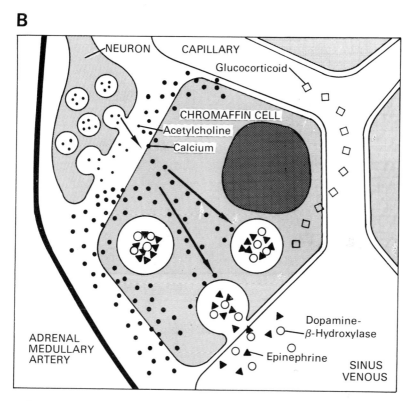

epinephrine to epinephrine reach the chromaffin cells from capillaries shown in (B). (B) Discharge of catecholamines from storage granules in chromaffin cells after nerve fiber stimulation resulting in the release of acetylcholine. Calcium enters the cells as a result, causing the fusion of granular membranes with the plasma membrane and exocytosis of the contents. Reproduced with permission from D. T. Krieger and J. C. Hughes, eds., "Neuroendocrinology." Sinauer Associates, Sunderland, Massachusetts, 1980.

B. Regulation of Biosynthesis

Tyrosine hydroxylase is the rate-limiting enzyme in the overall biosynthesis of epinephrine (Fig. 11-8). It is allosterically inhibited (heterotrophy) by norepinephrine. Presumably the initial enzyme contains an allosteric site with a K_i value which from time to time is exceeded by the amount of norepinephrine in the cytosol. This is undoubtedly of physiological significance because norepinephrine cannot be metabolized further without first entering the neurosecretory granule. Although perhaps not rate-limiting for the overall pathway, its concentration in cytosol could easily become effective. Also, the tyrosine hydroxylase

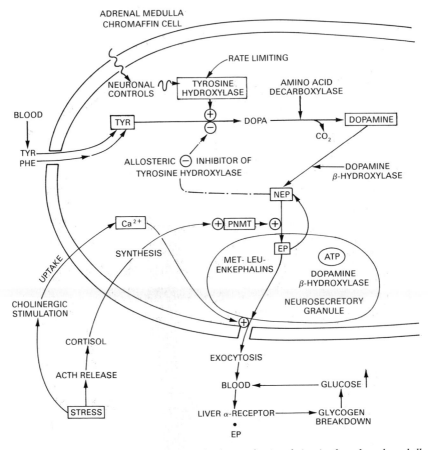

Figure 11-8. Biosynthesis, packaging, and release of epinephrine in the adrenal medulla chromaffin cell. PNMT, Phenylethanolamine N-methyltransferase; EP, epinephrine; NEP, norepinephrine. Arrows pointing upward following the name of a compound refer to an increase in the concentration of that substance. Neurosecretory granules contain epinephrine, dopamine β-hydroxylase, ATP, Met- or Leu-enkephalin, as well as larger enkephalin-containing peptides or norepinephrine in place of epinephrine. Epinephrine and norepinephrine are contained in different cells. Enkephalins could also be contained in separate cells, although that is not completely clear. Presumably, epinephrine once secreted into the bloodstream not only affects α receptors of hepatocytes to ultimately increase blood glucose levels as shown here, but also interacts with α receptors on vascular smooth muscle cells and on pericytes to cause cellular contraction and increase blood pressure.

rarely functions at maximal velocity and therefore, at least to a certain extent, is probably substrate controlled. At suitable concentrations, norepinephrine can bind to the allosteric site on tyrosine hydroxylase, producing a change in conformation and a rise in the K_m^{Tyr}.

Interestingly, ACTH, which so far we have considered in the context of the *zona fasciculata* and the *zona reticularis* of the cortex in the stimulation of steroid biosynthesis, also apparently binds to chromaffin cell membrane receptors and stimulates the intracellular level of cyclic AMP (see Fig. 10-11). Elevated cyclic AMP levels activate protein kinases which may phosphorylate some proteins in the cell. The activated protein kinase, alternatively, may translocate to the nucleus where reactions are stimulated, leading to an increased rate of synthesis of tyrosine hydroxylase.

Finally, the levels of tyrosine hydroxylase are also under neuronal controls. The dopa decarboxylase enzyme does not appear to be under specific hormonal or neural regulation. However, dopamine β-hydroxylase is a regulated enzyme. Like tyrosine hydroxylase, its synthesis is under neuronal control. Its level in the cell and consequently within the neurosecretory granules is also affected by ACTH by way of elevation of the intracellular level of cyclic AMP. The final enzyme in the pathway, PNMT, can be induced by cortisol mediated by a cytoplasmic glucocorticoid receptor, presumably at the transcriptional level (see Fig. 10-17). The extent of the increase in PNMT by cortisol is only about 50% with long-term stress. Under similar conditions, tyrosine hydroxylase, through the indicated regulators, can be increased threefold.

Tyrosine hydroxylase activity appears to have a half-life of about 3 days as judged from its exponential rate of decline following removal of long-term stress. Denervation of the adrenal gland by severing the splanchnic nerve prevents elevations of tyrosine hydroxylase and dopamine β-hydroxylase in stressed animals, whereas the activity of PNMT can still be induced by prolonged stress. Thus, nerve impulses, as indicated in Fig. 11-8, are required for the stimulation of tyrosine hydroxylase and of dopamine β-hydroxylase. In repeated or long-term stress in which epinephrine is secreted from the adrenal medulla in appreciable amounts, there is an elevation of the capacity for further catecholamine synthesis. This is accomplished by increases in the enzymes of the biosynthetic pathway discussed above.

C. Content of Neurosecretory Granules and Secretion

The neurosecretory granules have been found to contain epinephrine, ATP, dopamine β-hydroxylase, enkephalins, and enkephalin-contain-

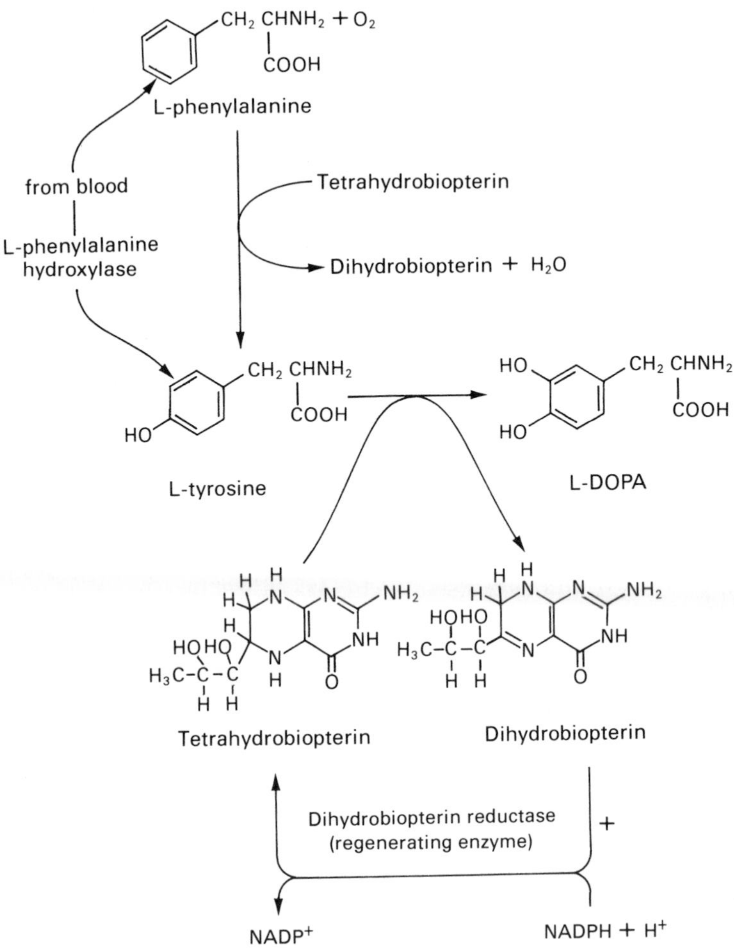

Figure 11-9. Biochemical steps in the synthesis of epinephrine by the chromaffin cell of the adrenal medulla.

ing peptides. The granules have an acidic interior, a condition which is known to stabilize epinephrine. The loss of dopamine β-hydroxylase from chromaffin when the content of granules has been exhausted provides a rationale for the interval required to produce epinephrine again in high levels. This is related to the time involved in the resynthesis of dopamine β-hydroxylase. The epinephrine released causes contraction of the vascular system already discussed and in the liver leads to glycogen breakdown. Both of these processes probably proceed by the mediation of α receptors.

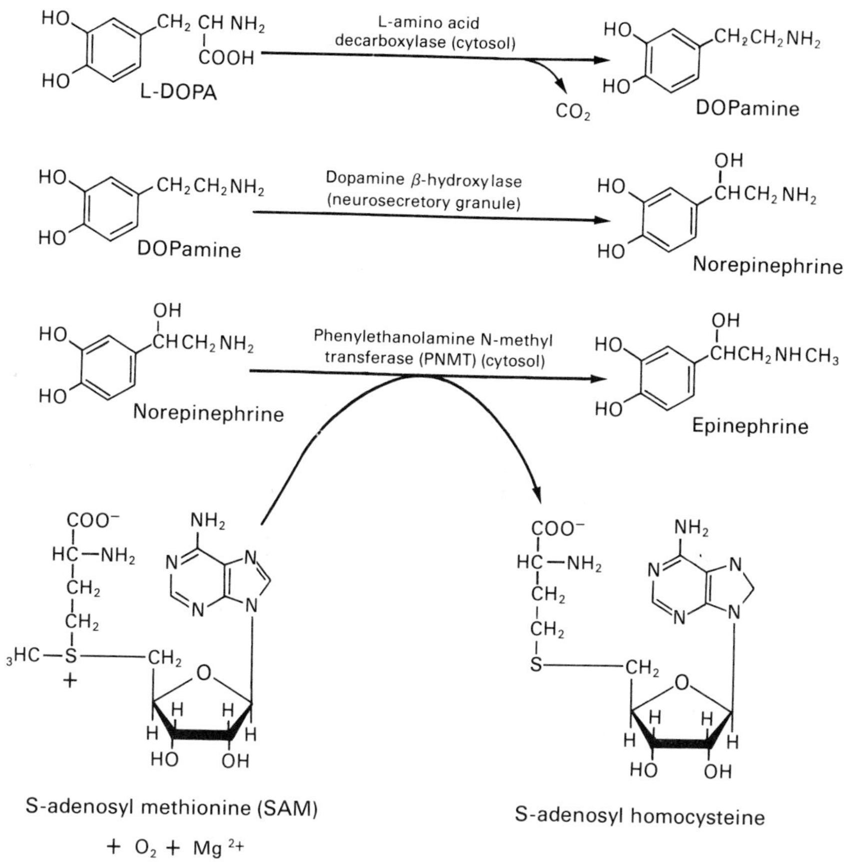

Figure 11-9 (Continued).

Enkephalins exert an analgesic effect in the central nervous system. The fate of these polypeptide hormones released into the bloodstream from the adrenal medulla is not clear. Obviously, there could be some problem in transporting them into the brain in view of the blood–brain barrier, and they do not function there.

The release of enkephalins from the adrenal medulla secretory granule is proportional to the release of epinephrine. Enkephalin is stored in the granule together with epinephrine. Epinephrine, as indicated before, must enter the chromaffin granule after its conversion in the cytosol by PNMT. This uptake into the neurosecretory granule is stimulated by Mg^{2+} and ATP coupled to an H^+ electrochemical gradient. The proton pumping Mg-ATPase and an anion transport site apparently

468

exist as parts of a macromolecular complex in the membrane of the chromaffin granule. The internal acidic milieu (pH 5.7) of the granule coincides with a pH optimum of dopamine β-hydroxylase of pH 5.5 and explains the need for compartmentation of this enzyme.

The chromaffin cells, maintained in cell culture conditions, are able to synthesize Met- and Leu-enkephalin *de novo* from radioactive amino acids. Reserpine (Fig. 11-10), a drug which has catecholamine-depleting activity, causes nearly complete removal of catecholamines from the chromaffin cells, but the synthesis of enkephalins is enhanced under these conditions, particularly that of Met-enkephalin. The adrenal medulla usually contains Met-enkephalin at several times the level of Leu-enkephalin. Free enkephalin pentapeptides are about 5% of the total enkephalin-containing peptides in adrenal medulla.

The details of the mechanism of the intracellular events preceding exocytosis of the neurosecretory granules are unclear. Once again, Ca^{2+} (see Chapter 1) is involved and is elevated in the cytosolic compartment following the release of acetylcholine from the sympathetic autonomic cholinergic neuron and the postsynaptic binding of the transmitter to the chromaffin cell membrane receptor. The exocytotic event appears to be an all-or-none process in which the total contents of the granule are released into the extracellular space and into the local blood circulation by entrance through *fenestrated* capillaries which overcome diffusion barriers in the normal arteriolar wall. Even though epinephrine and enkephalins may be contained in the same chromaffin cell, there is recent evidence that their synthesis may be under different controls. The empty granule is probably reabsorbed by the chromaffin cell (see Chapter 4) or is recycled from its fused state with the chromaffin membrane because empty granules can be found in the medulla cells after secretion has occurred. During exocytosis, all the products of processing of proenkephalin are released, including the largest and even a small amount

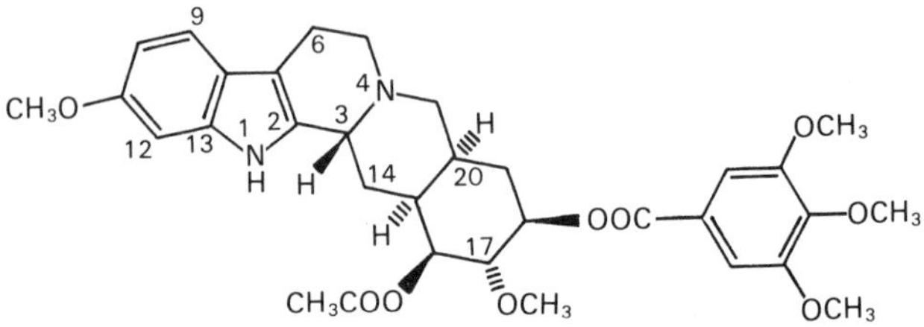

Figure 11-10. Structure of reserpine.

of proenkephalin itself. Three of the enkephalin-containing peptides are more active in isolated systems than the pentapeptides themselves, including peptide E, heptapeptide, and the octapeptide. Peptide E is a 25-amino acid residue chain which contains one copy of Tyr–Gly–Gly–Phe–Met– at the N terminal and one copy of Tyr–Gly–Gly–Phe–Leu– at the C terminus. These may not be processed to free enkephalin. Enkephalin receptors are present in many tissues where these hormones may act, but it appears that they do not act in the brain.

Prostaglandin E_2 (PGE_2) is bound specifically by particulate fractions of bovine, ovine, and human adrenal medulla cells. The binding is sensitive to treatment with phospholipases, glycosidases, trypsin, and sulfhydryl reagents. The dissociation constant of 2 nM PGE_2 indicates tight binding. The receptor site is quite specific for PGE_2 compared to other prostaglandins, and prostacyclin (PGI_2) has a lower affinity than PGE_2. The prostaglandins bind to this receptor site in the same order as they demonstrate potency to release epinephrine from chromaffin granules. Thus, PGE may play a role in controlling the activity of adrenal medulla secretions.

D. Catabolism of Catecholamines

As with most other hormones, epinephrine is active at its receptor site in the unmetabolized form. The routes of metabolic inactivation have been well established. These pathways of metabolism are shown in Fig. 11-11. The major reactions involve oxidation by monoamine oxidase (MAO), a mitochondrial enzyme in liver, kidneys, brain, and adrenergic nerve endings. The second major catabolic reaction is methylation. This is catalyzed by catechol O-methyltransferase (COMT), which is widely distributed, especially in liver and kidneys, but it is absent from nerve endings. Its location may be in the cytosol and possibly in the cell membrane. The aldehydes produced are converted to acids by aldehyde dehydrogenase. The aldehydes can be reduced also to form alcohols. COMT methylates catecholamines in the C-3 hydroxyl of the ring and to a vastly smaller extent the parahydroxyl group. There are variable amounts of MAO and COMT in different tissues, but the catecholamines eventually reach the liver and kidneys, which contain these enzymes. Consequently the urinary products appear in a fairly consistent pattern (Fig. 11-11). The majority of these excretion products are conjugated as glucuronides or sulfates, the latter being the more abundant form.

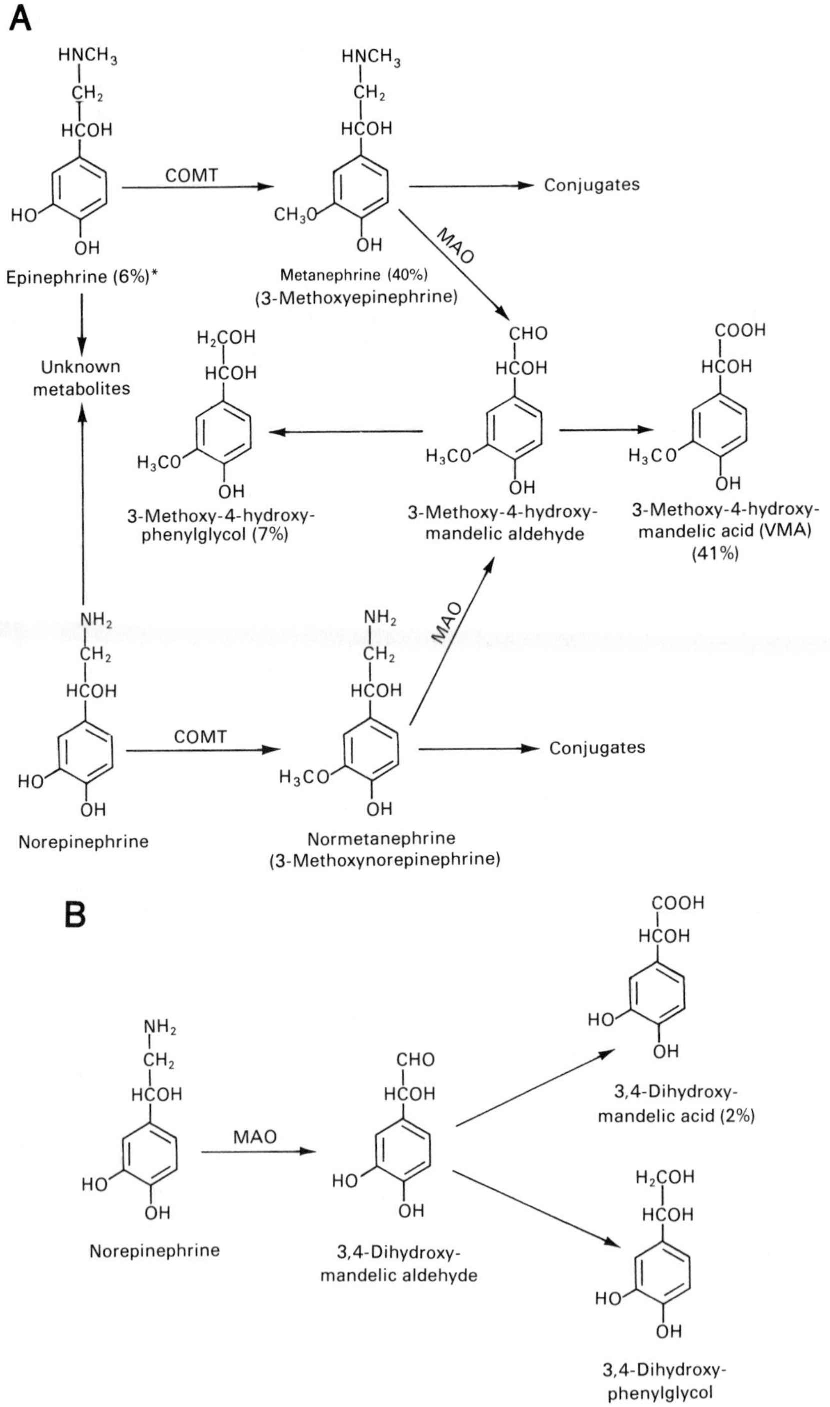
A
HNCH3
CH2
HCOH
HO
OH
Epinephrine (6%)*
COMT
HNCH3
CH2
HCOH
CH3O
OH
Metanephrine (40%)
(3-Methoxyepinephrine)
Conjugates
MAO
Unknown
metabolites
H2COH
HCOH
H3CO
OH
3-Methoxy-4-hydroxy-
phenylglycol (7%)
CHO
HCOH
H3CO
OH
3-Methoxy-4-hydroxy-
mandelic aldehyde
COOH
HCOH
H3CO
OH
3-Methoxy-4-hydroxy-
mandelic acid (VMA)
(41%)
NH2
CH2
HCOH
HO
OH
Norepinephrine
COMT
NH2
CH2
HCOH
H3CO
OH
Normetanephrine
(3-Methoxynorepinephrine)
MAO
Conjugates
B
NH2
CH2
HCOH
HO
OH
Norepinephrine
MAO
CHO
HCOH
HO
OH
3,4-Dihydroxy-
mandelic aldehyde
COOH
HCOH
HO
OH
3,4-Dihydroxy-
mandelic acid (2%)
H2COH
HCOH
HO
OH
3,4-Dihydroxy-
phenylglycol

V. ACTIONS OF EPINEPHRINE

A. General Effects of Catecholamines

Catecholamines act through pairs of outer cell membrane receptors which produce opposite actions. A similar phenomenon is characteristic of the prostaglandins (Chapter 15). A partial listing of opposite actions of catecholamines in various tissues is shown in Table 11-1. The opposing responses are generated by ligand binding to different receptors located on the same or different cell membrane, called α- and β-adrenergic receptors. α Receptors act by altering the pattern of ion flow into the cell, particularly with regard to Ca^{2+}, whereas the β receptor operates by stimulation of adenylate cyclase and the intracellular level of cyclic AMP (see, e.g., Fig. 10-11). The two receptor types are somewhat difficult to distinguish because either one usually can bind the same ligand (e.g., epinephrine). Many of the receptors have subclasses wherein each class may operate through a different mechanism. This is true for the α receptors. Two principal classes are α_1 and α_2 receptors. α_1 Receptors control Ca^{2+} ion flux, whereas α_2 receptors inhibit adenylate cyclase. α and β receptors can be resolved by a specific order of affinities for different compounds and especially by the use of specific inhibitors of each receptor type. α-Adrenergic receptors bind ligands (agonists) in the following order (starting with highest affinity): epinephrine > norepinephrine > phenylephrine > isoproterenol, whereas the order of agonist binding for α-adrenergic receptors is isoproterenol > epinephrine > norepinephrine > phenylephrine. The structures of these agonists are in Fig. 11-5. Thus, epinephrine can bind to both receptors and the actual physiological effect achieved may be a direct consequence of the available amount of the catecholamine in a particular location, since the binding constants for the various types of the adrenergic receptors may be quite different.

Figure 11-11. Catabolism of catecholamines in the blood and of norepinephrine in nerve endings. (A) The main site of catabolism of circulating epinephrine and norepinephrine is the liver. The conjugates formed there are mostly glucuronides and sulfates. Numbers in parentheses represent the percentage distribution occurring in normal urine; 4% is occupied by other compounds not shown here. (B) Catabolism of norepinephrine in adrenergic nerve endings. The acid and glycol enter the circulation and may be O-methylated subsequently in VMA and in 3-methoxy-4-hydroxyphenylglycol. MAO, Monoamine oxidase; COMT, catechol O-methyltransferase. Reproduced from W. F. Ganong, "Review of Medical Physiology," 9th Ed., p. 158. Lange Medical Publications, Los Altos, California, 1977.

Table 11-1. Responses of Effector Organs to Autonomic Nerve Impulses and Circulating Catecholamines[a]

Effector organs	Cholinergic impulse response	Receptor type	Adrenergic impulse response
Eye			
Radial muscle of iris	—	α	Contraction (mydriasis)
Sphincter muscle of iris	Contraction (miosis)		—
Ciliary muscle	Contraction for near vision	β	Relaxation for far vision
Heart			
S-A node	Decrease in heart rate; vagal arrest	β[b]	Increase in heart rate
Atria	Decrease in contractility, and (usually) increase in conduction velocity	β[b]	Increase in contractility and conduction velocity
A-V node and conduction system	Decrease in conduction velocity A-V block	β[b]	Increase in conduction velocity
Ventricles	—	β[b]	Increase in contractility, conduction velocity, automaticity, and rate of idiopathic pacemakers
Blood vessels			
Coronary	Dilatation	α β	Constriction Dilatation
Skin and mucosa	—	α	Constriction
Skeletal muscle	Dilatation	α β	Constriction Dilatation
Cerebral	—	α	Constriction (slight)
Pulmonary	—	α	Constriction
Abdominal viscera	—	α β	Constriction Dilatation
Renal		α	Constriction
Salivary glands	Dilatation	α	Constriction
Lung			
Bronchial muscle	Contraction	β	Relaxation
Bronchial glands	Stimulation		Inhibition (?)

	Cholinergic impulses: Response	Noradrenergic impulses: Receptor type	Noradrenergic impulses: Response
Stomach			
Motility and tone	Increase	β	Decrease (usually)
Sphincters	Relaxation (usually)	α	Contraction (usually)
Secretion	Stimulation		Inhibition (?)
Intestine			
Motility and tone	Increase	α,β	Decrease
Sphincters	Relaxation (usually)	α	Contraction (usually)
Secretion	Stimulation		Inhibition (?)
Gallbladder and ducts	Contraction		Relaxation
Urinary bladder			
Detrusor	Contraction	β	Relaxation (usually)
Trigone and sphincter	Relaxation	α	Contraction
Ureter motility and tone	Increase (?)		Increase (usually)
Uterus	Variable[c]	α,β	Variable[c]
Male sex organs	Erection		Ejaculation
Skin			
Pilomotor muscles	—	α	Contraction
Sweat glands	Generalized secretion	α	Slight, localized secretion[d]
Spleen capsule	—	α	Contraction
Adrenal medulla	Secretion of epinephrine and norepinephrine		—
Liver		α	Glycogenolysis
Pancreas			
Acini	Secretion		—
Islets	Insulin secretion	α	Inhibition of insulin secretion
		β	Insulin secretion
Salivary glands	Profuse, watery secretion	α	Thick, viscous secretion
Lacrimal glands	Secretion		—
Nasopharyngeal glands	Secretion		—
Adipose tissue	—	β	Lipolysis
Juxtaglomerular cells	—	β	Renin secretion

[a] Reproduced with permission from W. F. Ganong, "The Nervous System." Lange Medical Publications, Los Altos, California, 1977.

[b] The β receptors of the heart have been classified as β_1 receptors and most other β receptors as β_2 receptors.

[c] Depends on stage of menstrual cycle, amount of circulating estrogen and progesterone, and other factors. Responses of pregnant uterus different from those of nonpregnant.

[d] On palms of hands and in some other locations ("adrenergic sweating").

There are specific inhibitors or blockers of α- and β-adrenergic receptors (Fig. 11-5). α-Adrenergic antagonists are represented by phentolamine, phenoxybenzamine, and ergot alkaloids. Specific antagonists of β-adrenergic receptors are propranolol, dichlorisoproterenol, and pronethalol. Catecholamines, especially epinephrine, represent an emergency stimulus for alterations in carbohydrate metabolism to make available an energy source which can be burned quickly for "flight or fight" responses. Thus, the initial responses in various tissues are as follows: increases in glycogenolysis and gluconeogenesis in the liver, increased gluconeogenesis in skeletal muscle, increased inotropic effect (affecting force of muscular contraction in the heart), increased amylase secretion by the salivary gland, relaxation of the uterine musculature, conversion of triglycerides to free fatty acids and glycerol in adipose, elevations in blood pressure, heart rate, cardiac output (depending on amount of catecholamine), and dilation of bronchial musculature. Although norepinephrine is a pressor, its activity in this regard is much smaller than that of epinephrine.

B. Effects of Epinephrine on Glycogenolysis in the Liver

The breakdown of glycogen to glucose is accomplished by epinephrine operating at an α-adrenergic receptor on the hepatocyte membrane probably through a mechanism involving calcium ion fluxes. A scheme for the operation of the α receptor in hepatocyte glycogenolysis is shown in Fig. 11-12. As the result of a stressor, epinephrine binds to the α receptor. The nature of the second messenger is not clear, but changes in the turnover of phospholipids are involved. This action is thought to lead to an increase in cytosolic Ca^{2+} levels as a result generating inositol triphosphate and mobilizing calcium from the endoplasmic reticulum (or from mitochondria presumably deposited there as calcium phosphate). The elevated cytosolic Ca^{2+} level stimulates phosphorylase kinase which catalyzes the conversion of phosphorylase b to phosphorylase a, the active form, and glucose 1-phosphate is converted to glucose and secreted, raising the blood level for use as an emergency fuel. The synthesis of glycogen is also blocked under these conditions. In most species, particularly in man, β_2-adrenergic receptors are also important in epinephrine actions on the liver. Thus, epinephrine-induced glycogen breakdown may be thought of as being mediated by both α_1 and β_2 receptors for epinephrine.

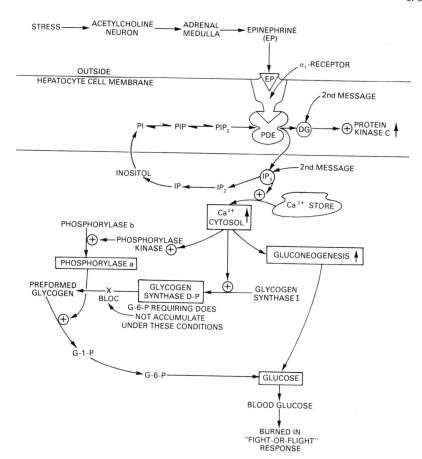

Figure 11-12. Possible scenario for the mode of action of epinephrine on the hepatocyte to generate glucose from increased glycogenolysis and gluconeogenesis. Epinephrine is released through the stress pathway by way of a two-neuronal system ending on an acetylcholinergic neuron innervating the adrenal medulla. The acetylcholine binds to membrane receptors on the chromaffin cell causing an increased cellular uptake of Ca^{2+}. This results in release of epinephrine (and other components) from granules through exocytosis. The released epinephrine binds to α receptors on hepatocytes (and on cells that bring about contraction and increased blood pressure), causing an elevation in cytosolic Ca^{2+} concentration. This may be brought about by enhanced metabolism of phosphatidylinositol (PI) and its phosphorylated derivatives: phosphatidylinositol-P (PIP), phosphatidylinositol bisphosphate (PIP$_2$), inositol triphosphate (IP$_3$), inositol diphosphate (IP$_2$), and inositol phosphate (IP). Generation of IP$_3$ serves as a second messenger for the release of Ca^{2+} from storage sites in the cell, most probably the endoplasmic reticulum. Elevated Ca^{2+} stimulates phosphorylase kinase activity, glycogen synthase I (the effect of Ca^{2+} may be indirect here), and gluconeogenesis, all of which lead to a generation of glucose and an increase in circulating glucose levels for use in fight or flight responses in adapting to the original stress. PDE, Phosphodiesterase; DG, diacylglycerol.

C. Ligand Detection of the Adrenergic Receptor Subclasses

The β receptor is a membrane site that acts to increase the rate of adenylate cyclase activity on the cytosolic side producing a stimulation in the level of intracellular cyclic AMP (see Chapter 1). The β receptors of the heart have been classified β_1-adrenergic receptors and the other receptors are classified as β_2-adrenergic receptors. Epinephrine and norepinephrine bind equally well to the β_1 receptor, whereas epinephrine is about a 10-fold better ligand than norepinephrine for the β_2 receptor.

The α receptors also are subdivided into α_1- and α_2-adrenergic receptors. These classes of receptors may be distinguished through the use of prazosin and yohimbine (Fig. 11-13). The action of the receptors may lead to a lowering of cyclic AMP (α_2 receptor; see Fig. 11-14) and may operate by altering the flux of Ca^{2+} within the cell (α_1 receptor; Fig. 11-12). The α_1 receptors refer to postsynaptic receptors or those located on effector cells and have a great affinity for the antagonist prazosin. The α_2 receptors refer to the presynaptic receptors, although it is apparently still unclear whether α_2 receptors actually are located on nerve terminals. They may also refer to postsynaptic effects which are coupled to adenylate cyclase in an inhibitory way, resulting in a lowering of intracellular cyclic AMP levels.

D. Regulation of Adrenergic Receptors

Adrenergic receptors are regulated by thyroid hormone and by glucocorticoids. In the hyperthyroid state, the heart β_1-adrenergic recep-

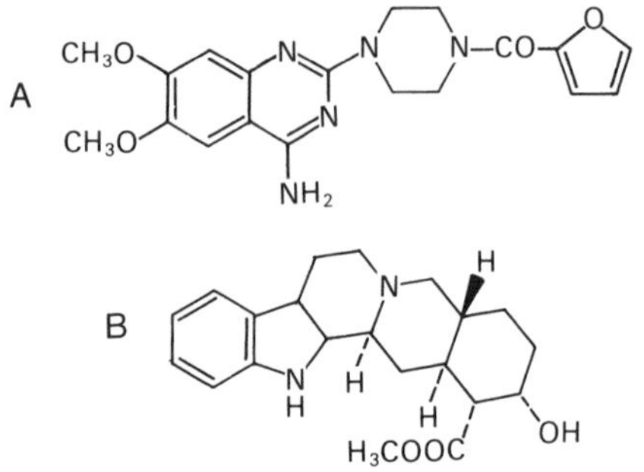

Figure 11-13. Structures of prazosin (A), an α_1-receptor antagonist, and yohimbine (B), an α_2-receptor antagonist.

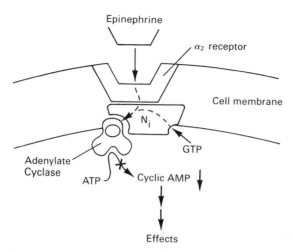

Figure 11-14. Outline of the function of an α_2 receptor for epinephrine. The hormone interacts with the α_2 receptor in the cell membrane and exerts an inhibition of adenylate cyclase activity. This requires the binding of GTP to the guanine nucleotide transducing agent, N_i, whose concerted action with the ligand receptor results in inhibition of the enzymatic reaction.

tor is elevated in concentration. In the absence of glucocorticoids, there is an increase in the number of β receptors without a detectable change in the number of α receptors.

"Desensitization" is another regulatory aspect of adrenergic receptors. Prolonged exposure to an agonist such as epinephrine leads to decreased responsiveness to a given target tissue. This desensitization occurs with both α and β receptors. The mechanisms of these responses are not clearly understood.

A model of the actual structure of the β receptor developed from experimental data is presented in Fig. 11-15.

Recent experiments have shown that certain cells in culture contain adenylate cyclase but lack β-adrenergic receptors. The membranes have been isolated from such cells and combined with extracts from other cells containing the receptor. The entire system can be reconstituted in the formerly receptor-deficient membrane. The reconstituted system reproduces the properties of a normal cell membrane in terms of the effects of agonists and antagonists in stimulating adenylate cyclase. Such experiments tend to strengthen our conception of the receptor system (as shown in Fig. 11-15).

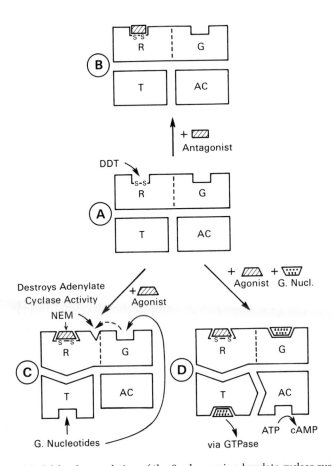

Figure 11-15. Model for the regulation of the β-adrenergic adenylate cyclase system by β-adrenergic agents and guanine nucleotides (G nucleotides). The system is composed of β-adrenergic receptors (R), transmitter molecules (T), and adenylate cyclase enzymes (AC). G nucleotide regulatory sites (G) are associated with R. (A) No bound ligands. R can be inactivated by the reducing agent, dithiothreitol (DTT), indicating the exposure of essential disulfide bonds. (B) β-Adrenergic antagonists bound to R; disulfide bonds of R are shielded. (C) β-adrenergic agonists bound to R; disulfide bonds of R are protected, but can be inactivated by N-ethylmaleimide (NEM), indicating the exposure of essential alkylatable groups of R. Interaction between G nucleotides and T is favored. (D) Binding of β-adrenergic agonists to R and G nucleotides to T and G:G induces protection of alkylatable groups of R. T induces activation of AC, resulting in the conversion of ATP to cyclic AMP. AC activation is terminated by hydrolysis of the G nucleotide bound to T by its GTPase. Reproduced from A. D. Strosburg, G. Vauquelin, O. Durieu-Trautmann, C. Delavier-Kutchko, S. Boltar, and C. Andre, *Trends Biochem. Sci.* **5,** 11–14 (1980).

VI. ENKEPHALINS

Opioid peptides have sprung into prominence in recent years. It has become clear that β-lipotropin and β-endorphin are produced in response to stress together with ACTH and secreted from the corticotroph of the anterior pituitary. Although enkephalins are smaller components incorporated into the endorphin structure, they appear to be the functional products of genes separate from that transcribing proopiomelanocortin message in the corticotroph (see Chapter 5). In fact, the major source of circulating enkephalins appears to be the adrenal medulla. These are secreted, like epinephrine, by the exocytosis of granules following cholinergic stimulation and calcium influx.

A precursor protein exists which contains multiple copies of the enkephalins. The individual enkephalins are released by the actions of trypsin-like enzymes. Proenkephalin, the precursor of these several individual enkephalins of the adrenal medulla contains one Leu- and six Met-enkephalin sequences. The structure of human adrenal proenkephalin mRNA and protein is shown in Fig. 11-16. This figure should be compared with Fig. 5-13, which shows the proopiomelanocortin (POMC) gene of the corticotroph. The structure of proenkephalin was obtained from a complete cDNA copy of the specific mRNA from a human pheochromocytoma. The precursor is 267 amino acids long. As shown in Fig. 11-17, five of the seven enkephalins are flanked on both sides by pairs of basic amino acid residues which probably serve as cutting sites for proteases. The precursor does not contain sequences of the opioid peptides, dynorphin, α-neoendorphin, or β-endorphin. It is apparent that in addition to the different enkephalin precursors in adrenal medulla and in hypothalamus, it is likely that the proteolytic processing to active enkephalins is also different.

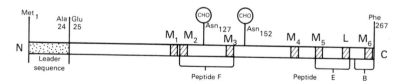

Figure 11-16. Low-resolution model of enkephalin precursor showing the distribution of Met-enkephalin sequences (M_1, M_2, M_3, through M_6) and Leu-enkephalin (L). The position of potential carbohydrate (CHO) attachment sites and the sequences corresponding to peptides F, E, and B of bovine adrenal medulla are shown. Reproduced from M. Comb, P. H. Seeburg, J. Adelman, L. Eiden, and E. Herbert, Primary structure of human Met- and Leu-enkephalin precursor and its mRNA. *Nature (London)* **295,** 663–666 (1982). © 1982 Macmillan Journals Limited.

5' – CUGGGGCCUGGGGGCCACCAGUGGGAAAAGAUAUUAAAAUCUCAUAAAUCCUCCGUAUCUUUUUUCCAUUUCAGGAACUUCUUUUGGAGUAACUUUCGCCUUCUUCG

UCGGAGGCAGAGCCCCGCAGCCUGGCCCGUGACCCCGCAGAGACGCUGAGGACCGCGACGAGUCGUGUCUGAACCCGGCUUUUCCAAUUGGCCUGCUCCAUCCGAACAGCGUCAACUCC

| 1 | | | | | | | | | 10 | | | | | | | | | 20 | | | | | | | | | 30 |
AUG GCG CGG UUC CUG ACA CUU UGC ACU UGG CUG CUG UUG CUC GGC CCC GGG CUC CUG GCG ACC GUG CGG GCC GAA UGC AGC CAG GAU UGC
met ala arg phe leu thr leu cys thr trp leu leu leu leu gly pro gly leu leu ala thr val arg ala glu cys ser gln asp cys

| | | | | | | | | 40 | | | | | | | | | 50 | | | | | | | | | 60 |
GCG ACG UGC AGC UAC CGC CUA GUG CGC CCG GCC GAC AUC AAC UUC CUG GCU UGC CUA AUG GAA UGU GAA GGU AAA CUG CCU UCU CUG AAA
ala thr cys ser tyr arg leu val arg pro ala asp ile asn phe leu ala cys val met glu cys glu gly lys leu pro ser leu lys

| | | | | | | | | 70 | | | | | | | | | 80 | | | | | | | | | 90 |
AUU UGG GAA ACC UGC AAG GAG CUC CUG CAG CUG UCC AAA CCA GAG CUU CCU CAA GAU GGC ACC AGC ACC CUC AGA GAA AAU AGC AAA CCG
ile trp glu thr cys lys glu leu leu gln leu ser lys pro glu leu pro gln asp gly thr ser thr leu arg glu asn ser lys pro

| | | | | | | | | <u>100</u> | | | | | | | | | 110 | | | | | | | | | 120 |
GAA GAA AGC CAU UUG CUA GCC|<u>AAA AGG</u>|UAU GGG GGC UUC AUG|<u>AAA AGG</u>|UAU GGA GGC UUC AUG|<u>AAG AAA</u>|AUG GAU GAG CUU UAU CCC AUG
glu glu ser his leu leu ala|lys arg|tyr gly gly phe met|lys arg|tyr gly gly phe met|lys lys|met asp glu leu tyr pro met

| | | | | | | | | 130 | | | | | | | | | 140 | | | | | | | | | 150 |
GAG CCA GAA GAA GAG GCC AAU GGA AGU GAG AUC CUC GCC|<u>AAG CGG</u>|UAU GGG GGC UUC AUG|<u>AAG AAG</u>|GAU GCA GAG GAG GAC GAC UCG CUG
glu pro glu glu glu ala asn gly ser glu ile leu ala|lys arg|tyr gly gly phe met|lys lys|asp ala glu glu asp asp ser leu

| | | | | | | | | 160 | | | | | | | | | 170 | | | | | | | | | 180 |
GCC AAU UCC UCA GAC CUG CUA AAA GAG CUU CUG GAA ACA GGG GAC AAC CGA GAG CGU AGC CAC CAC CAG GAU GGC AGU GAU AAU GAG GAA
ala asn ser ser asp leu leu lys glu leu leu glu thr gly asp asn arg glu arg ser his his gln asp gly ser asp asn glu glu

| | | | | | | | | 190 | | | | | | | | | 200 | | | | | | | | | 210 |
GAA GUG AGC|<u>AAG AGA</u>|UAU GGG GGC UUC AUG AGA GGC UUA|<u>AAG AGA</u>|AGC CCC CAA CUG GAA GAU GAA GCC AAA GAG CUG CAG|<u>AAG CGA</u>|UAU
glu val ser|lys arg|tyr gly gly phe met arg gly leu|lys arg|ser pro gln leu glu asp glu ala lys glu leu gln|lys arg|tyr

| | | | | | | | | 220 | | | | | | | | | 230 | | | | | | | | | 240 |
GGG GGC UUC AUG|<u>AGA AGA</u>|GUA GGU CGU CCA GAG UGG UGG AUG GAC UAC CAG|<u>AAA CGG</u>|UAU GGA GGU UUC CUG|<u>AAG CGC</u>|UUU GCC GAG GCU
gly gly phe met|arg arg|val gly arg pro glu trp trp met asp tyr gln|lys arg|tyr gly gly phe leu|lys arg|phe ala glu ala

| | | | | | | | | 250 | | | | | | | | | 260 | | | | | |
CUG CCC UCC GAC GAA GAA GGC GAA AGU UAC UCC AAA GAA GUU CCU GAA AUG GAA|<u>AAA AGA</u>|UAC GGA GGA UUU AUG AGA UUU UAA
leu pro ser asp glu glu gly glu ser tyr ser lys glu val pro glu met glu|lys arg|tyr gly gly phe met arg phe end

UAUCUUUUCCCACUAGUGGCCCCCAGGCCCCCAGCAAGCCUCCCUCCAUCCUCCAGUGGGAAACUGUUGAUGGUGUUUUAUUUGUCAUGUGUUGCUUGCCUUGUAUAGUUGACUUCAUUGU

CUGGCAUAACUAUACAACCUGAAAACUGUCACUUUCAGGUUCUGUGCUCGUUUUUGGAGUGUUUAAGCUCAGUAUUAGUGCUUAUUGCAGCGUAUCUCGUUUUUCAUGCUAAAAAUUAGUUUUUUUG

UUAUCUUGUCUCUUUAUUUUUUGACAAACAUCCAAUAAAAUGCUUACUUGUAUAUAGAGAGAAUAAUAAAACCUGUUUACCCCCAAGUGCAUAAAAAAAA – 3'

Figure 11-17. Primary structure of human Met- and Leu-enkephalin in precursor mRNA and protein. Reproduced from M. Comb, P. H. Seeburg, J. Adelman, L. Eiden, and E. Herbert, *Nature (London)* **295,** 663–666 (1982). © 1982 Macmillan Journals Limited.

As yet it is not clear what the role is of these adrenal medulla enkephalins. Ultimately, it can be considered that since the release of these hormones is triggered by stress, they likely play a role in stress adaptation.

VII. CLINICAL ASPECTS

A tumor of the adrenal medulla chromaffin cell, known as pheochromocytoma, is characterized by sporadic hypersecretion of epinephrine. Intermittent to permanent hypertension as well as death may result. Usually such tumors can be diagnosed and removed surgically. There are no known diseases associated with hypofunction of the chromaffin cells of the adrenal medulla.

Repeated stress causes many episodes of epinephrine release from the adrenal medulla and potentiates the ability of the medulla to produce more catecholamines by the induction of constituent enzymes of epinephrine synthesis. The same stimuli cause the release of glucocorticoids from the adrenal cortex. The catecholamines constantly elevate blood glucose by breaking down glycogen through the α_1-adrenergic receptor on the hepatocyte, and glucocorticoids elevate blood glucose levels by their catabolic effects on cell membrane of many peripheral tissues, resulting in inability to extract glucose from the blood. The elevated circulating glucose evokes insulin release from the β cell of the pancreas. Constant repetition of this scenario could lead to exhaustion of the β cell and precipitation of "stress-induced" diabetes. A hallmark of this diabetes is a deficiency of tissue stores of carbohydrate. In addition, the effects on blood pressure by catecholamines have been described and may lead to permanent hypertension. In the rat the magnitude of the response to catecholamines appears to be under genetic control and spontaneously hypertensive rats show the greatest increase in plasma catecholamines during exposure to specific stresses.

β-Adrenergic receptors have been postulated to play a crucial role in asthma. A defect in β_2 receptor may be associated with the cause of this disease; however, leukotrienes (see Chapter 15) also may be of considerable importance.

Recent reports indicate that the numbers of β-adrenergic receptor sites are decreased on the chronic lymphocytic leukemia lymphocyte surface. It is postulated that these membrane alterations interfere with basic mechanisms of communication, which may underlie the disease process characterized by loss of regulation of cell division.

References

A. Books

Ben-Jonathan, N., Bahr, J. M., and Weiner, R. I., eds. (1985). "Catecholamines as Hormone Regulators," Vol. 18, Serono Symposia. Raven, New York.

Lajtha, A., ed. (1984). "Handbook of Neurochemistry," 2nd ed., Vol. 6, Receptors in the Nervous System. Plenum, New York.

Snyder, S. H. (1976). *In* "Catecholamines, Serotonin and Chemistry" (G. J. Siegel, R. W. Albers, R. Katzman, and B. W. Agranoff, eds.), 2nd ed. Little, Brown, Boston, Massachusetts.

482

B. Review Articles

Ariens, E. J. (1979). Receptors: From fiction to fact. *Trends Pharmacol. Sci.* **1,** 11–15.

Blackmore, P. F., and Exton, J. H. (1985). Mechanisms involved in the actions of calcium-dependent hormones. *In* "Biochemical Actions of Hormones" (G. Litwack, ed.), Vol. 12, pp. 215–235. Academic Press, Orlando.

Catt, K. J., Harwood, J. P., Arguiliera, G., and Dufau, M. L. (1979). Hormonal regulation of peptide receptors and target cell responses. *Nature (London)* **280,** 109–116.

Exton, J. H. (1985). Role of calcium in α-adrenergic regulation of liver function. *In* "Calcium and Cell Physiology" (D. Marme, ed.), pp. 328–344. Springer-Verlag, Berlin and New York.

Farese, R. V. (1984). Phospholipids as intermediates in hormone action. *Mol. Cell. Endocrinol.* **35,** 1–14.

Hoffman, B. B., and Lefkowitz, R. J. (1980). Radioligand binding studies of adrenergic receptors: New insights into molecular and physiological regulation. *Annu. Rev. Toxicol.* **20,** 581–608.

Iversen, L. L., ed. (1973). Catecholamines. *Br. Med. Bull.* **29,** 91–178.

C. Research Papers

Beers, M. F., Johnson, R. G., and Scarpa, A. (1986). Evidence for an ascorbate shuttle for the transfer of reducing equivalents across chromaffin granule membranes. *J. Biol. Chem.* **261,** 2529–2535.

Charest, R., Blackmore, P. F., Berthon, B., and Exton, J. H. (1984). Changes in free cytosolic Ca^{2+} in hepatocytes following α-adrenergic stimulation. *J. Biol. Chem.* **258,** 8769–8773.

Comb, M., Seeburg, P. H., Adelman, J., Eiden, L., and Herbert, E. (1982). Primary structure of the human Met- and Leu-enkephalin precursor and its mRNA. *Nature (London)* **295,** 663–666.

Holz, R. W. (1980). Osmotic lysis of bovine chromaffin granules in isotonic solutions of salts of weak organic acids. *J. Biol. Chem.* **255,** 7751–7755.

Liston, D., Patey, G., Rossier, J., Verbank, P., and Vanderhaeghen, J.-J. (1984). Processing of proenkephalin is tissue-specific. *Science* **225,** 734–737.

La Gamma, E. F., Adler, J. E., and Black, I. B. (1984). Impulse activity differentially regulates Leu-enkephalin and catecholamine characters in the adrenal medulla. *Science* **224,** 1102–1104.

Noda, M., Furutani, Y., Takahashi, H., Toyosato, M., Hirose, T., Inayama, S., Nakanishu, S., and Numa, S. (1982). Cloning and sequence analysis of cDNA for bovine adrenal preproenkephalin. *Nature (London)* **295,** 202–206.

Pazoles, C. J., Creutz, C. E., Ramu, A., and Pollard, H. B. (1980). Permeant anion activation of Mg-ATPase activity in chromaffin granules. *J. Biol. Chem.* **255,** 7853–7869.

Udenfriend, S., and Kilpatrick, D. L. (1983). Biochemistry of the enkephalins and enkephalin-containing peptides. *Arch. Biochem. Biophys.* **221,** 309–323.

Androgens

HORMONES

I. INTRODUCTION

A. General Comments

The endocrine physiology of the male and the interplay of the several hormones associated with sex determination, fetal development, and, following birth, growth and sexual maturation are still another example of the effectiveness of endocrine differentiation. Its integrated operation is dependent upon the interaction of signals—both hormonal and neural—between the central nervous system, hypothalamus, pituitary, and the testes. The two major functions of the testes are steroid hormone production and gametogenesis.

The hormones of masculinity are comprised of the gonadotropins, LH and FSH, produced by the anterior pituitary and the androgenic steroid hormones, testosterone, androstenedione, dehydroepiandrosterone, and 5α-dihydrotestosterone produced by the gonads. Also, the female steroid hormones, estradiol and estrone, play an important role in the male in certain selected circumstances.

This chapter discusses the biology and biochemistry of the androgens and gonadotropins in the male. A portion of Chapter 14 is devoted to the hormonal aspects of fertilization and sex determination.

B. Characteristics of a Male

As discussed in Chapter 14 (Section IV,A,3), both males and females in the early embryonic state are morphologically identical. It is only after the onset of sex differentiation (during the fifth and sixth weeks of fetal development) that the inevitable consequences of expression of the genetic information resident in the XY (male) or XX (female) chromosomes normally manifest themselves to convert the "indifferent" gonad into the male testes or female ovaries.

The male testes have the dual function of being responsible for both the production and release of the germ cell, the spermatozoan, as well as the biosynthesis and secretion of the key androgenic steroid hormone testosterone. This steroid hormone and others produced from it play a dominant role in the differentiation, growth, and maintenance of the sexual reproductive tissues necessary for continuation of the species, growth and maintenance of secondary sex characteristics, and the anabolic effects of skeletal muscle growth and skeletal growth.

Sexually the male can be classified by six characteristics: (1) chromosomal composition and structure; (2) gonads that are functionally and structurally testes; (3) tonic androgen production in adequate amounts; (4) external and internal genitalia that are appropriate for a male; (5) rearing as a male; and (6) self-acceptance of a male role.

Thus, the male sexual identity is the summation of the four genetically determined organic characteristics as well as the two psychological characteristics of gender role and sex of rearing. Recent studies by B. McEwen indicate the key role of both androgens and estrogens early in fetal and postnatal development for the sexual development of the brain. Also, in certain male species androgens play a key role in mediating coital behavior patterns.

II. ANATOMICAL AND MORPHOLOGICAL RELATIONSHIPS OF THE MALE REPRODUCTIVE SYSTEM

A. Introduction

The male reproductive system is comprised of the gonads (two testes), excretory ducts (epididymus, vas deferens, and ejaculatory duct), and several accessory structures (prostate, seminal vesicles, bulbourethral glands, and penis). These are diagrammed in Fig. 12-1.

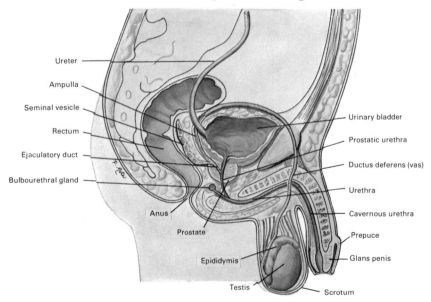

Figure 12-1. Male reproductive organs (midsagittal view).

The key steps of organogenesis of the sexually "indifferent" yet chromosomally determined male gonad are discussed in Chapter 14. The presentation of this chapter will begin with the generation of the morphologically identifiable testes.

B. The Testes

The male gonads or two testes are contained in the scrotum or pouch which is suspended outside the abdominal cavity between the thighs. The scrotum, besides housing the testes, plays an important role in temperature regulation necessary for normal testicular function. The formation of the male sex cells can optimally occur only at the scrotal temperature of 32.5°C. A key developmental step in the male, prior to birth, is the translocation of the gonads from the abdominal cavity into the scrotum; this process is androgen dependent. Failure of the testes to descend into the scrotum is termed cryptorchidism and results in sterility.

Each adult human testis is 4–5 cm long and is an ellipsoid of 35–45 g. Structurally each testis consists of the parenchyma or seminiferous tubules which are surrounded by a capsule comprised of three layers—the *tunica vaginalis*, the *tunica albuginea*, and the *tunica vasculosa* (see Fig. 12-2).

The *tunica albuginea* divides the parenchymal seminiferous tubules into lobules; these tubules are the site of production of the male sex cells, the spermatozoa; they have a total length of ~800 m (one-half mile). The seminiferous tubules are organized in a highly convoluted irregular pattern, with some blind pouches, terminating ultimately into the *tubulus recti* which in turn empties into the rete testis and the epididymal duct.

The seminiferous tubule walls are composed of germinal epithelium cells which are the site of the spermatogenesis process (discussed in Section II, E). The newly formed spermatozoa are transported through the lumen of the seminiferous tubules to the epididymus where they are stored.

The walls of the seminiferous tubules have a complex structure in that there is an array of many layers of epithelial germ cells interspersed with the Sertoli or "nurse" cells. The specialized Sertoli cells (see Fig. 12-3) line the basement membrane of the seminiferous tubules; their cytoplasm is in close contact with the innermost layer of the basement membrane which in a convoluted fashion is frequently surrounding the germ cells as they undergo their maturation process.

The Sertoli–Sertoli cell tight junctions (see Fig. 12-3) tend to form a blood–testis barrier (analogous to the blood–brain barrier) which di-

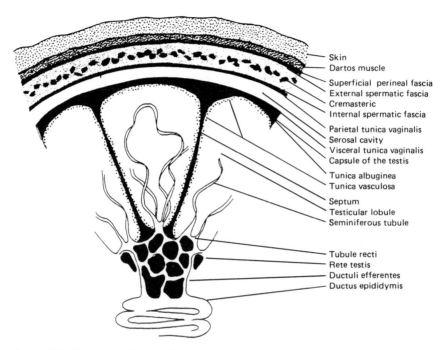

Skin
Dartos muscle
Superficial perineal fascia
External spermatic fascia
Cremasteric
Internal spermatic fascia
Parietal tunica vaginalis
Serosal cavity
Visceral tunica vaginalis
Capsule of the testis
Tunica albuginea
Tunica vasculosa
Septum
Testicular lobule
Seminiferous tubule
Tubule recti
Rete testis
Ductuli efferentes
Ductus epididymis

Figure 12-2. Schematic diagram of a testis surrounded by the scrotum. Modified from E. Steinberger, Structural consideration of the male reproductive system. *In* "Endocrinology" (L. J. DeGroot, G. F. Cahill, L. Martini, D. H. Nelson, W. D. Odell, J. T. Potts, E. Steinberger, and A. I. Winegrad, eds.), Vol. 3, p. 1502. Grune & Stratton, New York, 1979.

vides the germinal epithelium into an adluminal and basal compartment. As shown in Fig. 12-3, the basal compartment contains the immature spermatozoa or spermatogonia and the adluminal compartment the remainder of the germ cells. An important function of the blood–testis barrier is to prevent the back diffusion of autoantigens from the interior of the tubule to the bloodstream. The spermatozoa which carry surface antigens can stimulate an antibody response even in the host male. Thus, the Sertoli–Sertoli membrane barrier is an important protective mechanism. While the functions of the Sertoli cells in the adult male are not known with certainty, it is believed that they perform both a nutritive and phagocytic role, being responsible for the clearing of damaged germ cells from the seminiferous epithelium. Recently it has been demonstrated that FSH can stimulate the Sertoli cells to secrete into the seminiferous lumen an androgen binding protein (ABP).

As discussed in Chapter 14 (see Fig. 14-16), in the male fetus the Sertoli cell secretes the mullerian duct inhibitory factor which acts to

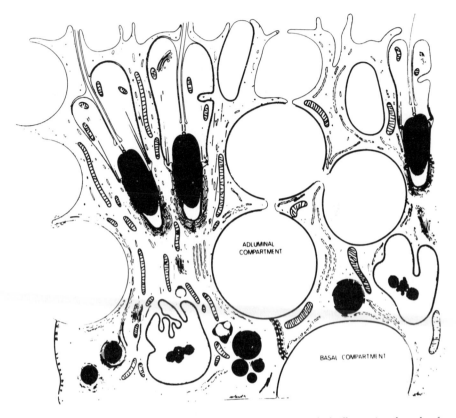

Figure 12-3. Schematic diagram of the wall of a seminiferous tubule illustrating the role of the Sertoli cells in forming a testis–blood barrier. Modified from E. Steinberger, Structural consideration of the male reproductive system. *In* "Endocrinology" (L. J. DeGroot, G. F. Cahill, L. Martini, D. H. Nelson, W. D. Odell, J. T. Potts, E. Steinberger, and A. I. Winegrad, eds.). Grune & Stratton, New York, 1979.

induce involution of the mullerian ducts and blocks the development of the uterus and fallopian tubes. Thus, the Sertoli cell has two major categories of biological action, depending upon whether it is operative in a fetal or adult testis.

The interstitial tissue which makes up 5% of the total testicular volume contains the primary endocrine cells of the testes, the Leydig cells. Leydig cells under the action of LH are the major site of production of testosterone. The Leydig cells are located in clusters that lie in the connecting tissue stroma between the seminiferous tubules. Shown in Fig. 12-4 is a schematic diagram of a Leydig cell; its structure is comparable to that of other steroid-secreting cells, particularly the lutein cells (see Fig.

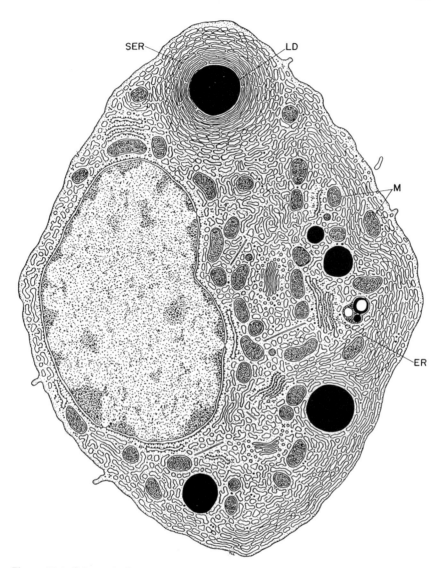

Figure 12-4. Schematic diagram of a Leydig or interstitial cell: LD, lipid droplet; M, mitochondria; ER, endoplasmic reticulum; SER, smooth-surfaced endoplasmic reticulum. Reproduced with permission from T. L. Lentz, "Cell Fine Structure," p. 253. Saunders, Philadelphia, Pennsylvania, 1971.

13-4D) of the corpus luteum. The membranes of the smooth endoplasmic reticulum are the site of conversion of pregnenolone into
testosterone.

C. The Duct System

The duct system connects each testis to the urethra and functions to
transport the mature spermatozoa during ejaculation. It is composed of
the epididymus, ductus deferens, and ejaculatory duct.

The epididymus is a small narrow structure attached to the surface of
the testis. Spermatozoa finish their maturation process as they pass
through the epididymus into the vas deferens.

The vas deferens is a 7- to 8-cm tubule connecting the epididymus
with the ejaculatory duct (see Fig. 12-1). Passage of sperm through the
vas deferens is accomplished by peristaltic contractions of smooth muscle in the duct wall.

The ejaculatory duct is located at the merger of the vas deferens and
seminal vesicles and extends through the prostate to the urethra.

D. Accessory Structures

The accessory structures include the seminal vesicles, prostate gland,
bulbourethral glands, and penis.

In adult males the two seminal vesicles are 10–20 cm in length and lie
distal to the ejaculatory duct. Under the actions of androgens they produce the mucoid secretions which constitute the major volume of the
ejaculate.

The prostate gland is a muscular organ containing 30–50 tubuloalveo-
lar glands which encompass the junction of the ejaculatory duct with the
urethra. The prostatic secretions which are highly responsive to androgens are rich in the enzyme acid phosphatase, which is a constituent
of the ejaculate.

The two bulbourethral glands, sometimes referred to as Cowper's
glands, which are 2–3 mm in diameter, secrete an alkaline mucoid solution into the urethra to neutralize the acidity and coat the urethral lining
immediately prior to the arrival of the ejaculate.

The penis, which is an external genital organ, carries the urethra to
the exterior of the body. Its erectile tissue is highly vascularized so that
when the penis is filled with blood, it is in an erect and firm state which
facilitates deposition of the spermatozoa in the female vaginal canal.

E. Spermatozoa and Semen

A mature human spermatozoon, which contains the haploid number of chromosomes including either the male, Y, or female, X, determining chromosome is ~50–60 μm long. Anatomically, the spermatozoon is composed of the head and tail (see Fig. 12-5). Under normal circumstances in the adult human ~30 million germ cells are produced per day and available for maturation over an 8- to 10-week interval into spermatozoa.

The ejaculate or seminal fluid, which normally consists of 2–3 ml, contains 100–300 million spermatozoa and a mixture of secretions from the various accessory genital glands. It is rich in fructose, ascorbic acid, prostaglandins, carnitine, and a variety of enzymes, including acid phosphatase, aminotransferases, muramidase, and dehydrogenases.

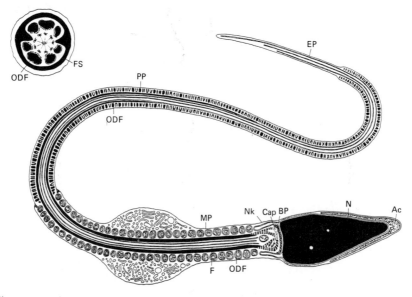

Figure 12-5. Schematic diagram of a spermatozoon. The spermatozoon consists of two principal regions: the head, containing the nucleus, and the tail, which can be subdivided into four regions: the neck (Nk), middle piece (MP), principal piece (PP), and end piece (EP). The head contains the nucleus (N) with its condensed chromatin enclosed by a nuclear envelope; the anterior portion of the nucleus is enclosed by the acrosomal cap (Ac) or acrosome. The middle piece contains elongated mitochondria wound helically around the flagellar fibers (F). As shown in the inset, the axial filament of the sperm flagellum is composed of two central single fibers surrounded by nine double fibrils (ODF). Reproduced with permission from T. L. Lentz, "Cell Fine Structure," p. 247. Saunders, Philadelphia, Pennsylvania, 1971.

III. CHEMISTRY, BIOCHEMISTRY, AND BIOLOGICAL RESPONSES

Table 12-1 tabulates the 9–10 hormones pertinent to male development and reproduction.

A. Steroid Hormones

1. Androgens

Androgens are steroid hormones that induce the differentiation and maturation of the male reproductive organs, the development of male secondary sex characteristics, and behavioral manifestations consistent with the male role in reproduction. The two most important steroid hormones of the adult male are testosterone and 5α-dihydrotestosterone. The structures of these compounds are presented in Fig. 12-6.

As reviewed in Chapter 2, the naturally occurring androgens are typically 19-carbon steroids. Testosterone is the principal male androgen produced and secreted by the testes. Also, a number of other androgen intermediates are released in low concentrations—particularly androstenedione and androstene-3β,17-diol. Table 12-2 summarizes the secretion rates, plasma levels, as well as the metabolic clearance rate of the principal sex steroids in the male.

The biochemical pathway for the production of androgens is discussed in Chapter 2. The side chain cleavage of cholesterol is confined to the mitochondria of the Leydig cells (see Fig. 2-21). The subsequent conversion of pregnenolone into testosterone requires five enzymatic reactions which are divided into two parallel pathways—one proceeding via 17-OH-pregnenolone, known as the Δ^5 pathway, and the other proceeding via 17-OH-progesterone, known as the Δ^4 pathway (see Fig. 2-23). The relative activities of the Δ^5 vs Δ^4 pathways vary among various mammalian species; in the rodent the Δ^4 pathway is predominant, while in the human testis the Δ^5 pathway is apparently dominant. All of these reactions occur in the microsomal fraction of the cell.

The hormonally active form of testosterone in the male is believed to be dihydrotestosterone (5α-DHT). Its major site of production are in the prostate, but there is also evidence for its production by the testes, skin, and submaxillary glands. The reduction of testosterone to DHT is mediated by the enzyme Δ-3-ketosteroid-5α-oxidoreductase, which requires as a cofactor NADPH. This enzyme is associated with both the microsomal as well as nuclear membranes of the prostate gland. Thus, DHT is

Table 12-1. Hormones Related to Male Development and Spermatogenesis

Hormone	Site of production	Principal target tissue	Principal biological function
Steroid hormones			
Testosterone	Leydig cells of testes	Many	Maintenance of functional male reproductive system and secondary male sex characteristics
5α-Dihydrotestosterone (DHT)	Prostate	Prostate	See Table 12–3
Androstenediol	Testes	Many	Not known with certainty
Dehydroepiandrosterone	Testes		Not known with certainty
Estradiol	Testes		
Peptide hormones			
LH	Adenohypophysis	Leydig cells	Stimulate steroidogenesis α production of testosterone
FSH	Adenohypophysis	Sertoli cells	Secretion of androgen binding protein
Gonadotropin releasing hormone (GnRH)	Hypothalamus		
Inhibin	Sertoli cells	Hypothalamus–pituitary	Feedback inhibition of FSH secretion
Prolactin	Adenohypophysis	Leydig cells	Potentiates the actions of LH

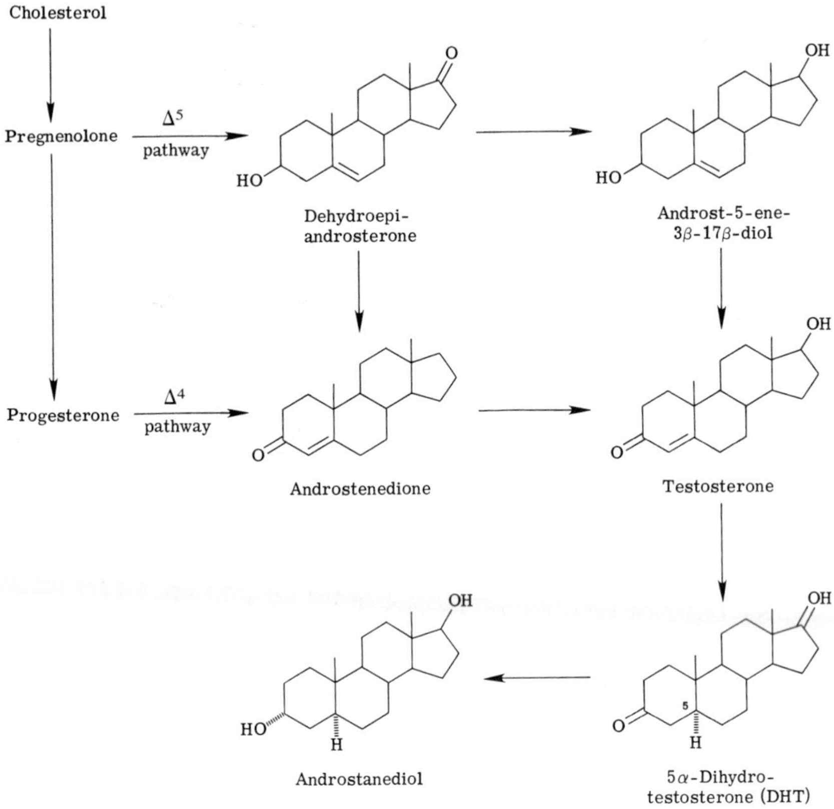

Figure 12-6. Metabolic pathway for the production of key androgenic steroids; in man the Δ^4 pathway is the major route of production of testosterone.

not transported systemically to its target tissues as are most classical steroid hormones; instead, it is generated intracellularly at its site(s) of action. Testosterone is further catabolized *in vivo* by two pathways: one operative in the liver to yield 17-ketosteroids, and the other in target tissues to produce androstanediols and androstanetriols.

In the liver, testosterone is converted to the two 17-keto compounds, androsterone and etiocholaneolone (see Fig. 2-32), which are in turn conjugated to either glucuronic acid or sulfate to yield a water-soluble form amenable to urinary excretion.

A minor pathway occurring in a number of androgen-responsive tissues (e.g., prostate) can convert DHT into androstanediols by reduction of the A ring double bond and the 3-ketone to a 3α-hydroxyl.

Table 12–2. Production Rates, Metabolic Clearance, and Plasma Levels of Sex Steroids in the Human Male

Steroid	Plasma concentration (ng/100 ml)	Testes secretion rate (μg/day)	Metabolic clearance rate[a] (liter/day)
Testosterone	700	5000	980
Androsterone-SO$_4$	43	—	—
Androstenedione	100	2500	2300
Androstane-3α,17β-diol	130	200	>1200
Dehydroepiandrosterone	504	—	—
Dihydrotestosterone (DHT)	30	50–100[b]	500
Estradiol	2–3[c]	10–15[c]	1700

[a] Metabolic clearance rate (MCR) is an estimation of the rate at which the steroid is irreversibly removed from the plasma by inactivation (further metabolism). The plasma flow through the liver is ~1500 liters/day. Abstracted from H. T. J. Makin, ed., "Biochemistry of Steroid Hormones." William Clowes & Sons, Ltd., London, 1975.

[b] Approximately 300–400 μg of DHT are estimated to be synthesized outside the testes.

[c] Most blood estradiol in the male is derived from peripheral aromatization of secreted testosterone.

The biological responses of the androgens are summarized in Table 12-3. They may be divided into four categories: (1) a growth-promoting or androgenic effect on the male reproductive tract; (2) a stimulatory or anabolic effect on body weight (skeletal muscle) and nitrogen balance; (3) development of male secondary sex characteristics; and (4) actions in the central nervous system and brain.

While it is clear that both testosterone and DHT are the predominant androgens, it has not been possible to unequivocally determine in which tissues which steroid is the primary or sole initiator; however, Table 12-3 includes some proposed assignments. Certainly it is not true that DHT is the only active androgen. Whether DHT or testosterone is the primary androgenic initiator presumably is a reflection of the tissue distribution of the 5α-reductase; however, as yet no comprehensive study has been reported.

The effects of androgens on the brain and central nervous system are complex and believed to occur as a consequence both of the metabolism of testosterone into DHT as well as estradiol. The 5α-reductase is present in the hypothalamus, midbrain, amygdala, hippocampus, cerebellum, and cerebral cortex. As yet the specific function of the localized DHT is not known; conceivably it may play a role in development of the brain and initiation of puberty. Also, testosterone, but not DHT, can be converted in specific neurons by aromatization into estradiol.

Table 12–3. Biological Responses of the Androgens

Response	Proposed androgenic mediation[a]
I. Androgenic actions on male reproductive tract	
Differentiation and growth of male reproductive tract: epididymus, prostate, seminal vesicles, vas deferens, bulbourethral glands	DHT
II. Androgenic stimulation of male secondary sex characteristics	
Growth of external genitalia (penis, scrotum)	
Deepening of voice through enlargement of larnyx and thickening of vocal cords	T
Hair, both growth and bodily distribution	
III. Anabolic actions	
Skeletal growth	
Skeletal muscle growth	T
Subcutaneous fat distribution	
Growth of accessory organs	
Prostate	DHT
Seminal vesicle	T, DHT
IV. Actions in the CNS and brain	
Differentiation of selected regions (hypothalamus, preoptic area, brain cortex)	Metabolism of T to E
Development of libido	T

[a] T, testosterone; DHT, dihydrotestosterone; E, estradiol. The proposed mediator assignments were made on the basis of the ligand selectivity of the receptor/binding protein present in the tissue in question.

2. Estrogens

As documented in Table 12-2, there are finite levels of estradiol and also estrone present in the male. Approximately 10–20% of this is generated by the testes; the remainder is produced in a variety of nonendocrine tissues including brain, liver, fat, and skin, all of which have low levels of the cytochrome P-450 aromatase necessary to transform androgens into estrogens (see Fig. 2-24). With the exception of the effects of testosterone-derived estradiol in the male brain, the biological role of the estrogens in the male is not well delineated.

B. Steroid Hormone Binding Globulin

Following their secretion from the tissue of origin, all steroid hormones are bound to one or more plasma proteins. For the sex steroids there is one plasma β-globulin protein that serves to transport both selected androgens as well as estrogens. This protein, termed steroid hormone binding globulin (SHBG), has been isolated and purified and is a glycoprotein protein with a molecular weight of 94,000. SHBG has a preference for steroids with a 17β-hydroxyl; accordingly, it binds testosterone, DHT, estradiol, but not progesterone or cortisol, with high affinity ($K_d = 1$–5×10^{-10} M). SHBG is synthesized by the liver, and its plasma levels, which are twofold greater in normal women than in men, are increased in pregnancy and hyperthyroidism.

The functions of SHBG are not clear. Since its ligands are reasonably water soluble, it cannot simply be a means of solubilization. Also, SHBG is not believed to participate directly in the mode of action of either androgens or estrogens. It has been suggested that an important function of SHBG is to provide a "reservoir" of bound hormone which could effectively dampen oscillations in the free concentrations. Because of the similarity of ligand binding sites on SHBG and the various androgen or estrogen receptors, it has also been hypothesized that the steroid plasma binding proteins may represent precursors of the target organ cellular receptors.

C. Peptide Hormones

1. Gonadotropins

The chemistry of luteinizing hormone (LH), which was formerly designated in the male as interstitial cell-stimulating hormone (ICSH), and follicle-stimulating hormone (FSH) is discussed in detail in Chapter 5. Both FSH and LH are secreted by the adenohypophysis; their release is governed in a complex fashion by gonadotropin releasing hormone (GnRH), the blood level of steroid hormones, and possibly other as yet uncharacterized factors.

(a) *Luteinizing Hormone.* The production and secretion of testosterone by the Leydig cell is under the control of LH in the adult male and by chorionic gonadotropin (hCG) in the developing male fetus. The secretion of LH is reciprocally related to the blood levels of testosterone and estradiol.

The actions of LH on the Leydig cell to stimulate testosterone are produced as a consequence of its interaction with a membrane receptor which stimulates cAMP production, and this in turn activates a cholesterol side chain cleavage pathway. A similar mechanism for LH is operative in the female corpus luteum and in both the male and female in the adrenal cortex where ACTH stimulates the production of the glucocorticoids.

(b) *Follicle-Stimulating Hormone.* FSH in the male in conjunction with testosterone acts on the Sertoli cells of the seminiferous tubule at the time of puberty to initiate sperm production. In the rat once the germinal epithelium differentiative process is established, testosterone alone can maintain viable sperm production; it is not yet certain whether this is also true in the primate. FSH interacts on the Sertoli cell with a membrane receptor which results in a concomitant increase in cAMP. This in turn then stimulates additional metabolic processes related to spermatogenesis.

d. GnRH. The secretion by the pituitary adenohypophysis of the gonadotropins FSH and LH is governed by the central nervous system–hypothalamus-mediated release of gonadotropin releasing hormone, GnRH. GnRH is a decapeptide (see Fig. 3-8) with a C-terminal glycinamide and an N-terminal pyroglutamyl residue. GnRH release by the hypothalamus stimulates the secretion and release from the adenohypophysis of LH and/or FSH.

2. Inhibin

The regulation of secretion of FSH from the adenohypophysis is only partly dependent on gonadal steroids; in addition, the protein hormone inhibin acts at the level of either the hypothalamus or pituitary to diminish the secretion of FSH. Inhibin is a hormone secreted in males by the Sertoli cells and in females by the ovarian follicles.

Inhibin is comprised of two dissimilar subunits: The α subunit is 18,000 Da and the β subunit is 14,000 Da. The primary amino acid sequences of inhibin were deduced from the complementary DNA sequences prepared from mRNA obtained from ovarian follicular fluid. The α and β subunits are cross-linked by one or more disulfide bridge(s). A more extensive description of inhibin is presented in Chapter 13 (see Fig. 13-8). As yet, it is not known whether the detailed structures of male- and female-derived inhibins are identical.

3. Prolactin

The blood levels of the adenohypophyseal hormone prolactin (PRL) in the male are only slightly lower than in the female. The chemistry of PRL is described in Chapter 5. The precise biological functions/ responsibility of PRL in the male are not yet known. However, the secretion of PRL is reduced under circumstances of androgen deficiency. It is known that there are PRL receptors on the plasma membrane of Leydig cells and that PRL can augment the stimulatory actions of LH on steroidogenesis. Some evidence also suggests that PRL has direct actions on the male reproductive tract, particularly the prostate and seminal vesicles, to increase the concentration of androgen receptors.

There are several reports of the clinical consequences of hyperprolactinemia in the male (usually a pituitary tumor); the common observation was testicular atrophy, a reduction in plasma testosterone levels, and a high incidence of impotence. All of these symptoms could be reversed by removal of the tumor.

IV. PHYSIOLOGICAL RELATIONSHIPS

A. Puberty and Sexual Development

1. General Comments

Puberty or the integral series of anatomical, physiological, and endocrinological changes occurring to produce a male competent for sexual reproduction occurs between 10 and 17 years of age in the human. The onset of puberty is believed to occur as a consequence of a change in the steady state of the prepubescent pituitary–gonadal system. It has been hypothesized that there is over years 6–10 a decrease in the feedback sensitivity of the central nervous system–pituitary axis, resulting in an increase in the secretion of GnRH, which in turn initiates the increased secretion of LH and FSH above the prepubescent low basal levels. Thus, LH secretion rises and reaches adult levels by age 15, while FSH secretion rises more slowly, achieving adult levels only by age 17. Also, in both males and females during the interval of puberty, there are intermittent bursts of both FSH and LH secretion which occur during sleep; their etiology is not known.

2. Hypothalamus–Pituitary–Leydig Cell Axis

The hypothalamus–pituitary–Leydig cell axis is diagrammed schematically in Fig. 12-7. The production and secretion of LH is governed by the medial-basal region of the hypothalamus. Destruction of the arcuate nucleus of the brain leads to a decreased secretion of both LH and testosterone. Neurons having their origins in the central nervous system impinge upon hypothalamic cells and secrete locally catecholamines, endorphins, and/or dopamine which results in the episodic production and release of GnRH into the hypophyseal portal system. The presence of GnRH on specific adenohypophyseal cell membrane receptors then results in the release of LH. The LH is transported systemically to the Leydig cells of the testes.

In the human, the Leydig cells differentiate and begin secretion of

500

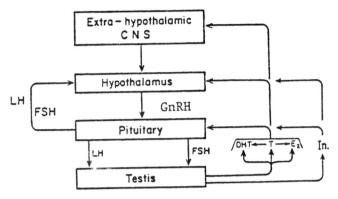

Figure 12-7. Schematic summary of the male hypothalamic–pituitary–testis axis. Modified from W. D. Odell and R. S. Swerdloff, Etiologies of sexual maturation: A model based on the sexually maturing rat. *Recent Prog. Horm. Res.* **32,** 245–288 (1976).

testosterone during the seventh week of fetal life; during the same time interval there also is an activation of the fetal pituitary secretion of LH. Then, following birth, the Leydig cells revert to a relatively undifferentiated state until they are activated at puberty.

LH-mediated stimulation of testosterone synthesis and secretion is initiated by the binding of LH to hormone-specific receptors on the outer membranes of the Leydig cell, which results in the concomitant production of cAMP inside the cell. Prolactin through binding to its Leydig cell membrane is also known to potentiate the actions of LH on testosterone production. During puberty, as a consequence of the increased secretion of LH, there results an increase in the secretion of testosterone by the Leydig cells.

The rate of testosterone biosynthesis and its secretion is positively correlated with the blood levels of LH. The secretion of the gonadotropin can be diminished by the increasing blood concentrations of sex steroids (both androgens and estrogens) which facilitate their binding to steroid receptors in the hypothalamus and pituitary; this is termed "suppressive negative feedback." As the sex steroid levels in the blood fall, LH levels can increase; this is termed the "recovery phase of negative feedback." The precise details of the feedback mechanisms are not yet clear. Since both androgens and estrogens are potentially subject to further metabolism in selected regions of the hypothalamus, it is possible that LH is a metabolite of the sex steroid rather than the parent steroid which is the initiating feedback signal. It is believed that the feedback effects on LH secretion are mediated by both influencing the amount of GnRH released by the hypothalamus as well as by changing the sensitivity of the adenohypophyseal-LH secreting cells to GnRH.

3. Hypothalamus–Pituitary–Sertoli Cell Axis

The hypothalamus–pituitary–Sertoli cell axis is diagrammed in Fig. 12-7. During puberty, due to the increased secretion of hypothalamic GnRH and FSH, there is a maturation of the Sertoli cells both in terms of their biochemical capability as well as their cellular anatomical development. Thus, the blood–testis barrier (see Fig. 12-3) forms at puberty and the Sertoli cells initiate a number of important functions, including (1) production of unique proteins, including androgen binding protein (ABP; see later); (2) nourishment of developing spermatozoa; (3) phagocytosis of damaged spermatozoa; (4) production of a bicarbonate and potassium-rich fluid used for transport of the mature sperm; and (5) production of estradiol from testosterone.

FSH actions on the seminiferous tubules are initiated by binding to specific receptors on the external plasma membrane of the Sertoli cells and result in the concomitant production inside the cell of cAMP. The mechanism(s) by which cAMP-increased protein kinase regulates Sertoli cell functions is not known.

The negative feedback loop from the Sertoli cell to the hypothalamus–pituitary to regulate FSH secretion is believed to be effected by the protein hormone, inhibin, which is postulated to be produced by the Sertoli cell. The chief evidence supporting the existence of an inhibin-like substance is that following orchiectomy (removal of the testes), FSH secretion rises. Further, this rise in FSH secretion cannot be blocked by either testosterone or estrogen administration—thus suggesting the presence of another endogenous regulating factor. As yet inhibin has not been isolated and biochemically characterized, so that details of its proposed regulating actions are not known.

B. Spermatogenesis

The process of gametogenesis in the male is termed spermatogenesis. In contrast to the comparable process in the female (oogenesis), which occurs exclusively in the embryonic phase, the process of spermatogenesis occurs from puberty throughout the bulk of adult life. Some of the other fundamental differences between the male process of spermatogenesis and female oogenesis are summarized in Table 12-4.

The overall process of the production of mature spermatozoa by the process of gametogenesis is dependent both on a specialized cellular anatomical relationship between the developing germ cells and the sur-

Table 12–4. Comparison of Male Spermatogenesis and Female Oogenesis

	Male spermatogenesis	Female oogenesis
Period of process:	After puberty throughout adulthood	Embryonic life
Number of functional germ cells produced in a lifetime:	Many trillions over a lifetime or about 30 × 10⁶/day	7,000,000 (twentieth week of fetus), 1–2 million at birth, 100–300 ova after puberty
Time required for production of a mature germ cell:	Approximately 60–65 days for sperm production followed by 10–14 days for epididymal transport	12–50 years for a mature ovum
Type of cell division:	"Even" division of cytoplasm	"Reductive" division yields production of one potential ovum and 3 polar bodies
Structural organization of the mature germ cell:	Has a specialized anatomical structure (see Fig. 12–10)	A relatively uncomplicated anatomical structure (see Fig. 13–4C)

rounding cells as well as the presence of the gonadotropins, FSH and LH. Figure 12-8 illustrates the complexity of the local cellular organization in a section of the testis. At least five cell types are involved in the overall process of spermatogenesis: (1) Sertoli cells; (2) Leydig cells; (3) developing germ cells; (4) myoepithelial cells; and (5) epithelial cells of the duct system.

The Sertoli cell is unusual in that it possesses receptors for both the steroid hormone, testosterone, as well as the peptide hormone, FSH. While both hormones are critical for the process of spermatogenesis, FSH is only mandatorily required for the maturation and testosterone-sensitizing process of the Sertoli cell that occurs during puberty. After puberty, if FSH is removed by hypophysectomy, spermatogenesis can be sustained in the rat by immediate administration of large doses of testosterone. In man, however, there is a continuing requirement for FSH along with testosterone or LH to obtain spermatogenesis.

The three most clearly documented actions of FSH on the Sertoli cell are (1) to stimulate the formation of tight junctions; (2) to inhibit the

Figure 12-8. Cellular organization of cells of the seminiferous tubules of a human testis. Leydig cells occur in clusters surrounded by several seminiferous tubules as well as capillaries. Reproduced with permission from A. K. Christensen, Leydig cells. *In* "Handbook of Physiology" (D. W. Hamilton and R. O. Greep, eds.), Sec. 7, Vol. V, pp. 57–94. Williams & Wilkins, Baltimore, Maryland, 1975.

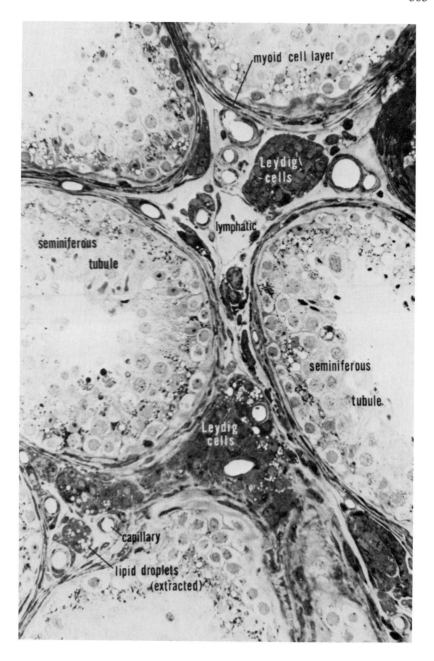

process of spermatogonium degeneration; and (3) to stimulate the production and secretion into the seminiferous tubule of ABP.

The production of ABP in the Sertoli cell is also stimulated by testosterone. In this regard, ABP is unique in that its biosynthesis is stimulated by both a peptide hormone and steroid hormone. ABP is a protein of molecular weight 90,000 which binds testosterone and DHT with high affinity ($K_d = 10^{-9}$ M). The presence of ABP ensures that the androgen concentration of the intraluminal fluid is high. The role of ABP is not known, although it may function to deliver testosterone to the seminiferous tubule and epididymus. ABP does not normally circulate in the blood.

The entire process of spermatogenesis takes place while the developing cell is completely embedded into the seminiferous tubule wall. The process involves several morphologically distinct and successive steps: (1) gonocyte–XY diploid; (2) spermatagonium–XY diploid; (3) primary spermatocyte–tetraploid XX,YY; (4) secondary spermatocyte–diploid either XX or YY; and (5) spermatid–haploid either X or Y. The total process in man requires ~64 days.

When embryonic gonocytes become committed to the future production of sperm cells, they are known as spermatogonia; they remain in this state until puberty. After puberty selected spermatogonia are converted into the primary spermatocyte which in turn can yield after meiosis two secondary spermatocytes. Secondary spermatocytes then divide again to generate two haploid spermatids. The cellular structures of a spermatocyte and spermatid are shown in Fig. 12-9.

Spermatogenesis is the process wherein the spermatid becomes gradually transformed into a mature spermatocyte. There is no evidence that either FSH or testosterone has a direct function on germ cell maturation. Rather, as emphasized in the model proposed by I. Fritz (Fig. 12-10), the androgen requirement for germinal cell differentiation results from the dependence of the germinal cells for interactions with its neighboring testicular somatic cells; in this model only the testicular somatic cells respond directly to FSH and androgen.

V. MOLECULAR ACTIONS

A. Production of Steroid Hormones

1. Steroid Biosynthesis—Actions of LH

The molecular actions of LH to stimulate steroidogenesis and the production of testosterone by the Leydig cell are analogous to that dis-

A

B

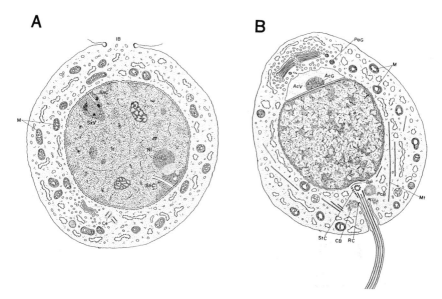

Figure 12-9. (A) Schematic diagram of a spermatocyte. The cytoplasmic structure of a spermatocyte as well as spermatogonium is unspecialized. The division of spermatozoa (giving rise to spermatocytes) and of spermatocytes is incomplete so that the daughter cells remain connected by intercellular bridges, IB. M, Mitochondria; SxV, sex vesicle; Ce, centriole. (B) Schematic diagram of a spermatid. Spermatogenesis is the process of differentiation of the spermatid into the mature sperm. As the spermatid develop, proacrosomal granules (PaG) coalesce to form a large dense acrosomal granule (AcG). Eventually the AcG spreads to cover the tip of the mature spermatozoon (see Fig. 12-5). The cell centrioles migrate from the Golgi zone, distally to give rise to the flagellum. Mt, mitochondria; AcV, acrosomal vesicle; StC, striated columns; CB, chromatoid body; RC, ring centriole; PcB, paracentriolar body. Reproduced with permission from T. L. Lentz, "Cell Fine Structure," pp. 243, 245. Saunders, Philadelphia, Pennsylvania, 1971.

cussed in Chapter 10 for the action of ACTH (see Fig. 10-11). This involves the production of cAMP as a consequence of the binding of LH to the Leydig cell plasma membrane. The cAMP then activates protein kinases which phosphorylate as yet unidentified proteins causing increased protein synthesis and ultimately increased rates of hydrolysis of cholesterol esters into cholesterol. Cholesterol is then subjected in the mitochondria to side chain cleavage to yield pregnenolone (see Fig. 2-21); this is the rate-limiting step in androgen biosynthesis.

2.) Actions of FSH

Other than the general description presented above, there is a paucity of information describing the molecular actions of FSH.

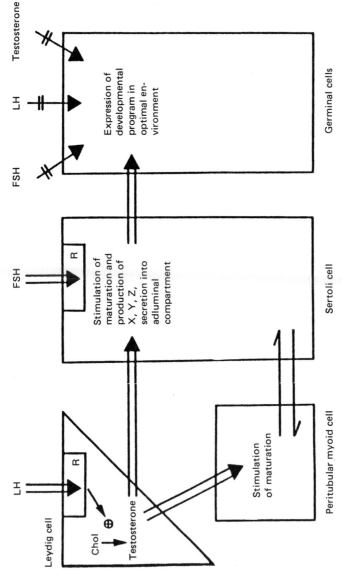

Figure 12-10. Schematic model of cellular sites of hormone action in the process of spermatogenesis. Abbreviations: Chol, cholesterol; R, receptor. This model illustrates the key interactions of the Leydig and Sertoli cells. In this scheme the diminution of estradiol production by the mature Sertoli cells permits testosterone formation to increase in response to LH. Production and secretion of X, Y, and Z by Sertoli cells refers to special products found in the tubular fluid of the seminiferous tubule, such as ABP. Modified from I. B. Fritz, Hormonal control of spermatogenesis. *In* "Biochemical Actions of Hormones" (G. Litwack, ed.), Vol. 5, pp. 249–281. Academic Press, New York, 1978.

B. Cellular Mechanisms of Action(s) of Androgens

1. Androgenic Receptors

The biological effects mediated by the androgenic steroids in the male reproductive system as well as in those tissues associated with the secondary sex characteristics (see Table 12-3) are all believed to occur as a consequence of the association of the appropriate androgen with a cytoplasmic receptor in a given target tissue. Table 12-5 tabulates the tissue distribution of androgen receptors/binding proteins. As discussed above, in some tissues dihydrotestosterone has been shown to be the initiating signal, while in other tissues it is believed to be testosterone.

The androgen receptor is localized in the cytoplasmic nuclear portions of the target cell. After association of the ligand with the protein receptor, the steroid–receptor complex associates with specific DNA domains and initiates specific gene transcription for proteins necessary for the biological response of the androgen in that particular target cell.

The most thoroughly studied system is the rat ventral prostate. The prostate cell nuclei have been shown to bind, on the average, ~2000–6000 molecules of DHT per cell nucleus. The DHT receptor has a mobility of both 7–12 S and 3–5 S in 5–20% sucrose gradients, suggesting a molecular weight for the oligomeric form of ~270,000 and a subunit molecular weight of ~70,000. The large units can be transformed into the smaller units by incubation at 20–30°C.

The anabolic actions of testosterone and its metabolites in nonreproductive tissue such as muscle, liver, kidney, and bone are as yet not as thoroughly studied. The major extragenital site of androgen action is in the skeletal muscle; the best studied system in this regard is the levator ani muscle. Current evidence indicates that in both the levator

Table 12–5. Tissue Distribution of Androgen Receptor[a,b]

I. Tissues where there are androgenic effects
    A. Male reproductive tract: testes, prostate, seminal vesicles, epididymus
    B. Secondary sex characteristic related: skin, hair follicle, cockerel comb, and wattles
    C. Brain: hypothalamus, pituitary, preoptic region, cortex
II. Tissues where there are anabolic effects: levator ani muscle, thigh muscle
III. Other tissues: kidney, uterus, submaxillary gland, bone marrow, pineal gland, sebaceous and preputial glands, androgen-sensitive tumors (Shionogi tumors)

---

[a] Abstracted from S. Liao, Molecular actions of androgens. *In* "Biochemical Actions of Hormones" (G. Litwack, ed.), Vol. 4, pp. 351–407. Academic Press, New York, 1977.
[b] Most of the entries are derived from studies carried out in either the rodent or mature chicken.

ani and kidney there is a cytoplasmic–nuclear receptor system for testosterone and that the anabolic actions of androgens are generated by mechanisms similar to that for the androgenic actions.

2. Antiandrogen Compounds

The principal antiandrogen compounds available include cyproterone acetate, α,α,α-trifluoro-2-methyl-4'-nitro-m-propionotoluide (flutamide), and 6α-bromo-17α-methyl-17β-OH-4-oxa-5α-androstane-3-one (BOMT) (see Fig. 12-11). The biological actions of these steroids result from their blocking active androgens from interacting with their target organ intracellular receptors.

Estrogens are also capable of generating antiandrogenic responses; these effects are largely mediated either by (1) inhibition of testicular androgen secretion via blocking the secretion of LH or (2) by a direct suppression of testosterone synthesis by Leydig cells.

3. Anabolic Steroids

Anabolic steroids are analogs of testosterone which mediate an array of responses in the skin, skeleton, and muscle, including nitrogen, potassium, and inorganic phosphorus retention as well as increased skeletal muscle mass. Chemically it has been possible to produce compounds that maximize the anabolic activity and minimize androgenicity. The examples of nandrolone decanoate, oxandrolone, and stanozolol are given in Fig. 12-11. The biochemical basis for their actions in muscle and skeleton are not known. Although these tissues do contain receptors for endogenous androgens, it has also been suggested that the anabolic steroids may function by competing with endogenous glucocorticoids for their receptors in these tissues.

VI. CLINICAL ASPECTS

A. Prostatic Cancer

Cancer of the prostrate is the second most frequently occurring cancer in the male in the United States. The pioneering work of the Nobel Laureate C. Huggins established the role of androgens in prostatic functions and suggested that a potentially effective management of the disease could be effected by surgical removal of the source of the testosterone (i.e., orchiectomy). This procedure was widely adopted starting in the period 1940–1956. Subsequently this procedure was replaced by

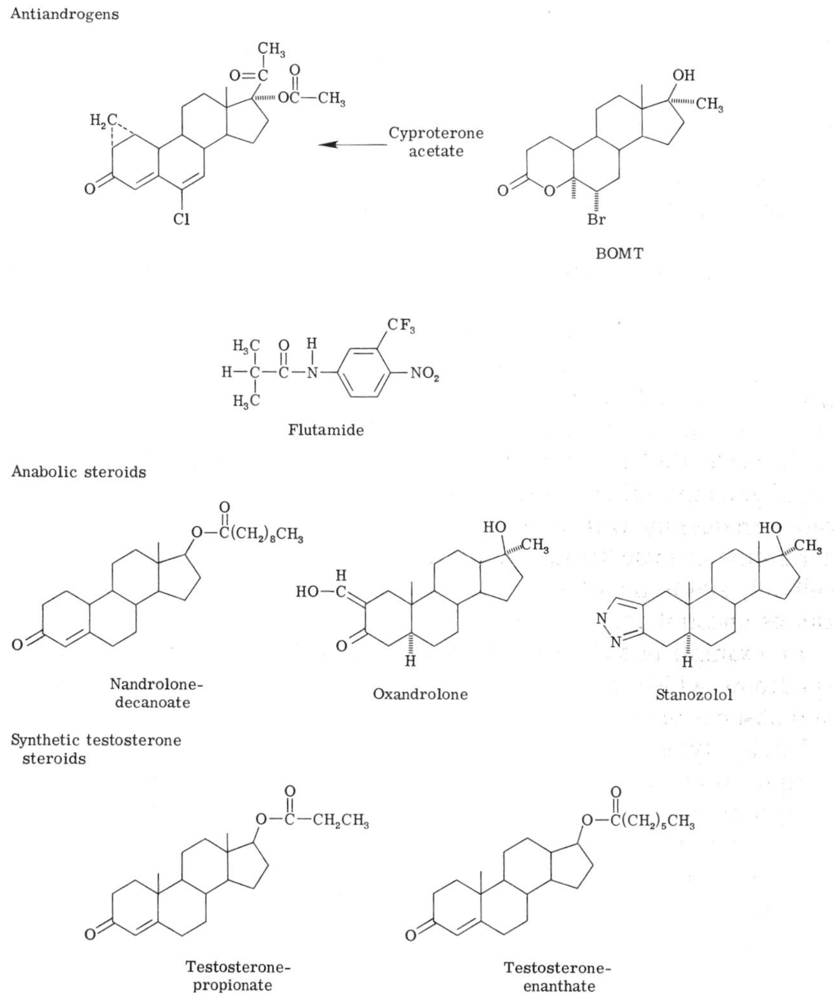

Antiandrogens

Cyproterone
acetate

BOMT

Flutamide

Anabolic steroids

Nandrolone-
decanoate

Oxandrolone

Stanozolol

Synthetic testosterone
steroids

Testosterone-
propionate

Testosterone-
enanthate

Figure 12-11. Structures of representative antiandrogens, anabolic steroids, and synthetic testosterone steroids.

treatment of the malignancy with large doses of the estrogen diethylstilbestrol. The logic was that if the growth of the tumor was dependent upon the presence of circulating androgens, this could be eliminated by estrogen feedback actions on pituitary gonadotropin secretions. Recent studies indicate that the use of an antiandrogen in combination with either small doses of estrogen or LHRH may be more efficacious in the treatment of prostate cancer, since adrenal as well as testicular androgens are blocked by this combination treatment.

B. Male Hypogonadism

Male hypogonadism is used to describe a spectrum of disorders of testicular function associated with inadequate sperm production and/or androgen secretion. The clinically observable end result may also occur as a consequence of a hypothalamic disorder, pituitary failure, or testicular disease.

Under circumstances of low gonadotropin levels, particularly LH, a wide spectrum of disorders including pituitary dwarfism, hypogonadotropic eunuchoidism (failure of appropriate gonadotropin secretion before and at puberty), and the Prader–Willi syndrome (often associated with cryptorchidism) may be encountered. Under circumstances of elevated gonadotropin production of Klinefelter's syndrome (a genetic disorder frequently with a chromosomal karotype of 47XXY), Noonan's syndrome or male Turner's syndrome (a genetic disorder), and Sertoli cell-only syndrome (the seminiferous tubules contain only Sertoli cells) can be encountered.

An example of a clinical syndrome due to absent LHRH is Kallman's syndrome which is associated with hypogonadotropic hypogonadism and absence of smell.

Finally, types IV, V, and VI of congenital adrenal hyperplasia (see Chapter 10) represent, respectively, a deficiency of the 3β-steroid dehydrogenase-Δ^5, Δ^4 isomerase (type IV), the 17α-hydroxylase (type V), and cholesterol side chain cleavage enzymes (type VI). In each instance there is a generalized inability of the steroidogenic tissue to biosynthesize androgens and accordingly there is no feedback suppression of gonadotropin secretion.

C. Cryptorchidism

Cryptorchidism, or the condition of one or two undescended testes, occurs at birth in 10% of males. Normally it is a self-correcting situation such that during the first year the testes will descend into the scrotum in all but 2–3% of males and after puberty only 0.3–0.4% of males will have either unilateral or bilateral undescended testes. If the cryptorchid state is not corrected by puberty, the exposure of the germinal epithelium to the internal body temperature will result in an impaired spermatogenesis.

D. Gynecomastia

Gynecomastia is defined as the inappropriate development of the male mammary glands. It occurs predominantly during puberty and adolescence as well as neonatal life and has been estimated to have an incidence rate of ~8 per 100,000. The pathophysiology of gynecomastia is complex and although estrogen is important for breast development (see Chapter 14), the disease is not simply explained by an estrogen excess. A further discussion of this disease state is beyond the scope of this book.

E. Male Contraception

Although the classical methods of male contraception, which include the use of condoms, interrupted coitus, and vasectomy (surgical removal of a small segment of the vas deferens), are reasonably effective, there has been a renewed interest in developing new endocrinological methods of male contraception. In principal, endocrinological approaches could have the potential of interrupting the male reproductive system in a more "natural" fashion to effectively produce a nonfertile but otherwise functionally competent state.

The use of steroids, such as testosterone enanthate or synthetic progestins, has been shown to inhibit pituitary gonadotropin secretion and thus create a condition of oligospermia or even azoospermia. Also, analogs of GnRH, which may be agonists and lead to down regulation of GnRH receptor sites or GnRH antagonists that block GnRH receptor binding, will both effectively inhibit testosterone production via the hypothalamic–pituitary axis and lead eventually to a suppression of spermatogenesis.

A third approach is to utilize drugs that act directly on the testis to inhibit spermatogenesis. Candidates here include the antiandrogen cyproterone and gossypol. Gossypol is an as yet chemically uncharacterized substance extracted from cottonseeds; it has been clinically evaluated in the People's Republic of China where it was found to block spermatogenesis without changing blood testosterone levels.

Finally, a fourth endocrinological approach is to utilize an agent that interrupts epididymal function. This has the advantage of avoiding potential adverse genetic effects, since germ cells do not divide in the epididymus. Candidates here include α-chlorohydrin, aminochlorhydrin, and a chlorinated sugar, 6-deoxy-6-chloro-D-glucose. While an effective and safe male endocrinologically based drug equivalent to the female "pill" has yet to be developed, it is to be anticipated that this will be an active area of future clinical investigations.

References

A. Books

Eik-Nes, K. B., ed. (1970). "The Androgens of the Testes." Dekker, New York.
Jeffcoate, S. L., ed. (1982). "Androgens and Anti-Androgen Therapy." Wiley, New York.
Mainwaring, W. I. P. (1977). "The Mechanism of Action of Androgens." Springer-Verlag, Berlin and New York.
Mann, T., and Mann, C. (1981). "Male Reproductive Function and Semen: Themes and Trends in Physiology, Biochemistry and Investigative Andrology." Springer-Verlag, Berlin and New York.

B. Review Articles

Baker, H. W. G., Bremner, W. J., Burger, H. G., deKretser, D. M., Dulmanis, A., Eddie, L. W., Hudson, B., Koegh, E. J., Lee, V. H., and Rennie, G. C. (1976). Testicular control of follicle-stimulating hormone secretion. *Recent Prog. Horm. Res.* **32**, 429–469.
Baranao, J. L. S., and Dylma, M. L. (1983). Gonadotropin-induced changes in the luteinizing hormone receptors of cultured Leydig cells. *J. Biol. Chem.* **258**, 7322–7330.
DeJong, F. H. (1979). Inhibin—fact or artifact. *Mol. Cell. Endocrinol.* **13**, 1–10.
Gomes, W. R., and VanDenmark, N. L. (1984). The male reproductive system. *Annu. Rev. Physiol.* **36**, 307–330.
Huggins, C. B. (1967). Endocrine-induced regression of cancers. *Science* **156**, 1050–1054.
Martin, L. (1982). The 5α-reduction of testosterone in the neuroendocrine structures: Biochemical and physiological implications. *Endocr. Rev.* **3**, 1–25.
Means, A. R., Dedman, J. R., Tash, J. S., Tindall, D. J., van Sickle, M., and Welsh, M. J. (1980). Regulation of the testis Sertoli cell by follicle-stimulating hormone. *Annu. Rev. Physiol.* **42**, 59–70.
Preslock, J. P. (1980). Steroidogenesis in the mammalian testis. *Endocr. Rev.* **1**, 132–139.
Rennie, P. S., Bruchovsky, N., and Cheng, H. (1983). Isolation of 35 androgen receptors from salt-resistant fractions and nuclear matrices of prostatic nuclei after mild trypsin digestion. *J. Biol. Chem.* **258**, 7623–7630.

C. Research Papers

Aragona, C., and Friesen, H. G. (1975). Specific prolactin binding sites in the prostate and testis of rats. *Endocrinology (Baltimore)* **97**, 677–684.
Bremner, W. J., and deKretser, D. M. (1976). The prospects for new, reversible male contraceptives. *N. Engl. J. Med.* **295**, 111–117.
Iqbal, M. J., and Johnson, M. W. (1979). Purification and characterization of human sex hormone binding globulin. *J. Steroid Biochem.* **10**, 535–540.
Kharroubi, A. T., and Slaunwhite, W. R. (1984). Hormonal regulation of prolactin receptors in male rat target tissues: The effect of hypothroidism and adrenalectomy. *Endocrinology (Baltimore)* **115**, 1283–1288.
Mason, A. J., Hayflick, J. S., Ling, N., Esch, F., Ueno, N., Ying, S.-Y., Guillenim, R., Niall, H., and Seeburg, P. H. (1985). Complementary DNA sequences of ovarian follicular fluid inhibin show homology with transforming growth factor B. *Nature (London)* **318**, 659–663.

National Coordinating Group on Male Antifertility Agents. Gossypol—A new antifertility agent for males. *Chin. Med. J. (Peking, Engl. Ed.)* [N.S.] **4,** 417–428.

Ramasharma, K., Sairam, M. R., Seidah, N. G., Chrétien, M., Manjunath, P., Schiller, P. W., Yamashiro, D., and Li, C. H. (1984). Isolation, structure and synthesis of a human seminal plasma peptide with inhibin-like activity. *Science* **223,** 1199–1202.

Rance, N. E., and Max, S. R. (1984). Modulation of the cytosolinrogen receptor in striated muscle by sex steroids. *Endocrinology (Baltimore)* **115,** 862–866.

Reyes, J., Allen, J., Tanphaichitr, N., Bellve, A. R., and Benos, D. J. (1984). Molecular mechanisms of gossypol action on lipid membranes. *J. Biol. Chem.* **259,** 9607–9615.

Viola, M. V., Fromowitz, F., Oraveg, S., Deb, S., Finekl, G., Lundy, J., Hand, P., Thor, A., and Schlom, J. (1986). Expression of *Vas* oncogene p21 in prostate cancer. *New Engl. J. Med.* **314,** 133–137.

Chapter 13

Estrogens and Progestins

I. INTRODUCTION

A. General Comments

The endocrine physiology in the female and the interplay of the many hormones associated with sex determination, conception, fetal development, birth, growth, puberty, the reproductive years (lactation), and finally the menopause beautifully illustrate the complexity and responsivity of this highly differentiated endocrine system. Its integrated operation is dependent upon the interaction of signals—both hormonal and neural—between the central nervous system (CNS), the pituitary, and the ovary (see Fig. 13-1).

The gonadotropins, follicle-stimulating hormone (FSH) and luteinizing hormone (LH), and the gonadotropin releasing hormones, particularly GnRH, are not believed to have any direct actions on bodily functions except through their specific actions on the pituitary and ovaries. In contrast to this limited sphere of action, the steroid hormones, estrogen and progesterone, have a wide range of actions in many tissues. Finally, specialized hormones such as relaxin, placental lactogen, and human chorionic gonadotropin are utilized at certain key intervals to achieve essential endocrinological responses. This chapter will discuss

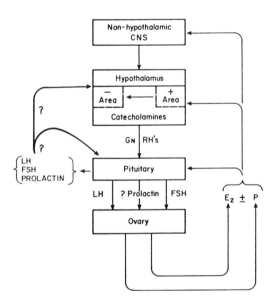

Figure 13-1. Schematic diagram of the female hypothalamic–pituitary–ovarian axis. Modified from W. D. Odell and D. C. Moyer, "Physiology of Reproduction." Mosby, St. Louis, Missouri, 1971.

the biology and biochemistry of the estrogens and progestins in the nonpregnant female; Chapter 14 will cover the hormonal relationships of pregnancy, lactation, and development, as well as the hormonal aspects of fertilization and sex determination.

B. Characteristics of a Female

As discussed in Chapter 14, the gonads of both males and females in the early embryonic stage are morphologically identical. It is only after the onset of sex differentiation (during the fifth and sixth weeks of fetal development) that the inevitable consequences of expression of the genetic information resident in the XX (female) or XY (male) chromosomes normally manifest themselves to convert the "indifferent" gonad into the fetal female ovary or male testis.

The female ovary has a dual function in being responsible for both the production and release of the germ cell or ova as well as the biosynthesis and secretion of the key steroid hormones, progesterone and estrogen. These steroid hormones play a dominant role in the differentiation, growth, and maintenance of the sexual reproductive tissues necessary for continuation of the species.

Sexually the female can be classified by six characteristics; (1) chromosomal composition and structure; (2) gonads that are functionally and structurally ovaries; (3) female sex hormone production (cyclically in the adult); (4) external and internal genitalia that are morphologically appropriate for a female; (5) rearing as a female; and (6) self-acceptance of a female role.

Thus, the female sexual identity is the summation of the four genetically determined organic characteristics as well as the two psychological characteristics of gender role and sex of rearing. Recent studies by B. McEwen indicate the key role of the sex steroid hormones (both estrogens and androgens) early in fetal and postnatal development for the sexual development of the brain.

II. ANATOMICAL AND MORPHOLOGICAL RELATIONSHIPS OF THE FEMALE REPRODUCTIVE SYSTEM

A. Introduction

The human female reproductive system is comprised of the gonads (two ovaries) and uterine tubes, a single uterus, a vagina, external genitalia, and the mammary glands. These are diagrammed in Fig. 13-2; the mammary glands are diagrammed in Fig. 14-4.

The key steps of organogenesis of the sexually indifferent yet chromosomally determined female gonad are discussed in Chapter 14. The presentation in this chapter will begin with the generation of a morphologically identifiable ovary.

B. The Ovaries

The adult human ovary is 4–5 cm in length and is almond shaped. Structurally each ovary consists of the cortex (outer) and medulla (inner) zones (see Fig. 13-3). Just below the surface layer of connective tissue is the site of generation of the follicles. Each primary follicle contains one central germ cell or oogonium which is surrounded by a layer of epithelial cells. Surrounding the follicular cells, but separated by a basement membrane, are the *theca externa* cells. The medulla comprises the central region of the ovary which is devoid of follicles. The normally functioning ovary undergoes a series of profound changes which are essential for female development, puberty, reproduction, and the menopause.

The ovarian follicle consists of a large round oocyte surrounded by

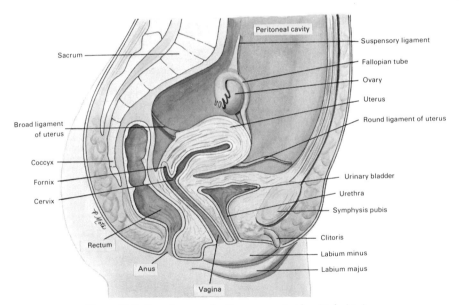

Figure 13-2. Female reproductive organs (midsagittal view).

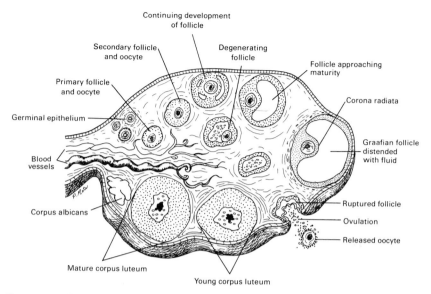

Figure 13-3. Schematic diagram of the ovary. The sequence of events necessary for the origin, growth, and rupture of a typical ovarian/graafian follicle and the concomitant formation and subsequent regression of the corpus luteum is presented. The sequence should be followed clockwise around the ovary beginning with the germinal epithelium at 10 o'clock.

follicular cells. Figure 13-4A presents a diagram of a typical follicular cell and Fig. 13-4B a diagram of a *theca interna* cell. Prior to ovulation, the *theca interna* cells and the follicular cells collaborate to biosynthesize estrogens.

The process of gametogenesis in the female is termed oogenesis. In contrast to the comparable process in the male (spermatogenesis), which is initiated in puberty and continues throughout the bulk of adult life, the process of germ cell production in the female occurs exclusively in embryonic life. During embryogenesis the oogonia or primordial germ cells available for a lifetime of ovulation are produced (see also Table 12-4 for other female/male comparisons). The polar bodies contain the same number of chromosomes as the primary or secondary oocytes; however, they have virtually no cytoplasm. During the meiotic division which generated the polar body, the bulk of the cytoplasm was apportioned to the oocyte. By the twentieth week of gestation there are ~7 million mitotic germ cells in each ovary. These germ cells then cease dividing by mitosis; some become atretic while others mature to the oogonia stage and proceed by meiotic division to the leptotene or ar-

A

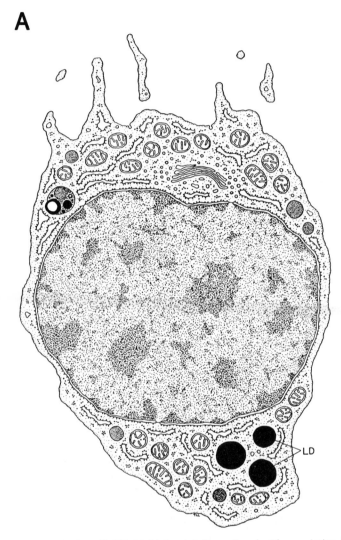

LD

Figure 13-4. (A) Follicular cell. LD, Lipid droplet. Reproduced with permission from T. L. Lentz, "Cell Fine Structure," p. 271. Saunders, Philadelphia, Pennsylvania, 1971. (B) Theca interna cell. LD, Lipid droplet. Reproduced with permission from T. L. Lentz, "Cell Fine Structure," p. 273. Saunders, Philadelphia, Pennsylvania, 1971. (C) Mature primary oocyte. G, Multiple Golgi complexes; CA, compound aggregates; AL, annulate lamellae; V, vesicles; Fl, wavy filaments; Nl, nucleolus. Reproduced with permission from T. L. Lentz, "Cell Fine Structure," p. 269. Saunders, Philadelphia, Pennsylvania, 1971. (D) Lutein cell of the corpus luteum. ER, Endoplasmic reticulum; M, mitochondria; LD, lipid droplet; SER, smooth endoplasmic reticulum. Reproduced with permission from T. L. Lentz, "Cell Fine Structure," p. 275. Saunders, Philadelphia, Pennsylvania, 1971.

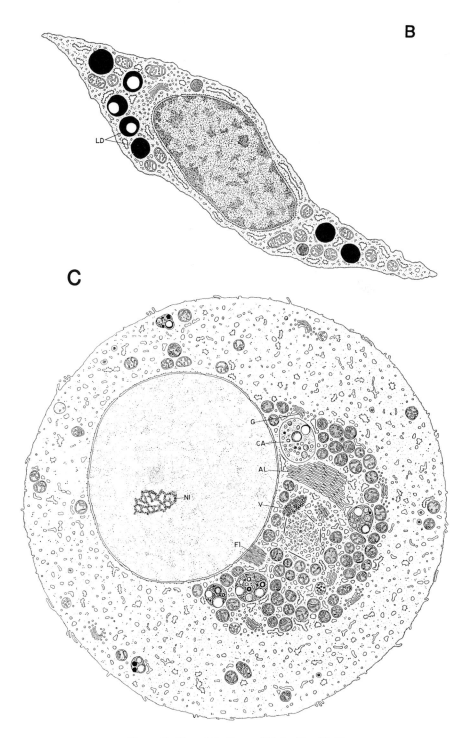

Figure 13-4B and C. See p. 522 for Fig. 13-4D.

D

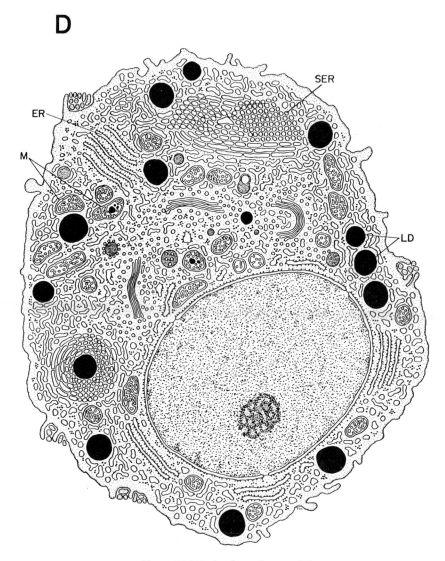

Figure 13-4D. See legend on p. 520.

rested prophase stage. These individual oogonia become surrounded by mesenchymal cells to form the primary follicles. By birth the number of follicles in an ovary number only 1–2 million; this number then decreases by further atresia and cell death so that by puberty there are only 100,000–300,000 oogonia in follicles to support the monthly ovulatory cycles over the next 35–40 years. These oogonia continue in the leptotene (arrested prophase) state until a limited number are selected by an as yet poorly understood endocrine process for further maturation which leads to ovulation and release of one mature ovum per month.

Ovulation of a single ovum each month requires only about a total of 400 oogonia over the 30 to 40-year period of reproductive fertility. At the time of the menopause the number of viable oogonia in the ovary is virtually zero. These events are summarized in Fig. 13-5. It is interesting that the ovum which is ultimately fertilized is the product of an intense selection procedure; there is a ratio of atresia-to-selection of ~20,000:1. Figure 13-4C presents a schematic diagram of a single oocyte.

During follicular development just prior to ovulation, the primary oocyte undergoes a meiotic or reductive division so that the number of chromosomes is reduced by one-half. This yields the secondary oocyte which contains 22 autosomes, one X sex chromosome, and the bulk of the cell cytosol; in addition, a polar body or polycyte is formed which also has 22 autosomes, one sex chromosome, and very little of the cell cytosol.

C. The Corpus Luteum

At the site of ovulation where the mature follicle ruptures and releases the ovum, the cells comprising the follicle under the actions of LH enlarge and differentiate into lutein cells (see Fig. 13-4D); as a consequence a yellowish substance (lutein) accumulates in the cytoplasm. The lutein cells are derived by maturation from both the *theca interna* and follicular cells. These cells are the principal site of production of progesterone and estrogen after ovulation. Subsequently capillaries grow into these cells, giving rise to the corpus luteum, a typical endocrine organ. In the human, the corpus luteum may range in size from 1.5 to 4 cm.

If the released oocyte is not fertilized within 1 to 2 days, then the corpus luteum will continue to increase in size for 10–12 days. This is then followed by virtual total regression of the gland to produce a small white ovarian scar known as the corpus albicans and concomitant cessation of progesterone and estrogen secretion (see Fig. 13-3).

If the released oocyte is fertilized, the corpus luteum continues to grow and function for the first 3 months of pregnancy. Then it slowly

524

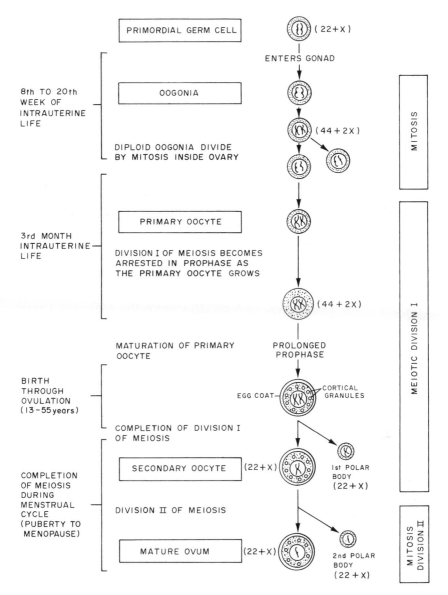

Figure 13-5. The meiotic processes in germ cells in women as relates to their age and sexual development. Modified from W. D. Odell, The reproductive system in women. *In* "Endocrinology" (L. J. DeGroot, G. F. Cahill, L. Martini, D. H. Nelson, W. D. Odell, J. T. Potts, E. Steinberger, and A. I. Winegrad, eds.), Vol. 3, p. 1385. Grune & Stratton, New York, 1979.

regresses, leaving a white scar on the ovary. The progesterone from the corpus luteum is essential for maintenance of the first 2 months of pregnancy; after this time the production of progesterone by the placenta is adequate for the continued maintenance of pregnancy.

D. The Fallopian Tubes

The uterine tubes are also variously referred to as fallopian tubes or oviducts. Each tube is 11–12 cm long and extends from the trumpet-shaped end, which is in contact with the ovary, down to the proximal end which penetrates the uterine wall (see Fig. 13-2). During the ovulatory process the many small finger-like projections or fimbriae of the ciliated cells (see Fig. 13-6A) on the inner surface of the fallopian tubes actively massage or undulate to aid in the translocation of the released mature oocyte down to the uterus. During the tubular passage of the oocyte, if it is not fertilized, it will eventually disintegrate and disappear; the biochemical/endocrine basis of these changes is not yet known.

If the oocyte becomes fertilized, it promptly completes its mitotic division and becomes a zygote. Usually the zygote will reach the uterus in 4–5 days where it will implant and continue to develop during pregnancy. If the zygote fails to reach the uterus, the woman is said to be subject to an ectopic pregnancy.

E. Uterus

In the nonpregnant adult woman the uterus is a muscular, thick-walled, pear-shaped organ 5 cm wide × 7.5 cm long × 2.5 cm thick. The cavity of the uterus communicates below with the vagina and above with the fallopian tubes.

The uterine wall is comprised of three chief layers: (1) the outer or perimetrium; (2) the middle or myometrium; and (3) the inner or endometrium.

The endometrium is a mucous membrane composed of two layers: the thin, basal layer and the outer functional layer. The functional layer changes dramatically under hormonal influence during the menstrual cycle and is lost almost completely during the process of menstruation. Figure 13-6B presents a schematic diagram of an endometrial epithelium cell. In the secretory phase of the menstrual cycle (14–28 days) the cells are quite tall and columnar with numerous microvilli.

The volume of the uterine cavity changes in capacity from 2–5 ml before pregnancy to 5000–7000 ml at the term of pregnancy; the increase

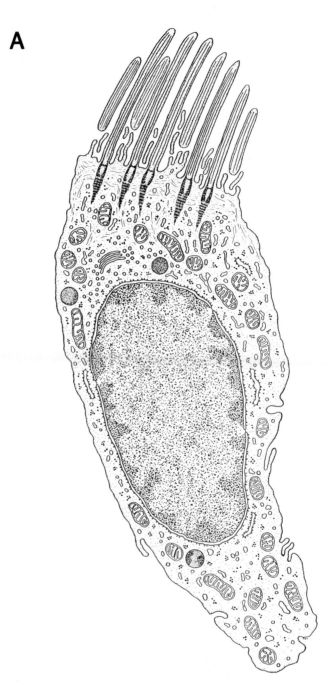

Figure 13-6. (A) A ciliated cell present on the inner surface of the fallopian tubes. Reproduced with permission from T. L. Lentz, "Cell Fine Structure," p. 279. Saunders, Philadelphia, Pennsylvania, 1971. (B) An endometrial epithelial cell of the human uterus. Gly, Glycogen granules; NE, nuclear envelope; Nl, nucleoli; NCS, nuclear channel system;

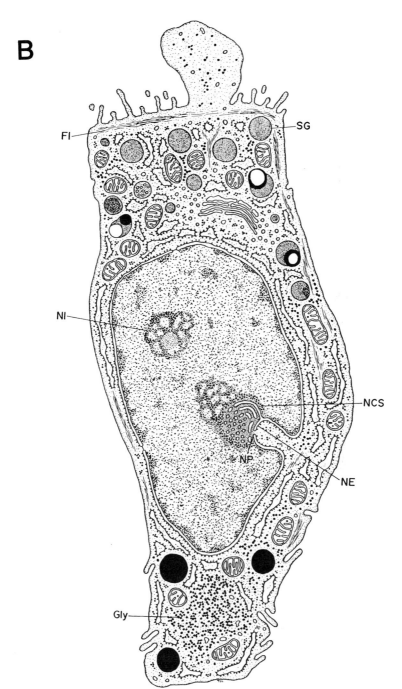

B

FI — SG

NI

NCS

NP

NE

Gly

NP, nuclear pore; SG, secretory granule; Fl, wavy filaments. Reproduced with permission from T. L. Lentz, "Cell Fine Structure," p. 281. Saunders, Philadelphia, Pennsylvania, 1971.

in uterine mass is from 60 g at puberty to 1000 g at the end of pregnancy, which is a 16-fold increase. The primary stimulus for the growth of the myometrium during pregnancy is estrogen produced by the placenta.

F. Vagina

The vagina is a 9-cm membranous tube which extends from the lower portion or cervix of the uterus downward and forward to the external opening in the vestibule (see Fig. 13-2). The wall of the vagina is composed of fibroelastic tissue and smooth muscle which is lined with a mucous membrane formed of squamous epithelial cells. These cells are quite responsive to estrogen and their physical appearance under the light microscope changes corresponding to the phase of the ovulatory cycle.

The Papanicolaou test, or Pap smear, which consists of a light microscopic examination of cells obtained painlessly from the vagina and cervix of the uterus, is an important diagnostic test which is of considerable clinical importance in the early diagnosis of cancer of the uterus. The foreign cancerous cells can easily be distinguished from the regular uniform appearance of the epithelial cells.

The description of the anatomical organization of the mammary glands and the placenta is presented in Chapter 14.

III. CHEMISTRY, BIOCHEMISTRY, AND BIOLOGICAL RESPONSES

Table 13-1 tabulates the 13–15 hormones pertinent to female development, reproduction, and lactation.

A. Steroid Hormones

1. Structural and Metabolic Relationships

The two most important steroid hormones of the adult female are estradiol and progesterone. In addition, estrone, estriol, and dehydroepiandrosterone play important roles in pregnancy. The structures of these compounds are presented in Fig. 13-7.

As reviewed in Chapter 2, the naturally occurring estrogens are typically 18-carbon steroids which have an aromatic A ring with a phenolic hydroxyl. The ovarian follicular cell in the nonpregnant female is the

Table 13–1. Hormones Related to Female Development, Reproduction, and Lactation

Hormone	Site of production	Principal target tissue	Principal biological function
Steroid hormones			
Estradiol-17β	Ovary and follicle	Uterine endometrium	Cell proliferation
Estrone	Placenta	—	—
Dehydroepiandrosterone sulfate (DHEA)	Fetal adrenal	—	—
Estriol (from DHEA sulfate)	Placenta	—	—
Progesterone	Corpus luteum	Uterine endometrium, mammary gland	Prepare for implantation of the blastocysts and development of mammary alveolar system
Peptide hormones (of both the nonpregnant and pregnant/lactating states)			
FSH	Adenohypophysis	Ovarian granulosa and thecal cells	Maturation of ovarial follicle and stimulation of estrogen production
LH	Adenohypophysis	Corpus luteum	Stimulate progesterone production
Inhibin	Follicle granulosa cell	Hypothalamus/pituitary	To participate in feedback inhibition of FSH secretion
Prolactin (of the pregnant/lactating states)	Adenohypophysis	Mammary tissue	Stimulate milk production
Human chorionic gonadotropin	Trophoblast and placenta	Maternal corpus luteum	Stimulate progesterone production
Human placental lactogen (HPL) [also known as human chorionic somatomammotropin (HCS)]	Trophoblast and placenta	Maternal tissue	To produce peripheral insulin resistance in the mother
Relaxin	Ovary	Uterine cervix	Softening of uterine cervix
Oxytocin	Neurohypophysis	Uterus and mammary tissue	Milk release
Gonadotropin releasing hormone (GnRH)	Hypothalamus	Adenohypophysis	Stimulation of release of FSH and LH
Other			
Prostaglandins	Fetus	Uterus	—

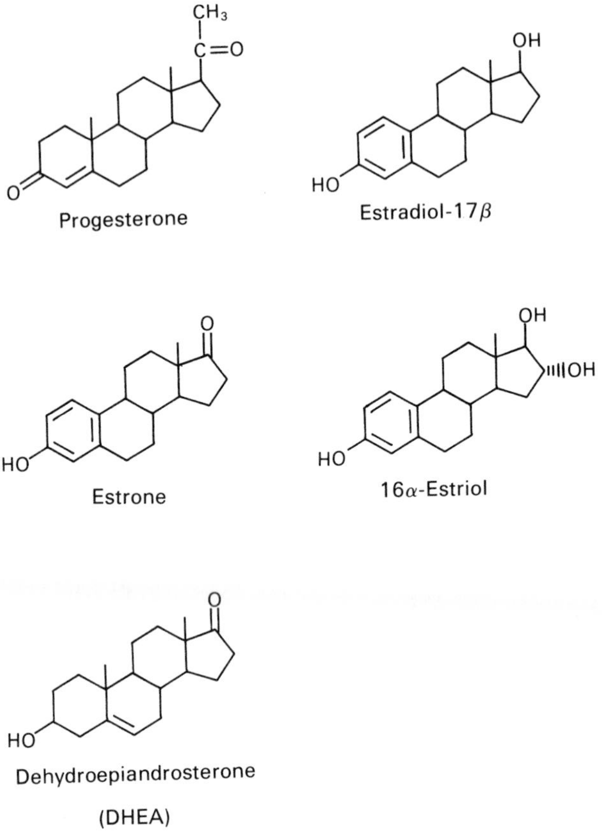

Figure 13-7. Structures of the important steroid hormones for the female (see also Figs. 2-21 and 2-24).

cellular site of production of estradiol. Also, substantial quantities of estrone may be secreted by the ovarian follicular cell as well as smaller quantities of estradiol-17α, 16α-estriol, and 6α-hydroxyestradiol-17β. Figure 2-24 reviews the pathway of biosynthesis of the principal estrogens in the nonpregnant female.

In the pregnant female the principal estrogen is estriol; it has a biological activity approximately equivalent to estradiol-17β. Estriol is synthesized in the placenta from the precursor dehydroepiandrosterone sulfate, which is provided by the adrenal cortex of the fetus (see Fig. 14-11).

As reviewed in Chapter 2, the naturally occurring progesterones have 21 carbons with an oxo functionality on both C-3 and C-20. The principal progestin produced by the corpus luteum is progesterone. Also, small quantities of 20β-hydroxyprogesterone, 10α-hydroxyprogesterone, and 17α-hydroxyprogesterone are secreted. Figure 2-21 reviews the pathways of biosynthesis of the principal progestins in the nonpregnant female (see also Fig. 13-7). Progesterone plays an indispensable role in the maintenance of pregnancy (see Fig. 14-10).

2. Secretion Rates

The secretion rates of the various steroids produced by the ovaries and corpus luteum have been estimated either by (1) careful determination of their concentration in the periphery and ovarian vein coupled with a measurement of the ovarian blood flow or (2) by use of radio-isotopes.

Table 13-2 tabulates the changes that occur in the secretion rate, plasma concentration, and metabolic clearance rates of the principal steroids produced by the ovarian follicles and corpus luteum throughout the various phases of the human menstrual cycle. It is apparent that

Table 13–2. Production Rates, Metabolic Clearance, and Plasma Levels of Steroid Hormones Produced by the Human Ovaries[a]

	Phase of menstrual cycle	Plasma concentration (ng/100 ml)	Ovarian secretion rate (mg/day)	Metabolic clearance rate[b] (liter/day)
Estradiol-17β	Early follicular	6	0.7	
	Late follicular	30–60	0.4–0.8	1300
	Midluteal	20	0.3	
Estrone	Early follicular	4	0.8	
	Late follicular	15–30	0.3–0.6	2200
	Midluteal	10	0.2	
Progesterone	Follicular	50–100	1.5	2200
	Midluteal	1000–1500	24	
17-OH-Progesterone	Early follicular	3	0.2	2000
	Late follicular	200	3–4	
Androstenedione	—	130–160	1.3	2000
Testosterone	—	35	—	700
Dehydroepiandro-sterone	—	400–500	2.0	1000

[a] Abstracted from G. E. Tagatz and E. Gurpide, Hormone secretion by the normal human ovary. *In* "Handbook of Physiology" (R. O. Greep and E. B. Astwood, eds.), Sect. 7, Vol. II, Part 1, pp. 603–613. Am. Physiol. Soc., Bethesda, Maryland, 1973.

[b] Metabolic clearance rate (MCR) is an estimation of the rate at which the steroid is irreversibly removed from the plasma by inactivation (further metabolism). The plasma flow through the liver (a frequent site of steroid catabolism) is ~1500 liters/day.

the actions of the gonadotropins, FSH and LH, have dramatic effects on the steroid-metabolizing enzymes of these tissues. In the plasma compartment the estrogens are transported by a specific plasma protein, the steroid hormone binding globulin (SHBG), and the progestins by the plasma protein termed the corticosteroid binding globulin (CBG). The biochemistry of CBG is described in Chapter 10 while SHBG is given in Chapter 12. Both proteins effectively reduce the "free" concentration of both classes of steroids.

B. Peptide Hormones

As summarized in Table 13-1, a family of peptide hormones is associated with female reproduction. Those strictly associated with pregnancy and lactation, for example, human chorionic gonadotropin, prolactin, human placental lactogen, oxytocin, and relaxin, will be discussed in Chapter 14.

1. Gonadotropins

The chemistry of FSH and LH is discussed in detail in Chapter 5. Both FSH and LH are secreted by the adenohypophysis; their release is governed in a complex fashion by gonadotropin releasing hormone (GnRH), the level of circulating steroid hormones, and possibly other as yet uncharacterized factors. The regulation of the secretion of FSH and LH as well as a description of their biological responses are given in Section IV, B.

2. GnRH

The secretion by the pituitary adenohypophysis of the gonadotropins FSH and LH is governed by the central nervous system (CNS) hypothalamus-mediated release of gonadotropin releasing hormone, GnRH. GnRH is a decapeptide (see Fig. 3-8) with an N-terminal pyroglutamyl residue and a C-terminal glycine amide. GnRH release by the hypothalamus results in an increased secretion of both FSH and LH by the appropriate cells of the adenohypophysis. The secretion of GnRH by the hypothalamus is governed by a complex interaction of CNS electrical signals as well as by the ambient concentration of estrogen and progesterone. Various chemically synthesized analogs of GnRH have been found to be useful in the clinical management of problems of female infertility and both female and male contraception.

3. Inhibin

Evidence has accumulated that the secretion of FSH from the adenohypophysis is regulated not only be gonadal steroids, but also by a protein hormone termed inhibin. Inhibin is a protein secreted in females by the ovarian follicles and in males by the Sertoli cells; it feeds back at either the hypothalamus or pituitary to diminish the secretion of FSH.

The team of R. Guillemin, H. Niall, and co-workers has established the structure of inhibin through application of recombinant DNA techniques to mRNA obtained from porcine follicular fluid. Inhibin is composed of two dissimilar subunits; the α subunit is a 134-amino acid residue (18,000 Da) and the β subunit is 116 residues (14,000 Da) (see Fig. 13-8). The mature inhibin α and β subunits contain seven and nine cysteine residues, respectively. Alignment of these residues indicates that both subunits have a similar distribution of cysteine residues; this suggests that both subunits may be derived from a common ancestral gene.

Both subunits of mature inhibin are derived from precursor prohormone species. Thus, the α subunit's primary transcript contains 364 amino acids, while the β subunit's primary transcript contains 424 amino acids. Both the mature α and β subunits lie at the extreme carboxyl end of their respective prohormone species. Each mature subunit is preceded by either two (α) or five (β) arginines which constitute the cleavage sites for proteolytic release of the mature subunits. It is known that the α and β subunits of biologically active inhibin are linked by disulfides bridges which suggests that their structure is more similar to immunoglobulins than the dimeric glycoprotein hormones TSH, FSH, or LSH.

Quite surprisingly, a structural homology was found between the amino acid sequence of inhibin and the primary amino acid sequence of human transforming growth factor-β (TGF-β). Both their peptide size as well as the distribution of nine cysteine residues were strikingly similar; also, 33 residues of the inhibin β subunit were identical to TGF-β. At this point, it is not clear why such homologous proteins should be engaged in seemingly unrelated activities. It is possible to speculate that by analogy with the growth factor activities of TGF-β that inhibin functions as an autocrine or paracrine growth regulator within gonadal tissue as well as regulating the secretion of FSH.

IV. PHYSIOLOGICAL RELATIONSHIPS

A. Puberty and Sexual Development

Puberty, or the time interval at which anatomical, physiological, and endocrinological changes occur to develop a female competent for sexu-

A

```
                                                                    1                                        10
                                                                    met trp pro gln leu leu leu leu leu leu ala pro
  1  TGTGGGGCAGACCCTGACAGAAGGGGCACAGGGCTGGGTGTGGGTTCACCGTTGGCAGGGCCAGGTGAGCT ATG TGG CCT CAG CTG CTC CTC TTG CTG TTG GCC CCA

          20                                      30                                       40
     arg ser gly his gly cys gln gly pro glu leu asp arg glu leu val leu ala lys val arg ala leu phe leu asp ala leu gly pro
108  CGG AGT GGG CAT GGC TGC CAG GGC CCG GAG CTG GAC CGG GAG CTT GTC CTG GCC AAG GTG AGG GCT CTG TTC CTG GAT GCC TTG GGA CCC

          50                                      60                                       70
     pro ala val thr gly glu gly gly asp pro gly val arg arg leu pro arg arg his ala val gly gly phe met arg arg gly ser glu
198  CCG GCA GTG ACT GGG GAA GGT GGG GAT CCT GGA GTC AGG CGT CTG CCC CGA AGA CAT GCT GTG GGG GGC TTC ATG CGC AGG GGC TCT GAG

          80                                      90                                      100
     pro glu glu glu asp val ser gln ala ile leu phe pro ala thr gly ala cys gly asp glu pro ala ala gly glu leu ala arg
288  CCC GAG GAG GAG GAT GTC TCC CAG GCC ATC CTT TTC CCG GCT ACA GGT GCC CGC TGT GGG GAC GAG CCA GCT GCT GGA GAG CTG GCC CGG

          110                                     120                                     130
     glu ala glu glu gly leu phe thr tyr val phe arg pro ser gln his thr his ser arg gln val thr ser ala gln leu trp phe his
378  GAG GCT GAG GAG GGC CTC TTC ACA TAT GTA TTC CGG CCG TCC CAG CAC ACA CAC AGC CGC CAG GTG ACT TCA GCT CAG CTG TGG TTC CAC

          140                                     150                                     160
     thr gly leu asp arg gln gln gly met ala ala ala asn asn ser ser gly pro leu leu asp leu leu ala leu ser ser arg gly pro val ala
468  ACG GGA CTG GAC AGA CAG GGG ATG GCA GCC GCC AAT AGC TCT GGG CCC CTG CTG GAC CTG CTG GCA CTA TCA TCC AGG GGT CCT GTG GCT

          170                                     180                                     190
     val pro met ser leu gly gln ala pro pro arg trp ala val leu his leu ala ala ser ala leu pro leu leu thr his pro val leu
558  GTG CCC ATG TCA CTG GGC CAG GCG CCC CCT CGC TGG GCT GTG CTG CAC CTG GCC GCC TCT GCC CTC CCT TTG TTG ACC CAC CCA GTC CTG

          200                                     210                                     220
     val leu leu leu arg cys pro leu cys ser cys ser ala arg pro glu ala thr pro phe leu val ala his thr arg ala arg pro pro
648  GTG CTG CTG CTG CGC TGT CCT CTC TGT :CC TGC TCA GCC CGG CCC GAG GCC ACC CCC TTC CTG GTG GCC CAC ACT CGG GCC AGG CCA CCC

                                      ⟶ α subunit       240-                                       250
     ser gly gly glu arg ala arg arg ser thr ala pro leu pro trp pro trp ser pro ala ala leu arg leu leu gln arg pro pro glu
738  AGC GGA GGG GAG AGG GCC CGA CGC TCC ACC GCC CCT CTG CCC TGG CCT TGG TCC CCC GCC GCG CTG CGC CTG CTG CAG AGG CCC CCG GAG

          260                                     270                                     280
     glu pro ala val his ala asp cys his arg ala ser leu asn ile ser phe gln glu leu gly trp asp arg trp ile val his pro pro
828  GAA CCC GCT GTG CAC GCC GAC TGC CAC AGA GCT TCC CTC AAC ATC TCC TTC CAG GAG CTG GGC TGG GAC CGG TGG ATC GTG CAC CCT CCC

          290                                     300                                     310
     ser phe ile phe his tyr cys his gly gly cys gly leu pro thr leu pro asn leu pro leu ser val pro gly ala pro pro thr pro
918  AGT TTC ATC TTC CAC TAC TGT CAC GGG GGC TGC GGG CTG CCG ACC CTG CCC AAC CTG CCC CTG TCT GTC CCT GGG GCC CCC CCT ACC CCT

          320                                     330                                     340
     val gln pro leu leu leu val pro gly ala gln pro cys cys ala ala leu pro gly thr met arg ser leu arg val arg thr thr ser
1008 GTC CAG CCC CTG TTG TTG GTG CCA GGG GCT CAG CCC TGC TGC GCT GCT CTC CCG GGG ACC ATG AGG TCC CTA CGC GTT CGC ACC ACC TCG

          350                                     360      364
     asp gly gly tyr ser phe lys tyr glu thr val pro asn leu leu thr gln his cys ala cys ile OC
1098 GAT GGA GGT TAC TCT TTC AAG TAC GAG ACG GTG CCC AAC CTT CTC ACC CAG CAC TGT GCC TGC ATC TAA GGGTGTCCCGCTGGTGGCCGAGCTCCC

1194 ACAGGCACCAGCCTGGAGGAAGGCAGAGTTCCCACCTCCCCTTTCCTTCCGCCTCTCCGCCTGGAGGCTCCCCTCCCTGTCCGCCCCTGTCCCATGGGTAATGTGACAATAAACAGCAT

1312 AGTGCAGATGACTCGGTGCGCAAAAAAAAA
```

Figure 13-8. Porcine inhibin amino acid sequence (derived from cDNA nucleotide sequence) for (A) the α subunit and (B) the β subunit. Nucleotides are numbered at the left and amino acids are numbered throughout. (A) The amino acid sequence underlined was used to design a long synthetic DNA probe. The 364 amino acids of the pro-α subunit includes a hydrophobic signal sequence, a proregion, and the mature α chain (amino acid residues 231–364). The two potential N-linked glycosylation sites are shown by open bars. The AATAA polyadenylation signal at the 3' end of the mRNA is underlined. (B) Two forms of the porcine β subunit were evaluated, namely, β_A and β_B. Nucleotide numbers on the left are for β_A cDNA sequences and amino acid numbers are for β_A precursor residues. The β_B sequence is shown underneath the β_A sequence and is aligned with it for maximum homology. Regions containing identical amino acid residues are boxed. Potential glycosylation sites are shown by open bars. Modified with permission from Figs. 1 and 2 of A. J. Mason, J. S. Hayflick, N. Ling. F. Esch, N. Ueno, S. Y. Ying, R. Guillemen, H. Niall, and P. H. Seeburg, *Nature (London)* **318,** 659–663 (1985). © 1985 Macmillan Journals Limited.

B

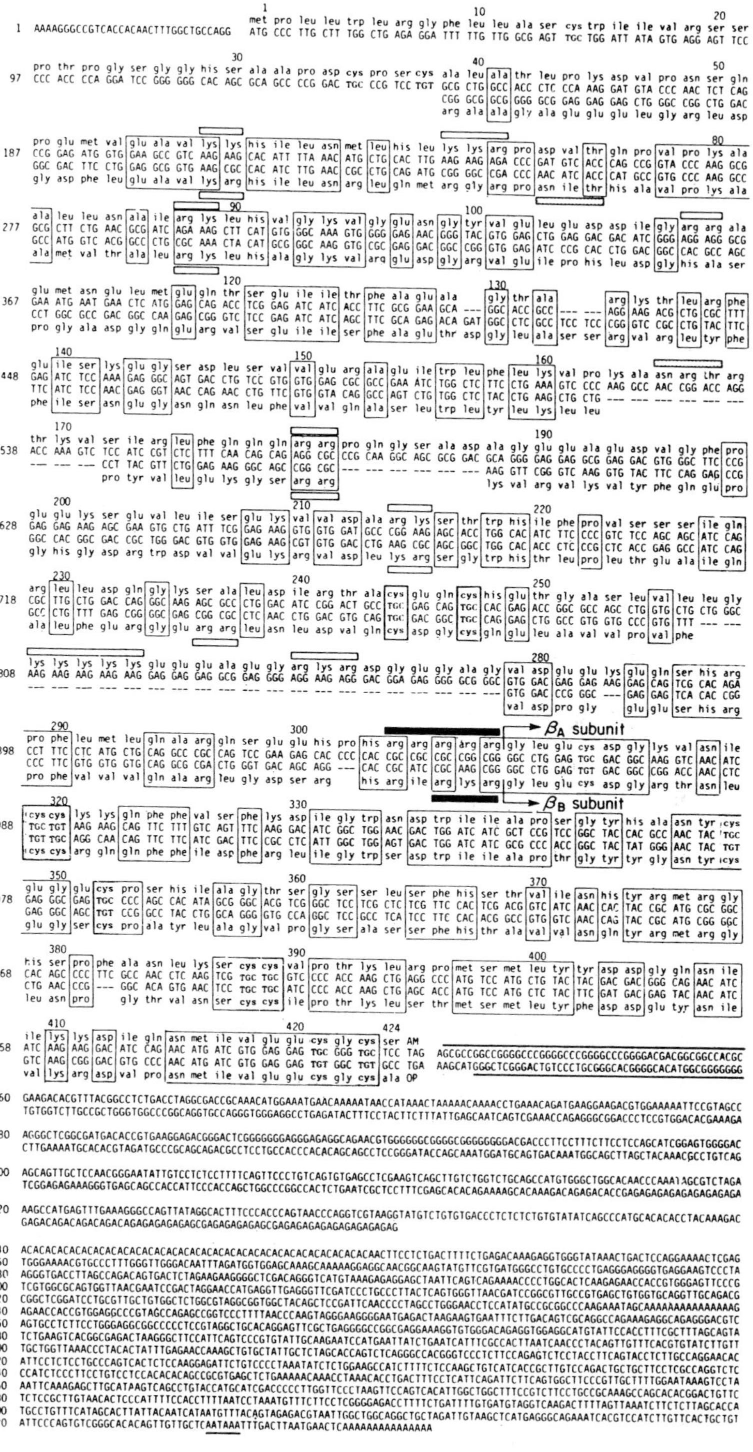

```
  1  AAAAGGGCCGTCACCACAACTTTGGCTGCCAGG
```

(Sequence figure: nucleotide sequence with three-frame amino acid translation, β_A subunit and β_B subunit indicated)

```
1360  GAAGACACGTTTACGGCCTCTGACCTAGGCGACGCAAACATGGAAATGAACAAAATAACCATAAACTAAAAACAAAACCTGAAACAGATGAAGGAAGACGTGGAAAAATTCCGTAGCC
      TGTGGTCTTGCCGCTGGGTGGCCCAGGTGCCAGGGTGGGAGGGTCTGAGATACTTTCCTACTTCTTTATTGAGCAATCAGTCGAAACCAGAGGGCGGACCCTCCGTGGACACGAAAGA
1480  AGGGCTCGGCGATGACACCGTGAAGGAGACGGGACTCGGGGGGGAGGGAGAGGCAGAACGTGGGGGGCGGGGGGGGACACCTTCCTTTCTTCCTCCAGCATCGGAGTGGGGAC
      CTTGAAAATGCACACGTAGATGCCCGCAGCAGACGCCTCCTGCCACCCACACAGCAGCCTCCGGGATACCAGCAAATGGATGCAGTGACAAATGGCAGCTTAGCTACAAACGCCTGTCAG
1600  AGCAGTTGCTCCAACGGGAATATTGTCCTCTCCTTTTCAGTTCCCTGTCAGTGTGAGCCTCGAAGTCAGCTTGTCTGGTCTGCAGCCATGTGGGCTGGCACAACCCAAATAGCGTCTAGA
      TCGGAGAGAAAGGGTGAGCAGCCACCATTCCCACCAGCTGGCCCGGCCACTCTGAATCGCTCCTTTCGAGCACACAGAAAAGCAACAAGAGAGACACCGAGAGAGAGAGAGAGAGAG
1720  AAGCCATGAGTTTGAAAGGGCCAGTTATAGGCACTTTTCCCACCCAGTAACCCAGGTCGTAAGGTATGTCTGTAGTGGACCCTCTCTCTGTGTATATCAGCCCATGCACACACCTACAAAGAC
      GAGACAGACAGACAGACAGAGAGAGAGACGAGAGAGAGGAGCGAGAGAGAGACGAGAGAGAGAGAGAGAG
1840  ACACACACACACACACACACACACACACACACACACACACACACACACACACACAACTTCCTCTGACTTTTCTGAGACAAAGAGGTGGGTATAAACTGACTCCAGGAAAACTCGAG
1960  TCGGAAAACGTGCCCTTTGGGTTGGGACAATTTAGATGGTGGAGCAAAGCAAAAAGGAGGCAACGGCAAGTATGTTCGTATGGGCCTGTGCCCCTGAGGGAGGGGGTGGAGGAAGTCCCTA
2080  AGGGTGACCTTAGCCACAGTGACTCTAGAAGAAAGGGGCTCGACAGGGTCATGTAAAGAGGGAGCTAATTCAGTCAGAAAACCCCTTGGCACTCAAGAGAACCACGTGGGGAGTTCCCG
2200  TCGTGGCGCAGTGGTTAACGAATCCGACTAGGAACCATGAGGTTGGAGGTTGAGGTTCAGTCAACATTTAGAGTAAGAGGAGATCCGGCCCTTCTGATCAGGGAAAAGGCGCTGCTGGAG
2320  CGGCTCGGATCCTGCGTTGCTGTGGCTCGGCGTAGGCGGTGGCTACAGCTCCGATTGCAAGCTCCGAATTCAACCCTAGCCTGGGAACCTCCATATGCCGCGGCCCTGACGGCATCGGAAGTGGGGAC
2440  AGAACCACCGTGGAGGCCCGTAGCCAGAGCCGGTCCCTTTTTAACCCAAGTGGGGAATGAGACTAAGAAGTGAATTTCTTGACAGTTGCAGCCCAGAAGAGATAGCAAAAAAAAAAAAAAG
2560  AGTGCCTCTTCCTGGGAAGCGGGGACCCCCTCCGTAGGCTGCACAGGAGTTCGCTGAGGGGCCGGCGAGGAAAAGGTGTGGGACAGAGGTGAGGGCATGTATCGCCACCTTTTCGCTTTAGCAGTA
2680  TCTGAAGTCACGGCGAGACTAAGGGCTTCCATTCAGTCCCGTGTATTGCAAGAATCCATGAAGTCAGACTTCAATAATCTTCTAACCTACAGTTGTTTCACGTGTATCTTGTT
2800  TGCTGGTTAAACCCTACACTATTTGAGAACCAAAGCTGTGCTATTGCTCTAGCACCAGTCTCAGGGCCACGGGTCCTTCTTCCAGAGTCTCCTACCTTCAGTACCTCTTGCCAGGAACAC
2920  ATTCCTCTCCTGCCCAGTCACTCTCAAGGAGATTCTGTCCCCTAAATATCTCTGGAAGCCATCTTTTCTCCAAGCTGTCATCACCGGCTTGTCCAGGACTGCTGCCTGCCAGGTCTC
3040  CCATCTCCCTTCCCTTCGTCCTCCACACACAGCCGCGTGAGCTCTGAAAAACAAAACTAAACACCTGACTTTCCTCATTCAGATTCTTCAGTGGCTTCCGGTTGCTTTGGAATAAAGTCCTA
3160  AATTCAAAGAGCTTGCATAAGCTACAGTTGACCATTCATCGACCCCCTTGGTTCCTCAGTCACATTTGGCTGGCACGACTTGCGTCCCTTCTTCCTGCCGCAAAGCCAGCACGACAGGACTGTTC
3280  TCTCCGCTTGTAACACTCCCATTTTTCAACCTTTTAATCCTAAATGTTTCTTCCTCGGGAGACCTTTTCTGATTTTGTGATGTAGGTCAAGACTTTTTAGTTAAATCTTCTCTTAGCACCA
3400  TGCCTGTTTCATAGCACTTATTACAATCATAATGTTACAGTAGAGAGACGTAATTGGCTGGCAGGCTACTGAGATTGTAAGCTCATGAGGGCAGAAATCACGTCCATCTTGTTCACTGCTGT
3520  ATTCCCAGTGTCGGGCACACAGTTGTTGCTCATGTAAAATTTGACTTAATGAACTCAAAAAAAAAAAAAAA
```

al reproduction, occurs over the time of 9–14 years of age in the human. Puberty in the female is initiated endocrinologically at age 9–10 by a gradually increasing CNS-mediated secretion of gonadotrophins; the menarche or first menstrual period normally occurs between ages 12 and 16. Until very recently the juvenile years before puberty were postulated to be endocrinologically relatively inert, but now due to increasing sensitivity of radioimmunoassay techniques for quantitating very low levels of various hormones, it is clear that significant changes in many individuals do occur. However, as yet there are no unifying hypotheses to explain these changes.

Puberty, then, is initiated by an increased pituitary output of the gonadotrophins, FSH and LH. It is not precisely clear what factors initiate this change. Possibly, throughout childhood the low levels of estrogen secreted by the ovaries of the pre-pubescent female are sufficient at the CNS–hypothalamus level to block the release of GnRH (see Fig. 13-1). Then as a consequence of a changing CNS–hypothalamus sensitivity to the prevailing blood estrogen levels, GnRH release is gradually increased, which results in an increased release of FSH and LH. In both females and males during the interval of puberty there are bursts of both FSH and LH secretion which occur during sleep; their etiology is not known. Associated with these changes is an increased sensitivity by the ovaries to FSH and LH which results in a gradually increasing metabolic production of estrogens and androgens. This in turn accelerates the growth of the uterus, vagina, accessory sex glands, genitalia, pelvis, breasts, and axillary and pubic hair. These changes then culminate after the menarche in the monthly cyclical process of ovulation and, in the absence of fertilization, menstruation.

B. The Female Reproductive Cycle

1. Background

Figure 13-9A details the cyclical change in FSH, LH, progesterone, estradiol, and morphological changes of the uterine endometrium which occur during the normal adult female menstrual cycle. The cycle can be

---

Figure 13-9. (A) Presentation of the cyclical hormonal changes throughout the human menstrual cycle; luteinizing hormone (LH), follicle-stimulating hormone (FSH), progesterone, 17-hydroxyprogesterone (17α-OHP), and estradiol (E_2). Modified from I. H. Thorneycroft, D. R. Mishell, Jr., and S. C. Stone, *Am. J. Obstet. Gynecol.* **111,** 947–951 (1971). (B) Schematic illustration of one human ovarian cycle keyed to the same time scale as (A). The sequential changes of the follicle/corpus luteum are shown in relation to the changes in the thickness of the endometrium.

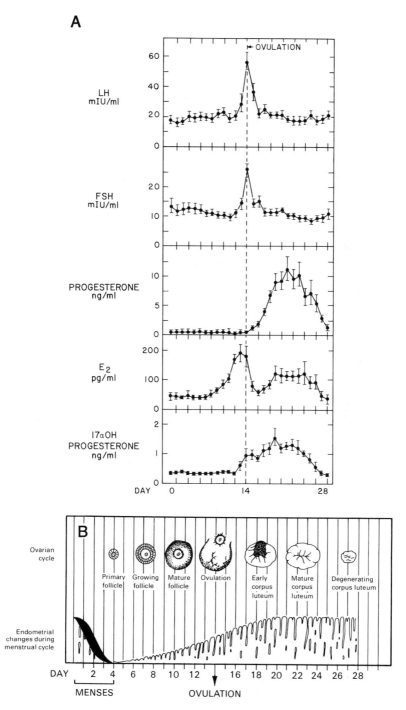

conveniently divided into two phases: pre- and postovulatory. The key events of the preovulatory phase are growth and maturation of the ovarian follicle and maturation of the uterine endometrium. The key event of the postovulatory phase is the growth, development, and involution of the corpus luteum and, in the absence of initiation of pregnancy, the shedding of the uterine endometrium. These changes are all orchestrated by the CNS–hypothalamus regulation of pituitary release of FSH and LH.

A 28-day cycle as shown in Fig. 13-9B is generally regarded as the mean length of normal cycles, but the range for different women extends from 25 to 35 days. The preovulatory phase is usually much more variable than the postovulatory or luteal phase; the latter is remarkably constant at 13 ± 1 days.

Table 13-3 summarizes the ovarian uterine and hormonal changes which occur throughout the menstrual cycle in relation to the morphological changes occurring in the ovaries and uterine endometrium.

2. Regulation of Secretion of FSH and LH

The multiple factors controlling the release of GnRH by the CNS–hypothalamus throughout the menstrual cycle are not clearly understood. As diagrammed in Fig. 13-9A, throughout the menstrual cycle there is a changing ratio of FSH to LH. From days 1 to 10 of the cycle FSH blood levels exceed LH levels; then at approximately day 10 there is a crossover, and FSH rapidly becomes elevated to a very large peak or surge on the day of ovulation; also, blood levels of FSH are increased at ovulation, but not to the extent achieved by LH. Then throughout the luteal phase the levels of FSH are low, while LH levels are relatively high on days 14–18, then fall to low levels in the absence of fertilization and implantation by day 28.

The secretions of FSH and LH are both believed to be governed by the same hypothalamic releasing factor, GnRH. This makes it difficult to explain or devise biochemical mechanisms that can rationalize the changing ratio of FSH to LH throughout the menstrual cycle. One suggestion is that the response of the adenohypophysis pituicyte cell which secretes FSH and LH in response to the hypothalamic-derived GnRH is determined by blood concentrations of estradiol and progesterone. There is evidence for the existence of receptors for both estrogen and progesterone in the adenohypophysis, the hypothalamus, as well as in higher brain centers. If changing occupancy of all these receptors by estrogen and progesterone can alter the "mix" of CNS–hypothalamic signals as well as modulate the pituicyte receptors for GnRH, this could have the consequence of modulating the ratio of FSH to LH which is secreted.

Table 13-3. Summary of Ovarian and Uterine Morphological Changes with Hormonal Activities in the Human Menstrual Cycle

Menstrual cycle		Uterine endometrium	Ovaries	Estrogen	Production of progesterone	FSH	LH
Days	Phase						
1–4	Menstrual	Shedding of outer layers	Initiation of follicular development	Low	Very low	Increasing	Low
5–12	Follicular	Reorganization and proliferation	Maturation of follicle	Increasing	Very low	High	Low
13–15	Ovulation	Further growth	Ovulation	High	Low	Low	High
16–25	Luteal	Highly vascularized and active secretion	Functional corpus luteum	First declining, then a secondary rise	Increasing	Low	High
26–28	Premenstrual	Initiation of degeneration	Regression of corpus luteum	Decreasing	Decreasing	Increasing	Decreasing

W. Odell has postulated the existence of both cyclic and tonic receptors for estrogen and progesterone in the hypothalamus. Thus, estrogen is proposed to be secreted by the developing follicle in a process likely mediated by progesterone, which is also secreted from the follicle; the secreted estrogen then acts via a "cyclic" receptor localized within the hypothalamus to stimulate the LH–FSH surge. In this model estrogen is postulated to be a positive feedback signal at this point in the cycle. After this cyclic area activity, which is only 2–4 hr in duration, the combination of progesterone and estrogen being secreted by the new corpus luteum acts via a postulated hypothalamic "tonic" center to suppress blood concentrations of LH and FSH to low levels.

Alternatively, there could also be a changing mix of CNS–hypothalamus electrical signals that modulate the secretion of GnRH. Indeed, some support for the important role of the CNS–hypothalamus in modulating the pituicyte secretion ratio of FSH and LH can be derived from the study of animals that are anestrus or that ovulate only in response to coitus. In this instance, mechanical stimulation of the vagina develops specific CNS electrical signals which results in pituicyte secretion of FSH and LH. This response can be duplicated by selective electrical stimulation of precise anatomical regions of the preoptic–superchiasmatic area of the hypothalamus and inhibited by CNS-active drugs, such as pentobarbital or atropine. A third possibility is that there could be a selective feedback inhibitor for FSH (which has not yet been biochemically characterized), operative at the pituitary level, which would permit the selective increase in LH secretion necessary for ovulation.

3. Hormonal Events in the Ovary and Corpus Luteum

The dominant hormonal changes of the menstrual cycle, particularly on the uterine endometrium, are mediated by the steroid hormones secreted by the ovaries and corpus luteum (see Table 13-3). Associated with the cyclical changes in the gonadotropins described in the preceding section are related changes in the blood levels of estrogen and progesterone. In the early preovulatory or follicular phase, estradiol levels remain low until ~7–8 days before the LH surge. Then estradiol increases and reaches a peak 1 day before the LH surge; next, there is a drop of estradiol at days 14–16 followed by a rise to a second peak at day 22–23.

Progesterone secretion by the ovaries in the preovulatory period is very low and accordingly the blood levels are low. Some additional progesterone is produced by the adrenals (see Fig. 2-22). The blood levels of progesterone rise dramatically after the LH surge and ovulation and peak at days 18–24 of the cycle; this is coincident with maximum steroid metabolism activity of the corpus luteum. The blood levels of both progesterone and estradiol fall after day 24 until initiation of menstruation. If fertilization and implantation of the zygote occurs (see later), hCG rescues the corpus luteum and stimulates the continued production of progesterone until the placenta becomes functional (see Chapter 14).

The mechanisms that govern the initiation of follicular growth as well as the selection of one follicle for the necessary maturation prior to ovulation are not clearly understood. This involves the sequence of maturation diagrammed in Fig. 13-10. Important factors are the amount of FSH and the ratio of FSH/LH; also, the availability of estrogen and possibly androgens is critical. In the immature female hypophysectomized rat model, estrogens clearly promote ovarian growth, reduce follicular atresia, induce granulosa cell hyperplasia, and increase the ovarian response to FSH. In contrast, androgens in the same model promote follicular atresia. Thus, if LH were to stimulate androgen (androstenedione) production in certain follicles or if there is a difference in different secondary follicles of the ratio of estradiol to the androgen combined with a favorable cellular receptor concentration for FSH, then one "selected" follicle would be stimulated to develop into a graafian follicle. The graafian follicle, in turn, would be subject to the influence of the gonadotropins and eventually ovulate.

Shown in Fig. 13-10A is a pictorial representation of the developmental stages of the follicular maturation and corpus luteum development in the ovary. In the selected secondary follicle on days 1–3 of the cycle, the oocyte becomes progressively larger and the surrounding granulosa cells proliferate further. The granulosa cells produce principally only estradiol. The cells adjacent to the follicle become enlarged and arranged in concentric circles; this cellular array is termed the theca. The theca cells are active in steroid metabolism and can produce both estradiol and androstenedione. As the follicle cell develops (days 6–10), the granulosa cells produce, as a consequence of the trophic actions of FSH, increasing amounts of estradiol. Blood levels of estradiol increase slowly (days 3–7) and then more rapidly to reach an apex (days 11–13) just prior to the LH surges. This has the effect of establishing the high levels of estradiol required for the positive feedback at the CNS–hypothalamus and pituitary level. Simultaneously receptors for LH are appearing in increasing concentration on both the thecal and granulosa cells in preparation for ovulation. Very late (days 11–13) in the follicular phase, after the crossover between the blood levels of FSH and LH (LH now > FSH), the thecal cells are stimulated by LH to begin producing progesterone. By

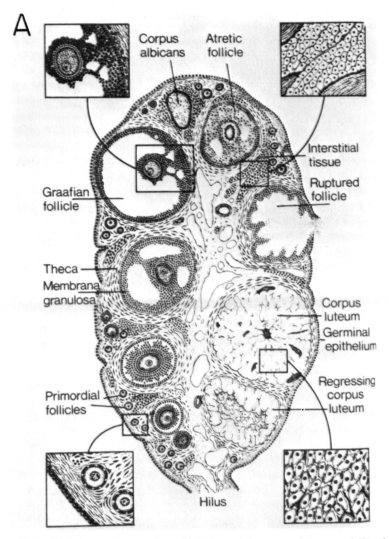

A

Corpus albicans
Atretic follicle
Interstitial tissue
Ruptured follicle
Graafian follicle
Theca
Membrana granulosa
Corpus luteum
Germinal epithelium
Regressing corpus luteum
Primordial follicles
Hilus

Figure 13-10. (A) Scheme of maturation of follicles and the corpus luteum and (B) role of intraovarian androgens in promoting follicular atresia. Reproduced from C. D. Turner and J. T. Bagnara, The biology of sex and reproduction. *Gen. Endocrinol.* **5,** 400 (1971). (B) P. K. Siiteri and F. Febres, Ovarian hormone synthesis, circulation and mechanism of action. *In* "Endocrinology" (L. J. DeGroot, G. F. Cahill, L. Martini, D. H. Nelson, W. D. Odell, J. T. Potts, E. Steinberger, and A. I. Winegrad, eds.), Vol. 3, p. 1401. Grune & Stratton, New York, 1979.

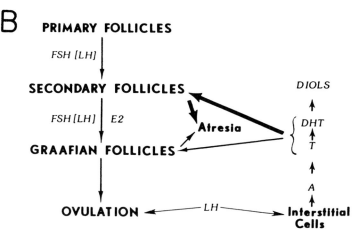

Figure 13-10B.

day 11–12 of the cycle the general maturation of the secondary follicle is complete and it is referred to as a graafian follicle. During this 12-day developmental process, the primary follicle has increased in size some 400 times from 50 to 29,000 μm, while the oogonium has increased some 10 times from 15 to 150 μm.

Recently, evidence has been accumulating that oxytocin is synthesized in an extraposterior pituitary location, the corpus luteum (Fig. 13-11). It may represent the luteolytic substance which has been conjectured on for some time. The data are summarized into an overview in Fig. 4-22. The corpus luteum can produce oxytocin or an oxytocin-like peptide which is secreted. This production is under the control of a substance from the uterus (X). $PGF_{2\alpha}$ can also stimulate production of oxytocin in the corpus luteum, and its effect is blocked by ovariectomy or hysterectomy. Secreted oxytocin apparently binds the luteal membrane receptors, leading to alterations in the cell which depress steroid (progesterone) synthesis and promote luteolysis. Because the luteal production of oxytocin is blocked by hysterectomy (and pregnancy), it is likely that a factor stimulating the luteal process derives from the uterus (it could be $PFG_{2\alpha}$, arachidonic acid, or something else). Interestingly, the luteal oxytocin induces the formation of oxytocin receptors in the uterine myometrium. Oxytocin obviously may account for the fall in the LH spike during the ovarian cycle.

After ovulation, both the thecal and granulosa cells of the follicle undergo rapid mitosis. Capillaries are generated from the theca that invade the granulosa cells, thus creating a new endocrine organ, the

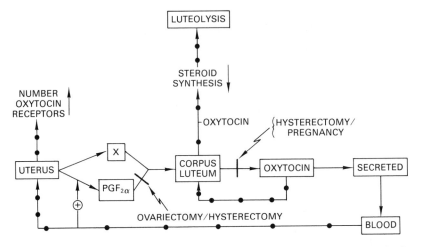

Figure 13-11. Extraposterior pituitary production of oxytocin and its postulated role in luteolysis. $PGF_{2\alpha}$, Prostaglandin 2α.

corpus luteum. The corpus luteum reaches its maximum size within 2–8 days, and if fertilization and zygote implantation does not occur by 8–9 days, then it undergoes regression and degeneration, leading ultimately to the production of the corpus albicans. The corpus luteum under the stimulus of LH actively produces progesterone.

4. Changes in the Uterine Endometrium

The endometrium and vaginal epithelium undergo very striking morphological changes throughout the 28 days of the menstrual cycle (see Fig. 13-9B). During the first half of each menstrual cycle, which is often denoted the follicular or preovulatory phase, the estrogen concentrations gradually increase to reach a maximum 24 hr before ovulation, while the progesterone concentrations are relatively low. These changes in estrogen, with a low progesterone value, stimulate the endometrium to increase in thickness from 1 to 3–5 mm. Then 36 hr after ovulation, which signals the initiation of the luteal or postovulatory phase, the progesterone concentration rises sharply due to its secretion from the corpus luteum. Simultaneously estrogen levels are maintained at levels two-thirds of their previous maximum. This balance of progesterone and estrogen induces further specific morphological change in the endometrium. Glycogen-containing granules appear in the glandular cells; additionally, the glands of the endometrium become increasingly tortuous. This phase of the cycle is also termed the secretory phase since the lumens of the endometrial glands are filled with secretions. Also, the endometrium becomes highly vascularized with the ingrowth of new spiral arteries from the arcuate vessels of the myometrium. The growth of these spiral arteries is stimulated by estrogen. In the event that fertilization and implantation do not occur, then the stromal edema decreases, glandular secretions diminish, and the endometrium is invaded by lymphocytes. The concentration of estrogen and progesterone both fall sharply at days 27–28 of the cycle as a consequence of the involution of the corpus luteum. At the time of the rapid fall in estrogen and progesterone at the end of the luteal phase, the spiral arteries become constricted. Accordingly, blood flow through the capillaries supported by these arteries diminishes. Eventually blood stasis and stromal degeneration follow and the endometrial tissue is sloughed off.

C. Menopause

The menopause is defined as the cessation of ovulation by the ovaries. This occurs in women between age 40 and 50 due to the utilization of the fixed number of follicles that were established in the fetal ovary. Each month of ovulation several follicles disappear by the process of atresia and normally only one matures to contribute an ovum. Thus, at some interval in the fourth decade there are no more follicles available to support this cyclical process. The endocrinological consequences of cessation of ovulation are varied and a variety of medical problems may develop, depending upon the exact nature of the reproductive hormonal balance achieved.

In the postmenopausal woman the average blood concentration of FSH and LH remains elevated for the remainder of life. The postmenopausal secretion of immunoreactive LH is sevenfold higher and FSH threefold higher than a premenopausal woman. While the postmenopausal ovary is not totally devoid of the ability to secrete steroids, the production level is markedly reduced in comparison to a younger ovulating woman. In menopausal women the major circulating estrogen is estrone; this is formed almost exclusively by aromatization of androstenedione by the adrenals as well as adipose tissue and muscle. Figure 13-12 diagrams the feedback relationship to the CNS–hypothalamus–pituitary system of the postmenopausal woman. The control of LH and FSH secretion in postmenopausal women is mediated via a short feedback loop wherein FSH and LH themselves act on the hypothalamus in conjunction with steroids which are largely derived from the adrenals.

546

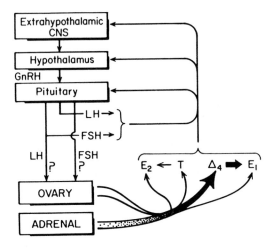

Figure 13-12. The CNS–hypothalamus–pituitary feedback relationships of the postmeno-pausal woman. Modified from W. D. Odell, Ovarian hormone synthesis, circulation, and mechanisms of action. *In* "Endocrinology" (L. J. DeGroot, G. F. Cahill, L. Martini, D. H. Nelson, W. D. Odell, J. T. Potts, E. Steinberger, and A. I. Winegrad, eds.), Vol. 3, p. 1490. Grune & Stratton, New York, 1979.

V. BIOLOGICAL AND MOLECULAR ACTIONS

A. Cellular Mechanisms of Action of the Reproductive Hormones

1. GnRH

An elucidation of all the factors governing the release of GnRH as well as a biochemical description of their action are only now emerging. The problem has not been readily approachable through the classical biochemical techniques of fractionation, purification, and so on due to the complex but critically important anatomical relationships existent between the CNS, the hypothalamus, which secretes GnRH, and the adenohypophysis of the pituitary, which is the site of action of GnRH.

The release of GnRH from the hypothalamus is determined by an integration of visual, olfactory, pineal, stress, as well as endocrine factors. The hypothalamus acts as a clearinghouse to determine whether GnRH should be released. Figure 13-13 presents a model describing the regulatory factors governing the secretion by the adenohypophysis of FSH and LH in the female. The release of FSH and LH is a highly regulated process determined by (1) negative feedback, (2) positive feed-back, and (3) neural components.

Any detailed explanation of this system must provide an explanation for the integration of the neural impulses of the CNS with the feedback actions of progesterone and estrogen acting on the hypothalamus. The observation that hypothalamic catecholamines turn over in response to changes in the levels of gonadal hormones is suggestive that the metabolism of catecholamines may be involved in GnRH release. A second

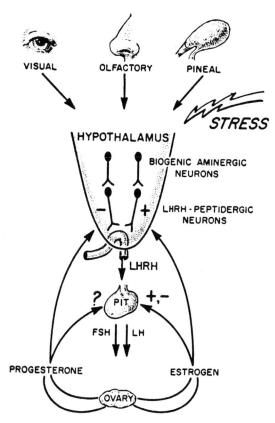

Figure 13-13. Schematic model describing the regulated secretion of FSH and LH by the adenohypophysis in the adult human female. The model emphasizes the interactions of both the neural and hormonal feedback controls. Depending upon dose, time course, and prior hormonal status, estrogens can either stimulate or inhibit LH secretion through effects at either the pituitary or hypothalamus. Progesterone activity also stimulates or inhibits LRH, but has little effect at the level of the pituitary. Modified from J. Martin and S. Reichlin, "Clinical Neuroendocrinology." Davis, Philadelphia, Pennsylvania, 1977.

) providing a mechanism that allows for differing
nd LH to be released from the pituitary by only one
nRH, at differing time points in the menstrual cycle.
k of LH may be due to release of a large bolus of
·y granules containing the stored peptide hormones.

2. The Gonadotropins (FSH and LH)

The principal biochemical actions of FSH and LH are, respectively, to induce the production of estrogen (by the ovarian thecal cell) and of progesterone (by the corpus luteum). Their generally accepted mechanism of action is not dissimilar from the actions of the peptide hormone ACTH in stimulating steroidogenesis in the adrenal cortex.

Receptors for both FSH and LH are present in the cell surface of their respective target cells. Both FSH and LH stimulate intracellularly the production of cAMP by adenyl cyclase. Ovarian cells also contain receptors for prostaglandins and catecholamines, both of which can mimic some of the actions of LH and cAMP. The cAMP then, as shown in Fig. 13-14, activates a protein kinase which stimulates cholesterol side chain cleavage, eventually increasing the production of estradiol and progesterone. C. Channing and co-workers have shown that there is a good correlation between receptor occupancy by LH, stimulation of cAMP, activation of protein kinase, and progesterone production.

Further work is required to describe at the biochemical level the complex series of steps associated with maturation of the ovarian follicle, lutenization of the granulosa cells, and formation of a functional corpus luteum. It has been proposed by C. Channing that the cyclical nature of the menstrual cycle is largely governed by temporal changes in the cell surface receptors of the ovarian follicles for FSH and LH. These changes in turn drive in a cyclical fashion the biosynthetic and mitotic activity of the follicular granulosa cells and the steroid-producing thecal cells.

In the early phases of the cycle of granulosa cell development (days 2–6 of the cycle), the granulosa cell is quite dependent upon FSH. At this point, it has largely FSH receptors and only a limited number of LH receptors; it is rapidly dividing, growing, and acquiring the enzymatic capacity to aromatize androgens to estradiol. At this point the production of estradiol is a collaboration between the surrounding thecal cells, which convert cholesterol to androgens, and the granulosa cell, which converts the androgen to estradiol. This granulosa-produced estrogen then collaborates with FSH to speed up the replication rate of the granulosa cells. Thus, although there is now (days 8–10 of the cycle) a falling plasma concentration of FSH, there is an increased capacity to respond to FSH (due to the increased concentration of FSH receptors) and to

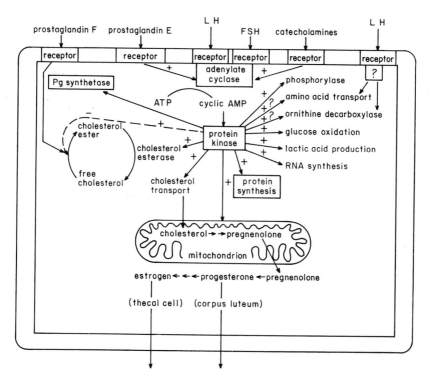

Figure 13-14. Model to describe the steroidogenic actions of FSH and LH on the ovary. Modified from P. K. Siiteri and F. Febres, Ovarian hormone synthesis, circulation, and mechanisms of action. *In* "Endocrinology" (L. J. DeGroot, G. F. Cahill, L. Martini, D. H. Nelson, W. D. Odell, J. T. Potts, E. Steinberger, and A. I. Winegrad, eds.), Vol. 3, p. 1405. Grune & Stratton, New York, 1979.

produce estradiol. Concurrently there is an increased concentration of LH receptor on the thecal and granulosa cell in preparation for ovulation and formation of the luteal phase of the cycle. Channing and co-workers have evidence for the existence of two low-molecular-weight peptides (1000 and 2000) derived from follicular fluid that inhibit the maturation of the oocyte. Also, there is evidence for the involvement of inhibin which in the female is secreted by the granulosa cells and which likely inhibits FSH secretion by the pituitary. Then as the late follicular phase ensues (days 11–13), the aromatization capacity of the granulosa cells becomes maximal and the blood level of estrogen rises dramatically (see Fig. 13-8), which leads to a positive feedback loop at the hypothalamus–pituitary axis and initiates the midcycle surge in LH secretion (days 13–14).

Thus, LH (1) initiates the production of progesterone by both the thecal and granulosa cells, (2) inhibits mitosis by the granulosa cells, and (3) stimulates the production of prostaglandin $F_{2\alpha}$ and proteolytic enzymes by the granulosa cells, which collectively lead to rupture of the follicle and ovulation (day 15).

After ovulation under the continued action of LH, the thecal and granulosa cells are transformed into the corpus luteum, which is the site of production and secretion of large quantities of progesterone and moderate quantities of estradiol.

3. Estrogen

a. Background. The dominant actions of estrogen occur in the female reproductive tract, although there are also significant biological actions mediated in the hypothalamus and brain as well as in a variety of other visceral organs. Table 13-4 tabulates the tissue distribution of the estrogen receptor. Summarized in Table 13-5 is a tabulation of the temporal events initiated in the immature or ovariectomized rat uterus as a consequence of estradiol administration. It is not clear whether all the actions reported in Table 13-6 are mediated as a consequence of estrogen interaction with target organ-specific receptors for the steroid hormone. The presence of the estrogen receptor in a tissue is presumptive of the biological actions of estrogen at that location.

One particularly well-studied system, however, is the developmental role of estrogen acting in the liver of the adult hen to induce the biosynthesis of vitellogenin. J. Tata and co-workers have documented the detailed role of estrogen, acting through its receptor, and specific gene activation to produce vitellogenin. Vitellogenin, which is a phosphoprotein, is then transported through the blood (it also cotransports Ca^{2+}

Table 13–4. Tissue Distribution of Estrogen Receptors

Reproductive tract	Testis
Uterus (mammals)	Epididymis
Vagina (mammals)	Prostate gland
Placenta (mammals)	Seminal vesicles
Oviduct (chicken)	Mullerian duct (chick embryo)
Ovary	
Corpus luteum	
Mammary tissue (mammals)	
Neuroendocrine system	Visceral organs
Pituitary	Liver
Hypothalamus	Kidney
Brain (preoptic area, septum, amygdala, cortex)	Lung

Table 13–5. Temporal Actions of Estrogens in the Rat Uterus[a]

Time after estradiol administration	Sequence of responses
30 min	Stimulation of RNA polymerase II
1 hr	Stimulation of glucose and phospholipid metabolism
1.5 hr	Stimulation of RNA polymerase I
2–5 hr	Stimulation of general protein synthesis
5–7 hr	Acceleration of water imbition
10–20 hr	Stimulation of net protein, RNA, and DNA synthesis
20–30 hr	Acceleration of cell division

[a] Modified from Fig. 1 of B. S. Katzenellenbogen and J. Gorski, Estrogen action on syntheses of macromolecules in target cells. *In* "Biochemical Actions of Hormones" (G. Litwack, ed.), Vol. 3, p. 187. Academic Press, New York, 1975.

required for the eggshell) to the ovary where it is cleaved to yield the final egg yolk proteins phosvitin and lipovitellin.

b. Estrogen Receptors. V. Sica and F. Bresciani as well as G. Puca have succeeded in isolating and purifying via classical methods the bovine uterine receptor for estradiol. The procedure which involved several chromatography steps, including an affinity column of estradiol-17-hemisuccinyl-ovalbumin-Sepharose 4B, yielded a 15,600-fold, purified, homogeneous protein of molecular weight 70,000. This protein has a Stokes radius of 3.9 nm, a 5–20% sucrose gradient mobility of 4.2 S, an axial ratio of 3.0 (indicative of a prolate ellipsoid), and a single ligand binding site for estradiol. The 70,000 Da form of the estrogen receptor is believed to represent a subunit of the native receptor which has an apparent molecular weight of 430,000 and a 5–20% sucrose gradient mobility of 8 S. These results suggest that the native receptor is an aggregate of six subunits, each of 65,000–70,000 molecular weight.

Table 13–6. Biological Actions of Progesterone

Thermogenesis (in woman)
Regulation of egg movement through fallopian tubes
Preparation of the uterus to receive the blastocyst
Alteration of electrical activity in the brain
Control of uterine contraction (at parturition)
Generation of the secretory system of breasts (during pregnancy)

With the skillful application of recombinant DNA technology, it has recently been feasible to achieve a previously impossible goal, namely, acquisition of the primary amino acid sequence of two steroid receptors, the glucocorticoid receptor (Chapter 10) and the estrogen receptor (this chapter).

G. Greene, E. Jensen, and P. Chambon and co-workers have reported (see Fig. 13-15) that the human estrogen receptor present in MCF-7 human breast cancer cells is comprised of a single polypeptide chain of

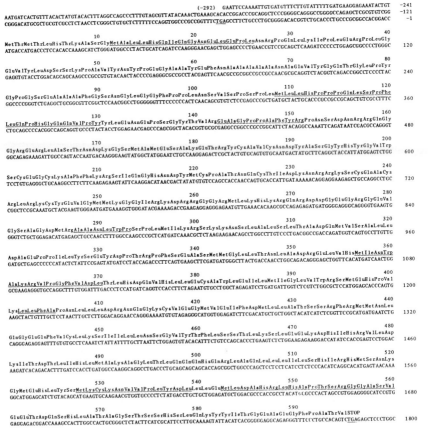

Figure 13-15. Human estrogen receptor amino acid sequence (derived from a cDNA nucleotide sequence) from MCF-7 human breast cancer cells. The complete open reading frame consisting of nucleotides 1–1785 is underlined. Peptide sequences originally obtained from highly purified MCR-7 estrogen receptor are underlined. Modified with permission from Fig. 1 of G. L. Greene, P. Gilna, M. Waterfield, A. Baker, Y. Hort, and J. Shine, *Science* **231**, 1150–1154 (1986). Copyright 1986 by the AAAS.

595 amino acids (molecular weight of 66,200). This amino acid sequence was deduced from sequencing 2042 cDNA base pairs (bp) derived from a 6.2-kilobase polyadenylated mRNA for the estrogen receptor. When this 2042-bp cDNA was inserted into a pBR vector containing a metallothionein promoter and SV40 enhancer sequence and was used to transform Chinese hamster ovary cells (CHO), it was found that the CHO cells (which contain no endogenous estrogen receptor) now produce a new protein of 66,000 molecular weight capable of specifically binding estradiol as a ligand.

Ultimately, it is anticipated that identification of the properties and locations of functional domains on the estrogen receptor protein can assist in establishing the precise mechanism by which the receptor regulates gene transcription. Immunochemical analyses of both the estrogen and glucocorticoid receptors have already identified the existence of a steroid hormone binding domain and a DNA binding region. When the amino acid sequences of the estrogen receptor and glucocorticoid receptor were compared (see Fig. 13-16), a striking homology was observed in a region rich in arginine, lysine, and cysteine. This region occurred ~300–350 amino acid residues from the COOH terminus of both receptors. Also, intriguingly, both receptors showed a good homology with the putative v-*erb*-A oncogene protein product. This suggests that these two steroid receptors and v-*erb*-A may share a common ancestral gene. It will be interesting to learn whether the mechanisms by which steroid receptors regulate gene transcription have features in common with the mechanism by which the v-*erb*-A promotes cell transformation.

4. Progesterone

a. Background. In contrast to estradiol, the biological actions of progesterone are largely restricted to the female reproductive tract and mammary tissue. Table 13-6 tabulates many of the known biological actions of progesterone. Receptors for progesterone have been found in the uterus, mammary tissue, placenta, and the anterior pituitary.

b. Progesterone Receptors. W. Schrader, E. Baulieu, and D. Toft have separately isolated and purified the chick oviduct progesterone receptor to apparent homogeneity; intriguingly, as summarized in Table 13-7, they obtained somewhat different results with respect to the biochemical properties of their isolated receptor. According to Schrader, the chick oviduct progesterone receptor is composed of two nonidentical protein subunits, while Baulieu has evidence for only one subunit form.

Analysis of oviduct cytosol by 5–20% sucrose gradient analysis typically presents a complex picture of progesterone receptor forms. If the cytosol is obtained from estrogen-primed chick oviducts and analyzed in

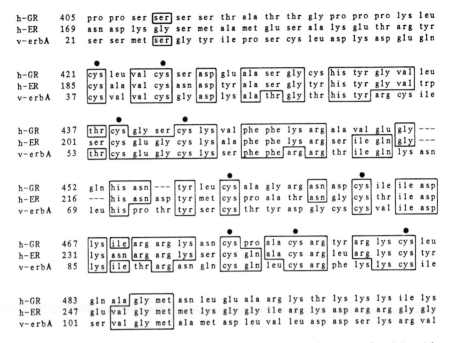

Figure 13-16. Amino acid sequence alignment of the cysteine-, lysine-, and arginine-rich regions of the human estrogen receptor (h-ER), the human glucocorticoid receptor (h-GR), and the putative v-*erb*-A oncogene product. Amino acid residues 185–250 from ER were aligned with residues 421–486 from GR and 37–104 from the protein p75$^{gag-erb-A}$. Common residues are boxed and gaps are indicated by dashes. Matching cysteine residues are indicated by dots above the sequences. In this region, there were 40 matches (61%) between ER and GR. Similarly, there were nine cysteines of ER conserved and 9 out of 10 GR and v-*erb*-A cysteines conserved. Modified with permission from Fig. 1 of G. L. Greene, P. Gilna, M. Waterfield, A. Baker, Y. Hort, and J. Shine, *Science* **231**, 1150–1154 (1986). Copyright 1986 by the AAAS.

a low ionic strength environment, there are equivalent amounts of a 6 S and 8 S species, whereas if the cytosol is obtained from unprimed oviducts, there are equivalent amounts of 4 S and 6 S forms. The current interpretation by Schrader and colleagues of these data is that the 6 S form is a dimer consisting of one A subunit and one B subunit. The 8 S form is postulated to be an aggregate of the 4 S species, while the 4 S form is a mixture of the individual A and B monomers. Distinct functional properties of the monomeric and aggregated forms of the receptor have yet to be identified; as yet it has not been possible to reconstitute the 6 S form from pure A and B receptor forms.

Evidence has been presented for a temperature-dependent activation of the chick oviduct 6 S A:B dimer form of the receptor. Thus, in terms of

Table 13–7. Biochemical Properties of the Progesterone Receptor[a]

	Schrader isolation		Baulieu isolation[b]
	Subunit		
	A	B	
Molecular weight			
Intact form	183,000		240,000–280,000
Subunit form	71,000	114,000	85,000
Stokes radius (nm)	4.6	6.4	7.0
Frictional ratio (f/fo)	1.74	1.9	—
Isoelectric point (pH)	4.5	5.0	—
Sedimentation coefficient (5–20% sucrose gradients)	3.6	4.2	8.9

[a] Data obtained from W. V. Vedeckes, W. T. Schrader, and B. W. O'Malley, The chick oviduct progesterone receptor. *In* "Biochemical Actions of Hormones" (G. Litwack, ed.), Vol. 5, p. 335. Academic Press, New York, 1978.

[b] Data obtained from J. M. Renoir, C. Yang, P. Formstechen, P. Lustenberger, A. Wolfson, G. Redeweh, J. Mester, H. Fog, and E. Baulieu, Chick oviduct progesterone receptor. Purification of a molybdate-stabilized form and preliminary characterization. *Eur. J. Biochem.* **127,** 71–79 (1983).

the two-step model for hormone action (see Chapter 1), only occupied 6 S receptor, which has been warmed to 25°C for 30 min, can gain access or bind to the nucleus. Unoccupied 6 S progesterone receptor which has been exposed to a 25°C environment for 30 min has no affinity for nuclei or chromatin. The nature of the biochemical change occurring via the "activation" process is not known.

The chick oviduct cell has only 1000–2000 high-affinity (K_d = 3 × 10^{-11}) sites for the progesterone–receptor complex. Once in the nucleus of the oviduct cell, the steroid receptor A:B complex dissociates into its subunits. The A subunit is believed to possess a preference for binding to DNA, while the B subunit is believed to bind to some specific, but not yet characterized acceptor proteins associated with the chromatin. The DNA binding properties of the A subunit are masked in the A:B dimer form of the receptor.

B. Mechanism of Progesterone and Estrogen Receptor Action (as Exemplified by the Chick Oviduct System)

One system contributing extensively to our current understanding of the mode of action of steroid hormones is the chick oviduct. W. Schrader,

B. O'Malley, and colleagues as well as R. Palmiter and R. Schimke have carried out a detailed biochemical analysis of estrogen- and progesterone-mediated induction of ovalbumin, conalbumin, and other egg white proteins in the chick oviduct. Figure 13-17 presents a schematic diagram of the hormone-mediated events in the immature chick oviduct. As shown here, estrogen plays a key role in priming the immature oviduct to be responsive to subsequent treatment with either estrogen or progesterone. Then secondary stimulation with either progesterone or estrogen leads to a rapid biosynthesis of ovalbumin and other egg white proteins.

The synthesis of DNA complementary to ovalbumin messenger RNA (cDNA probes) has permitted a detailed study of gene expression in the chick oviduct system. By employing this cDNA probe to analyze the consequences of primary estrogen treatment or secondary estrogen or progesterone treatment, extensive data have been accumulated which strongly support the primary hypothesis that steroid hormones act by gene activation.

Figure 13-18 presents a model integrating the various structural and functional properties of the progesterone receptor in the chick oviduct. Progesterone, or P, which is bound to a serum binding protein in the

HORMONAL STATE	OVIDUCT GROWTH	OVIDUCT WEIGHT	STATE OF DIFFERENTIATION	HORMONE–INDUCED PROTEINS	
				ESTROGEN	PROGESTIN
UNSTIMULATED		0.01g	UNDIFFERENTIATED CELLS	NONE	NONE
	P↓ NO GROWTH ↓E				
PRIMARY STIMULATION		2g	TUBULAR GLANDS / GOBLET CELLS / — LUMEN	{OVALBUMIN OTHERS} – – – – – – – – AVIDIN	NONE
	DISCONTINUE ESTROGEN ↓				
WITHDRAWAL		0.25g	REGRESSED STRUCTURE	NONE	NONE
	P↓ OR ↓E				
SECONDARY STIMULATION		0.5g	TUBULAR GLANDS / GOBLET CELLS / — LUMEN	{OVALBUMIN OTHERS} – – – – – – – – AVIDIN	{OVALBUMIN OTHERS}

Figure 13-17. Schematic model describing the mode of action of estrogen and progesterone in the chick oviduct. Modified from W. V. Vedekis, W. T. Schrader, and B. W. O'Malley, The chick oviduct progesterone receptor. *In* "Biochemical Actions of Hormones" (G. L. Litwack, ed.), Vol. 5, p. 359. Academic Press, New York, 1978.

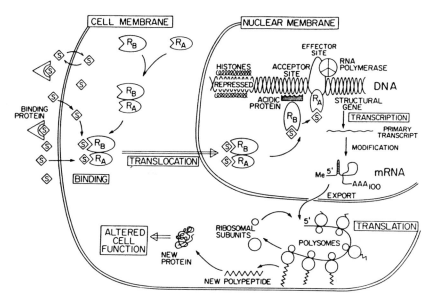

Figure 13-18. Proposed model for progesterone action in the chick oviduct. Modified from R. E. Buller, R. J. Schwartz, W. T. Schrader, and B. W. O'Malley, *J. Biol. Chem.* **251,** 5178–5186. Williams & Wilkins, Baltimore, Maryland (1976).

blood, enters the cell by diffusion. Then P binds to the 6 S A:B dimer form of the receptor, which after activation it associates with the nuclear chromatin. Here the dimer dissociates and the B subunit is postulated to "search" the chromatin until it interacts with the appropriate acceptor protein(s). The biochemical consequences of the A receptor subunit interacting with the chromatin acceptor proteins are not yet clear. The A subunit then interacts with some effector or initiation site for RNA synthesis which leads to messenger RNA synthesis and ovalbumin biosynthesis.

C. Hormonal Effects on Ovulation and the Menstrual Cycle

1. Steroid Receptors

The mammalian uterus structure and function is determined in large part as a consequence of its exquisite sensitivity to progesterone and estrogen. In general, progesterone and estradiol exert opposing effects on the estrogen and progesterone receptor system. These relationships are diagrammed in Fig. 13-19. The presence of estradiol increases via protein synthesis pathways the concentration of receptors for both pro-

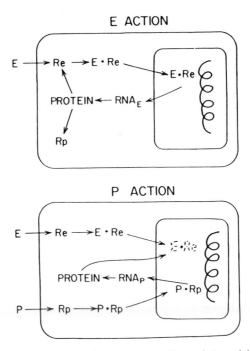

Figure 13-19. Proposed mechanism of progesterone (P) regulation of the nuclear levels of the estrogen (E) receptor (Re). During estrogen secretion the estradiol–receptor complex interacts with chromatin to stimulate estrogen-dependent RNA (RNA$_E$) and protein synthesis, two products of which are progesterone and estrogen receptors. Progesterone action is mediated by the progestene receptor (Rp) system, resulting in a progesterone-dependent RNA (RNA$_P$) and protein synthesis. A product of progesterone action is proposed to be the estrogen receptor regulating factor which is responsible for the degradation of estrogen–receptor complex in the target cell nucleus. Modified from R. W. Evans and W. W. Leavitt, Progesterone inhibition of uterine nuclear estrogen receptor: Dependence on RNA and protein synthesis. *Proc. Natl. Acad. Sci. U.S.A.* **77**, 5856–5860 (1980).

gesterone and estradiol, while progesterone generally leads to a down regulation of receptor binding sites for these steroids. An additional regulatory component relates to the blood levels of the steroid hormones and whether after formation of the steroid–receptor complex it is mandatorily translocated to the nucleus where gene activation occurs.

In the golden hamster there is ample evidence of a positive relationship between the increase in estrogen secretion occurring during the follicular phase of the estrous cycle and the elevation of the uterine nuclear estrogen receptor and the progesterone cytosol receptor (see Fig. 13-20). The details of the biochemical changes contributing to receptor changes during ovulation are not clear. Probably the ovulatory surge

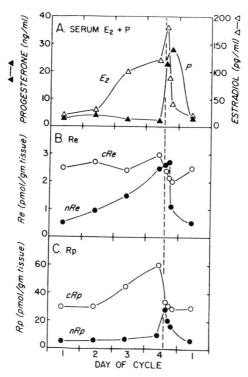

Figure 13-20. Serum steroid relationships during the 4-day hamster estrous cycle. The dashed vertical line indicates the time of the critical period for the ovulatory surge of the gonadotropins. Symbols: c, Cytosol; E_2, estradiol-17β; n, nuclear; P, progesterone; Re, estrogen receptor; Rp, progesterone receptor. Modified with permission from W. W. Leavitt, Hormonal regulation of estrogens and progesterone receptor system. *In* "Biochemical Actions of Hormones" (G. Litwack, ed.), Vol. 10, p. 329. Academic Press, New York, 1983.

of gonadotropin stimulates a transitory rise in serum estradiol which effects translocation of the estrogen receptor to the nucleus; however, the occupied estrogen receptor fails to accumulate due to suppression by the preovulatory levels of progesterone. Then when the serum concentrations of estradiol fall, the cytosol estrogen translocation diminishes and nuclear levels of the estrogen receptor fall precipitously as a consequence of unopposed progesterone action. Thus, changes in the cytosol and nuclear levels of the estrogen receptor are a balance between first the combined actions of the simultaneous presence of progesterone and estradiol, and second the unopposed action of progesterone during estrogen withdrawal.

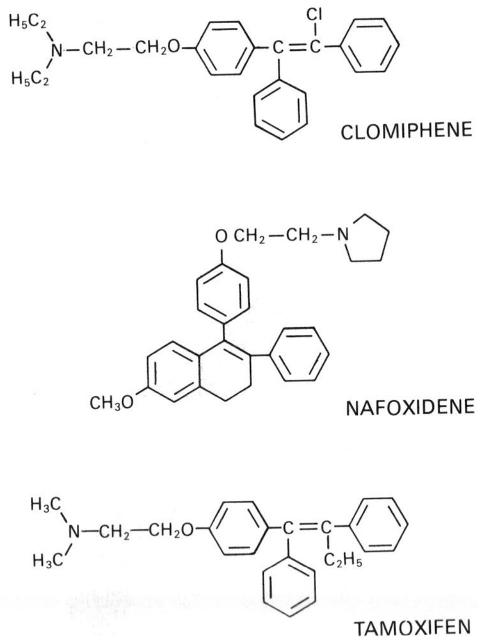

Figure 13-21. Structures of the principal antiestrogen compounds currently available.

2. Antiestrogen Compounds

The principal antiestrogen compounds available include nafoxidene clomiphene and tamoxifen, which are all derivatives of triphenylethylene (see Fig. 13-21). The biochemical basis of the action of these compounds is not clear, since they do bind to the estrogen receptor and translocate with it to the nucleus of the cell.

VI. CLINICAL ASPECTS

A. Female Contraception

Of the various methods available for contraception, the use of oral steroids and the "rhythm" method are strictly based on endocrinological principles.

The rhythm method of contraception is predicated on the following facts: (1) The human ovum can be fertilized for only about 24 hr after ovulation; (2) spermatozoa are competent to fertilize an ovum only up to

48 hr after coitus; and (3) ovulation usually occurs 12–16 days before the onset of menstruation. Therefore if a woman has accurately established the length of her menstrual cycles, she can calculate her personal fertile period by subtracting 18 days from her previous shortest cycle and 11 days from her previous longest cycle. Then in each subsequent cycle, the couple should abstain from coitus during this calculated fertile interval. The failure rate in one United States study assessing the effectiveness of the rhythm method was reported to be 30 pregnancies per 100 woman years. The principal reason for failure is the irregularity of the menstrual cycle even in women with previous regular cycles. Since progesterone causes an increase in basal body temperature, the effectiveness of the rhythm method can be increased by abstinence for 48 hr after the rise in body temperature. Under these circumstances, the failure rate was only 6.6 pregnancies per 100 woman years (Marshall, 1968).

The steroid contraceptive pill is the most widely used method of contraception; worldwide some 50 million women take some form of oral contraceptive. Figure 2-11 presents the structure of some of the presently employed synthetic oral contraceptives. The most common formulation consists of tablets containing both a progestin and an estrogen which are given continuously for 3 weeks. Normally a "blank" pill is taken for the fourth week to permit the process of menstruation to occur and to establish the "regularity" of taking the daily pill. Contraceptive steroids prevent ovulation by interfering with the release of GnRH by the hypothalamus and LH and FSH by the pituitary and thus block the midcycle surge of gonadotropins which mediate ovulation. The failure rate, provided that no tablets are omitted, is less than 0.2% per 100 woman years at the end of 1 year.

Contraception by "interception" can be accomplished by administration of high doses of estrogen or diethylstilbestrol in the early postovulatory period. This treatment, known as the "morning after pill," when continued for 5 days prevents implantation of the zygote or morula and can be quite effective (a failure of only 0.3%). However, because of the side effects associated with the high doses of estrogen (nausea, breast soreness, menstrual irregularities), interception is only recommended as an emergency treatment.

B. Hirsutism

Hirsutism or the heavy, abnormal growth of hair in the female is a medical problem of endocrine origin.

Hair may be classified as either terminal hair (coarse and pigmented) or vellus hair (fine, soft, and unpigmented). The hair follicle may produce either terminal or vellus hair in response to appropriate stimuli. In hirsutism there is an androgen-dependent transition to the production of terminal hair. Androgens neither increase the number of hair follicles nor increase the mitotic rate of the cells of the connective tissue of the papillae of the hair follicle. Instead, androgens mediate an increase in the number and size of the cells of the papilla which leads to an increase in hair growth rate and diameter.

Most common hirsutism results from inappropriately high plasma levels of testosterone and its precursors. If the elevated plasma level of testosterone is extensive over a prolonged time interval (e.g., years), virilization (masculinization) may also occur. The most common causes of elevated levels of testosterone in the female are congenital adrenal hyperplasia (see Chapter 10) or the presence of a tumor in the adrenal cortex, hyperplasia of the androgen-producing cells (the stromal and thecal cells) of the ovaries or ovarian tumor, and occasionally polycystic ovary disease. Hirsutism may result from the inappropriate production of testosterone or the testosterone precursors dehydroepiandrosterone, 3α-androstanediol, or androst-4-ene-3,17-dione (see Fig. 2-23).

C. Anovulation

The inability of a woman to become pregnant may in some instances be due to a lack of ovulation. There are four chief ways to induce ovulation; these include administration of clomiphene (a nonsteroidal compound with weak estrogen activity), gonadotropins (LH and or FSH), or ergolins (such as bromoergocriptine), or by the surgical procedure of ovarian wedge resection. Clomiphene is an antiestrogen compound which blocks the binding of estrogen to its receptor. Clomiphene's effectiveness as an inducer of ovulation is believed to occur as a circulating estradiol. This permits GnRH to be secreted, leading to the pituitary release of LH and FSH. Polycystic ovary disease is the most common form of anovulation and is often associated with hirsutism. The hirsutism results from an excessive androgen production that is in some unknown way linked with the inability to ovulate.

D. Primary Amenorrhea

Amenorrhea is the absence of expected menstrual periods. When the menarche has not occurred by age 16, it is appropriate to seek an explanation. If there has been no change in the growth of breasts, appearance of pubic hair, or changes in vaginal smears, this suggests a tentative diagnosis of primary amenorrhea. The disorder can be due either to extragonadal or gonadal problems. One retrospective analysis found that gonadal dysgeneses and primary gonadal failure in phenotypic females who were genetic males accounted for about 40% of the patients with primary amenorrhea. An additional 20% have a gonadal dysfunction (e.g., polycystic ovaries), or "resistant ovary syndrome." In about 40% of cases, the etiological basis for the amenorrhea could be attributed to dysplasia of the mullerian ducts or hypogonadotropic states.

E. Menopause

Cessation of reproductive activity is associated with a number of bodily changes resulting from changes in the circulating levels of estrogen, progesterone, FSH, and LH. A major problem can be the development of the bone disease osteoporosis. Osteoporosis is a thinning of the skeleton which, if it occurs over a long enough time interval, incurs the definite risk of increased accidental or spontaneous fracture. In the view of many, the onset of osteoporosis is initiated by the absence of estradiol (see Chapter 9).

References

A. Books

Gurpide, E., ed. (1977). "Biochemical Actions of Progesterone and Progestins," Vol. 286. N. Y. Acad. Sci., New York.
Odell, W. D., and Moyer, D. C. (1971). "Physiology of Reproduction." Mosby, St. Louis, Missouri.

B. Review Articles

Bresciani, F., Sica, V., and Weisz, A. (1979). Properties of estrogen receptor purified to homogeneity. In "Biochemical Actions of Hormones" (G. Litwack, ed.), Vol. 6, pp. 461–480. Academic Press, New York.
Channing, C. P., and Tsafriri, A. (1977). A mechanism of action of lutenizing hormone and follicle-stimulating hormone on the ovary, in vitro. Metab., Clin. Exp. 26, 413–468.
DeJong, F. H., and Sharpe, R. M. (1976). Evidence for an inhibin-like activity in bovine follicular fluid. Nature (London) 263, 71–72.
Grossman, C. J. (1984). Regulation of the immune system by sex steroids. Endocr. Rev. 5, 435–455.
McEwen, B. S. (1981). Neural gonadal steroid actions. Science 211, 1303–1311.
O'Dell, W. D. (1978). Reproductive system in women. In "Textbook of Endocrine Physiology" (L. J. DeGroot, ed.), Vol. 3, pp. 1383–1400. Grune & Stratton, New York.
Westoff, C. F. (1976). Trends in contraceptive practice: 1965–1973. Fam. Plann. Perspect. 8, 54–57.

C. Research Papers

Bally, A., Atger, M., Atger, P., Cerbon, M., Alizon, M., Hai, M. T. V., Logeat, F., and Milgröm, E. (1983). The rabbit uteroglobin gene: Structure and interaction with the progesterone receptor. J. Biol. Chem. 258, 10384–10389.

564

Birnbaumer, M., Schrader, W. T., and O'Malley, B. W. (1983). Assessment of structural similarities in chick oviduct progesterone receptor subunits by partial proteolysis of photoaffinity-labeled proteins. *J. Biol. Chem.* **258,** 7331–7337.

Dean, D. C., Gope, R., Knoll, B. J., Riser, M. E., and O'Malley, B. W. (1984). A similar 5'-flanking region is required for estrogen and progesterone induction of ovalbumin gene expression. *J. Biol. Chem.* **259,** 9967–9970.

Dougherty, J. J., Puri, R. K., and Toft, D. O. (1984). Polypeptide components of two 8S forms of chicken oviduct progesterone receptor. *J. Biol. Chem.* **259,** 8004–8009.

Greene, G. L., Gilna, P., Waterfield, M., Baker, A., Hort, Y., and Shine, J. (1986). Sequence and expression of human estrogen receptor complementary DNA. *Science* **231,** 1150–1154.

Maggi, A., Schrader, W. T., and O'Malley, B. W. (1984). Progesterone-binding sites of the chick oviduct receptor: Presence of a weaker ligand site destroyed by phosphatase treatment. *J. Biol. Chem.* **259,** 10956–10966.

Marshall, J. A. (1968). A field trial of the basal body temperature method of regulating births. *Lancet* **2,** 8–10.

Mason, A. J., Hayflick, J. S., Ling, N., Esch, F., Ueno, N., Ying, S. Y., Guillemin, R., Niall, H., and Seeburg, P. H. (1985). Complementary DNA sequences of ovarian follicular fluid inhibin show precursor structure and homology with transforming growth factor-β. *Nature (London)* **318,** 659–663.

Muller, R. E., Traish, A. M., and Wotz, H. H. (1983). Estrogen receptor activation precedes transformation. *J. Biol. Chem.* **258,** 9227–9236.

Renoir, J. M., Chang-Ren, Y., Formstecher, P., Lustenberger, P., Wolfson, A., Redeweh, G., Mester, J., Foy, H., and Baulieu, E. (1983). Chick oviduct progesterone receptor: Purification of a molybdate-stabilized form and preliminary characterization. *Eur. J. Biochem.* **127,** 71–79.

Sasson, S., and Notides, A. (1982). The inhibition of the estrogen receptor's positive cooperative estradiol binding by the antagonist clomiphene. *J. Biol. Chem.* **257,** 11540–11545.

Scholl, S., and Lippman, M. E. (1984). The estrogen receptor in MCF-7 cells: Evidence from dense amino acid labeling for rapid turnover and a dimeric model of activated nuclear receptor. *Endocrinology (Baltimore)* **115,** 1295–1301.

Sherman, M. R., Moran, M. C., Tuazon, F. B., and Stevens, Y. W. (1983). Structure, dissociation, and proteolysis of mammalian steroid receptors. *J. Biol. Chem.* **258,** 10366–10377.

Walter, P., Green, S., Greene, G., Krust, A., Bornert, J. M., Jettsch, J. M., Staub, A., Jensen, E., Scrace, G., Waterfield, M., and Chambon, P. (1985). Cloning of the human estrogen receptor cDNA. *Proc. Natl. Acad. Sci. U.S.A.* **82,** 7889–7893.

Chapter **14**

Hormones of Pregnancy and Lactation

I. INTRODUCTION

A. General Comments

The ultimate purpose of reproduction is to reproduce a new male or female in order to maintain or prolong the species. As described in

HORMONES

566

Chapters 12 and 13 for the male and female, respectively, there is extensive anatomical and endocrinological specialization which, besides defining the individual's fundamental male or female status, collectively emphasizes their functional complementarity. It is the successful union both in an anatomical as well as an endocrinological sense which is essential for procreation (i.e., the meeting of a competent sperm with the ovum). Thus, the fundamental unit of reproductive biology is not the individual, but the triad of the mother, father, and offspring.

This chapter describes the human endocrinology that is unique to the process of pregnancy and lactation. It is beyond the scope of the chapter to describe the cell biology and endocrinology—involving growth factors and paracrine substances—of growth and development of the fetus and placenta.

B. Sequence of Events in Reproduction

The process of conception or fertilization of an ovum by a spermatozoon initiates a complex series of developmental and metabolic events for both the fetus and the mother which are controlled by an array of endocrine factors. In this regard a primordial endocrine event occurring shortly after the merging of the spermatozoon with the ovum to yield the zygote is the determination of the sex or gender of the offspring. This leads next to the development of the placenta as a mechanism for delivering nutrients to the developing fetus. Eventually through further endocrine intervention parturition or birth occurs which then initiates the process of lactation.

II. ANATOMICAL AND MORPHOLOGICAL RELATIONSHIPS

A. Placenta

After fertilization, the zygote immediately initiates cell division by mitosis and passes through the 2-, 4-, 8-cell stage until a tiny cluster of cells known as a morula is formed. After 3–4 days the morula reaches the uterus where it continues to grow. The morula now differentiates to create an outer shell, designated the trophoblast and an inner mass of cells that will ultimately become the embryo (see Fig. 14-1). This fluid-filled ball or blastocyst adheres to the surface of the uterine endometrium and begins the implantation process by secretion of proteolytic enzymes which digest a cavity in the endometrium. The portion of the endometrium to which the blastocyst adheres and implants is termed the *decidua basalis*.

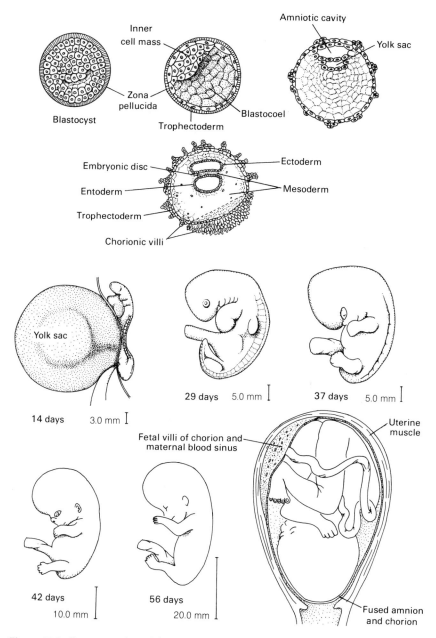

Figure 14-1. Representation of the various stages of development from blastocyst to early fetus.

568

Following implantation, the trophoblast of the blastocyst proliferates new villi rapidly. These villi infiltrate the endometrial decidua, tapping blood vessels with the creation of a labyrinth circulatory network. Simultaneously the embryonic blood vessels develop in the trophoblast and as soon as it is vascularized, it is termed the chorion (see Fig. 14-2). Subsequently another fetal membrane, the amnion, develops around the growing embryo; the amnion is connected to the chorion by the body stalk (see Fig. 14-2). The villi in this region enlarge to form the *chorion frondosum*, which ultimately develops into the fetal portion of the placenta. The smooth outer surface of the chorion is termed the *chorion laeve*. The body stalk then ultimately develops into the umbilical cord. Thus, the fully developed placenta consists of the maternal—*decidua basalis*—and the fetal—*chorion frondosum*—respectively. As diagrammed in Fig. 14-3, the fetal and maternal placenta have entirely separate circulatory systems; there is no direct communication between these two tissues.

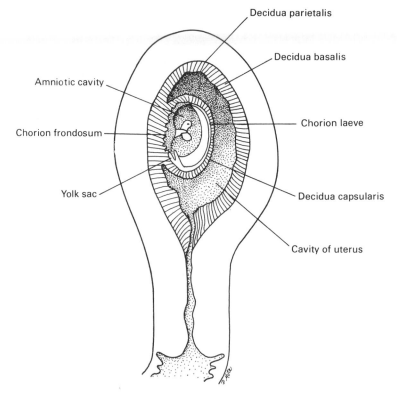

Figure 14-2. Midsagittal section of a uterus with developing embryo. The embryo is ~1 month old.

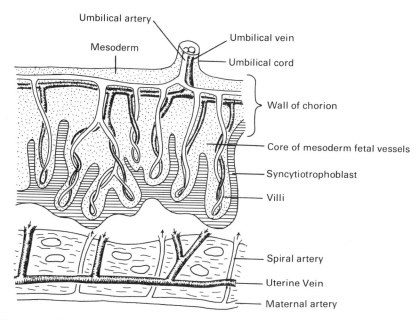

Figure 14-3. Diagram of the maternal and fetal circulating circulatory systems which emphasizes the entirely separate nature of the two systems.

One obvious function of the placenta is to provide the fetus with oxygen and all nutrients and to carry away excretory products. A second major role of the placenta is to serve as an endocrine gland to maintain pregnancy. In this respect the placenta takes over the endocrine function of the ovary and the anterior pituitary.

Cholesterol from the mother is metabolized by the placenta into progesterone. In the interim until placental production of progesterone is firmly established, the trophoblast secretes human chorionic gonadotropin, or hCG, which maintains the production of progesterone by the maternal corpus luteum. To form the other steroid hormones, placentally derived progesterone is transported to the fetal liver and fetal adrenal and then returned to the placenta for transformation into estrogens and a group of androgens, including testosterone.

B. Mammary Glands

The breasts or mammary glands are functionally related to the female reproductive system in that they secrete milk for nourishment of the newborn; anatomically the breasts are related to the skin (see Fig. 14-4).

Each breast is comprised of 15–20 lobes which overlay the major chest

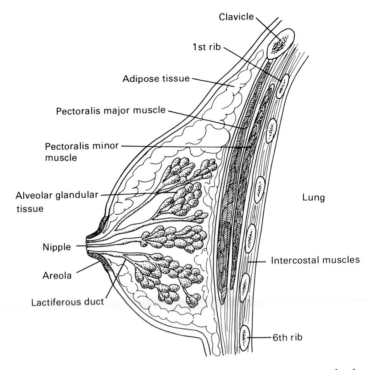

Figure 14-4. Ducts and glandular tissue of the human mammary gland.

muscle, the pectoralis. They lie between the second and sixth rib. Each lobe consists of glandular lobular tissue that is individually drained by intralobular ducts which empty in turn into the main lactiferous ducts. The breast tissue is responsive during pregnancy to estrogen, progesterone, prolactin, and oxytocin. The process of lactation is one of the most complex endocrine-mediated events in the body. The maturation of the mammary glands is initiated when the developing zygote is implanted in the uterus. Estrogens are responsible for the growth of the duct system, while progesterone mediates generation of the secretory system; then prolactin stimulates the production of milk.

In the first trimester of pregnancy there is initially a rapid growth and branching from the terminal portions of the gland followed by the appearance of true glandular acini. The hollow alveolus becomes lined with a single layer of myoepithelial cells ultimately enclosing the glandular alveolus in a loose network surrounded by capillaries so that the lumen of the alveolus is connected to an interlobular duct (see Fig. 14-5). In the second trimester of pregnancy the alveolar secretion begins. In

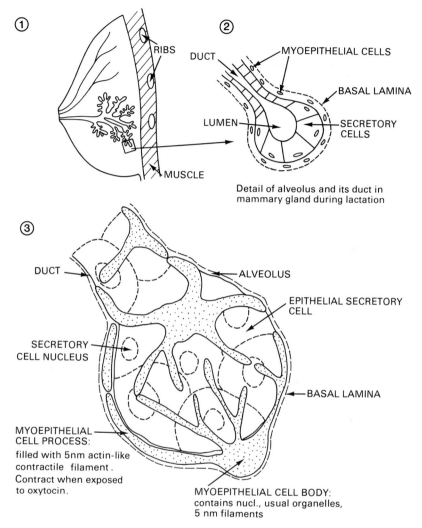

Figure 14-5. Schematic diagram of mammary gland alveolus and its duct. (Drawn by Dr. L. Paavola, Department of Anatomy, Temple University Medical School; provided by G. Litwack.)

the third trimester, particularly in the ninth month, breast enlargement occurs as a consequence of the hypertrophy of parenchymal cells and distention of the alveoli with colostrum.

Figure 14-6 presents a diagram of the mammary gland cell. The glandular epithelial cells are cuboidal in appearance and have small micro-

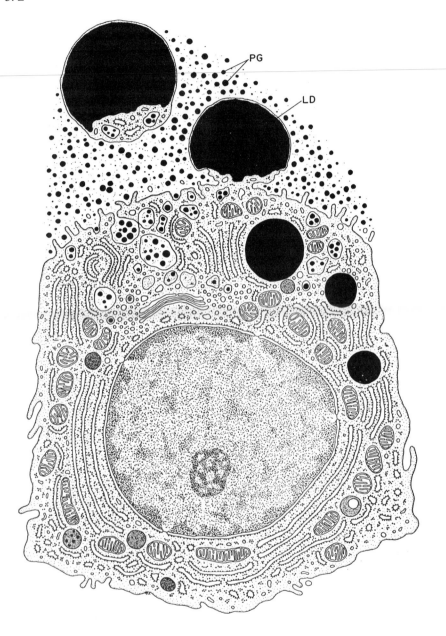

Table 14–1. Composition of Milk

Component	Bovine (%)	Human (%)
Water	87	87.5
Total solids	13	12.5
Carbohydrate	4.5–5.0	7.0–7.5
Lipid	3.5–5.0	3.0–4.0
Protein	3.0–4.0	1.0–1.5
Ash	0.75	0.2

Specific components of human milk[a]

Ash	Lipids	Carbohydrates	Proteins
Ca^{2+}	Triglycerides with fatty	Lactose	Caseins (80% of protein
HPO_4^{2-}	acids		nitrogen)
K^+	Oleic (32%)		β-Lactoglobulin (50% of
Na^+	Palmitic (15%)		whey protein)
Mg^{2+}	Myristic (20%)		Immunoglobulins (IgA)
Cl^-	Stearic (15%)		Albumin
	Other (6%)		α-Lactalbumin
	Cholesterol (4%)		Lactoperoxidase
	Phospholipids (8%)		Xanthine oxidase
			Alkaline phosphatase

[a] Abstracted from H. Vorherr, To breast-feed or not to breast-feed. *Postgrad. Med. J.* **51**, 127–139 (1972).

villi on the membrane surface facing the ducts. These cells are the site of biosynthesis of the various milk proteins and milk fats.

In the human, the rate of milk production is normally 500 ml/day by 1 week postpartum; after 3 weeks milk production increases to 800–1000 ml/day. Table 14-1 tabulates the composition of milk. The colostrum or milk obtained in the several days immediately following parturition differs from milk in its biological and physical properties. The principal difference is a higher protein content (up to 5% or 20% in the human and bovine, respectively); the additional proteins are largely immunoglobulins and include all the antibodies present in the maternal blood.

Figure 14-6. Diagram of a mammary gland epithelial cell. The glandular epithelial cells of the mammary gland are cuboidal. Scattered microvilli occur on the free surface. The lateral borders are bound together by junctional complexes and interdigitate, while a few villous processes occur basally. The nucleus is situated toward the base of the cell and contains a nucleolus. Two particulate components are found in the milk of the mammary gland: small dense protein granules (PG) and large lipid droplets (LD). Reproduced by permission from T. L. Lentz, "Cell Fine Structure," p. 287. Saunders, Philadelphia, Pennsylvania, 1971.

III. CHEMISTRY, BIOCHEMISTRY, AND BIOLOGICAL RESPONSES

A. Pregnancy

1. Introduction

The endocrine changes accompanying pregnancy are remarkable. A pregnant woman in the late phase of the third trimester produces on a daily basis some 250–300 mg of progesterone, 15–20 mg of estradiol-17β, 50–100 mg of estriol, 75–100 mg of cortisol, 3–8 mg of deoxycorticosterone (DOC), and 1–2 mg of aldosterone. In addition, there is a massive production of human placental lactogen (in excess of 1 g/day), human chorionic gonadotropin and human chorionic thyrotropin, chorionic ACTH, as well as increased plasma levels of the angiotensins and renin. Figure 14-7 summarizes the temporal changes of many of these hormones through gestation.

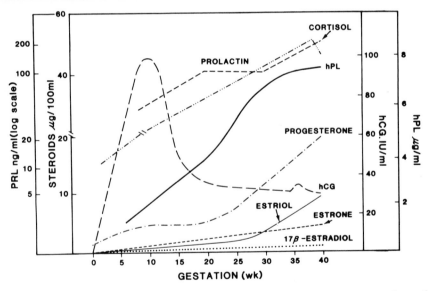

Figure 14-7. Temporal changes during human pregnancy in the serum concentrations of several hormones. hPL, Human placental lactogen; hCG, human chorionic gonadotropin; PRL, prolactin. Modified from C. Aragona and H. G. Friesen, Lactation and galactorrhea. *In* "Endocrinology" (L. J. DeGroot, G. F. Cahill, L. Martin, D. H. Nelson, W. D. Odell, J. T. Potts, E. Steinberger, and A. I. Winegrad, eds.), Vol. 3, pp. 1614–1617. Grune & Stratton, New York, 1979.

2. Peptide Hormones

a. Human Chorionic Gonadotropin. Human chorionic gonadotropin, hCG, is a glycoprotein of molecular weight 57,000 with two subunits, designated α and β. The α chain consists of 92 amino acid residues, while the β chain consists of 147 amino acid residues. The primary amino acid sequences are presented in Fig. 5-11 (α chain) and Fig. 5-12 (β chain). Figure 5-14B presents a schematic model for the attachment of the some 20–30 carbohydrate residues to the protein. There is a strong structural homology between hCG and LH and TSH, particularly for the α subunits. Although hCG has both N-glycosidic as well as O-glycosidic linked carbohydrates, the pituitary-derived LH and TSH contain only N-glycosidic linked carbohydrates.

Also, there is a structural homology for the β subunit, which defines the biological and immunological reactivity between hCG and LH. Table 14-2 summarizes the structural homology of several of the released pituitary and placental hormones. hCG produced by the synctiotrophoblast, which is diagrammed in Fig. 14-3, is concerned with the attachment of the embryo to the maternal placenta; thus technically hCG is produced by the fetus. The rate of production of hCG is maximal by the tenth week of pregnancy, then it falls slowly to a nadir at 17 weeks and remains at a low but readily measurable level for the duration of the pregnancy.

Table 14–2. Structural Homology of Pituitary and Placental Hormones

Hormone	Molecular weight	Number of amino acids in the chains		Carbohydrate containing
		α	β	
Glycoproteins				
FSH (follicle-stimulating hormone)	32,000	(236)		+
LH (luteinizing hormone)	30,000	98	119	+
hCG (human chorionic gonadotropin)	57,000	92	139	+
TSH (thyroid-stimulating hormone)	28,000	96	113	+
Somatomammotropins				
PRL (prolactin)	23,000	(198)		−
GH (growth hormone)	22,000	(191)		−
hPL (human placental lactogen)	22,000	(191)		−

The precise function and biological effects of hCG in pregnancy are not known. Its dominant action is to function as a luteotropin, that is, to stimulate the production of progesterone by the corpus luteum. This ensures a continual supply of the ovarian progesterone until the placenta has developed to the point (usually at 6–8 weeks) when it can generate adequate quantities of progesterone when the corpus luteum of pregnancy atrophies. By analogy with LH (Chapter 5) and TSH (Chapter 6), the β subunit of hCG is believed to interact specifically with a membrane receptor to stimulate production of progesterone from cholesterol.

  b. Human Placental Lactogen. Human placental lactogen (hPL), which is sometimes referred to as human chorionic somatomammotropin (HCS), is a 190 amino acid polypeptide (single chain) of molecular weight 21,500. Its amino acid sequence is presented in Fig. 14-8. It has a degree of molecular similarity to both human growth hormone (see Fig. 5-5) and human prolactin (see Fig. 5-6). Little information is available concerning the production and secretion of hPL by the trophoblasts and placenta. The major biological roles of hPL are not well described; its effects on mobilization and metabolism of maternal fat stores have been

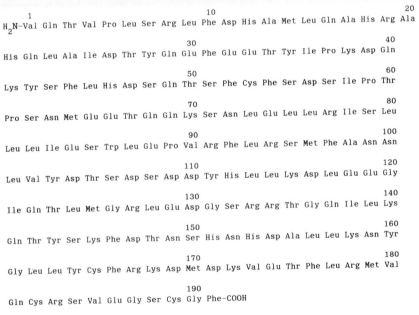

Figure 14-8. Primary amino acid sequence of human placental lactogen (or human chorionic somatomammotropin). Modified from C. H. Li, J. S. Dickson, and D. Chung, Amino acid sequence of human chorionic somatomammotropin. *Arch. Biochem. Biophys.* **155,** 95–110 (1973).

described. Also, hPL is an insulin antagonist and in this role is postulated as being involved in the regulation of maternal blood glucose levels to ensure optimal availability of blood glucose to meet the caloric requirements of the fetus. Also, hPL has been suggested as being one of the contributory agents to the development of diabetic ketoacidosis in pregnant women who have had no prior history of diabetes.

    c. Relaxin. Relaxin (RLX) is the name given to a bioactive protein that has been isolated and purified from the corpus luteum of porcine ovaries of pregnant animals. Its biological action is believed to be to promote relaxation of the birth canal and softening of the cervix and ligaments of the *symphysis pubis* in preparation for parturition. As shown in Fig. 14-9, the primary structure of porcine RLX consists of two peptide chains (designated α and β) of 22 and 31 amino acid residues, respectively. The α and β chains are covalently linked by two interchain disulfide bonds with an intradisulfide link also in the A chain. Thus, RLX is structurally very similar to insulin (see Fig. 7-6) and it is therefore also related to the "insulin-like" growth factors (IGF) (see Chapter 19). The sequence of the pig, rat, and shark RLX have been determined and there is a low degree of homology, in contrast to the high homology among the insulins from these same three species.

    RLX is primarily produced by the corpus luteum, but there is some evidence of its presence also in the follicles as well as in human placenta in the female. Given the commonality of hormones in the series, it is not surprising that RLX activity has also been detected in rooster seminal

```
              1            5              10             15
α Chain    Arg-Met-Thr-Leu-Ser-Glu-Lys-Cys-Cys-Gln-Val-Gly-Cys-Ile-Arg-

                        20
           -Lys-Asp-Ile-Ala-Arg-Leu-Cys


              1            5              10             15
β Chain    Glu-Ser-Thr-Asn-Asp-Phe-Ile-Lys-Ala-Cys-Gly-Arg-Glu-Leu-Val-

                        20                   25             30
           -Arg-Leu-Trp-Val-Glu-Ile-Cys-Gly-Ser-Val-Ser-Trp-Gly-Arg-Thr-


           -Ala-Leu
```

Figure 14-9. Primary amino acid sequence of the α and β chains of porcine relaxin. There is a known structural homology between relaxin, insulin, nerve growth factor, and insulin-like growth factor I (see Fig. 19-8). Modified from Figure 1 of G. D. Bryant-Greenwood, Relaxin as a new hormone. *Endocr. Rev.* **3,** 62–90 (1982). © by The Endocrine Society (1982).

fluid and in the prostate. In common with insulin and IGF, RLX is also synthesized as a prohormone.

The hormonal actions of RLX are manifest on the collagenous interpubic ligament (to cause elongation and thus separation of the pubic bones at parturition), the uterus (to mediate uterine quiescence and to increase uterine collagenase activity), and in the cervix (in concert with estrogen, progesterone, and prostaglandins to soften the fibrous connective tissue at the time of parturition). Little specific information is available concerning the mode of action of RLX; it is to be presumed that like other peptide hormones, it interacts with specific external membrane receptors on its target cells.

d. Oxytocin. Oxytocin is a nonapeptide secreted by the neurohypophysis. An extensive discussion of its chemistry and mode of action is presented in Chapter 4. Milk letdown and milk ejection from the mammary tissue are the chief biological responses. There is also some preliminary evidence to support the action of oxytocin on the uterine endometrium at parturition to stimulate its contraction. High concentrations of oxytocin can be detected in fetal blood.

e. Other Peptide Hormones. Evidence, both chemical and immunochemical, has been presented indicating that human placental tissue produces and secretes human chorionic thyrotropin (an analog of TSH) and chorionic ACTH. Preliminary evidence also suggests the possibility of placental production of GnRH and TRH releasing hormones. These factors may play a role in placental secretion of hCG and chorionic thyrotropin.

3. Steroid Hormones

a. Introduction. The steroid hormones generated specifically as a consequence of the circumstances of pregnancy are produced in a number of tissues; these include the maternal and fetal placenta, the maternal adrenal and fetal adrenals, and maternal ovaries and liver. The steroids produced at these sites are tabulated in Table 14-3.

There is a changing pattern of production of steroid hormones throughout the trimesters of pregnancy, so that as the fetus differentiates and develops, the fetal adrenals and liver have an increasing responsibility for steroid metabolism. Immediately following conception through 12–13 weeks of the pregnancy, the principal source of progesterone and estrogen is the corpus luteum. By week 7 and until parturition, the placenta produces significant quantities of both estrogens (in the forms of estradiol-17β, estriol, estrone, and estetrol) and progesterone. Both the placental and corpus luteum production of progesterone are stimulated by hCG.

Table 14–3. Steroid Hormones of Pregnancy and Their Site of Production

Mother	Placenta	Fetus
		Estriol
		Estradiol, estetrol
		Δ^5-Pregnenolone
		Progesterone
		Progesterone, 16-OH-progesterone
		17-OH-Progesterone
Adrenal cortex	Dehydroepiandrosterone sulfate	Pregnenolone sulfate
	Cortisol	17α-OH-Pregnenolone sulfate
		Dehydroepiandrosterone sulfate
		16α-Dehydroepiandrosterone sulfate
		Δ^5-Pregnenolone sulfate
Ovaries (corpus luteum)	Progesterone	
	17-OH-Progesterone	—
	Estrone	—
	Estradiol	—
Liver	Cholesterol (maternal source)	Cholesterol (fetal source)
		Estriol

Since the placenta does not have the complete array of steroid-metabolizing enzymes to convert cholesterol into estradiol, progesterone, or other steroids, during the second and third trimester both the maternal adrenal cortex and fetal adrenal cortex serve as major sources of precursors for placental steroidogenesis. In this regard dehydroepiandrosterone sulfate from the maternal adrenals is converted by the placenta to estrogens. The fetal adrenal cortex becomes enzymatically competent to produce steroids by day 50 of the pregnancy. In this fetal compartment many of the steroids are sulfate conjugates. The fetal adrenal also assumes a major responsibility for the production of C-19 androgens and sulfoconjugated Δ^5 C-21 steroids such as pregnenolone sulfate in the second and third trimesters.

b. Production of Progesterone. Throughout the course of pregnancy there are three principal forms of the C-21 progestins present: progesterone, 16α-OH-progesterone, and 17α-OH-progesterone. Figure 14-10 summarizes their separate pathways of biosynthesis.

Progesterone is produced largely by the corpus luteum up to 5–6 weeks of gestation; then by week 12 of gestation the placenta becomes the dominant site of biosynthesis. Thus, the plasma level of progesterone rises from 1–2 ng/ml at conception to over 100 ng/ml by parturition.

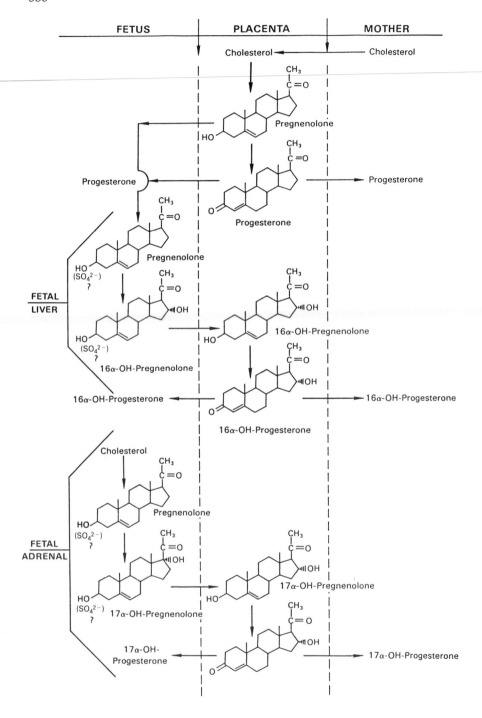

The placenta contains all the enzymes required for the conversion of maternally derived cholesterol into progesterone.

17α-Hydroxyprogesterone levels in the plasma rise from 0.5 ng/ml at conception to a plateau of 50–60 ng/ml at weeks 6–36 of gestation. Up to the first 8–12 weeks of gestation the maternal ovary is the principal site of 17α-OH-progesterone. After the first trimester, the placenta uses the precursor 17-OH-Δ^5-pregnenolone produced from Δ^5 C-21 sulfoconjugates in the fetal adrenal cortex to produce 17-OH-progesterone.

16α-Hydroxyprogesterone plasma levels rise gradually from 0.5 ng/ml at conception to a level of 120–140 ng/ml by 32 weeks of gestation. The precise biosynthetic pathway of 16α-OH-progesterone is not known; it is believed that the fetal liver produces Δ^5-pregnenolone-16-OH-sulfate and that this is converted by the placenta into 16α-OH-progesterone which is then available to both the mother and fetus. There is no known specific biological response attributable to 16α-OH-progesterone.

c. Production of Estrogens. Throughout the course of pregnancy there are four principal forms of the C-18 estrogens present. At parturition the relative serum concentrations are as follows: estradiol (10–30 ng/ml), estriol (5–10 ng/ml), estrone (5–8 ng/ml), and estetrol (2–4 ng/ml). Estetrol is 15,16(OH)$_2$-estradiol. Figure 14-11 summarizes their pathways of biosynthesis.

By the end of the first trimester the placenta is the principal site of biosynthesis of estradiol and estrone. Estriol is produced largely from the placental conversion of 16-OH-dehydroepiandrosterone sulfate derived successively from the fetal liver and adrenals. Finally, estetrol is believed to be largely produced in the fetal compartment from placentally generated estriol.

Since the fetus plays a key role in the production of estetrol and estriol, the measurement of the maternal blood levels of these steroids has been proposed to provide some insight into the fetal well-being. Thus, deteriorating fetoplacental health in the third trimester is often associated with falling unconjugated maternal serum estriol or estetrol concentrations.

Figure 14-10. Pathways and anatomical compartmentalization of the production of the C-21 progestins, particularly progesterone, 17α-OH-progesterone, and 16α-OH-progesterone in the human fetal–placental unit. These figures were derived in part from J. E. Buster and J. R. Marshall, Conception, gamete and ovum transport, implantation, fetal placental hormones, hormonal preparation for parturition and parturition control. *In* "Endocrinology" (L. J. DeGroot, G. F. Cahill, L. Martini, D. H. Nelson, W. D. Odell, J. T. Potts, E. Steinberger, and A. I. Winegrad, eds.), Vol. 3, pp. 1601, 1602. Grune & Stratton, New York, 1979.

582

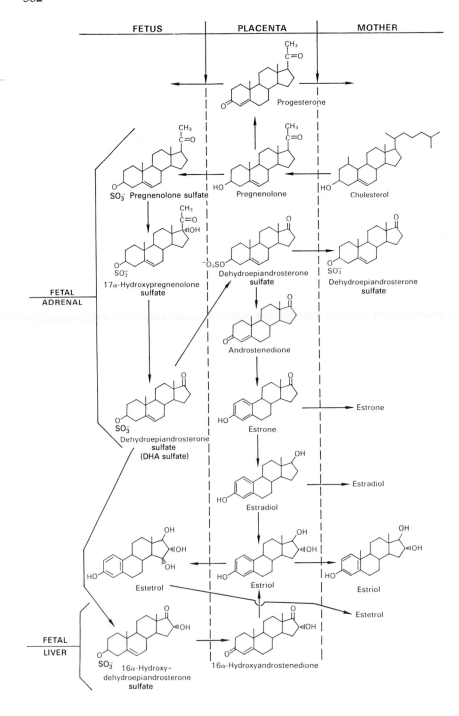

d. Production of Androgens. The principal C-19 androgen in the pregnant female is dehydroepiandrosterone sulfate; prior to conception the maternal serum level is 1600 ng/ml and this decreases throughout gestation to a value of 800 ng/ml at parturition. As described in Fig. 14-12, the principal source of androgens in the female is from the maternal adrenal cortex; here cholesterol is converted to pregnenolone and then finally to dehydroepiandrosterone sulfate. The fall in blood levels of dehydroepiandrosterone sulfate is believed to reflect an increased metabolic clearance rate due to a significant uptake of this steroid by the placenta for conversion into estrogens.

e. Vitamin D Steroids. Associated with fetal growth and development in the third trimester is the requirement for significant amounts of calcium for skeletal development. This calcium is ultimately derived from either the dietary calcium or skeletal calcium reserves of the mother. The calcium is actively transported across the placenta. It is intriguing, therefore, that the placenta and also the fetal kidney have the enzymatic capability to convert 25-OH-vitamin D_3 into $1,25(OH)_2$-vitamin D_3; this later seco-steroid is a hormonally active form of vitamin D_3 (see Chapter 9) that is known to be required for both intestinal as well as bone calcium processes.

4. Prostaglandins

The local production of prostaglandins PGE_2 and $PGF_{2\alpha}$ by the placenta is associated with the onset of labor and parturition. The structures of PGE_2 and $PGF_{2\alpha}$ are given in Fig. 16-2. The enzymatic capability for the production of these prostaglandins resides in the decidua. The released prostaglandins then act on the myometrium to stimulate an adenyl cyclase.

B. Parturition

In human pregnancy, a normal birth can occur after 34–36 weeks of gestation. The process of labor and birth represents the culmination of a complex series of endocrinological events in the mother and fetus.

After 34 weeks of gestation there is a large increase in the fetal ex-

---

Figure 14-11. Pathways and anatomical compartmentalization of the production of the C-18 estrogens: estradiol, estrone, estriol, and estetrol in the human fetal–placenta unit. These figures were derived from J. E. Buster and J. R. Marshall, Conception, gamete and ovum transport, implantation, fetal placental hormones, hormonal preparation for parturition and parturition control. *In* "Endocrinology" (L. J. DeGroot, G. F. Cahill, L. Martini, D. H. Nelson, W. D. Odell, J. T. Potts, E. Steinberger, and A. I. Winegrad, eds.), Vol. 3, pp. 1595–1612. Grune & Stratton, New York, 1979.

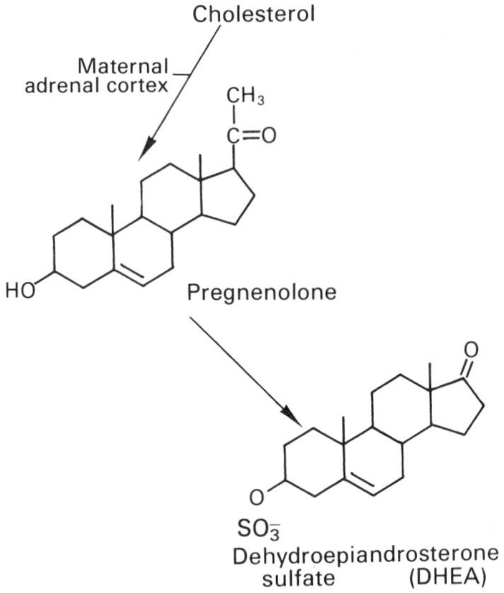

Figure 14-12. Pathways for the production of androgens related to pregnancy.

posure to glucocorticoids, particularly cortisol. Contributing to the rise in cortisol is a sharp decrease in corticosteroid binding globulin (CBG), also called transcortin, in fetal serum. This protein normally has bound to it the greatest proportion of circulating cortisol. The resulting increase in "free" hormone triggers major biochemical changes in the placenta, as shown in Fig. 14-13.

Throughout pregnancy, the placenta has been secreting large amounts of progesterone which has a profound effect on mammary gland development and blockage of the action of prolactin on differentiated mammary gland cells, so that they are not manufacturing milk proteins. Although still controversial, some evidence suggests that the large amount of available progesterone binds to the glucocorticoid receptor in mammary gland instead of cortisol and prevents the activity of the glucocorticoid receptor which may be required, in addition to prolactin, for expression of milk proteins. Also, blocked by progesterone is the release of oxytocin from the neurohypophysis. This is an important control, since oxytocin exerts strong action on uterine contractions. When free cortisol levels rise near term, the large output of progesterone by the placenta is depressed by a fall in the secretion of hCG from the trophoblast and may be blocked presumably by a glucocorticoid receptor-mediated mechanism perhaps similar to the action of glucocorticoids on the thymus (Fig. 10-13). The sharp fall in progesterone levels relieves the brake on the maternal

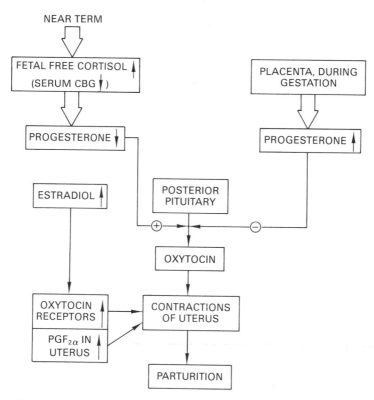

Figure 14-13. Probable roles of glucocorticoid hormone in normal termination of pregnancy. + indicates stimulation; − indicates inhibition.

neurohypophysis exerted throughout pregnancy and results in release of oxytocin. Cortisol also acts on the placenta to stimulate estrogen production. Concomitantly the amount of $PGF_{2\alpha}$ is increased and the uterus may be the primary source of this prostaglandin. Both estrogen and $PGF_{2\alpha}$ sensitize the uterus to the action of oxytocin. Thus, the oxytocin released from the neurohypophysis causes smooth muscular contractions of the uterus which culminates in the expulsion of the fetus. Cortisol appears to be the main trigger in starting the process.

The cortisol may also play a role in induction of the fetal pulmonary surfactant, a substance essential to lung alveolar stability as well as in the storage of glycogen in the fetal skeletal and cardiac muscle and the liver. This later event may assist the fetus to avoid the stresses of hypoxia during labor.

The biochemical and endocrinological changes specifically associated with the birth process are not yet precisely formulated. Certainly prostaglandins produced in the cell membranes of the deciduum, fetal steroids, fetal oxytocin, as well as maternal catecholamines and oxytocin all participate in this key event.

C. Lactation

1. Introduction

The endocrine changes associated with lactation are no less remarkable than those encountered in pregnancy. In fact, it is not realistic to separate the process of lactation from that of pregnancy; while they are temporally related to one another, there are key endocrine events related to lactation that occur early in pregnancy.

For lactation to ultimately occur, it is necessary during pregnancy to effect duct, lobule, and alveolar growth. It has been concluded from experiments using combinations of oophorectomized, hypophysectomized, and adrenalectomized rats that no less than six pituitary hormones, as well as placental lactogen, estrogen, progesterone, glucocorticoids, thyroxine, and insulin are all involved in some aspect of mammary growth and development. However, it is beyond the scope of this chapter to consider in detail these developmental changes.

Summarized below is an enumeration of the effects of hormones necessary for the actual process of lactation.

2. Peptide Hormones

a. Prolactin. The principal peptide hormone of lactation is the pituitary hormone prolactin. Prolactin is a 22,550-molecular weight protein composed of a single polypeptide chain of 198 amino acids. Its primary amino acid structure is given in Fig. 5-6. There is a strong structural homology between prolactin and growth hormone.

In females the biological action of prolactin is to mediate proliferation and differentiation of the breast and thus to permit, after appropriate stimuli, the secretion of milk (discussed in detail later). The physiological role of prolactin in the male is not known. However, newborn infants of both sexes have plasma levels of prolactin that exceed the highest levels of the mother either during pregnancy or lactation.

b. Other Peptide Hormones. Insulin (see Chapter 7) has been shown to be required for proper functioning of the mammary gland during lactation. Although the biochemical bases of its actions have not been elucidated, it seems likely that insulin will stimulate glucose uptake by mammary cells which will facilitate lipogenesis.

Parathyroid hormone (PTH) (see Chapter 9) is also necessary for optimal lactation. Parathyroidectomy of lactating animals depresses lactation; however, it is not known whether the reduction in lactation is due to perturbation in the actions of PTH (1) directly on the mammary tissue, (2) on mobilization of bone calcium to provide calcium for milk secretion, or (3) as an expression of its action in stimulating the renal production of 1,25-dihydroxyvitamin D_3 [1,25(OH)$_2$D$_3$]. The 1,25(OH)$_2$D$_3$ in turn would mediate the intestinal absorption of adequate amounts of calcium to support its secretion in milk (see Table 14-1) and avoid the deleterious consequences of extensive bone calcium mobilization.

c. Other Hormones. The thyroid hormone thyroxine (see Chapter 6) is believed to be important in man for proper milk secretion. Hypothyroid subjects are sometimes associated with galactorrhea, which is the secretion of milk from the breast under nonphysiological circumstances.

With respect to the involvement of steroid hormones in lactation, surprisingly neither estrogen nor progesterone is essential for established milk secretion; oophorectomy does not abolish milk production. In the mouse, rat, and goat, adrenal steroids have been shown to be essential for the induction and maintenance of milk secretion.

IV. CELL BIOLOGY AND MOLECULAR ACTIONS

A. Hormonal Aspects of Fertilization and Sex Differentiation

1. Capacitation

Within 5–15 min after depositing sperm in the vagina, motile spermatozoa are present in the fallopian tubes. Estrogen, secreted late in the follicular phase, causes the endocervical glands to secrete a mucus which favors sperm transport and motility. The process of fertilization is initiated by the union of a competent spermatozoon with an ovum of the same species.

Capacitation of a spermatozoon is required before a successful union with an ovum can be achieved. Capacitation involves the removal of an outer coating from the surface of the spermatozoon; this is followed by the removal of the acrosome or tip of the spermatozoon (see Fig. 14-14 and also Fig. 12-5). This latter process, which has been termed the acrosome reaction, allows the acrosomal hyaluronidase enzymes to come into contact with the substances surrounding the ovum so that the sper-

588

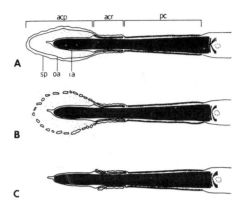

Figure 14-14. Capacitation of a spermatozoon before (A), during (B), and after (C) acrosomal reaction. acp, Acrosomal cap region; acr, acrosomal collar region; ia, inner acrosomal membrane; oa, outer acrosomal membrane; pc, postnuclear cap region; sp, plasma membrane of the spermatozoon. Modified from R. Yanagimachi and Y. Noda, Electron microscope studies of sperm incorporation into the golden hamster egg. *Am. J. Anat.* **128,** 429–462 (1970).

matozoon may penetrate and unite. While estrogens do not have an effect on the capacitation process, progesterone can inhibit the capacitation from occurring in the uterus.

2. Conception

Normally fertilization takes place in the distal one-third of the fallopian tubes. The species specificity of the fertilization process is determined by a receptor-like mechanism present in the vitelline membrane of the ovum. W. Lennarz and associates have isolated a glycoprotein from sea urchin egg membranes that will only cross-react with a species-specific protein, termed bindin, present on the surface of a homologous sea urchin spermatozoon.

The attachment of a single spermatozoon to any region of the *zona pelucida* on a single ovum is the formal process of fertilization; the entire spermatozoon then enters the ovum, so that there is both a nuclear and cytoplasmic contribution to the zygote.

After the sperm penetration, the fertilized ovum forms the second polar body (see also Fig. 13-5). This is then followed by the formation of female and male pronuclei; fusion of these haploid nuclei then creates, for the first time, the diploid nuclei of a totally new and unique individual. Some 30 hr later the first mitotic cleavage occurs, yielding a zygote with two cells; then within another 10 hr the mitotic cleavage occurs again, producing a 4-cell state. Within 50–60 hr of fertilization the morula arises, followed by the blastocyst at 3–4 days (see Fig. 14-1).

3. Sex Determination

Union of the spermatozoon with the ovum not only restores the diploid number of chromosomes (46 in man), but also determines the genetic sex of the new individual. Since the oocyte always has an X chromosome, the sex of the offspring is determined by the fertilizing spermatozoon; if it is an X-bearing spermatozoon, the gender is female (XX) while if it is a Y-bearing spermatozoon, the gender will be male (XY).

Under normal circumstances of the union of the human spermatozoon with the secondary oocyte, there is the creation of a zygote with 46 chromosomes. However, in some instances there are chromosomal abnormalities which may result in the offspring having an incorrect number of either autosomal chromosomes or sex chromosomes. Some of these abnormalities are summarized in Table 14-4. It is beyond the scope of this chapter to consider in detail the wide array of endocrine and nonendocrine disorders resulting from perturbations of genetic mechanisms of sexual development. The interested reader is referred to the text by M. Grumbach.

There are several other parameters besides the genetic sex which are utilized in describing the total definition of sex of an individual. These are summarized in Table 14-5. "Gonadal sex" is a reflection of the morphology of the gonads and the hormones they elaborate and is of dominant practical importance in defining the sex of an individual. "Phenotypic sex" is a reflection of the appearance of the external genitalia (i.e., the penis and vulva) as well as the secondary sex characteristics including the beard and breasts, while "somatic sex" reflects the difference in the structures of the internal sex organs. Finally, "psychological sex" is a reflection of the social environment and behavioral aspects in which an individual may be raised.

In the instance of individuals who are transsexuals, transvestites, and

Table 14–4. Chromosomal Karotypes Related to Human Disorders

Clinical condition	Total number of chromosomes	Sex chromosome	Number of autosomal chromosomes
Normal male	46	XY	44
Normal female	46	XX	44
Turner's syndrome	45	X	44
Klinefelter's syndrome	47	XXY	44
Super female	47	XXX	44
Mongolism (female)	47	XX	45
Mongolism (male)	47	XY	45

Table 14–5. Parameters Involved with the Definition of Sex

Parameter	Description
Physiological sex	
Genetic or gender	Interaction of sex chromosomes XY = ♂, XX = ♀
Gonadal	Comparison of ovaries with testes
Somatic	Comparison of the internal sex organs in the male and female
Phenotypic	Comparison of the external genitalia and secondary sex characteristics: male: penis, beard; female: vulva, breasts
Birth certificate	A legal document usually certified by the physician present at birth, but which may not correctly state the gonadal or genetic sex of the individual
Nonphysiological sex	
Psychological	A reflection of the social dimensions around the individual as she/he is reared which may also reflect behavioral attitudes of key individuals in the environment

homosexuals, their physiological sex may not agree with their psychological sex. Thus, when an individual experiences a normal development and sexual differentiation and is exposed to a normal psychosocial environment, then her/his genetic, gonadal, somatic, phenotypic, and psychological sexes will match. However, disturbances in any one of these parameters can result in aberrant gender identification and pose serious clinical, endocrinological, and psychological problems.

4. Sex Differentiation

The ultimate purpose of sex differentiation is to produce a female or male of the species. While the genetic sex of the new offspring is determined at fertilization, no morphological differences in the reproductive system of the embryo can be detected until the initiation of sexual differentiation and appearance of characteristic gonadal sex attributes at approximately the fourth week of development.

The gonadal anlage or gonadal precursor cells can be identified in the 4-week-old embryo and is preformed from the coelomic epithelium and from condensation with its underlying mesenchyme. At this stage, since it is impossible to distinguish whether the embryo will differentiate into ovaries or testes, it is designated as an "indifferent gonadal anlage." The indifferent anlage has two putative genital ducts: the mullerian ducts, which can ultimately become the internal reproductive tract of the adult female, and the wolffian ducts and mesonephros, which can become the adult male internal reproductive system. If the embryo is destined to become a male, the mullerian ducts degenerate, while if the embryo is destined to become a female, the wolffian ducts degenerate.

There is an inherent tendency for the indifferent gonadal anlage to undergo differentiation to yield ovaries provided that the correct X chromosome is present: The production of the male gonads, the testis, is believed to be related to the H-Y antigen, a cell surface protein coded for by a gene(s) uniquely located on the Y chromosome. The chronology of these relationships are diagrammed schematically in Fig. 14-15. The indifferent gonads begin to develop in the male at 43-50 days and in the female slightly later at 50–60 days.

The H-Y antigen has been demonstrated in the mouse embryo to be present as early as the 8-cell stage. It must be considered to be a male hormone in that it is postulated to be the "inducer" substance which directs the appearance of the male gonads from the wolffian ducts (see Fig. 14-16). Clear biological evidence for this postulate has come from studies in pregnant cows bearing male and female twins. When a vascular anastomosis between the female and male embryo occurs (these are referred to as "freemartins"), there occurs a testis-like differentiation of the gonads of the female twin. Although the gonads of the fetal female freemartin have only a very low proportion of XY cells (they are intrinsically XX), they do contain as much H-Y antigen as the normal bovine male fetal testes, which supports the concept that the testicular organization of the XX gonad is due to the H-Y antigen derived from the XY cells of the partner male twin.

The H-Y antigen is an oligomeric protein of molecular weight greater than 280,000; the monomeric subunit is ~18,000 Da; the polymeric form is known to contain disulfide bridges. The only gonadal cell believed to release the H-Y antigen is the primitive Sertoli cell. There are postulated to be two receptors for the H-Y antigen. One receptor is relatively nonspecific and ubiquitous, and it provides the stable binding sites on the external cell membrane in all male cells; it may be related structurally to the major histocompatibility complex cell surface antigens (HLA). The second receptor is only present in gonadal cells of both the male and female; it binds the H-Y antigen with a higher affinity than the first receptor site.

Figure 14-17 diagrams the steps of human sex determination which lead to the conversion of the indifferent gonad anlage into either a testis or ovary. This process of gonad differentiation is determined by the individual's genetic sex and it is the subsequent male or female gonadal secretions that determine the somatic and phenotypic sex. Figure 14-18 diagrams the reciprocal changes occurring in the male and female with respect to either the wolffian or mullerian duct development.

In the absence of the H-Y antigen, female sex differentiation will lead to conversion of the indifferent gonad anlage into ovaries and to the regression of the wolffian ducts. Thus, the development of the female

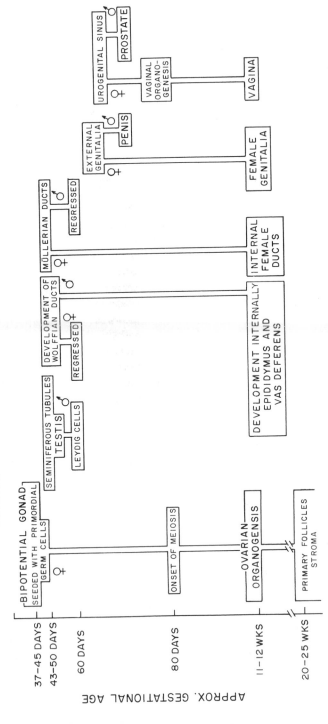

Figure 14-15. Chronology of the development of the external and internal male and female sex organs. Modified from F. A. Conte and M. M. Grumbach, Pathogenesis, classification, diagnosis, and treatment of anomalies of sex. In "Endocrinology" (L. J. DeGroot, G. F. Cahill, L. Martini, D. H. Nelson, W. D. Odell, J. T. Potts, E. Steinberger, and A. I. Winegrad, eds.), Vol. 3, p. 1318. Grune & Stratton, New York, 1979.

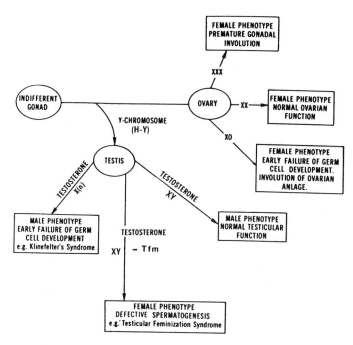

Figure 14-16. Current concepts of genetic and hormonal mechanisms associated with sexual differentiation. Also indicated are the consequences of genetic alteration in the normal complement of human chromosomes (44XX, normal female), (44XY, normal male). It is proposed that on the X-chromosome there is a gene, T_{fm}, which confers testosterone responsiveness to all cells in the organism which may be sensitive to testosterone action. Reproduced with permission from E. Steinberger, Genetics, anatomy, fetal endocrinology. *In* "Endocrinology" (L. J. DeGroot, G. F. Cahill, L. Martini, D. H. Nelson, W. D. Odell, J. T. Potts, E. Steinberger, and A. I. Winegrad, eds.), Vol. 3, p. 1315. Grune & Stratton, New York, 1979.

reproductive tract requires no hormonal stimulation from either ovaries or testes.

Differentiation of the male indifferent gonad anlage occurs as a consequence of the presence of the H-Y antigen and produces functional testes. With the appearance of the fetal testes (by week 7 of embryo life), two hormones are secreted—antimullerian hormone and testosterone. The existence of a mullerian duct inhibiting factor (or the antimullerian hormone) has been inferred from studies where castrated male fetuses or normal female fetuses treated with androgens did not result in regression of the mullerian ducts. This observation led to the suggestion that there must be two testes-derived hormones required for complete masculinization of the internal reproductive tract: testosterone and a factor

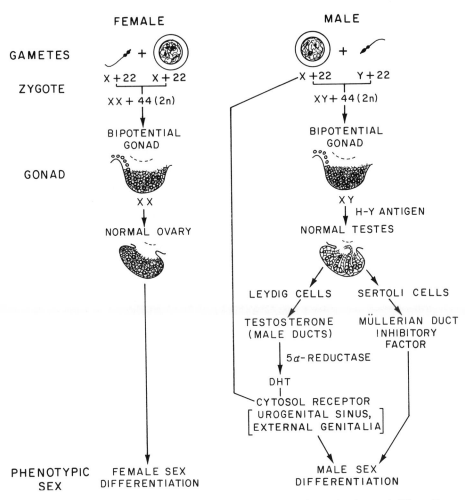

Figure 14-17. Schematic diagram of male and female sex determination and differentiation. Modified from M. M. Grumbach, *In* "Biologic Basis of Pediatric Practice" (R. E. Cooke, ed.), p. 1060. McGraw-Hill, New York, 1967.

designated antimullerian hormone. This suggestion is supported by both clinical studies of the syndrome of testicular feminization as well as by studies employing antiandrogens (see Fig. 12-11) where it has been observed that these compounds block the ability of the testes to induce the differentiation of the wolffian duct, but did not block the ability of the testes to induce the regression of the mullerian ducts. Antimullerian hormone has not yet been well characterized biochemically; it is sug-

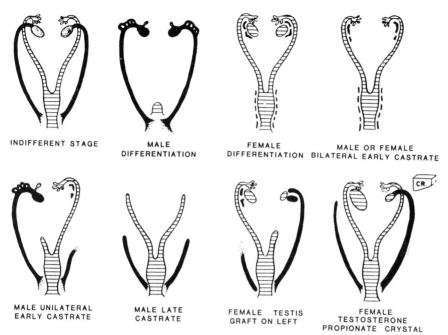

Figure 14-18. Schematic diagram of male (wolffian duct) and female (mullerian duct) differentiation. Testosterone stimulates wolffian duct development, but has no effect on mullerian duct inhibitory factor. Modified from M. M. Grumbach and J. Van Wyk, *In* "Textbook of Endocrinology" (R. H. Williams, ed.), 5th ed. Saunders, Philadelphia, Pennsylvania, 1974.

gested that it is a fucosylated protein with two subunits, where the subunit molecular weight is ~72,000. The antimullerian hormone is believed to be produced by the Sertoli cells of the fetal testes. Its biological function is believed to be to induce involution of the paired mullerian ducts, which prevents the development of the fallopian tubes and uterus (see Fig. 14-18).

The Leydig cells of the testes (see Chapter 12) are the principal site of steroidogenesis leading to the production of testosterone. Testosterone, after further metabolism in target cells by the 5α-reductase enzyme to dihydrotestosterone, functions as a steroid hormone to cause differentiation of the wolffian ducts into the epididymis, seminal vesicles, and vas deferens (see Fig. 14-2).

Interestingly, the gene for the cytoplasmic androgen binding protein, which is present in all androgen-dependent tissues, has been shown by C. Migeon to be present on the X chromosome. Thus, an X-linked gene controls androgen response of somatic cell types by generating the messenger RNA coding for the nuclear cytosol receptor protein.

B. Pregnancy

1. Placental Transfer of Hormones

While the maternal–placental unit provides all the nutrients, electrolytes, water, vitamins, and thermogenesis and respiratory and excretory functions required for fetal growth, an important endocrinological problem has been to elucidate the relative independence/dependence of the fetus from the mother with respect to the plethora of peptide and steroid hormones. Since there is no direct circulatory connection between the maternal placenta and fetal placenta, transfer of hormones cannot occur by "direct" pathways. It has been determined that the placenta is impermeable to all polypeptide and thyroid hormones. However, steroid hormones and the catecholamines epinephrine and norepinephrine are capable of transfer across the placenta. Thus, as described in Figs. 14-10 and 14-11, the fetus, mother, and placenta work cooperatively to produce and transfer the required amounts of progesterone and estrogen to the maternal–placental unit to maintain pregnancy. Presumably the transfer of the new steroid hormone occurs by a simple diffusional process.

2. Fetal Endocrinology

In view of the general lack of hormone transfer to the fetus from the mother, it is clear that the growing fetus must develop its endocrine system in coordination with its own growth and development. It is essential by the time of parturition that all endocrine systems be operative and competent to assume responsibility for their respective domains. However, growth of the fetus appears to be largely controlled by inherent tissue factors and genetics rather than by placental hormones. Selected aspects of fetal metabolism are affected to a degree by the fetal pituitary and placental hormones. Table 14-6 summarizes the endocrine functions of the fetus.

With the exception of the catecholamines, the fetus is capable of functioning autonomously. The basal secretion rates of all the anterior pituitary hormones are quite high by the end of the second trimester; by the third trimester their secretion is somewhat reduced, probably due to inhibitory feedback control. The production of cortisol is known to occur in the human fetus by the tenth week of gestation; both cortisol and dehydroepiandrosterone sulfate have been shown to increase after ACTH stimulation. Both glucagon and insulin secretion are reduced in

Table 14–6. Summary of the Endocrine Functions in the Fetus[a]

Hormone	Neuroendocrine transducer		Gland function	Tissue response
	Basal secretion	Feedback control		
GH	↑	—	—	Prob. ↓
PRL	↑	—	—	Prob. N
ACTH	Prob. ↑	Yes	—	N
FSH-LH	Prob. ↑	Yes	—	N
TSH	Prob. ↑	Yes	—	N
AVP	N	—	—	N
Cortisol	—	—	↑	N
Thyroid hormones	—	—	↑	N
Catecholamines	Prob. ↓	—	Prob. ↓	N
Insulin	—	—	↓	Prob. N
Glucagon	—	—	↓	Prob. ↓
PTH	—	—	↓	↓
Calcitonin	—	—	↑	Prob. N

[a] N, normal; ↑, increased; ↓, decreased; Prob., probably. Reproduced with permission from D. A. Fisher, *In* "Endocrinology" (L. J. DeGroot, G. F. Cahill, L. Martini, D. H. Nelson, W. D. Odell, J. T. Potts, E. Steinberger, and A. I. Winegrad, eds.), Vol. 3, p. 1655, Table 133-8. Grune & Stratton, New York, 1979.

the fetus; this may be a reflection of the relative constancy of the fetal blood sugar. Finally, the relatively high fetal serum calcium levels effectively suppress parathyroid hormone secretion and promote calcitonin secretion. Also, the fetal kidney is believed to be able to produce the dihydroxylated metabolites of vitamin D_3.

C. The Breasts and Lactation

1. Hormonal Regulation of Breast Development

There have been extensive studies dealing with the hormonal control of mammary growth and function. The three principal hormones required for mammary gland maturation are prolactin, insulin, and cortisol.

The effects of prolactin on the mammary gland are described in Fig. 14-19. This figure shows the steps in differentiation of a milk-secreting cell from a stem precursor cell. There are two distinct phases—the proliferative phase and the differentiative phase.

In the proliferation phase, stem cells divide into precursors or other

598

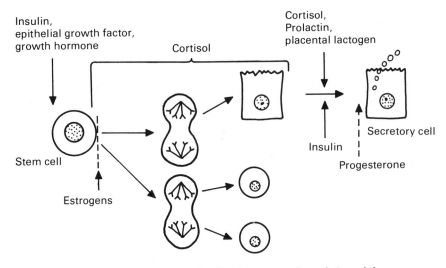

Insulin,
epithelial growth factor,
growth hormone

Cortisol

Cortisol,
Prolactin,
placental lactogen

Stem cell

Estrogens

Insulin

Secretory cell

Progesterone

Figure 14-19. Effects of prolactin on the development and regulation of the mammary gland secretory cell. Modified from R. W. Turkington, Multiple hormone actions: The mammary gland. *In* "Biochemical Actions of Hormones" (G. W. Litwack, ed.), Vol. 2, p. 55–80. Academic Press, New York, 1972.

cell types. Proliferation is regulated by insulin, epidermal growth factor (EGF), and growth hormone, all of which act as mitogenic stimuli. Prolactin (PRL) may sensitize the stem cell to the action of insulin and may act like a mitogen itself. Apparently, PRL also increases the formation of its own receptors in cell membranes and may increase the level of cyclic AMP binding proteins in cytosol. Thyroid hormone, as will be summarized shortly, regulates the amount of PRL available to the mammary gland for these actions. Since TSH and PRL are both controlled by TRH, which is negatively adjusted by the level of circulating thyroid hormone, the higher the level of thyroid hormone, the smaller the signal will be for the release of both TSH and PRL. Therefore the thyroid status of the female may be of importance in determining the amounts of PRL available for the processes described in Fig. 14-20.

In the differentiative phase, a number of hormones are involved. Glucocorticoids (hydrocortisone = cortisol) are important and appear to play a role in this process. Prolactin and insulin are critical. The secretory cell can appear in the absence of prolactin (in organ culture), but they will not produce milk constituents. Apparently the mRNAs for the milk proteins are under the control of PRL, but cortisol probably plays a role here. Cortisol may be required for PRL to elevate the mRNAs for milk proteins. If glucocorticords are required, in this way one could arrive at a

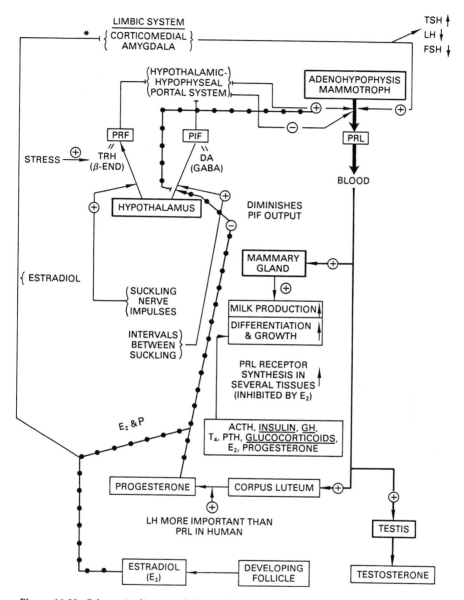

Figure 14-20. Schematic diagram of the regulated secretion of prolactin from the pituitary and summary of its biological actions. + indicates stimulation; − indicates inhibition.

very reasonable explanation of the effect of high progesterone levels during pregnancy and the blockade of milk production. Since progesterone is a competitor of glucocorticoids at the receptor level, the high level of progesterone during pregnancy might compete with cortisol and paralyze the glucocorticoid receptor. Only at the end of pregnancy, when there is an abrupt fall in the level of placental progesterone, would the cortisol become effective in occupying ligand binding sites of the glucocorticoid receptor and generating the prolactin-induced effects on milk protein mRNAs.

It is important to emphasize that both estrogen and progestin also stimulate the development of the mammary gland, estradiol-stimulating duct development, as well as causing a lowering of PIF (dopamine) to generate PRL release, progesterone-stimulating alveolar development, and a lowering of the level of PIF (Fig. 14-20). In addition, estradiol may stimulate the release of PRL at the anterior pituitary through a mechanism involving the corticomedial amygdala of the limbic system. Thus, although PRL is being secreted in pregnancy and the mammary gland is developing, milk is not being synthesized due to the high levels of progesterone which may block the glucocorticoid receptor. At term, free progesterone levels fall and the mammary cells become functional, as shown in Fig. 14-20.

2. Hormonal Regulation of Lactation

  a. Effects on Milk Proteins. The principal target organ for prolactin in the female is the mammary gland. Figure 14-21 shows a postulated mechanism of action for prolactin to describe its biological actions in stimulating the synthesis of milk constituents. It is generally argued that there are membrane receptors for PRL, but as yet it has not been possible to demonstrate that PRL activates adenylate cyclase. Eventually after PRL interacts with its membrane receptor, nuclear activation occurs and the messenger RNA levels increase for the milk proteins, casein, α-lactalbumin, β-lactoglobulin, and so on (see Table 14-1).

  b. Effects of Suckling on Prolactin Secretion. The regulation of prolactin release and its subsequent actions is diagrammed in Fig. 14-22. Normally in the male and female the PRL serum concentration is 5–10 ng/ml or 0.2–0.4 nM; at this level PRL receptors in the mammary tissue are about half saturated.

Starting with the hypothalamus, PRL is postulated to be released from the mammotrope by a pair of presumptive releasing factors, PIF and PRF. PIF appears to be related to or identical to dopamine (DA), which inhibits the secretion of PRL. The positive releasing factor is PRF, which may be identical to TRH (see Chapter 5 for structures of releasing fac-

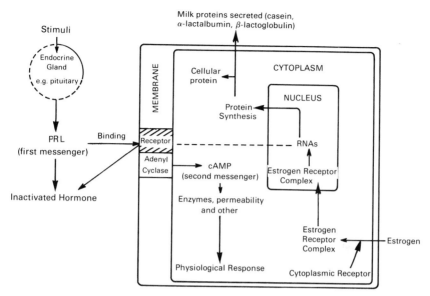

Figure 14-21. Model for the mechanism of action of prolactin. Modified from C. Aragona and H. G. Friesen, Lactation and galactorrhea. *In* "Endocrinology" (L. J. DeGroot, G. F. Cahill, L. Martini, D. H. Nelson, W. D. Odell, J. T. Potts, E. Steinberger, and A. I. Winegrad, eds.), Vol. 3, pp. 1613–1627. Grune & Stratton, New York, 1979.

tors), and TRH causes PRL to be released from the mammotrope of the anterior pituitary. Note that other hormones influence PRL secretion by altering the levels of the modifying hypothalamic releasing factors or by acting directly on the anterior pituitary. Progesterone and estrogen inhibit release of PIF (dopamine), thus increasing the secretion of PRL by diminishing a negative constraint. Estradiol acts indirectly on the mammotrope to effect the release. Apparently this is accomplished by direct action of estradiol on the corticomedial amygdala of the limbic system, higher than the hypothalamus. Such an effect could act subsequently on hypothalamic releasing factors. In stress, β-endorphin is produced via β-LPH in the corticotrope and later stimulates the release of PRL at the level of the mammotrope. One of the end hormones in stress, cortisol from the adrenal gland, feeds back negatively on the mammotrope to inhibit further release of PRL.

In lactation, a dominant overriding signal is the suckling nerve impulse which travels through the spinal column, reaching the brain in a millisecond time frame, and stimulates the prompt release of PRF (TRH), which in turn acts on the mammotrope to release PRL. Such an effect could be delivered by serotonergic neurons and additionally by

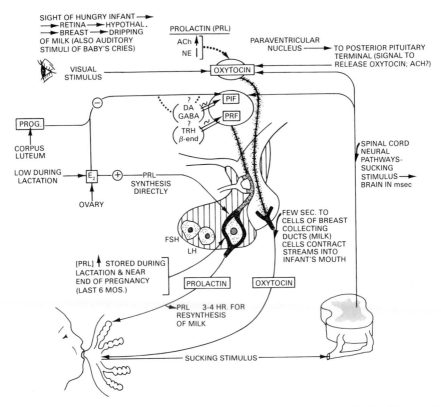

Figure 14-22. Integrated model to describe the neuroendocrine control of suckling and lactation. This figure is redrawn in part from C. Ezrin, J. O. Godden, R. Volpe, and R. Wilson, "Systematic Endocrinology." Harper & Row, Hagerstown, Maryland, 1973.

stimulation of β-endorphinergic neurons which also could release PRL as shown by its effect in the stress mechanism.

The main events in the suckling stimulus are featured in Fig. 14-22. The first few minutes of suckling prepares PRL for release into the circulation. This interval is referred to as the "pituitary depletion stage." The amount prepared depends on the previous nonsuckling period. After "preparation," PRL is secreted into the circulation in a steady minute-by-minute fashion independently of the prior nonsuckling interval. Steady secretion continues until the pool of prepared PRL is exhausted. During intervals between suckling, PIF (dopamine) is stimulated which reduces PRL release.

In addition to endogenous inhibitors of PRL release, that is, PIF or

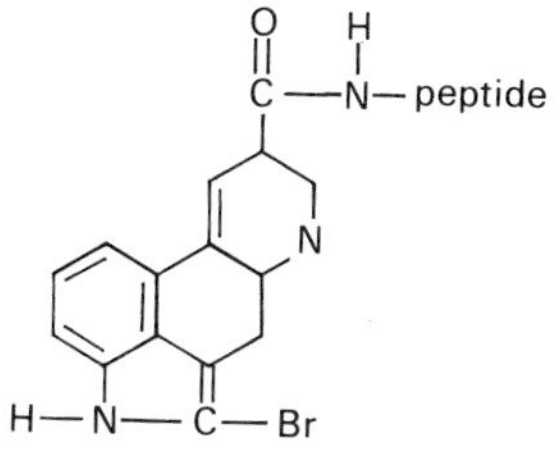

Figure 14-23. Structure of bromocryptine or 2-bromo-α-ergocryptine, an inhibitor of pituitary prolactin secretion.

dopamine, the drug 2-bromo-α-ergocryptine (bromocryptine) is an inhibitor used experimentally and clinically. Its structure is given in Fig. 14-23. The drug appears to cause decreased synthesis of PRL and an increase in the degradation rate of PRL; thus, the drug finds use in terminating milk production at weaning; if it is administered abruptly, its use may prevent development of mastitis and infection in the mammary gland due to stasis of milk. It has been used experimentally to determine if mammary tumors, whose growth might be stimulated by PRL, could be regressed.

V. CLINICAL ASPECTS

A. Pregnancy—Gestational Neoplasms

Gestational neoplasms are the group of related tumors that can occur as a consequence of pregnancy. Morphologically gestational tumors can be categorized as (1) a hydatidiform mole occurring after a molar pregnancy, and a (2) choriocarcinoma which can occur following any kind of gestation. A hydatidiform mole is a gestational neoplasm that occurs as the trophoblast initiates the implantation process in the uterine endometrium. Normal fetal vascularity is lost and the trophoblastic cells surrounding the villi show varying degrees of proliferation. Choriocarcinoma represents the more malignant histological type of gestational neoplasm. The incidence of gestational neoplasms is low: 1 in 2000 to 1 in 15,000. Further, of 900 patients studied at the New England Trophoblastic Disease Center, 71% had a molar pregnancy and in the remaining 29% there was no evidence of metastases; an overall cure rate of 93% was achieved.

In instances of molar pregnancy there frequently is massive production of human chorionic gonadotropin, hCG. Thus, plasma determination of hCG is quite useful for diagnosis as well as for evaluation of the success of management of the disease.

B. Anomalies of Sex Determinants

There is an extremely wide spectrum of endocrine disorders which may arise from perturbations in the many processes contributing to sexual organization. Thus, there are clinical problems present at each level of sex definition, that is, genetic sex, gonadal sex, somatic sex, and phenotypic sex (see Table 14-3). It is beyond the scope of this chapter to consider other than a few of these disorders.

Klinefelter's syndrome or seminiferous tubule dysgenesis results from an XXY chromosome. Such individuals are characterized by the presence of small testes, gynecomastia (partial breast development), azoospermia, and elevated gonadotropins.

Subjects with Turner's syndrome have a single X chromosome; they are usually small in stature and exhibit undeveloped secondary sex characteristics and amenorrhea.

Individuals with an XXX chromosome are designated as a "super female." This chromosomal aberration occurs approximately once in 1600 female births.

There is a wide spectrum of hermaphrodites which reflects the various problems that can arise from incorrect gonadal differentiation. A true hermaphrodite is an individual who possesses both testicular and ovarian tissue.

C. Breast Cancer and Galactorrhea

1. Breast Cancer

Breast cancer is the leading cancer in the female. Annually there are ~100,000 new cases of breast cancer in the United States and almost 50% of them will ultimately be fatal. Mammary tissue requires more endocrine factors for its structural development and regulation of its lactation function than virtually any other tissue; this includes estrogen and progesterone, prolactin, vasopressin, insulin, growth hormone, glucocorticoids, thyroxine, 1,25-dihydroxyvitamin D_3 and oxytocin. While it is conceivable that any or all of these hormones could mediate cell growth of a breast tumor, to date only estrogen, progesterone, and prolactin have been linked to malignant breast growth. The dramatic demonstration by G. Beatson in 1896 that mammary cancer regressed after bilateral oophorectomy in premenopausal women initiated the view that mammary tumors could be controlled by manipulating the endocrine environment. E. Jensen has shown a good correlation between the presence of an estrogen receptor in breast tumors and the likelihood of response to endocrine therapy. Approximately 66% of all breast tumors have significant levels of estrogen receptor. Such information is now utilized as part of the diagnostic evaluation of women with breast cancer; those premenopausal individuals who are estrogen receptor-positive become candidates for castration. Postmenopausal women who are estrogen receptor-positive are candidates for treatment with anti-estrogens such as tamoxifen.

Regrettably in the human, endocrine therapy rarely achieves total extinction of the tumor and other management procedures including chemotherapy or surgical procedures must often be instituted.

2. Galactorrhea

Galactorrhea is defined as a persistent discharge from the breast of a milk-like fluid that is not associated with parturition and lactation. Galactorrhea may occur as a consequence of a wide variety of endocrine and nonendocrine disorders; these endocrine-related instances include pituitary tumors which produce prolactin, the Chiari–Frommel syndrome (which is defined as galactorrhea and amenorrhea persisting more than 6 months postpartum) in the absence of nursing, galactorrhea following oral contraceptive usage, and primary hypothyroidism.

Serum levels of prolactin are usually elevated in galactorrhea. If the cause of the elevated plasma level of prolactin is an inappropriate secretion by the adenohypophysis, then the possibility of a pituitary tumor must be considered. In this instance surgical removal or chemotherapy with drugs such as L-dopamine or the ergot alkaloid bromocryptine may be initiated. These two compounds interfere with prolactin secretion by the pituitary. The structure of bromocryptine is given in Fig. 14-23.

References

A. Books

Cowie, A. T., and Tindal, J. S. (1971). "The Physiology of Lactation," p. 107. Edward Arnold, London.

Grumbach, M. M. (1979). Genetic mechanisms of sexual development. *In* "Genetic Mechanisms of Sexual Development" (I. H. Porter and H. L. Vallet, eds.), pp. 33–74. Academic Press, New York.

Hafez, E. S. E. (1973). Gamete transport. *In* "Human Reproduction: Conception and Contraception" (E. S. E. Hafez and T. N. Evans, eds.), p. 85. Harper & Row, New York.

Yokoyama, A., Mizuno, H., and Nagasawa, H., eds. (1978). "Physiology of Mammary Glands." University Park Press, Baltimore, Maryland.

606

B. Review Articles

Bryant-Greenwood, G. D. (1982). Relaxin as a new hormone. *Endocr. Rev.* **2,** 62–90.
Ohno, S. (1976). Major regulatory genes for mammalian sexual development. *Cell* **7,** 315–321.
Seron-Ferré, M., and Jaffe, R. B. (1981). The fetal adrenal gland. *Annu. Rev. Physiol.* **43,** 141–162.
Topper, Y. (1970). Multiple hormone interactions in the development of mammary gland *in vitro. Recent Prog. Horm. Res.* **26,** 287–303.

C. Research Papers

Bethea, C. L. (1984). Stimulatory effect of estrogen on prolactin secretion from primate pituitary cells cultured on extracellular matrix and in serum-free medium. *Endocrinology (Baltimore)* **115,** 443–451.
Crish, J. F., Soloff, M. S., and Shaw, A. R. (1986). Changes in relaxin precursor mRNA levels in the rat ovary during pregnancy. *J. Biol. Chem.* **261,** 1909–1913.
Haeuptle, M., Aubert, M. L., Dijane, J., and Kraehenbuhl, J. P. (1983). Binding sites for lactogenic and somatogenic hormones from rabbit mammary gland and liver. *J. Biol. Chem.* **258,** 305–314.
Hudson, P., Haley, J., John, M., Cronk, M., Crawford, R., Haralambidis, J., Tregear, G., Shine, J., and Niall, H. (1983). Structure of a genomic clone encoding biologically active human relaxin. *Nature (London)* **301,** 628–631.
Jelliffe, D. B. (1975). Unique properties of human milk. *J. Reprod. Med.* **14,** 133.
Li, C. H., Dickson, J. S., and Chung, D. (1973). Amino acid sequence of human chorionic somatomammotropin. *Arch. Biochem. Biophys.* **155,** 95–110.
Liggins, G. C. (1979). Initiation of parturition. *Br. Med. Bull.* **35,** 145–150.
Meyer, W. J., III, Migeon, B. R., and Migeon, C. J. (1975). Locus on human X chromosome for dihydrotestosterone receptor and androgen insensitivity. *Proc. Natl. Acad. Sci. U.S.A.* **72,** 1469–1472.
Mitchell, J., Cross, P., Hobkirk, R., and Challes, J. R. G. (1984). Formation of unconjugated estrogens from estrone sulfate by dispersed cells from human fetal membranes and decidua. *J. Clin. Endocrinol. Metab.* **58,** 850–856.
Picard, J. Y., Tran, D., and Josso, N. (1978). Biosynthesis of labeled antimullerian hormone by fetal testes. *Mol. Cell. Endocrinol.* **12,** 17–24.
Royer, F., Simmler, M. C., Johnsson, C., Vergnaud, G., Cooke, H. J., and Weissenbach, J. (1986). A gradient of sex linkage in the pseudoautosomal region of the human sex chromosomes. *Nature (London)* **319,** 291–295.
Schmell, E., Earles, B. J., Breaux, C., and Lennarz, W. J. (1977). Identification of a sperm receptor on the surface of eggs of the sea urchin *Arbacia punctulata. J. Cell Biol.* **72,** 35–46.
Tran, D., and Josso, N. (1982). Localization of antimullerian hormone in the rough endoplasmic reticulum of the developing bovine Sertoli cell using immunocytochemistry with a monoclonal antibody. *Endocrinology (Baltimore)* **111,** 1562–1567.
Walsh, F., Stanczyk, Z., and Navy, M. J. (1984). Daily hormonal changes in the maternal, fetal, and amniotic fluid compartments before parturition in a primate species. *J. Clin. Endocrinol. Metab.* **58,** 629–639.
Whitaker, M. D., Klee, G. G., Kao, P. C., Randall, R. V., and Heaer, D. W. (1984). Demonstration of biological activity of prolactin molecular weight variants in human sera. *J. Clin. Endocrinol. Metab.* **58,** 826–830.

Chapter 15

Hormones of the Kidney

I. INTRODUCTION

A. Background

The kidney plays an indispensable role for the maintenance of life in higher organisms not only from the perspective of maintaining the constancy of many components of the extracellular fluid and filtering out of nitrogenous wastes, but also as a major endocrine organ. The kidney as an endocrine gland is the site of production of renin and the following hormones: (1) erythropoietin, which is a peptide hormone essential for the process of erythropoiesis or red blood cell formation by the bone marrow; (2) 1,25-dihydroxyvitamin D_3, the hormonally active form of vitamin D which is essential for calcium homeostasis; and (3) the kallikreins, a group of serine proteases which act on blood proteins to produce bradykinin, a potent vasodilator. Renin is an enzyme with proteolytic activity which acts on a plasma protein, α_2-globulin, to produce the hormonal angiotensins which in turn act at the adrenal cortex to stimulate the biosynthesis and secretion of the mineralocorticoid aldosterone. In addition, the kidney serves as an endocrine target organ for a number of hormones. Table 15-1 summarizes the endocrine aspects of the kidney both as an endocrine secretory gland as well as an endocrine target organ.

An important physiological function of the kidney was observed by J. Peters in 1835, "The kidneys appear to serve as the ultimate guardians of the constitution of the internal environment." In this regard, it is clear that the kidney occupies a unique position within the physiological network of the living organism in that it functions as the ultimate organ for the monitoring and conservation of body water, of all its electrolyte constituents, as well as many small organic molecules. In addition, the kidney plays an important physiological role in maintaining correct acid–base balance. It is thus perhaps not surprising to see concentrated in the kidney such an array of hormone production sites as well as sites of hormone action. It seems likely that the exquisite anatomical organization of the kidney (see later) offers significant advantages to the organism in terms of the regulation of production of key hormones as well as the regulation of the biological responses to various hormones which affect the homeostasis of key bodily electrolytes.

B. Scope of This Chapter

It is not pedagogically feasible to present a succinct description of the kidney functioning both as an endocrine secretory gland and target organ as well as the site of key intermediary metabolic events. After a review of the anatomy of the kidney, this chapter will present separately the renal aspects of the renin–angiotensin–aldosterone—atrial natriuretic factor—sodium reabsorption system, the kallikrein–kinin system, and the erythropoietin–erythropoiesis system. A portion of the renin–angiotensin–aldosterone system, particularly that involving the bio-

Table 15–1. Hormones That Are Produced or Have Major Actions in the Kidney

Hormones produced by the kidney	Major target organ(s)	Function
Erythropoietin	Bone marrow	Stimulate red blood cell formation
1,25-Dihydroxyvitamin D_3 (+ other vitamin D metabolites)	Intestine, bone, kidney	Maintenance of calcium homeostasis
Renin (an enzyme)[a]	Blood to mediate production of the hormonal angiotensins	To mediate production of aldosterone (by the adrenal cortex)
Prekallikreins	Serum protein α_2-globulins	To produce kinins (e.g., bradykinin) which are potent vasodilators
Prostaglandins	Kidney	Juxtaglomerular apparatus

Hormones acting on the kidney		
Aldosterone		
Atrial natriuretic factor (atriopeptin)		
1,25(OH)$_2$-vitamin D_3		
Vasopressin		
Prostaglandins		
Cortisol		
Insulin		
Glucagon		
Thyroxine		
Catecholamines (epinephrine, norepinephrine)		

[a] Technically renin, an enzyme, does not fit the classical or modern definition of a hormone (see Chapter 1).

synthesis and secretion of aldosterone, is included in Chapter 10. The roles of the kidney in calcium and phosphorus homeostasis, including its production of key vitamin D metabolites and its actions as a target organ for parathyroid hormone, calcitonin, and 1,25-dihydroxyvitamin D_3, are covered in Chapter 9. Also, it is not the purpose of this chapter to provide a detailed description of the physiological participation of the kidney in the formation of urine, that is, glomerular filtration and determination of electrolyte and acid–base balance. Rather, the focus will be limited to endocrinological aspects of these topics.

II. ANATOMICAL, MORPHOLOGICAL, AND PHYSIOLOGICAL RELATIONSHIPS

A. Introduction

The kidneys, along with the ureters, urinary bladder, and male or female urethra, comprise the anatomical units responsible for the multiplicity of endocrine, metabolic, and filtering actions of the kidney. Figure 10-1 presents a gross anatomical overview of the urinary system.

With the completion of the metabolic and filtration actions of the kidneys, the urine, containing a wide variety of bodily wastes, is conveyed via the two ureters (one per kidney) to the urinary bladder for temporary storage. Then, at the time of micturition or emptying of the urinary bladder, the urine is voided through the urethra. The normal output of urine per day in the adult may range from 600 to 2500 ml. Table 15-2 lists the principal electrolytes of the intracellular and extracellular fluids and urine.

Table 15–2. Principal Constituents of Major Body Fluids in the Normal Adult

Constituent	Intracellular compartment	Extracellular compartment (meq/liter)[a]	Urine[b] (g)[c]	[Urine] [plasma]
Cations				
Sodium	11	142	2–4	1.0
Potassium	162	4	1.5–2	10–15
Calcium	2	5	0.1–0.3	
Magnesium	28	2	0.1–0.2	
Anions				
Chloride	3	101	17.1	1.5
Bicarbonate	10	27		1.5
Phosphate (HPO_4^{2-})	102	2	0.15–2.5	25
Sulfate (SO_4^{2-})	20	1	0.6–1.8	50
Other				
Protein	65	16	—	
Urea			30.0	35
Creatinine			1.0	70
Organic acids	3	6	—	—
Glucose (mg/100 ml)		80–110	6–8	—

[a] The values reported for the extracellular compartment are also applicable to plasma.
[b] Calculated assuming a daily urinary output of 2 liters.
[c] Amount excreted in a 24-hr interval by a normal man consuming an average mixed diet.

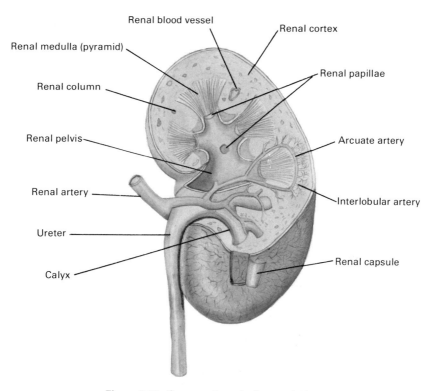

Renal blood vessel

Renal cortex

Renal medulla (pyramid)

Renal papillae

Renal column

Renal pelvis

Arcuate artery

Renal artery

Interlobular artery

Ureter

Renal capsule

Calyx

Figure 15-1. Cross section of a human kidney.

B. Gross Structure

The two kidneys in man are located in a posterior position in the abdominal cavity; they present a "bean-like" appearance and are enclosed in a fibrous capsule. In the central portion of the concave border is the hilus which contains all the blood vessels and nerves for the kidney as well as the ureter. Diagrammed in Fig. 15-1 is the cross-sectional appearance of the kidney. There are three general regions: the renal pelvis, the renal cortex, and the renal medulla. The renal pelvis, which is attached to the upper end of the ureter, receives or collects the urine from all regions of the kidney. The renal medulla, which is the inner portion of the kidney, is composed of cone-shaped renal masses termed renal pyramids. The renal cortex constitutes the outer portion of the kidney.

612

C. Microscopic Structure

The fundamental operational unit of the kidney is the nephron (see Fig. 15-2). Each human kidney contains ~1 million nephrons. The nephron is the anatomical structure responsible for the formation of the urine as a consequence of the filtration of the blood and concomitant

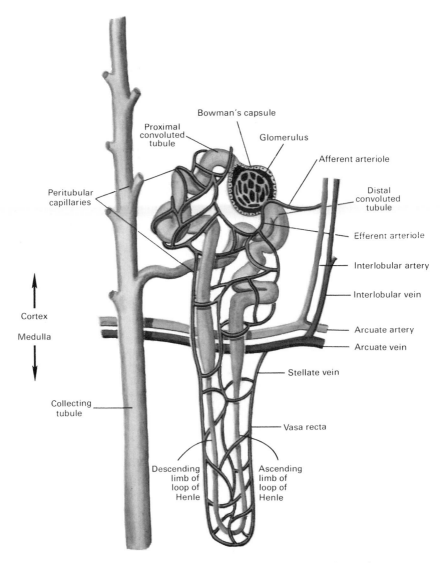

Figure 15-2. Schematic diagram of a nephron with its associated vascular system.

associated selective absorption and secretion of constituents in the newly created urine.

Each nephron consists of a renal tubule (largely in the medulla) and renal corpuscle (located in the cortex). The renal corpuscle (see Fig. 15-3), in turn, is comprised of a glomerulus enclosed by a capsule termed Bowman's capsule. The glomerulus is an exquisite anatomical structure containing a group of capillaries interposed between two arterioles. The vessel transporting blood to the glomerulus is known as the afferent arteriole; it divides into 40–60 capillary loops which then ultimately reunite to form the exit pathway for the blood known as the efferent arteriole. As noted in Fig. 15-2, the efferent arterioles subsequently arborize to form a network of capillaries surrounding the renal tubule. Associated with the cells of the efferent arteriole (see Fig. 15-3) is a cluster of cells termed the juxtaglomerular or JG cells. The JG cells are the site of production of the enzyme renin.

The capsule of Bowman constitutes the beginning of the renal tubule. Specialized cells, termed podocytes, in Bowman's capsule form slits or pores of such a molecular dimension that restrict and effectively prevent the passage of macromolecules in the blood into the top of the nephron; thus, only small molecules pass into the filtrate.

The renal tubule (see Fig. 15-2) anatomically is structured to permit countercurrent distributive processes both between its proximal and distal regions and the loop of Henle as well as the arborized network of capillaries.

An important distinction to note is that the far distal region of each renal tubule is anatomically connected to the afferent arteriole of its own glomerulus. The point of attachment of each distal tubule to its glomerulus is the macula densa; the cells of the macula densa interact with the juxtaglomerular cells. Thus, this anatomical specialization allows for physiological, metabolic, and hormonal communication to occur between the distal tubule (containing the exiting urine) and afferent arteriole (containing the entering blood which will be filtered).

The distal convoluted tubule empties into a branch of the collecting ducts which ultimately lead to a main collecting duct connecting in turn to a network of renal papillae coursing through the renal pyramids to the renal pelvis.

Figures 15-4 and 15-5, respectively, present the cellular organization of a juxtaglomerular cell and a glomerular epithelial cell. These are anatomically closely related to one another.

Figure 15-6 compares the cellular and subcellular structure of cells from the proximal tubule, the loop of Henle, the distal tubule, and the collecting duct.

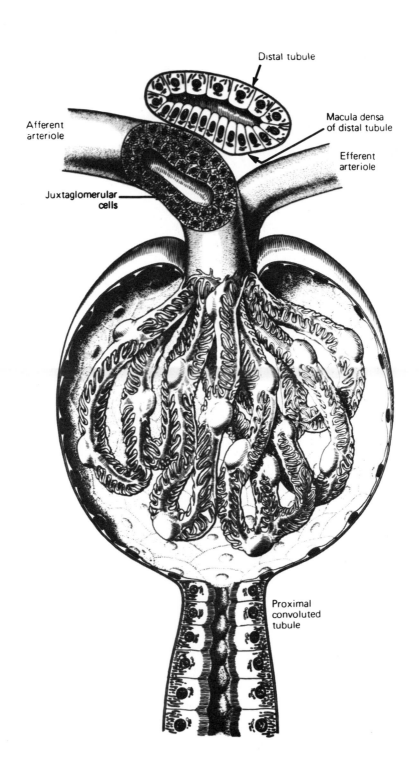

Distal tubule

Macula densa
of distal tubule

Efferent
arteriole

Afferent
arteriole

Juxtaglomerular
cells

Proximal
convoluted
tubule

D. Physiological Processes

The kidney is the principal organ responsible for homeostasis of a wide spectrum of electrolytes as well as conservation of body water. The kidney carries out its homeostatic actions sequentially by a selective glomerular filtration (mediated by a high blood pressure in the glomerulus), tubular secretion, and tubular reabsorption; these are all processes that collectively regulate the concentration of the metabolic end products, the osmotic pressure, the ionic composition, and the volume of the internal environment. Figure 15-7 is a schematic diagram of a typical kidney nephron indicating the sites of reabsorption of the various ionic substances. The key to the achievement of homeostasis is the process of countercurrent distribution. Countercurrent distribution occurs as a consequence of the anatomical organization of the nephron and is supported by the processes of passive diffusion, tubular reabsorption, and tubular secretion. Both of the latter processes utilize energy-dependent active transport mechanisms. The end result of these activities is the formation of the residual urine containing bodily wastes (both ionic, organic, and nitrogenous); however, in the process of forming the urine from the glomerular filtrate, the tubule has returned many essential nutrients and electrolytes to the blood. A comparison of the extracellular concentrations versus urine concentrations of major urine constituents is presented on Table 15-2.

III. HOMEOSTASIS OF FLUID, ELECTROLYTES, AND BLOOD PRESSURE

The maintenance of salt homeostasis and circulatory volume and blood pressure requires the integrated actions of the renin–angiotensin–aldosterone system, the adrenergic nervous system, vasopressin, and the atrial natriuretic factor (ANF), also known as atriopeptin. Each of

---

Figure 15-3. Cross section of a renal corpuscle. The upper part shows the vascular pole with afferent and efferent arterioles and the macula densa. Note the juxtaglomerular cells in the wall of the afferent arteriole. Podocytes cover glomerular capillaries. Their nuclei protrude on the cell surface. Podocyte processes can be seen. Note the cells of the parietal layer of Bowman's capsule. The lower part of the drawing shows the urinary pole and the proximal convoluted tubule. Modified from L. C. Junqueira and J. Carneiro, "Basic Histology," 4th ed., p. 400. Lange Medical Publications, Los Altos, California, 1983.

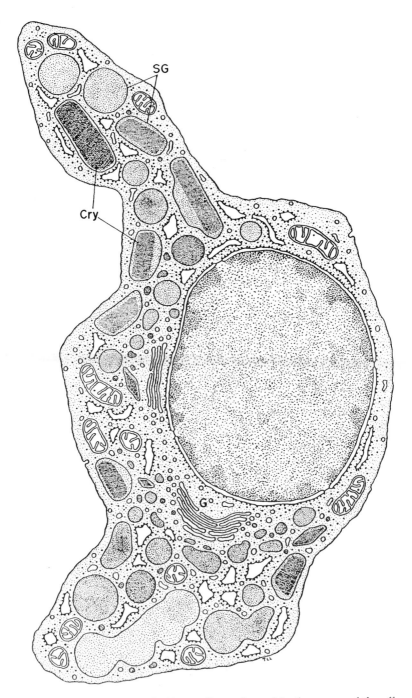

Figure 15-4. Juxtaglomerular cell. These cells are located in the course of the afferent arteriole just before its entrance into the glomerulus; they are the site of secretion of renin. They are highly irregular in shape with conspicuous secretory granules (SG) and a crystalline (Cry) internal structure. Modified from T. L. Lentz, "Cell Fine Structure," p. 237. Saunders, Philadelphia, Pennsylvania, 1971.

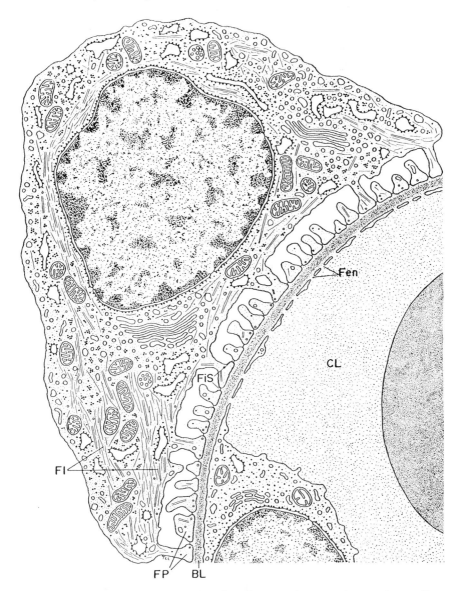

Figure 15-5. Glomerular epithelial cell and capillary. BL, basement lamina; CL, capillary lumen; Fen, fenestrae or pores; FP, secondary foot processes or pedicals; Fl, filaments. Fluid from the glomerular capillaries is filtered through the surrounding space of Bowman's capsule. It must therefore pass through the filtration slits between foot processes of the podocytes. The fluid in Bowman's capsule is an ultrafiltrate of plasma containing small molecules, but relatively free of large protein molecules. Modified from T. L. Lentz, "Cell Fine Structure," p. 227. Saunders, Philadelphia, Pennsylvania, 1971.

A

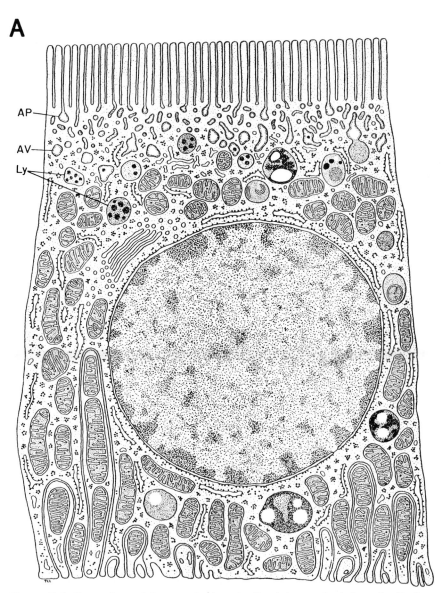

Figure 15-6. Comparison of the organization of cells of the renal tubule and collecting duct. (A) Proximal tubule epithelial cell. The apical surface of the cell has a few blunt microvilli and the cytoplasm is filled with elongated mitochondria. AP, Apical pits; AV, apical vesicles; Ly, lysosomes. Reproduced with permission from T. L. Lentz, "Cell Fine Structure," p. 229. Saunders, Philadelphia, Pennsylvania, 1971. (B) Epithelial cell of loop of Henle. A sparse number of microvilli variable in length occur on the linimal surface. Reproduced with permission from T. L. Lentz, "Cell Fine Structure," p. 231. Saunders, Philadelphia, Pennsylvania, 1971. (C) Distal tubule epithelial cell. Large numbers of elongated mitochondria (M) with many cristae fill the cellular processes; they may be essential for energy production required for ion transport. V, vesicles. Reproduced with permission from T. L. Lentz, "Cell Fine Structure," p. 233. Saunders, Philadelphia, Pennsylvania,

B

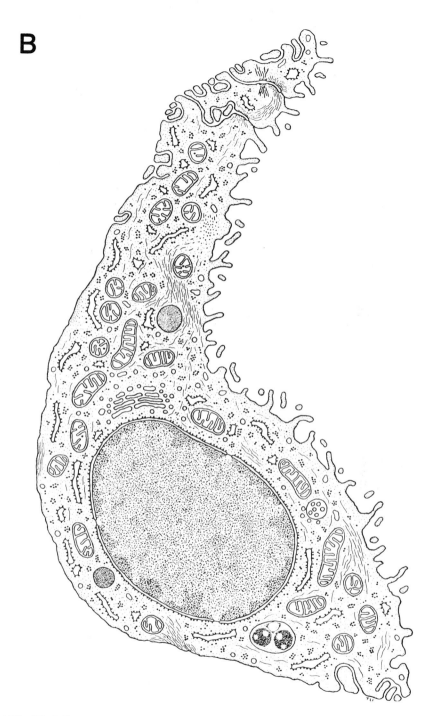

1971. (D) Collecting duct epithelial cell. The collecting duct is comprised of cuboidal to columnar cells. Reproduced with permission from T. L. Lentz, "Cell Fine Structure," p. 235. Saunders, Philadelphia, Pennsylvania, 1971.

C

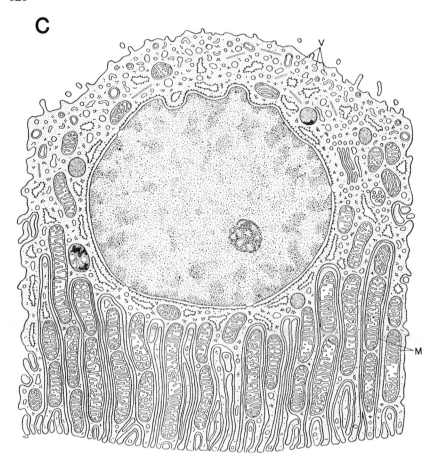

Figure 15-6C. See legend on pp. 618 and 619.

these hormone systems is capable of mediating important biological effects in the kidney.

The volume of the extracellular fluid (ECF) is governed by the extracellular fluid sodium concentration; the Na^+ concentration of the ECF is determined by regulating the extent of excretion of sodium in the urine. The principal, although not exclusive, factors governing the excretion of sodium are the steroid hormone aldosterone and the glomerular fitration rate.

The glomerular filtration of the kidney can be markedly increased by the actions of atriopeptin, thus increasing the extraction of blood sodium. Also, atriopeptin acts on smooth muscles present in large arteries

D

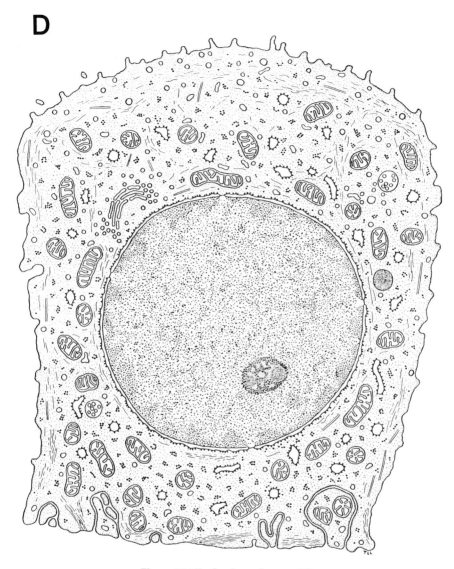

Figure 15-6D. See legend on p. 619.

and vascular beds to effect relaxation and thus reduction of blood pressure.

The function of aldosterone is to directly stimulate absorption of sodium by the renal tubules; this has the consequence of increasing the extracellular fluid volume. Thus, in the renin–angiotensin system the

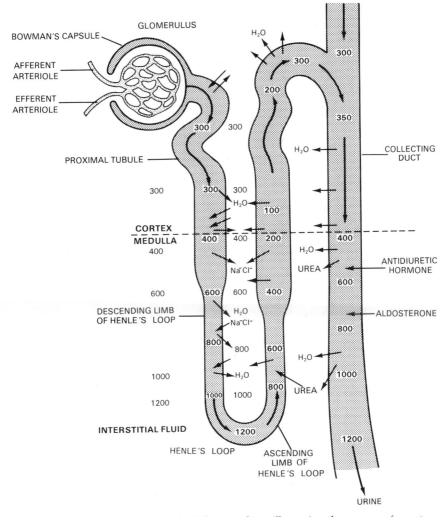

Figure 15-7. Schematic diagram of a kidney nephron illustrating the process of counter-current exchange. The numbers indicate gradients in osmolarity which result as a consequence of simple diffusion and transport or exchange. The filtrate as it enters the loop of Henle becomes further concentrated by diffusion of water into the hypotome interstitium. In the ascending limb of the loop of Henle, Na^+ is actively transported out of the filtrate (thereby diluting it) into the interstitium, where it is concentrated. The osmolarity of the interstitial fluid can increase from 300 to 1100 mOsm/kg H_2 as the papilla is approached. Then as the distal tubule passes back past the glomerulus, additional Na^+ may be reabsorbed in exchange for H^+ or K^+ ions; eventually water is reabsorbed in the distal tubule and collecting duct. Also indicated are the sites of reabsorption of various constituents. Aldosterone and antidiuretic hormone act principally on the collecting duct. Modified from R. F. Pitts, "Physiology of the Kidney and Body Fluids," 3rd ed., p. 134. Copyright © 1974 by Year Book Medical Publishers, Inc., Chicago.

rate of secretion of aldosterone by the adrenal cortex is regulated by the extracellular fluid volume.

As discussed in Chapter 10, bilateral adrenalectomy is fatal; this results from the absence of aldosterone which, in turn, leads to an increased loss of sodium in the urine, a concomitant retention of potassium in the extracellular fluid, and loss of water from both extracellular and intracellular compartments. If this process continues, death inevitably follows.

Figure 15-8 summarizes the role of the renin–angiotensin system in determining the synthesis and secretion of aldosterone by the adrenal cortex and the steroid's subsequent actions back in the kidney to stimulate sodium reabsorption and effect an increased blood pressure. The key element of this system is an enzyme, renin, which is secreted by the juxtaglomerulus in response to a decreased intravascular volume detected by baroreceptors (pressure receptors) located in the right atrium of the heart and large veins near the heart. The baroreceptors send impulses to the brain which are integrated with impulses received from osmoreceptors located in the hypothalamus (see Fig. 4-11). This will result in neural signals being sent to the posterior pituitary, which secretes vasopressin, and the kidney, which results in the secretion of renin.

Renin acts on a plasma α_2-globulin, which ultimately results in the production of the octapeptide hormone angiotensin II. Angiotensin II is the tropic stimulatory factor acting on the *zona glomerulosa* of the adrenal cortex to stimulate synthesis and secretion of aldosterone (see Chapter 10). After systemic transport to the kidney, aldosterone functions to induce the production of proteins/enzymes necessary to effect the renal tubular reabsorption of sodium.

Biochemistry and Physiology

1. Renin

Renin is a glycoprotein-containing enzyme of ~42,000 Da. Renin may be isolated both from kidney and mouse submaxillary glands. Isolation of the pure protein required a 3 million-fold purification. The primary sequence of human renin has been deduced through cloning and sequence analysis of cDNA prepared from human kidney poly(A^+) RNA (see Fig. 15-9). Renin is biosynthesized in a preproform consisting of 406 amino acids; the pre sequence comprises 20 amino acids, the pro sequence of 46 amino acids leaving 347 amino acid residues for the secreted form of renin.

Renin as an enzyme belongs to the class of aspartyl proteinases.

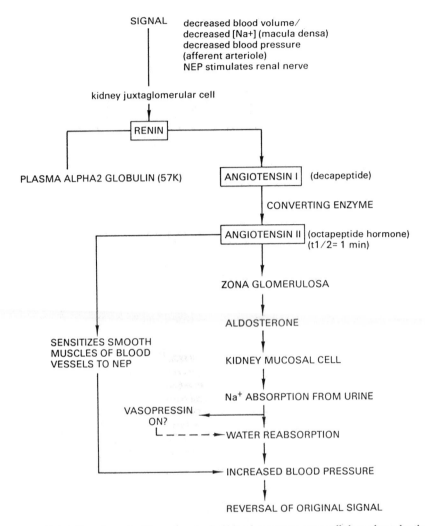

Figure 15-8. Mineralocorticoids and control of blood pressure–extracellular volume by the kidney–adrenal axis.

Figure 15-9. Primary amino acid sequence of human prepro renin as deduced from sequence analysis of a cDNA prepared from poly(A+) RNA obtained from a human kidney. The deduced amino acid residues are indicated below the nucleotide triplets. The mature peptide begins at the Leu residue labeled [1]. The numbers in the braces refer to amino acid positions within the mature renin. The single and double arrowheads indicate the probable ends of the leader sequence and prosequence, respectively. The two catalytically important aspartic acid residues and potential N-glycosylation sites as well as the AATAAA sequence at the 3′ end are underlined. Modified with permission from T. Imai,

```
                                      -42 AACCTCAGTGGATCTCAGAGAGAGCCCCAGACTGAGGGAAGC  -1

  1  ATG GAT GGA TGG AGA AGG ATG CCT CGC TGG GGA CTG CTG CTG CTG CTC TGG GGC TCC TGT    60
     Met Asp Gly Trp Arg Arg Met Pro Arg Trp Gly Leu Leu Leu Leu Leu Trp Gly Ser Cys
      1                       {-60}       10                        {-50}          20

 61  ACC TTT GGT CTC CCG ACA GAC ACC ACC ACC TTT AAA CGG ATC TTC CTC AAG AGA ATG CCC   120
     Thr Phe Gly Leu Pro Thr Asp Thr Thr Thr Phe Lys Arg Ile Phe Leu Lys Arg Met Pro
                         {-40}        30                    {-30}              40

121  TCA ATC CGA GAA AGC CTG AAG GAA CGA GGT GTG GAC ATG GCC AGG CTT GGT CCC GAG TGG   180
     Ser Ile Arg Glu Ser Leu Lys Glu Arg Gly Val Asp Met Ala Arg Leu Gly Pro Glu Trp
                    {-20}        50                    {-10}               60

181  AGC CAA CCC ATG AAG AGG CTG ACA CTT GGC AAC ACC ACC TCC TCC GTG ATC CTC ACC AAC   240
     Ser Gln Pro Met Lys Arg Leu Thr Leu Gly Asn Thr Thr Ser Ser Val Ile Leu Thr Asn
                {-1}{1}           70                    {10}               80

241  TAC ATG GAC ACC CAG TAC TAT GGC GAG ATT GGC ATC GGC ACC CCA CCC CAG ACC TTC AAA   300
     Tyr Met Asp Thr Gln Tyr Tyr Gly Glu Ile Gly Ile Gly Thr Pro Pro Gln Thr Phe Lys
                    {20}            90              {30}                 100

301  GTC GTC TTT GAC ACT GGT TCG TCC AAT GTT TGG GTG CCC TCC TCC AAG TGC AGC CGT CTC   360
     Val Val Phe Asp Thr Gly Ser Ser Asn Val Trp Val Pro Ser Ser Lys Cys Ser Arg Leu
                    {40}            110               {50}                120

361  TAC ACT GCC TGT GTG TAT CAC AAG CTC TTC GAT GCT TCG GAT TCC TCC AGC TAC AAG CAC   420
     Tyr Thr Ala Cys Val Tyr His Lys Leu Phe Asp Ala Ser Asp Ser Ser Ser Tyr Lys His
                    {60}            130               {70}                140

421  AAT GGA ACA GAA CTC ACC CTC CGC TAT TCA ACA GGG ACA GTC AGT GGC TTT CTC AGC CAG   480
     Asn Gly Thr Glu Leu Thr Leu Arg Tyr Ser Thr Gly Thr Val Ser Gly Phe Leu Ser Gln
                    {80}            150               {90}                160

481  GAC ATC ATC ACC GTG GGT GGA ATC ACG GTG ACA CAG ATG TTT GGA GAG GTC ACG GAG ATG   540
     Asp Ile Ile Thr Val Gly Gly Ile Thr Val Thr Gln Met Phe Gly Glu Val Thr Glu Met
                    {100}           170               {110}               180

541  CCC GCC TTA CCC TTC ATG CTG GCC GAG TTT GAT GGG GTT GTG GGC ATG GGC TTC ATT GAA   600
     Pro Ala Leu Pro Phe Met Leu Ala Glu Phe Asp Gly Val Val Gly Met Gly Phe Ile Glu
                    {120}           190               {130}               200

601  CAG GCC ATT GGC AGG GTC ACC CCT ATC TTC GAC AAC ATC ATC TCC CAA GGG GTG CTA AAA   660
     Gln Ala Ile Gly Arg Val Thr Pro Ile Phe Asp Asn Ile Ile Ser Gln Gly Val Leu Lys
                    {140}           210               {150}               220

661  GAG GAC GTC TTC TCT TTC TAC TAC AAC AGA GAT TCC GAG AAT TCC CAA TCG CTG GGA GGA   720
     Glu Asp Val Phe Ser Phe Tyr Tyr Asn Arg Asp Ser Glu Asn Ser Gln Ser Leu Gly Gly
                    {160}           230               {170}               240

721  CAG ATT GTG CTG GGA GGC AGC GAC CCC CAG CAT TAC GAA GGG AAT TTC CAC TAT ATC AAC   780
     Gln Ile Val Leu Gly Gly Ser Asp Pro Gln His Tyr Glu Gly Asn Phe His Tyr Ile Asn
                    {180}           250               {190}               260

781  CTC ATC AAG ACT GGT GTC TGG CAG ATT CAA ATG AAG GGG GTG TCT GTG GGG TCA TCC ACC   840
     Leu Ile Lys Thr Gly Val Trp Gln Ile Gln Met Lys Gly Val Ser Val Gly Ser Ser Thr
                    {200}           270               {210}               280

841  TTG CTC TGT GAA GAC GGC TGC CTG GCA TTG GTA GAC ACC GGT GCA TCC TAC ATC TCA GGT   900
     Leu Leu Cys Glu Asp Gly Cys Leu Ala Leu Val Asp Thr Gly Ala Ser Tyr Ile Ser Gly
                    {220}           290               {230}               300

901  TCT ACC AGC TCC ATA GAG AAG CTC ATG GAG GCC TTG GGA GCC AAG AAG AGG CTG TTT GAT   960
     Ser Thr Ser Ser Ile Glu Lys Leu Met Glu Ala Leu Gly Ala Lys Lys Arg Leu Phe Asp
                    {240}           310               {250}               320

961  TAT GTC GTG AAG TGT AAC GAG GGC CCT ACA CTC CCC GAC ATC TCT TTC CAC CTG GGA GGC  1020
     Tyr Val Val Lys Cys Asn Glu Gly Pro Thr Leu Pro Asp Ile Ser Phe His Leu Gly Gly
                    {260}           330               {270}               340

1021 AAA GAA TAC ACG CTC ACC AGC GCG GAC TAT GTA TTT CAG GAA TCC TAC AGT AGT AAA AAG  1080
     Lys Glu Tyr Thr Leu Thr Ser Ala Asp Tyr Val Phe Gln Glu Ser Tyr Ser Ser Lys Lys
                    {280}           350               {290}               360

1081 CTG TGC ACA CTG GCC ATC CAC GCC ATG GAT ATC CCG CCA CCC ACT GGA CCC ACC TGG GCC  1140
     Leu Cys Thr Leu Ala Ile His Ala Met Asp Ile Pro Pro Pro Thr Gly Pro Thr Trp Ala
                    {300}           370               {310}               380

1141 CTG GGG GCC ACC TTC ATC CGA AAG TTC TAC ACA GAG TTT GAT CGG CGT AAC AAC CGC ATT  1200
     Leu Gly Ala Thr Phe Ile Arg Lys Phe Tyr Thr Glu Phe Asp Arg Arg Asn Asn Arg Ile
                    {320}           390               {330}               400

1201 GGC TTC GCC TTG GCC CGC TGAGGCCCCTCTGCCACCCAGGCAGGCCCTGCCTTCAGCCCTGGCCCAGAGCTGGA  1273
     Gly Phe Ala Leu Ala Arg
                    {340}406

1274 ACACTCTCTGAGATGCCCCTCTGCCTGGGCTTATGCCCTCAGATGGAGACATTGGATGTGGAGCTCCTGCTGGATGCGT  1352

1353 GCCCTGACCCCTGCACCAGCCCTTCCCTGCTTTGAGGACAAAGAGAATAAAGACTTCATGTTCAC
```

H. Miyazaki, S. Hirose, H. Hori, T. Hayashi, R. Kageyama, H. Ohkubo, S. Nakanishi, and K. Murakami, Cloning and sequence analysis of cDNA for human renin precursor. *Proc. Natl. Acad. Sci. U.S.A.* **80**, 7405–7409 (1983).

Human renin exhibits amino acid sequence homology with mouse sub-maxillary gland renin (68% of residues identical) and human pepsinogen (34% of residues identical). The aspartyl residue at positions 38 and 226 are believed to be catalytically important. X-Ray crystallographic studies of aspartyl proteinases indicate that the molecule is bilobal, with two approximately equal domains separated by a long and deep cleft that serves as the substrate binding site. The two catalytically important aspartyl residues are centrally located in the cleft. Model building using the renin amino acid sequence suggests that the common structural features of aspartyl proteinases are also present in renin.

Summarized in Table 15-3 are the factors governing the secretion of renin. Thus, several mechanisms related to a decreased extracellular fluid volume or decreased arterial blood pressure stimulate the secretion of renin by the juxtaglomerular cells.

2. Angiotensins I and II

The natural substrate for renin is the plasma protein, an α_2-globulin which is termed angiotensinogen. Angiotensinogen is a glycoprotein of 57,000 Da, which is synthesized and secreted into the bloodstream by the liver. The biosynthesis of angiotensinogen is increased by glucocorticoids, estrogens, and some oral contraceptives.

The details of the conversion of angiotensinogen into angiotensin I (a decapeptide) and angiotensin II (an octapeptide) are summarized in Fig. 15-10. In the circulatory system renin hydrolyzes the –Leu–Leu– bond of angiotensinogen at residues 10 and 11 to yield the decapeptide angiotensin I. This peptide has limited biological activity. Angiotensin I is converted by a converting enzyme (molecular weight ~ 200,000), dipep-

Table 15–3. Factors Governing the Secretion of Renin by the Juxtaglomerular Cells of the Kidney

Factors inhibiting secretion	Factors stimulating secretion
Increased renal arterial pressure	Decreased renal arterial pressure
Increased extracellular fluid volume	Decreased extracellular fluid volume
Catecholamines occupying α_2-adrenergic receptor[a]	Catecholamines occupying β-adrenergic receptor[a]
Increased Na^+ concentration at the macula densa	Decreased Na^+ concentration at the macula densa
Increased K^+ concentration (hyperkalemia)	Decreased K^+ concentration (hypokalemia)

[a] See Chapter 11.

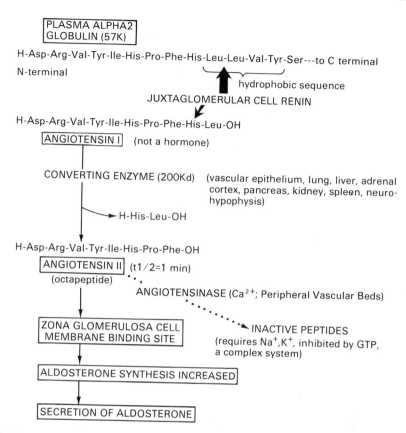

H-Asp-Arg-Val-Tyr-Ile-His-Pro-Phe-His-Leu-Leu-Val-Tyr-Ser---to C terminal

N-terminal

hydrophobic sequence

JUXTAGLOMERULAR CELL RENIN

H-Asp-Arg-Val-Tyr-Ile-His-Pro-Phe-His-Leu-OH

ANGIOTENSIN I (not a hormone)

CONVERTING ENZYME (200Kd) (vascular epithelium, lung, liver, adrenal cortex, pancreas, kidney, spleen, neurohypophysis)

H-His-Leu-OH

H-Asp-Arg-Val-Tyr-Ile-His-Pro-Phe-OH

ANGIOTENSIN II (t1/2=1 min) (octapeptide)

ANGIOTENSINASE (Ca^{2+}; Peripheral Vascular Beds)

ZONA GLOMERULOSA CELL MEMBRANE BINDING SITE

INACTIVE PEPTIDES (requires Na$^+$,K$^+$, inhibited by GTP, a complex system)

ALDOSTERONE SYNTHESIS INCREASED

SECRETION OF ALDOSTERONE

Figure 15-10. Details of angiotensin I, II, and III formation. Dark arrows indicate major pathways. The numbers correspond to the position of amino acid residues in angiotensinogen. Modified from E. L. Smith *et al.*, "Principles of Biochemistry: Mammalian Biochemistry," p. 159. McGraw-Hill, New York, 1983.

tide-1-carboxypeptidase, which removes an His–Leu dipeptide to yield the octapeptide hormone angiotensin II.

Angiotensin-converting enzyme is a zinc-containing protein. Its most important actions are (1) to convert angiotensin I → II, and (2) to inactivate bradykinin (a very potent vasodilator). The principal site of conversion of angiotensin I to II is in the vascular epithelium of the lung. A potent orally active synthetic inhibitor of the converting enzyme is the drug captopril or 1-(D-3-mercapto-3-methylpropanoyl)-2-proline. The converting enzyme is also called kininase II because of its action on bradykinin (see later). Angiotensin III, a nonapeptide, is produced by

Table 15–4. Biological Actions of the Angiotensins

Activity	Angiotensin
Stimulation of aldosterone biosynthesis and secretion by the adrenal	II = III >>> I
Elevation of blood pressure via vasoconstriction	II > III
Stimulation of release of catecholamines by adrenal medulla	II
Stimulation of thirst by action on central nervous system	II > III

action of an N-terminal peptidase action on angiotensin I. Table 15-4 summarizes the biological actions of the angiotensins.

All the biological actions of the angiotensins are mediated through binding to high-affinity membrane receptors. The actions of angiotensin II on the *zona glomerulosa* of the adrenal cortex to stimulate aldosterone secretion are described in Chapter 10. In addition, angiotensin II is the most potent pressor agent known.

All the components of the renin–angiotensin system necessary to produce angiotensin II are also present in the brain, where the latter substance may function as a neurotransmitter.

3. Aldosterone Actions on Renal Tubular Sodium Reabsorption

In humans, the principal biologically active mineralocorticoids are aldosterone, cortisol, and to some limited extent deoxycorticosterone; their structures are presented in Fig. 10-8. The mineralocorticoids mediate their actions on ion balance principally in the kidney, but also in the salivary glands, gut, and sweat glands.

In the kidney the actions of the mineralocorticoids result in an increased cortical collecting tubule reabsorption of sodium with a concomitant secretion of potassium and hydrogen (as ammonium). Only a fraction of the filtered sodium is actually reabsorbed as a consequence of aldosterone action; however, this fraction can effect significant consequences on electrolyte balance.

The precise mechanism by which aldosterone acts to stimulate the reabsorption of Na^+ from the urine is not known. However, there are experiments suggestive of the mechanism; these ideas are set forth in Fig. 15-11.

After aldosterone is secreted from the *zona glomerulosa* of the adrenals, it enters the circulation and reaches the kidney mucosal cells which concentrate aldosterone because of the cellular content of soluble cytoplasmic aldosterone receptors. Once inside the cell (Fig. 15-11, step 1), the hormone binds to high-affinity soluble receptors (step 2) by a

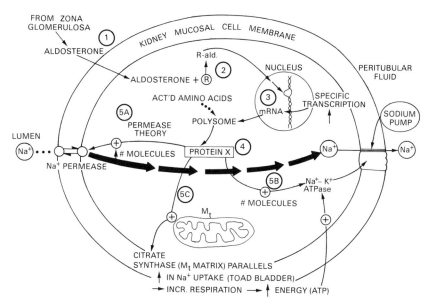

Figure 15-11. Possible mechanisms of action of aldosterone.

reaction similar to the one described for cortisol in the liver cell (see Chapter 10). The complex of aldosterone receptor presumably is activated and translocated to the nucleus where it stimulates the rate of transcription of certain mRNAs (step 3). It is not clear exactly what cellular enzymes are coded for by the increased amounts of mRNA. One or more specific enzymes must be synthesized as a result of these reactions (step 4). Protein X may be one or more of three possible enzymes. Step 5A (Fig. 15-11) indicates that the level of a postulated sodium ion permease enzyme may be increased. This change would increase the number of atoms of Na^+ entering the mucosal cell from the urine and suggests that the facilitated entrance of Na^+ may be the rate-limiting step in Na^+ reabsorption. Another possibility is an increase in the number of molecules of Na^+,K^+-ATPase which is responsible for pumping Na^+ from the cell cytoplasm on the peritubular side of the cell into the peritubular fluid (step 5B). Obviously, such a change would increase the removal of Na^+ from the cell on its way to the blood circulation and would influence positively the reactions of Na^+ leading up to this step by mass action. Finally, a third possibility (step 5C) involves an increase in the amount of citrate synthase in the mitochondrial matrix. As the name implies, this enzyme catalyzes the synthesis of citrate from oxalacetate and acetyl CoA. An increase in the level of this enzyme obviously would increase the rate of synthesis of citrate which, after traversing the mitochondrial oxidative pathway, would give rise to correspondingly more ATP.

Studies of aldosterone action in the toad bladder, which has proved to be a good experimental model for the mammalian kidney mucosal cell, show that this tissue responds to the steroid hormone aldosterone with an increase in the activity of citrate synthase in parallel with increases of Na^+ uptake. Thus, stimulated respiration in mitochondria would avail a more plentiful supply of ATP to drive the Na^+,K^+-ATPase pump on the peritubular side of the cell.

4. Atrial Natriuretic Factor

It had been known for some 30 years that the cardiocytes of heart atrial muscle contain electron-dense granules which resembled granules found in peptide hormone-producing cells. In the 1970s in a series of physiological experiments conducted by A. J. de Bold and co-workers, it was observed that dietary changes in sodium and water were found to alter the granularity of myocytes in rat atria, thus suggesting a link with electrolyte and fluid balance. This led ultimately to the isolation and characterization in 1985 of a new peptide hormone termed either atrial natriuretic factor (ANF) or atriopeptin.

The ANF gene codes for a prepro hormone of 152 amino acids (see Fig. 15-12). Loss of the 24-amino acid hydrophobic leader sequence generates the 126-amino acid prohormone which is stored in the perinuclear granules of the atrial myocytes. A single glycosylation site exists at residues 87–89. Although it is not yet known with certainty, the principal form of ANF released into the circulating system is believed to be the low-molecular-weight carboxy terminal fragment of 31 amino acids which results from proteolysis of the Arg–Arg residues at positions 101–102. However, as indicated in Fig. 15-12, a number of slightly shorter ANF peptides have been isolated. Biologically active ANF is believed to possess a disulfide linkage between the cysteine residues at positions 129 and 145.

The secretion of ANF is stimulated by any of the following: (1) atrial stretch caused by volume expansion; (2) constrictor agents that result in an elevated blood pressure; (3) high salt diets; or (4) atrial tachycardia.

Table 15-5 summarizes the principal physiological actions of ANF, while Fig. 15-13 presents an integrated diagram of the ANF hormonal system.

The most striking renal effect of ANF is the prompt and sustained increase in glomerular filtration rate (GFR), which is triggered without increasing renal blood flow. This effect frequently occurs in the presence

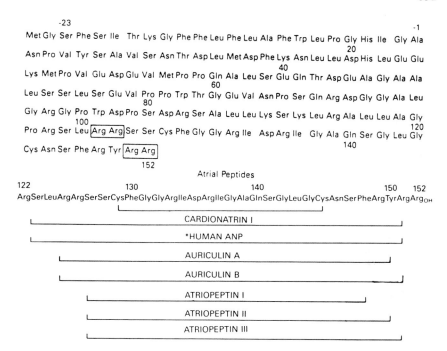

Figure 15-12. Amino acid sequence of rat atrial natriuretic factor (ANF) precursor (top) and of atrial peptides isolated by several laboratories (bottom). The biologically active ANP is believed to lie within the peptide extending from residue 122 to the COOH terminus at residue 152; this peptide contains the disulfide linking the cysteine 129 and 145 residues. The signal peptide is postulated to extend from residue −1 to −23. Modified with permission from T. Maack, M. J. F. Camargo, H. D. Kleinert, J. H. Laragh, and S. A. Atlas, Atrial natriuretic factor: Structure and functional properties. *Kidney Int.* **27,** 607–615 (1985).

Table 15–5. Physiological Actions of Atrial Natriuretic Factor

Site of action	Effect produced
Kidney	Increased glomerular filtration rate (GFR) leading to increased Na^+ excretion
Smooth muscle	Muscle relaxation of arteries and pre-constricted renal vasculature
Systemic circulation and blood pressure	Reduction in blood pressure
Renin–angiotensin–aldosterone system	Suppression of renal renin secretion

632

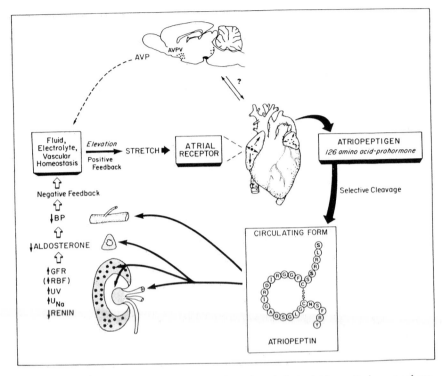

Figure 15-13. Schematic diagram of the atrial natriuretic factor/atriopeptin hormonal system. The prohormone is stored in granules located in perinuclear atrial cardiocytes. An elevated vascular volume results in cleavage and release of atriopeptin, which acts on the kidney (glomeruli and papilla) to increase the glomerular filtration rate (GFR), to increase renal blood flow (RBF), to increase urine volume (UV) and sodium excretion (U_{Na}), and to decrease plasma renin activity. Natriuresis and diuresis are also enhanced by the suppression of aldosterone and its actions and the release from the posterior pituitary of arginine vasopressin (AVP). Diminution of vascular volume provides a negative feedback signal that suppresses circulating levels of atriopeptin. Reproduced with permission from P. Needleman and J. E. Greenwald, Atriopeptin: A cardiac hormone intimately in fluid, electrolyte, and blood pressure homeostasis. *New Engl. J. Med.* **314**, 828–834 (1986).

of a decreased arterial pressure and thus is likely mediated via selective constriction of the efferent arterioles. This leads to an increased urine volume and natriuresis.

ANF also suppresses renal renin secretion which will reduce ultimately the delivery of aldosterone to the renal tubule. This action of ANF then effectively reduces the extent of aldosterone-mediated renal tubular sodium reabsorption, thus supporting the natriuresis process.

There is also evidence that ANF blocks adrenal aldosterone secretion as well as the vasoconstrictive actions of angiotensin II.

The second major biological action of ANF peptides is their powerful relaxation of preconstricted renal vasculature and large arteries and other vascular beds. This action of ANF has been shown to be associated with an increase in cyclic guanosine monophosphate (cGMP) in the vascular smooth muscle. It is believed that the increase in cGMP is the result of a direct action of ANF on the guanylate cyclase rather than through effects on phosphodiesterase.

Infusion of ANF into rats or dogs results in an immediate drop in blood pressure which persists for the duration of the infusion. This response has been attributed to an induced fall in cardiac output or venous return, but the mechanism of this reponse is not known.

5. Water Balance

Osmoreceptors (Fig. 4-11) located in the hypothalamus (and also in the carotid artery) are capable of sensing the concentrations of solutes, particularly sodium ion. This leads to a secretion of vasopressin. At the same time the thirst center in the hypothalamus, which is closely related to the osmoreceptor, is stimulated and ensuing water consumption would facilitate the end result of the stimulated thirst center. The original signal of higher $[Na^+]$, or water loss, would negate the positive signal (increase in Na^+ or blood volume) to the aldosterone-producing system so that Na^+ reabsorption in the kidney would be low.

New evidence places a second system in the neurohypophysis, involving the formation of angiotensin II, a hormone, in that location which could elevate cyclic AMP levels and cause additional release of vasopressin. Normally, the production of angiotensin II is viewed to occur primarily in the blood circulation. Besides this, there is new evidence of a polypeptide hormone called neurotensin found in the hypothalamus which acts as a hypotensive agent (its action would be similar to the effect of lowering the circulating concentration of Na^+).

Dilution of body fluids results from activation of the osmoreceptor, the thirst center, and inactivity of the aldosterone-producing mechanism. The response of the system is a fall in the level of Na^+ so that the original signals from the osmoreceptors and the thirst centers are quenched.

6. Renal Relationships of Potassium and Sodium

Although sodium is the principal extracellular cation and potassium the principal intracellular cation, the metabolism and homeostasis of these monovalent cations is closely interrelated. It is essential to life that serum potassium levels be maintained within normal limits (3.8–5.4 meq/liter) so that the normal intracellular potassium concentration of 150–160 meq/liter of intracellular water can be supported. Table 15-6 summarizes those hormones related to the kidney which participate in the regulation of blood pressure.

The homeostatic control of potassium is not as stringently regulated as for sodium. An important endocrine contribution to potassium homeostasis is the major stimulatory effects of potassium on aldosterone secretion. Aldosterone in turn acts on the renal tubules to restore plasma potassium to normal by enhancing the renal tubular excretion of potassium. Also, the falling levels of plasma K^+ are known to stimulate renin secretion, which in turn will lead ultimately to the normal actions of aldosterone on increasing sodium reabsorption. It is to be emphasized that there is no stoichiometric relationship between sodium reabsorption and potassium excretion; thus, potassium excretion may increase prior to an effect on sodium and normally the aldosterone effect on potassium diminishes before its actions on sodium terminate.

Finally, potassium can stimulate the secretion of insulin. This leads in turn to the promotion by insulin of both glucose and potassium entry into cells, which also has the consequence of lowering blood K^+.

Table 15–6. Summary of Hormonal Effectors in the Kidney Which Participate in the Regulation of Blood Pressure

Factors increasing blood pressure	Consequences
Aldosterone	Mediates renal tubular energy-dependent Na^+ reabsorption leading to an increased plasma osmolarity which leads to water reabsorption by distal tubule and collecting ducts
Vasopressin	Increases permeability of distal renal tubules which facilitate water movement into the cell
Angiotensin	—
Renin (renal or ectopic)	Increases production of angiotensin II and aldosterone

Factors decreasing blood pressure	Consequences
Bradykinin	Modulates extensive vasodilation resulting in hypotension
Atrial natriuretic factor	Promotes increase in glomerular filtration, natriuresis, and water diuresis; also can suppress plasma renin levels and relax blood vessels

IV. KALLIKREINS AND KININS

A. Introduction

The kallikreins are a group of serine proteases which act on plasma α_2-globulins known as kininogens to release kinins such as bradykinin. Bradykinin is the most potent vasodilator substance known. There is increasing evidence of an integrated interaction of the kallikrein–kinin system and prostaglandin with the renin–angiotensin system to effect systemic arterial pressure and renal blood flow. Figure 15-14 summarizes the possible interrelationships between the kallikrein–renin system.

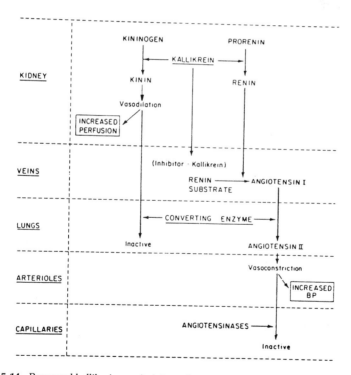

Figure 15-14. Proposed kallikrein–renin interactions to maintain systemic arterial pressure and renal blood flow. Reproduced with permission from J. E. Sealey, S. A. Atlas, and J. A. Laragh, Linking the kallikrein and renin systems via activation of inactive renin: New data and a hypothesis. *Am. J. Med.* **65,** 994–999 (1978).

B. Biochemistry and Physiology

Two classes of kallikreins have been identified: (1) those present in organs, principally the kidney but also the salivary gland and pancreas, and (2) those present in the plasma. The plasma kallikreins have a molecular weight of 107,000 while the glandular kallikreins are smaller, with a molecular weight of 27,000–43,000. All of the kallikreins are serine proteases. The plasma kallikrein is normally found as a proenzyme termed prekallikrein. Prekallikrein is activated to kallikrein by one of the blood clotting factors, factor XII, or Hageman factor. In turn, Hageman factor is activated by the plasma kallikrein. The renal kallikrein has been localized by immunohistochemical techniques to be present in the distal convoluted tubule. Here it is believed to play a role in increasing renal blood flow and possibly in mediating the conversion of prorenin to renin.

The kallikreins utilize their protease activity to release peptide kinins from their precursor substrate forms. There are two classes of kallikrein substrate: (1) those with a high molecular weight present in the plasma and which release the nonapeptide bradykinin, and (2) those with a low molecular weight present in tissues which release the decapeptide kallidin. Kallidin, or lysyl-bradykinin, has an additional lysine at the amino terminus of bradykinin.

There are at least three interconnections between the kallikrein–kinin system, the renin–angiotensin–aldosterone system, and renal prostaglandins: (1) the enzyme kallikrein appears to be involved in the conversion of prorenin to renin; (2) the enzyme activities of kininase II and the angiotensin I-converting enzyme are properties of the same protein; and (3) the production (and renal excretion) of prostaglandins is increased by production of renal kinins, while kallikrein decreases the production of the prostaglandins.

All of the kinins have very similar biological actions; they are potent stimulators of renal blood flow, mediate hypotension, and increase urine flow and sodium excretion. Bradykinin has been shown to stimulate the synthesis of prostaglandin PGA_2, probably via converting an inactive phospholipase into an active phospholipase which releases the arachidonic acid necessary for prostaglandin synthesis from membrane phospholipids.

V. PROSTAGLANDINS

The factors leading to the synthesis of prostaglandins in the kidney as described in Fig. 15-15 are called into play after the renin–angiotensin

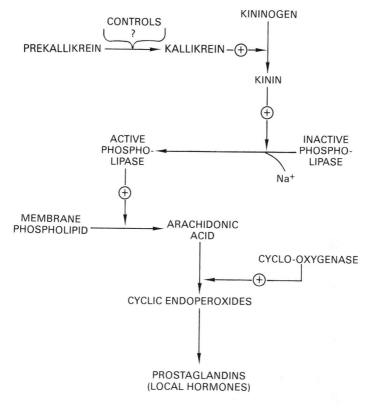

Figure 15-15. Outline of the actions of the kallikrein–kinin system in kidney.

system has been in operation. Certain signals to set the system in motion can occur via the autonomic nervous system. Examples of this kind of signal would be intellectual activity or fright, either of which are hypertensive stimuli. Increased adrenergic activity (norepinephrine release) results and stimulation of the secretion of renin by the juxtaglomerular apparatus of the kidney follows. This leads to an elevation in blood pressure, as outlined in Fig. 15-8, through the angiotensin system and aldosterone release. Ultimately, the increase in blood pressure follows from sodium ion reabsorption and subsequent increase in fluid volume of the circulatory system. The increased blood pressure is sensed by the kidney medulla, resulting in an increased blood flow. The increased blood flow through the kidney medulla must set the events of Fig. 15-15 into play and also results in the release of PGA_2 (PGE_2 can be released also) by the interstitial cells. The PGA_2 is circulated to the kidney cortex where it antagonizes the hypertension produced by the reabsorption of Na^+.

PGA$_2$ must contact the peritubular Na$^+$,K$^+$-ATPase pump either directly or through a transducer to change the conformation of this enzyme in such a way that its affinity for ATP or Na$^+$ is greatly decreased (in the enzymatic reaction, an increase in the K_m Na$^+$ or K_m ATP would be expected). By such a mechanism each molecule of the peritubular Na$^+$ pump would show a diminished rate of pumping Na$^+$ to the peritubular fluid. Consequently, more Na$^+$ would be lost into the urine. The action of PGA$_2$ antagonizes the initial hypertensive stimulus by decreasing blood volume through a direct effect on reducing the amount of Na$^+$ reabsorption by the kidney cortex mucosal cells. When the [Na$^+$] falls in the blood, the plasma volume will be decreased and this decreases the blood pressure.

VI. ERYTHROPOIETIN

A. Introduction

The kidney is the organ primarily responsible for regulating the production of erythropoietin in response to perceived changes in oxygen availability. The protein hormone erythropoietin, which is produced in the kidney, exerts a major stimulatory effect on hemoglobin synthesis by increasing the number of erythrocytes or red blood cells making hemoglobin. Hemoglobin is a tetrameric protein of 64,000 Da; each subunit (16,000 Da) contains one heme group which can coordinatively bond to one molecule of oxygen or carbon dioxide. Hemoglobin is biosynthesized in the erythrocyte, and thus the concentration of oxygen carriers in the blood will be dependent upon the blood concentration of erythrocytes.

The circulating erythrocytes as well as the total mass of their precursor erythropoietic cells (in the bone marrow) constitute the erythron. The erythron may be thought of as a dispersed organ whose prime function is the transport of oxygen and carbon dioxide as well as maintenance of the blood pH. The mature erythrocyte in mammals is nonnucleated and is relatively devoid of other subcellular organelles; thus, the hemoglobin content of an erythrocyte is determined prior to its maturation and release from the bone marrow.

The normal adult's blood contains $\sim 2 \times 10^{13}$ erythrocytes (2.5–3.0 kg); they are biosynthesized at a rate of $\sim$2 million per second. The human erythrocyte has a lifetime in the circulatory system of $\sim$120 days. Thus, there is a need for the continued production and secretion of erythropoietin to maintain adequate blood levels of hemoglobin.

B. Chemistry and Biochemistry

Experimental evidence for the existence of a humoral factor which induces an increase in the number of red blood cells was first provided in 1950 by K. Reissman. Subsequently in 1957 E. Goldwasser and colleagues demonstrated that the kidney was a primary source of erythropoietin. The principal sources of erythropoietin employed for its biochemical characterization are human plasma from anemic subjects or human urine.

The primary amino acid sequence of human erythropoietin has been determined via classical amino acid sequencing techniques, while the structure of the prepro erythroprotein has been deduced from sequence analysis of the erythropoietin gene. The mature, secreted protein has 166 amino acid residues (molecular weight 18,399) (see Fig. 15-16). The

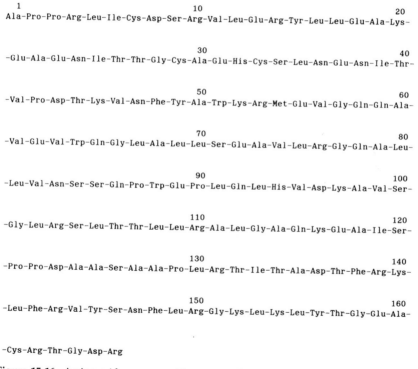

```
1                          10                              20
Ala-Pro-Pro-Arg-Leu-Ile-Cys-Asp-Ser-Arg-Val-Leu-Glu-Arg-Tyr-Leu-Leu-Glu-Ala-Lys-

                              30                              40
-Glu-Ala-Glu-Asn-Ile-Thr-Thr-Gly-Cys-Ala-Glu-His-Cys-Ser-Leu-Asn-Glu-Asn-Ile-Thr-

                              50                              60
-Val-Pro-Asp-Thr-Lys-Val-Asn-Phe-Tyr-Ala-Trp-Lys-Arg-Met-Glu-Val-Gly-Gln-Gln-Ala-

                              70                              80
-Val-Glu-Val-Trp-Gln-Gly-Leu-Ala-Leu-Leu-Ser-Glu-Ala-Val-Leu-Arg-Gly-Gln-Ala-Leu-

                              90                              100
-Leu-Val-Asn-Ser-Ser-Gln-Pro-Trp-Glu-Pro-Leu-Gln-Leu-His-Val-Asp-Lys-Ala-Val-Ser-

                              110                             120
-Gly-Leu-Arg-Ser-Leu-Thr-Thr-Leu-Leu-Arg-Ala-Leu-Gly-Ala-Gln-Lys-Glu-Ala-Ile-Ser-

                              130                             140
-Pro-Pro-Asp-Ala-Ala-Ser-Ala-Ala-Pro-Leu-Arg-Thr-Ile-Thr-Ala-Asp-Thr-Phe-Arg-Lys-

                              150                             160
-Leu-Phe-Arg-Val-Tyr-Ser-Asn-Phe-Leu-Arg-Gly-Lys-Leu-Lys-Leu-Tyr-Thr-Gly-Glu-Ala-

-Cys-Arg-Thr-Gly-Asp-Arg
```

Figure 15-16. Amino acid sequence of human erythropoietin. The Asn at position 83 is known to be glycosylated. This figure was derived from information presented in P. H. Lai, R. Everett, F. F. Wang, T. Arakawa, and E. Goldwasser, Structural characterization of human erythropoietin. *J. Biol. Chem.* **261**, 3116–3121 (1986).

proerythropoietin was deduced to possess a 27-amino acid signal peptide. As yet computer analysis of the amino acid sequence of erythropoietin has not revealed any discernible homology with any other proteins.

C. Renal Production

The proposed role of the kidney in erythropoiesis is supported both by experimental and clinical studies. In the latter case it is known that anemia or hemoglobin deficiency is often associated with renal insufficiency. Experimental evidence includes the following: (1) Renal ablation or nephrectomy of rats results in a markedly diminished plasma concentration of erythropoietin; (2) erythropoietin appears in fluid circulated through isolated kidneys subjected to oxygen deficiency; and (3) erythropoietin activity can be extracted from kidney mitochondria.

Although there are now multiple lines of evidence that the kidney is the primary source of production of erythropoietin, it is not yet known with certainty which anatomical unit of the kidney is responsible for the generation of this peptide hormone. Preliminary evidence obtained in studies with hypoxic dog kidneys utilizing a horseradish peroxidase-labeled antibody to erythropoietin suggests a localization with the epithelial cells of the glomerular tufts.

D. Mode of Action

The principal site of action of erythropoietin is the erythron. The blood concentration of erythropoietin is ~1–10 × 10^{-10} M; its concentration in plasma is elevated 50–100 times in severely anemic individuals as a consequence of hypoxia.

Erythropoietin has been shown to be essential for the differentiation and development of stem cells (see Fig. 15-17). There appear to be three general classes of cells which constitute the pathway of red cell production: the pluripotent stem cell, a population of erythroid-committed precursor cells, and the maturing erythron. The pluripotent cells also have the capability when grown *in vitro* to proliferate into lymphoid, megakarocytic, as well as the erythroid cells (see Fig. 9-14). At some point, not yet clearly defined, under *in vivo* conditions the stem cell becomes responsive to erythropoietin and develops into a pronormoblast cell. Four cell divisions later (over a 72-hr interval), the mature normoblast cells appear; over this same time interval the bulk of the hemoglobin is biosynthesized. The orthochromatic normoblast then, over a 10-min interval, expels its nucleus to generate the enucleated reticulocyte. The re-

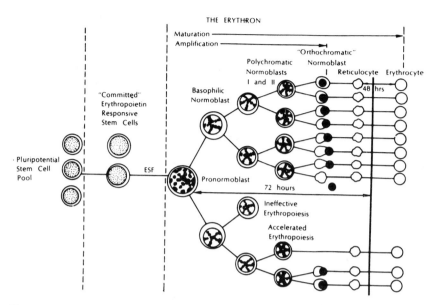

Figure 15-17. Schematic outline of the differentiation and maturation events occurring in the erythron during erythropoiesis. Erythropoietin stimulates stem cells to develop into pronormoblasts which, in turn, differentiate into enucleated reticulocytes and finally into the mature erythrocyte. A single pronormoblast amplifies by four cell divisions to give four different types of pronormoblasts, each with a different morphology. Also shown (bottom) is "ineffective erythropoiesis" in which normoblast formation stops with cell death in the bone marrow and accelerated erythropoiesis as seen in polycythemia. Modified from L. L. Lessin and M. Bessis, Body fluids and their constituents. *In* "Hematology" (W. J. Williams, E. Beutler. A. J. Ersler, and R. W. Rundles, eds.), p. 104. McGraw-Hill, New York, 1977.

ticulocyte then enters the general circulation and over the next 48 hr matures into an erythrocyte.

Erythropoietin does not appear to increase hemoglobin, or more specifically globin synthesis, by affecting individual cells, but acts to increase the total number of cells actively making hemoglobin. This emphasizes the mitogenic or growth factor-like property of erythropoietin. It causes the stem cells to divide and differentiate into the more mature erythroid cells. The earliest reported effect of erythropoietin is to stimulate RNA synthesis. At least three general biochemical mechanisms have been proposed to describe the actions of erythropoietin on cell differentiation and globin gene expression.

The responsiveness of the precursor stem cell may be due to the presence of membrane receptors for erythropoietin which may respond via several pathways: (1) The increase in activity of expression of the globin gene would parallel that of the family of other genes related to differentiation of the stem cell into a normoblast. (2) Erythropoietin may stimulate in a normoblast modification of a particular protein which interacts with chromatin to permit transcription of the globin gene. Here erythropoietin is mediating differentiation of the normoblast cell with respect to its ability to produce globin. (3) Interaction of erythropoietin with its membrane receptor on a normoblast cell may generate a specific "cytoplasmic factor" which is necessary to mediate the transcription of the globin genes. It is not possible, on the basis of the available data, to make a choice between these models.

VII. CLINICAL ASPECTS

A. Hypertension

Hypertension is a disorder that may occur throughout life; it is defined as the continued elevation of blood pressure beyond defined limits. In adults the criterion of an elevated blood pressure is ≥95 mm Hg (diastolic) or ≥160 mm Hg (systolic). Hypertension has a worldwide incidence of 9–18% of the adult population. The maintenance of normal blood pressure is the end result of an integrated system in which the hormones, particularly atrial natriuretic factor, renin–angiotensin–aldosterone, vasopressin, and kallikrein–kinin, as well as the prostaglandins and dietary intake of salt play an integral role. In addition, the catecholamines, estrogens, glucococorticoids, and thyroxines can be implicated under some circumstances in a causative or contributory manner to the state of hypertension.

In the presence of continuing uncontrolled hypertension there is frequently a high incidence of heart disorders (congestive failure, coronary heart disease), stroke, kidney disease, and/or aneurisms of the aorta.

There are three general causative factors which may lead to the development of hypertension: (1) primary aldosteronism which results in an unrestrained production of aldosterone by the adrenals (see Chapter 10); (2) a pheochromocytoma which is a tumor that produces catecholamines (see Chapter 11); and (3) renovascular hypertension which results in a lowered blood supply to one kidney with a normal blood flow to the second kidney. An important component of diagnosis of the etiology of hypertension is a determination of the level of sodium excretion in relation to the plasma levels of renin and also the daily amount of aldosterone excreted in the urine. Such an analysis may provide formulation of a rational basis of treatment which can include inhibitors of the renin–angiotensin system; such antagonists as saralasin, β-blocking drugs such as propanolol, or dietary restriction of salt intake are employed. It is beyond the scope of this presentation to consider in detail this topic.

B. Bartter's Syndrome

Bartter's syndrome is both a metabolic and a renal disorder that results in abnormally low levels of potassium in the blood (hypokalemia) and a metabolic alkalosis. Typically a patient with Bartter's syndrome will have elevated plasma levels of renin and aldosterone and a hyperplasia of the juxtaglomerular apparatus, but a normal blood pressure. There are also some abnormalities in the renal levels of prostaglandins and the kallikrein–kinin system. The etiology for this syndrome has not yet been provided.

C. Erythropoietin

There are no known major disease states or endocrine disorders with a high incidence attributable to erythropoietin. There can in some circumstances be a tumor which results in the ectopic production of erythropoietin.

References

A. Books

Fisher, J. W., ed. (1977). "Kidney Hormones," Vol. 2. Academic Press, New York.

Peters, J. P. (1835). "Body Water." Baillière, London.

Pitts, R. F. (1974). "Physiology of the Kidney and Body Fluids," 3rd ed. Yearbook Publ., Chicago, Illinois.

B. Review Articles

Cantin, M., and Genest, J. (1985). The heart and atrial natriuretic factor. *Endocr. Rev.* **6**, 107–127.

Goldwasser, E. (1975). Erythropoietin and the differentiation of red blood cells. *Fed. Proc., Fed. Am. Soc. Exp. Biol.* **34**, 2285–2292.

Inagami, T., Chang,. J., Dykes, C. W., Takii, Y., Kisarage, M., and Misono, K. S. (1983). Renin: Structural features of an active enzyme and inactive precursor. *Fed. Proc., Fed. Am. Soc. Exp. Biol.* **42**, 2729–2734.

Needleman, P., and Greenwald, J. E. (1986). Atriopeptin: A cardiac hormone intimately involved in fluid, electrolyte, and blood pressure homeostasis. *New Engl. J. Med.* **314**, 828–834.

Schambelan, M., and Biglieri, E. G. (1976). Hypertension and the role of the renin–

644

angiotensin–aldosterone system in renal failure. *In* "The Kidney" (B. M. Brenner and F. C. Rector, Jr., eds.), pp. 1486–1521. Saunders, Philadelphia, Pennsylvania.

C. Research Papers

Capponi, A., Leu, P. D., Jornot, L., and Vallotton, M. B. (1984). Correlation between cytosolic free calcium and aldosterone production in bovine adrenal glomerulosa cells: Evidence for a difference in the mode of action of angiotensin II and potassium. *J. Biol. Chem.* **259**, 8803–8869.

Chao, J., Tanaka, S., and Mangolurs, H. S. (1983). Inhibiting effects of sodium and other monovalent cations on purified versus membrane-bound kallikrein. *J. Biol. Chem.* **258**, 6461–6465.

Edelman, I. S. (1979). Mechanism of action of aldosterone: Energetic and permeability factors. *J. Endocrinol.* **81**, 49–53.

Edelman, I. S., and Marver, D. (1980). Mediating events in the action of aldosterone of steroid. *Biochemistry* **12**, 219–224.

Lai, P., Everett, R., Wang, F., Arakawa, T., and Goldwasser, E. (1986). Structural characterization of human erythropoietin. *J. Biol. Chem.* **261**, 3116–3121.

Levy, S. B., Lilley, J. J., Frigon, R. P., and Stone, R. A. (1977). Urinary kallikrein and plasma renin activity as determinants of renal blood flow. *J. Clin. Invest.* **60**, 129–138.

Lin, F., Suggs, S., Lin, C., Browne, J. K., Smalling, R., Egrie, J. C., Chen, K. K., Fox, G. M., Martin, F., Stabinsky, Z., Badrawi, S. M., Lai, P. H., and Goldwasser, E. (1985). Cloning and expression of the human erythropoietin gene. *Proc. Natl. Acad. Sci. U.S.A.* **82**, 7580–7584.

Misono, K. S., and Inagami, T. (1982). Structure of mouse submaxillary gland renin: Identification of two disulfide-linked polypeptide chains and complete amino acid sequence. *J. Biol. Chem.* **257**, 7536–7540.

Nasjletti, A., and Malik, K. U. (1979). Relationships between the kallikrein–kinin system and prostaglandins. *Life Sci.* **25**, 99–110.

Sealey, J. E., Atlas, S. A., and Laragh, J. H. (1978). Human urinary kallikrein converts inactive to active renin and is a possible physiological activator of renin. *Nature (London)* **275**, 144–145.

Truscello, A., Geering, K., Gaggeler, H. P., and Rossier, B. C. (1983). Effects of butyrate on histone deacetylation and aldosteine-dependent Na$^+$ transport in the toad bladder. *J. Biol. Chem.* **258**, 3388–3395.

Weingerger, M. H., Grim, C. E., Hollifield, J. W., Ken, D. C., Granguly, A., Kramer, N. J., Yune, H. Y., Wellman, H., and Donohue, J. P. (1979). Primary aldosteronism: Diagnosis, localization, and treatment. *Ann. Intern. Med.* **30**, 386–395.

Wiggins, R. C. (1983). Kinin release from high-molecular-weight kininogen by the action of Hageman factor in the absence of kallikrein. *J. Biol. Chem.* **258**, 8963–8970.

Wong, T. W., and Goldberg, A. R. (1983). *In vitro* phosphorylation of angiotensin analogs by tyrosyl protein kinases. *J. Biol. Chem.* **258**, 1022–1025.

Prostaglandins

HORMONES

I. INTRODUCTION

A. Background

The prostaglandins (PG) represent a class of substances produced in a wide variety of cells. These act on the cells which produce them, on neighboring cells, or usually over short distances and can be classified as "autocrine" hormones. Some PGs, such as prostacyclins (PGI_2), may be regarded as acting like the more traditional endocrine hormones in the sense that they are synthesized in blood vessel cells, survive in the bloodstream for a period of time, and can exert effects somewhat distant from their sites of synthesis. However, we usually think of PGs and their relatives as being potent local hormones (autocrine and paracrine) acting over a short lifetime.

PGs and their relatives, PGI_2, thromboxanes (TX), and leukotrienes (LT), derive from fatty acids stored in cellular membranes as phospholipids or as triglycerides. Fatty acid precursors, typically arachidonic acid, are released by a phospholipase or by a lipase in the cell membranes following a stimulatory event. This event usually will be a signal to activate the enzyme liberating arachidonic acid from lipids in the membrane. A series of synthetic reactions catalyzed by enzymes takes place in the membrane, culminating in the release of the PG product from the membrane into the cellular cytoplasm. The released PG may bind to its receptor located within the plasma membrane or other internal membrane or it may be released to the cell exterior and ultimately produce an effect by binding to a receptor in the cell membrane of a neighboring cell. There is little information available on the mechanism by which PGs are secreted from cells.

PGs and their relatives are for the most part different from the more traditional endocrine hormones which usually are secreted from a gland of synthesis and act on a distant target cell after extensive transport in the circulation. It may be useful to think of this group as "locally acting hormones" or "autocrines." This emphasizes the trend of breaking down the traditional view of hormones as substances produced by and acting exclusively like the endocrine gland hormones. As our information develops further, we may have to broaden our definitions to encompass all molecules acting as signals and operating through receptors.

PGs are produced by many different cells in the body. It is not yet clear whether all cells are capable of producing them, but this seems a distinct possibility. Table 16-1 lists several tissues from various animals which are known to release PGs in response to various kinds of stimuli.

Table 16–1. Stimulated Release of Prostaglandins from Various Tissues[a]

Species	Tissues	Stimulus
Rabbit	Eye (anterior chamber)	Mechanical
	Spleen	Catecholamines, serotonin
	Epigastric fat pad	Hormones
	Somatosensory cortex	Neural, analeptics, etc., reticular formation
	Spleen	Catecholamines
	Adrenal	Acetylcholine
Dog	Spleen	Neural, neural catecholamines, neural colloids, colloids
	Bladder	Distension
	Cerebral ventricles	Serotonin
Rat	Phrenic diaphragm	Neural, biogenic amines
	Epididymal fat pad	Neural, biogenic amines
	Stomach	Neural stretch, neural, neural secretagogues
	Skin	Inflammation
	Liver	Glucagon
	Lung	Air embolus, infusion of particles
Guinea pig	Lung (whole, perfused)	Anaphylaxis, particles, histamine, tryptamine, serotonin, passage air embolus, distension
	Lung (chopped)	Stirring
Human	Thyroid	Medullary carcinoma
	Uterus	Parturition, distension
	Platelets	Thrombin
Frog	Intestine	Distilled water
	Skin	Isoproterenol
	Spinal cord	Neural analeptics

[a] Reproduced with permission from P. W. Ramwell and I. Rabinowitz, *in* "Effects of Drugs on Cellular Control Processes" (B. R. Rabin and R. B. Freedman, eds.), pp. 207–235. Macmillan, New York, 1972.

Ultimately the release of PGs from cells may be a product of the action of other hormones or neurotransmitters (i.e., the signal to the cell to synthesize PGs).

PGs exert a wide variety of effects on different target tissues. They affect behavior through direct actions on individual neurons, substructures of the brain, such as the cerebellar and reticular formation (the latter is responsible for screening various kinds of environmental signals), and they act on the hypothalamus and the pituitary. Vasomotor and temperature-regulatory centers are affected by PGs. Autonomic and neuromuscular junctions are also affected. As is evident in other chapters, PGs act on anterior pituitary trophic hormone target tissues such as thyroid, adrenal, ovary, and testis; on exocrine hormone targets such as pancreas and gastric mucosa; and on endocrine target tissues such as renal tubules, bone, and adipocytes. They act on smooth muscles of the reproductive, alimentary, and respiratory tracts and on cardiovascular smooth muscles. Some of these effects will be elaborated in this chapter. PGs act on red blood cells, leukocytes, and on platelets, the last of which will be described here. The role of PGs in pain will be mentioned, consistent with the inflammatory actions of certain PGs (see Chapter 10).

B. Structural Classes of PG Relatives

Although there is a huge complexity of structures under the heading of PGs and their relatives, it may be helpful to describe briefly the differences between the major classes. All of these compounds are derived from fatty acids, often arachidonic acid, an open chain, 20-carbon structure. The PGs, including TX and PGI_2, all arise by mediation through a cyclic endoperoxide. On the other hand, LTs are formed directly from a fatty acid metabolite and do not involve a cyclic endoperoxide intermediate.

PGs resemble hairpins with a 5-membered ring and two chains extending from the ring. Substituents on the 5-membered ring determine the subclass and activity of the PGs. TXs have a 6-membered ring with two chains extending from the ring. The 6-membered ring has one or more oxygens associated with it. PGI_2 has two adjacent rings, one of which contains an oxygen with one chain extending from each ring. Often TX and PGI_2 are found to have opposing biological activities. LTs are essentially modified open chain fatty acids which may be conjugated to glutathione or glutathione degradation products. There is a wide array of related structures with characteristic activities or inactivity if such structures result from metabolism. The characteristics of general structures mentioned above are shown in Fig. 16-1.

C. Classification of PGs

Although the many structures in this group of compounds may seem bewildering at first (Fig. 16-2), there are some simple generalizations which can be set forth to allow a facile understanding of structure–function relationships. PGs arise from a cyclic endoperoxide generated by the enzyme system, PG synthetase. This is probably a complex of enzymes required to produce the key intermediate, the cyclic endoperoxide derivative of arachidonic acid or other fatty acids. The inter-

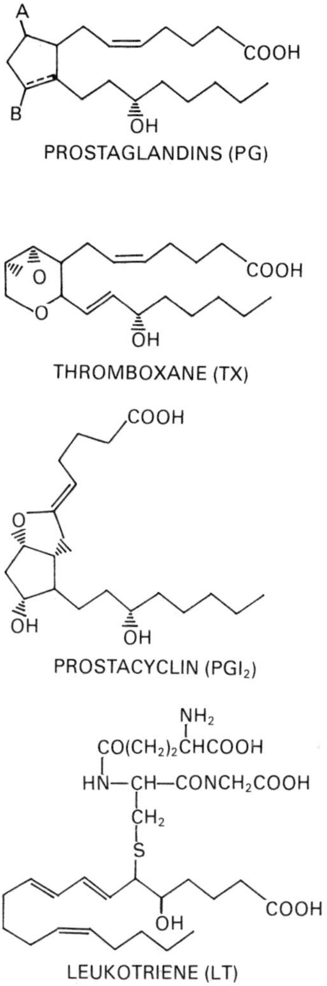
A
COOH
B
OH
PROSTAGLANDINS (PG)
O
COOH
O
OH
THROMBOXANE (TX)
COOH
O
OH
OH
PROSTACYCLIN (PGI2)
NH2
CO(CH2)2CHCOOH
HN—CH—CONCH2COOH
CH2
S
COOH
OH
LEUKOTRIENE (LT)

Figure 16-1. General features of major classes of PG relatives.

mediate is acted on by various isomerases to produce PG subclasses. The cyclic endoperoxide is also a precursor of PGI_2 and TX. On the other hand, the most recently discovered group of compounds in this class, LT, is derived mainly from arachidonic acid without mediation of a cyclic endoperoxide (Fig. 16-1). An overview of the formation of all the PG relatives is presented in (Fig. 16-2). The one double-bond members of some of the classes, such as PGE_1 or $PGF_{1\alpha}$, are not shown here, but are illustrated elsewhere in the chapter. Of the many groups of com-

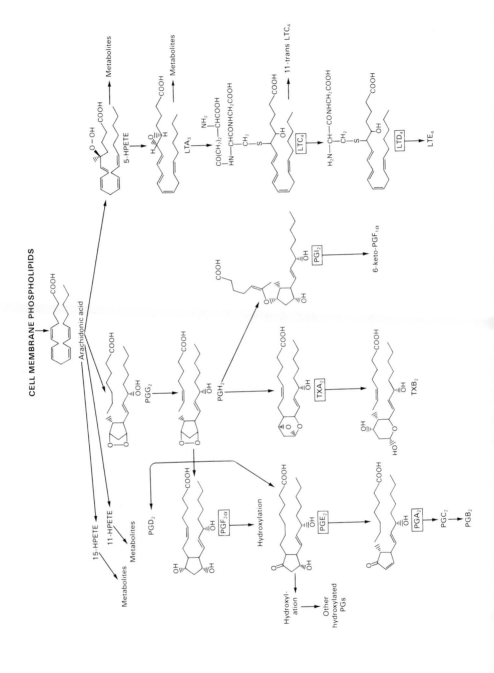

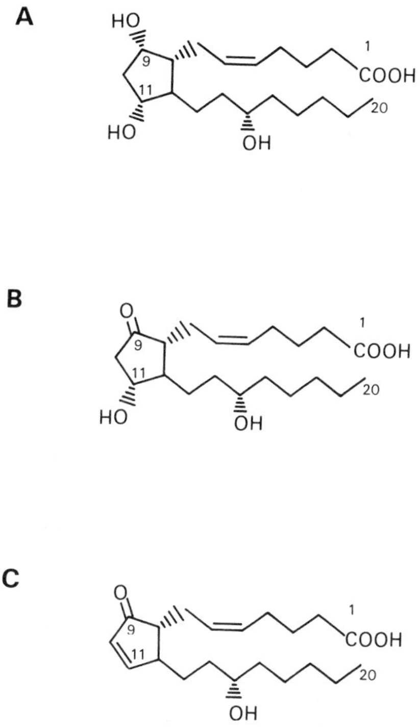

Figure 16-3. General structures of three major classes of PGs. (A) General structure of PGF series. (B) General structure of PGE series. (C) General structure of PGA series.

pounds, the PGs are composed of only three abundant groups: PGF, PGE, and PGA. F stands for phosphate buffer-soluble (phosphate begins with an "F" in Swedish) structures which the most hydrophilic or polar of the PGs. The F series has the general structure shown in Fig. 16-3A. All the PGs have the 5-membered ring shown here. The F series (most polar) has two hydroxyls in the C-9 and C-11 positions constituting the most hydrophilic of the classical PGs. The E series (PGE) is intermediate in solubility (is ether soluble, thus E) and has one hydroxyl and one ketone substituting the 5-membered ring (Fig. 16-3B). The A series (PGA) is least polar or hydrophilic, most lipophilic, and has no

Figure 16-2. Routes of synthesis to some of the PGs, PGI$_2$, TX, and LT from arachidonic acid. Note that all of the classes of PG relatives are synthesized through a cyclic endoperoxide intermediate except for the LTs and related structures which are essentially modified fatty acids. Reproduced with permission from N. A. Nelson, R. C. Kelly, and R. A. Johnson, *Chem. Eng. News* Aug. 16, p. 30 (1982). Copyright 1982 American Chemical Society.

652

hydroxyl groups substituting in the 5-membered ring, but rather a ketone group and an unsaturation (Fig. 16-3C). These classes of PGs have
characteristic actions depending on the 5-membered ring substituents,
as shown in Table 16-2.

Inspection of Table 16-2 provides an easy means to relate structure
with activity. Since PGF is the most "water soluble," it has hydroxyl
groups on both C-9 and C-11. As will be seen later, PGF plays a role in
termination of pregnancy. This association will make it possible to remember that the F series is active in muscular contraction (i.e., as in
uterine contractions of parturition).

The PGE series is intermediate between PGF and PGA. Consequently,
it shares both activities of those groups as well as their characteristic ring
substituents. The structure therefore can be deduced as one in which the
ring has both a hydroxyl (typical of PGF) and a ketone (typical of PGA)

Table 16–2. Principal Classes of the Classical Prostaglandins and Their Actions[a]

Structure	Compound	Effect on blood pressure	Effect on nonvascular smooth muscle (uterus/intestine)
↑ [increasing polarity]			
	(PO$_4$ soluble)	Transient increase	Very active
	(ether soluble)	Decrease	Very active
		Decrease	Inactive
↓ [increasing lipophilicity]			

[a] Reproduced in part from J. B. Lee, in "Principles of Endocrinology" (R. H. Williams, ed.), 5th ed., p. 855. Saunders, Philadelphia, Pennsylvania, 1975.

and has both activities of stimulating muscular contraction and of decreasing blood pressure. Finally, PGA is least polar (a ketone and a double bond in the ring) and has the opposite activity of PGF; it reduces blood pressure and has little effect on nonvascular muscle contraction.

In designating the PGs, two kinds of subscripts may appear at the end of the abbreviation (e.g., $PGF_{2\alpha}$). The subscript, which is a number, denotes the number of double bonds in the structure. The Greek letter, α, following the subscript number refers to the steric position of the C-9 substituent as being α (extending behind the plane of the ring, away from the reader). This becomes apparent in the structure of $PGF_{2\alpha}$. If 2 is added to this number (4 in the case of $PGF_{2\alpha}$), we get the number of double bonds which must have been present in the fatty acid precursor of $PGF_{2\alpha}$, that is, eicosatetraenoic acid (20:4 ω 6) or arachidonic acid. The information in parentheses, in this case (20:4 ω 6), presents information about the fatty acid. Thus, 20 is the number of carbons in the structure, 4 is the number of double bonds, and ω 6 indicates that there are six methyls in the chain from the end until a double bond appears (Fig. 16-4).

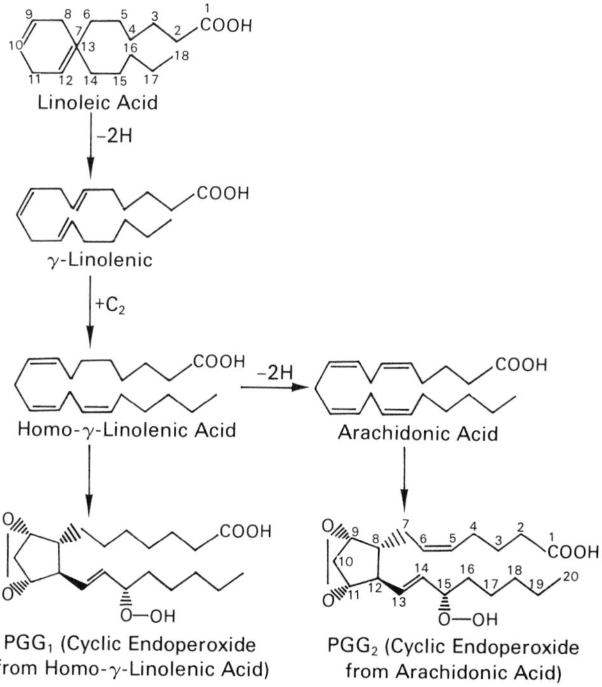

Figure 16-4. Interconversions of fatty acids leading to the production of major endoperoxide intermediates in the synthesis of PGs.

D. General Aspects of PGs

The synthesis of PGs and relatives from membrane lipids, release of the finished products into the cytoplasm, and actions are summarized by Fig. 16-5. Thus, when PG synthesis is stimulated in a cell, a fatty acid precursor, often arachidonic acid, is released from the membrane lipids by phospholipase A_2. It is acted on by the membrane PG synthetase complex which produces a cyclic endoperoxide intermediate (Fig. 16-4). This intermediate can give rise to PGE_2, $PGF_{2\alpha}$, and PGI_2 in cells that contain PGI_2 synthetase, or to TX, TXA_2, in cells that contain TX synthetase (Fig. 16-2). When homo-γ-linolenic acid (20:3) (Fig. 16-4) is the parent fatty acid, a different cyclic endoperoxide is produced. This intermediate can give rise to PGE_1 and $PGF_{1\alpha}$. Thus, the PGs or relatives occurring in a given cell depend on the precursor and especially upon the enzymes present in the biosynthetic pathways.

II. CHEMISTRY

Conformation of PGs and Thromboxanes (TX)

The conformational analysis of $PGF_{2\alpha}$ has been accomplished by the use of X-ray diffraction techniques. Two independent structures appear as familiar hairpin configurations, as shown in Fig. 16-6. In contrast, TX molecules as represented by TXB_2 (Fig. 16-2) do not adopt the PG hairpin configuration as shown in Fig. 16-7. These configurations specify obvious differences between the architecture of the PG and TX receptors.

III. BIOCHEMISTRY

A. Biosynthesis

The biosynthetic mechanism can be typified by the PG synthetase system in sheep seminal vesicle microsomes (Fig. 16-8). Obviously this system consists of a complex of enzymes. To produce the cyclic hydroperoxy intermediate, there are two oxygenation steps which may be catalyzed by the same or separate enzymes. Conversion of the hydroperoxy intermediate to the C-15-hydroxylated form occurs through the agency of glutathione peroxidase, and this reaction can be stimulated to occur nonenzymatically by a combination of tryptophan and hemo-

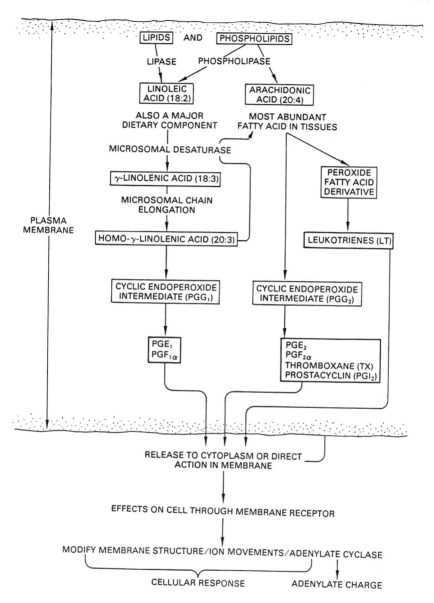

Figure 16-5. Overview of PG and relatives syntheses and actions.

656

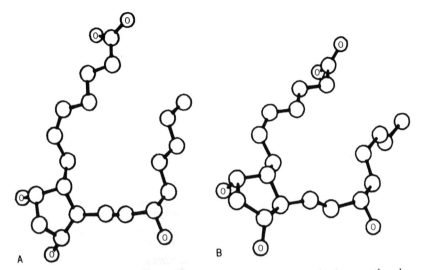

Figure 16-6. The two conformers of $PGF_{2\alpha}$. The views are the projections on the planes defined by atoms C-12, C-15, and O-15. Reproduced from D. A. Langs, M. Erman, and G. T. Detita, *Science* **197**, 1003–1005 (1977). Copyright 1977 by the AAAS.

globin. This group of reactions has been referred to as Fraction I. Succeeding reactions are catalyzed by glutathione-requiring isomerases which may be identical to ligandin, a GSH *S*-transferase, which has been demonstrated to have Δ^{5-4}-3-ketosteroid isomerase activity and requires glutathione anion as a catalytic cofactor. The action of aspirin (acetylsalicylic acid) or indomethacin is to acetylate the PG endoperoxide synthetase. This results in loss of the cyclooxygenase activity, but not of the peroxidase activity. Apparently one acetylation per molecule of 68,000 Da is sufficient to complete the reaction. It is likely that the hydroxyl group of a serine in the N-terminal portion is acetylated.

The biosynthetic system is further elaborated in Fig. 16-9. A parallel set of reactions can be developed for substrates other than arachidonic acid. These reactions, pictured in Figs. 16-9 and 16-10, account for the major PGs, TXs, PGI_2. Recently, a possible mechanism has been suggested for the formation of TXA_2 and PGI_2 from PGH_2, as shown in Fig. 16-11.

A newly discovered class of compounds, called the leukotrienes (LT), derive from arachidonic acid, but do not proceed through a cyclic endoperoxide. Instead, this class of compounds derives by modification of arachidonic acid or other fatty acids, as shown in Fig. 16-12.

As can be seen from Fig. 16-12, there are at least seven known LTs.

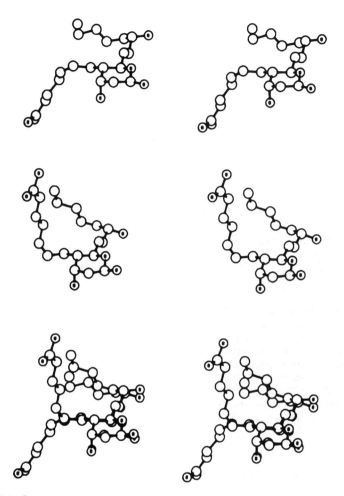

Figure 16-7. Stereograms of the α tail (top) and β tail (middle) conformers of TXB₂, and a composite (bottom) of the two conformers. Reproduced from D. A. Langs, S. Fortier, M. G. Erman, and G. T. Detita, *Nature (London)* **281,** 237–238 (1979). © 1979 Macmillan Journals Limited.

Importantly, LTC₁, LTC₄, and LTC₅ contain glutathione, and LTD₄ contains cysteinylglycine. The D series contains sulfur amino acid residues, as well. None of these very active compounds arise via a cycloendoperoxide, but all arise from the direct peroxidation of the fatty acid substrate on C-5. These compounds are very active bronchoconstrictors in the lungs and airways and are undoubtedly of vital importance in the etiology of asthma.

658

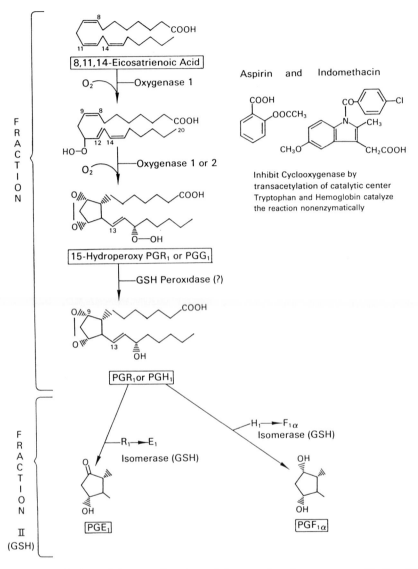

Figure 16-8. Outline of the overall actions of the complex of enzymes constituting PG synthase (synthetase).

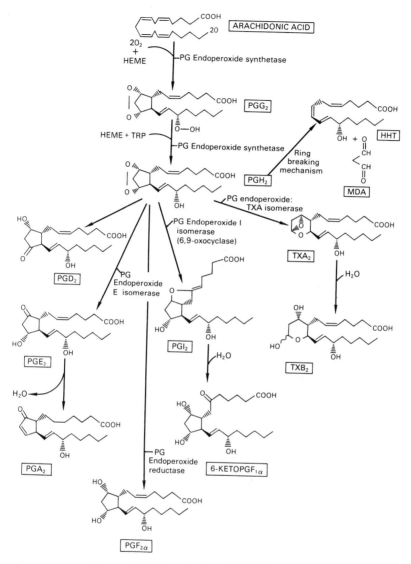

Figure 16-9. Biosynthesis of PG, PGI$_2$, and TX.

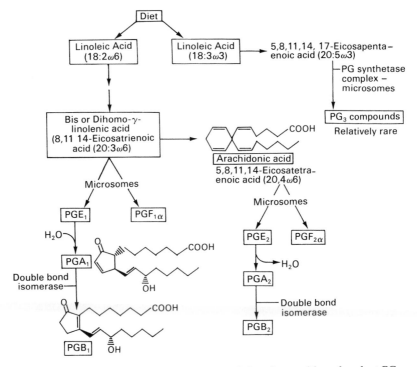

Figure 16-10. Overview of the biosynthesis of abundant and less abundant PGs.

B. Metabolism

The PGs are metabolized in many positions, for example, PGE₂ (Fig. 16-13A). TXA₂, assumed to be the major active TX in the human platelet, is metabolized to the less active TXB₂ (Fig. 16-13B). PGI₂ is metabolized to the 6-keto-PGF₁α (Fig. 16-13C). In the cases of PGI₂ and TXA₂, metabolism concerns the opening of an oxygen-containing ring. Futher metabolic steps are indicated as for the PGs.

C. Binding Proteins and Receptors

1. Serum Binding

Human serum has been shown to bind PGs presumably by strong noncovalent interactions. PGs bind tightly in inverse relation to their polarity. Thus, the order of tightness of binding is PGA > PGE₁ > PGF₂α. Since it is known that PGA₁ is cleared slowly in comparison to other PGs, its strong interaction with serum may explain its slow turnover.

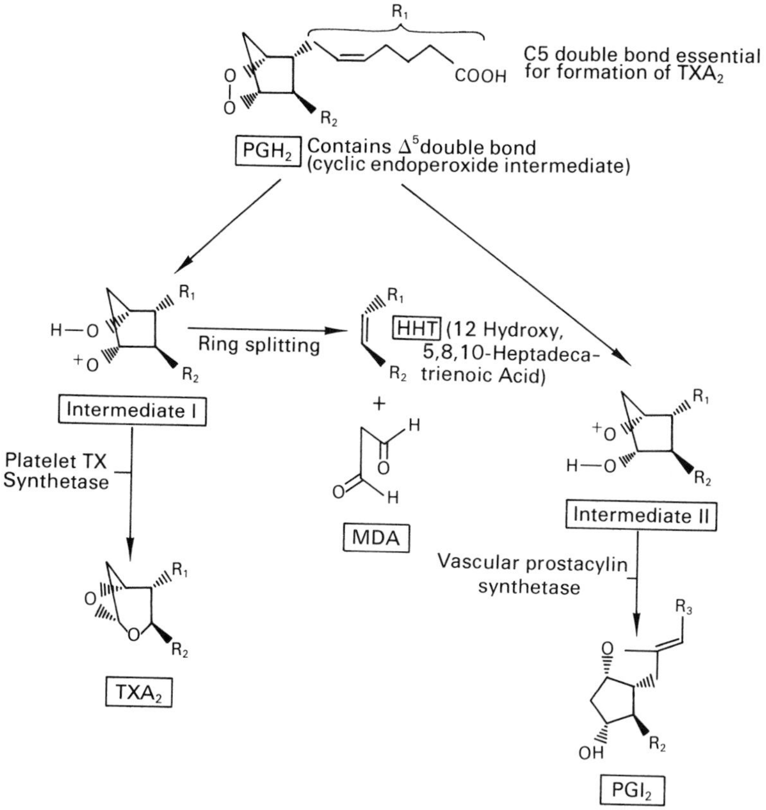

Figure 16-11. Possible mechanism for the formation of TXA$_2$ and PGI$_2$ from PGH$_2$.

2. Receptors

It is generally agreed that there are specific receptors for PGs and relatives in cell membranes. Receptors for PGs are present in the cell membranes of cells which are responsive to PG, usually measured by their ability to stimulate adenylate cyclase or to raise the level of intracellular cyclic AMP. In cells that are unresponsive to PG, cell membrane receptors are not measurable. These findings are consistent with what is found with other hormone receptors, hormone-responsive cells contain receptors and hormone-unresponsive cells either do not contain measurable receptors or they contain receptors which are altered in such a way as to render them virtually ineffective (e.g., in mutants).

Although the information is incomplete, there appear to be at least two types of receptors located in various cell membranes, one for PGEs

662

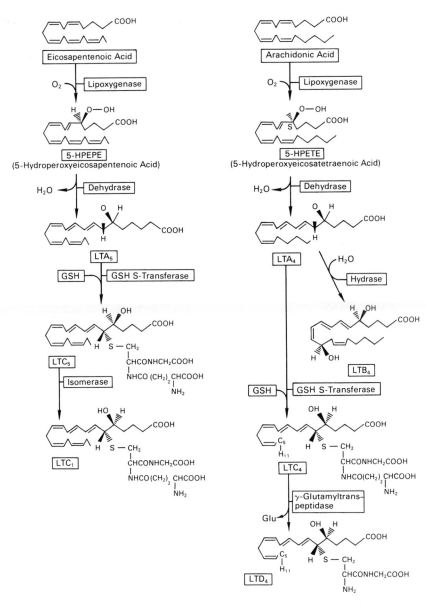

Figure 16-12. Biosynthesis of LT. Subscripts are number of double bonds.

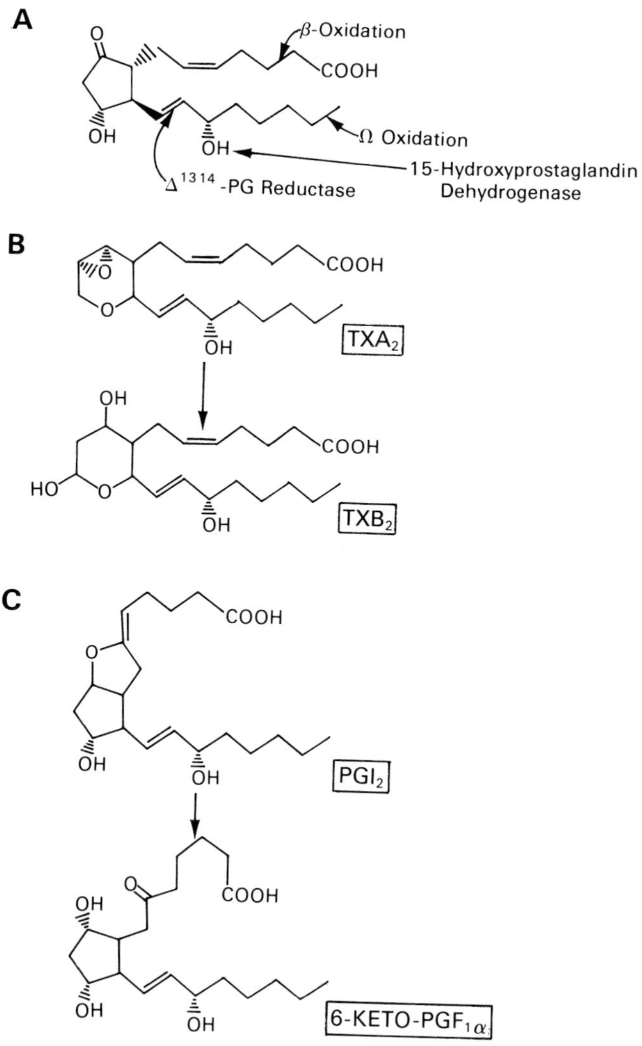

Figure 16-13. (A) Positions in which PGs are metabolized. (B) Metabolism of TX. (C) Metabolism of PGI$_2$.

whose second messenger is cyclic AMP and one for PGF$_{2\alpha}$ whose second messenger may be cyclic GMP. Some evidence indicates that the receptor for PGI$_2$ on platelet membranes is similar or identical to the PGE receptor. Thus, the significance of PGI$_2$ in the platelet mechanism obtains from the fact that PGI$_2$ is available in the bloodstream, in essence

664

a circulating hormone at least to a limited extent. PGE is more unstable, being destroyed rapidly. The specificity of binding of PG analogs is stringent enough to fulfill the requirements for a receptor and, in several cases, there has been reasonable agreement between the ability of various PGs to produce a biological response and ability to stimulate adenylate cyclase so that PG receptors and adenylate cyclase can be connected in PG action. Also, reports are available suggesting that levels of PG producing a biological response correlate with data of binding to the membrane receptor.

The PGE_1 receptor appears to be present in liver, corpus luteum, uterus, adipocytes, and thymocytes.

Partial characterization of the $PGF_{2\alpha}$ receptor from bovine corpus luteum has been achieved by solubilizing the receptor from membranes with sodium deoxycholate. A Stokes radius of 61 Å and a sedimentation coefficient of 4.8 S have been reported. After correction for bound detergent, a molecular weight of 107,000 was calculated. As the result of structure–function studies, it is possible to speculate on the interaction of the receptor with $PGF_{2\alpha}$ (Fig. 16-14).

There is probably a distinct receptor for TX, based on structural differences revealed by X-ray analysis, from PGs and there are probably distinct receptors for LTs. Partial purification of separate receptors for LTC_4 and LTD_4 has been reported.

IV. BIOLOGICAL ACTIONS

Many hormonal and other signaling mechanisms which operate through plasma membrane receptors may involve the PGs. At this

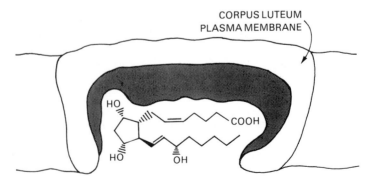

Figure 16-14. Speculation on the groupings in $PGF_{2\alpha}$ critical to receptor binding.

point, some systems have been worked out sufficiently to describe them at reasonable length and others have not. However, it is important to convey the extent of the contribution of PGs and therefore a number of systems are described below, some very briefly.

A. $PGF_{2\alpha}$ as an Agent for Therapeutic Abortion

At termination of a normal pregnancy, parturition is started by an increased availability of fetal free cortisol generated by programmed changes in the fetal hypothalamus. The nature of the "clock" is unknown. With increased ACTH and a fall in the level of serum transcortin, the circulating level of free cortisol is sharply increased. This leads to a marked decrease in placental production of progesterone, a stimulation of estradiol synthesis, $PGF_{2\alpha}$ synthesis, and oxytocin release, all of which bring about contractions of the uterus to expel the fetus. $PGF_{2\alpha}$ has been used as an agent for therapeutic abortion by intraamniotic injection, sometimes in combination with oxytocin. The uterine myometrium appears to contain $PGF_{2\alpha}$ receptors. How the interaction of $PGF_{2\alpha}$ with receptor generates muscular contraction is not clear, although stimulation of the Ca^{2+} uptake channel would be an attractive possibility. Increased levels of Ca^{2+} in the cytoplasm would be expected to cause muscular contraction by derepressing the contractile mechanism.

B. Pancreas

Some experiments performed with isolated, perfused rat pancreas suggest that PGE_2, in the micromolar range, can stimulate the release of glucagon and insulin. Since glucagon release precedes that of insulin, the latter may be released secondarily by glucagon rather than in direct response to PGE_2. The effective concentrations of PGE_2 are in a range close to that observed in extracts of rat pancreas. It seems possible that PGE may be a transducer for several known secretagogues of glucagon.

C. Transduction System

The action of some releasing hormones on anterior pituitary cells in some cases has involved PGE_1. This transduction system is particularly evident in TSH action (Fig. 6-12) in the thyroid gland to increase intracellular cyclic AMP and may be a component of stimulation of steroidogenesis by ACTH in the adrenal gland. It may be a component of the action of luteinizing hormone on the corpus luteum.

D. Ectopic Bone Resorption

A transplantable mouse fibrosarcoma secretes a potent bone resorption-stimulating factor which has been identified as PGE_2. Animals bearing this tumor have elevated levels of serum PGE_2 and Ca^{2+} which can be lowered by administration of inhibitors of PG synthetase, such as indomethacin.

E. Autonomic Nervous System

Stimulation of sympathetic nerves causes release of PGEs. PGEs inhibit adrenergic transmission by depressing responses to the adrenergic transmitter at a postjunctional level. PGEs may also inhibit transmitter release from nerve terminals. Opposite effects are seen with PGFs which often heighten responses of effectors to norepinephrine. $PGF_{2\alpha}$ can facilitate release of epinephrine from the adrenal medulla.

F. PGI_2 in Fibroblasts

Recent reports with 3T3 mouse fibroblasts or human foreskin fibroblasts show that these cells synthesize PGI_2 (Fig. 16-15). The stimulation of cyclic AMP in human fibroblasts is produced by PGs in the order $PGI_2 > PGH_2 = PGE_1 >> PGE_2$, while PGD_2 is inactive. The stimulation by PGH_2 occurred through its transformation to PGI_2.

G. PGs and the Pain Mechanism

The pain mechanism is essential for survival, since acute pain is a warning mechanism for threatening conditions. Chronic pain is a more complicated subject, but both conditions may be grouped together for the purposes of our discussion. There is relatively little known about the pain mechanism.

The nociceptors, when excited by potentially harmful stimuli, cause pain by way of their afferent nerve fibers (Fig. 16-16). Probably every organ in the body contains these receptors. There are two classes of nociceptive afferents: those found among thin myelinated Aδ fibers, and those among the nonmyelinated C fibers. The Aδ fibers are associated with sharp, focused pain, whereas the C fibers are associated with dull, burning, diffuse pain.

Chemical substances excite nociceptors or sensitize them to other stimuli (Fig. 16-16A), resulting in the generation of pain. Endogenous substances in this category are PGE and bradykinin. These are referred

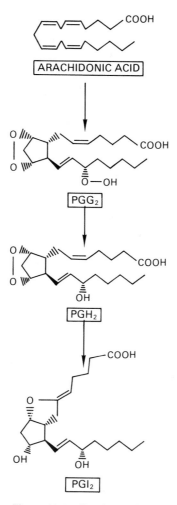

Figure 16-15. Synthesis of PGI₂.

to as "algesic substances" or agents producing pain. Substance P is considered in this category as it is thought to be a transmitter of the pain signal being released from the nociceptor (afferent) nerve terminal. Nociceptor firing occurs at levels of stimuli below those producing a frank sensation of pain, thus these impulses probably summate spatially and temporally in the central nervous system before pain is perceived. Nociceptor firing rate and perception of pain both increase with the strength of the stimulus. PGs and other algesics can apparently cause

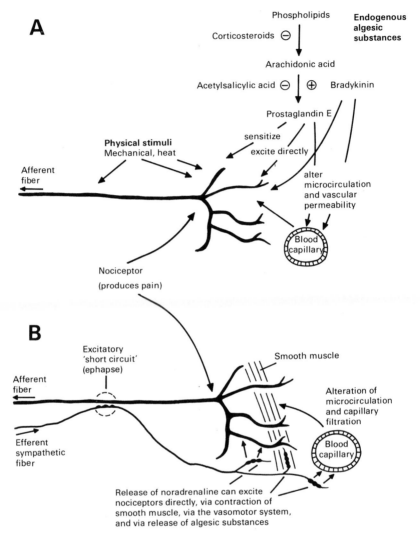

Figure 16-16. Pain transmission and the nociceptor. (A) Diagram showing the nociceptor and its environment. The nociceptor, represented anatomically as the terminal arborization of an afferent fiber, has its excitability influenced by physical stimuli and endogenous algesic substances. The action of these substances also can be indirect, operating on the microcirculation. Various substances, such as bradykinin, facilitate PG synthesis and can intensify the action of algesic substances. Analgesics can inhibit PGE synthesis, explaining part of their actions. (B) Diagram of the nociceptor and its environment and possible sympathetic mechanisms which may influence the excitability of the nociceptors. Sympathetic efferents can stimulate nociceptors when regulation is disturbed. Reproduced from M. Zimmerman, *Triangle Sandoz J. Med. Sci.* **20**, 7 (1981). Copyright 1981, Pergamon Press, Ltd.

pain when applied to the skin of humans. PGE_2 can lower the threshold of nociceptors to other stimuli, such as heat. It seems clear that PGEs operating through a receptor to stimulate adenylate cyclase and the level of cyclic AMP have a direct relation to the generation of pain. A speculative overall scheme tying together a number of observations is presented in Fig. 16-17.

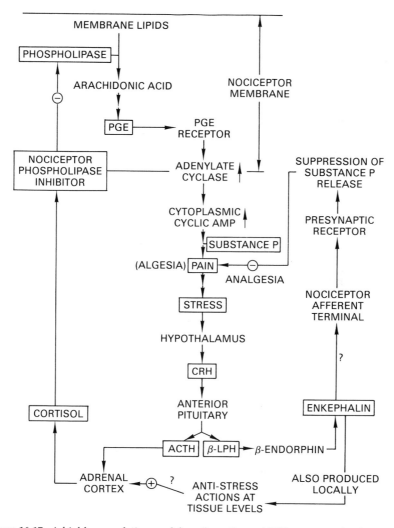

Figure 16-17. A highly speculative model on the actions of PGEs versus enkephalin and glucocorticoids on pain production.

Pain is produced by an irritant, trauma, or nervous stimulation causing the release of fatty acids from membrane phospholipids, and PGEs are formed by the PG synthetase system. These dissolve in a cellular membrane and bind to the PGE receptor which causes a stimulation of adenylate cyclase to form elevated amounts of cyclic AMP. It is not clear whether cyclic AMP is actually required for production of pain or release of substance P, or whether PGE merely changes the properties of the nociceptor membrane which results in increased firing. The elevated cyclic AMP, if involved, somehow produces pain which, if persistent, results in a stress response via the hypothalamus (CRH) to release ACTH and then cortisol from the adrenal gland. In addition to ACTH, β-lipotropin is formed in equivalent amounts (see Fig. 5-13), which is processed to enkephalin via β-endorphin, and enkephalin binds to a cell membrane receptor which may compete with the PGE receptor in some way or produce a second messenger opposing the action of cyclic AMP.

Elevated levels of circulating cortisol may produce a polypeptide, called "lipocortin" ($\sim$40,000 Da), in the same cells that originally produced the elevated PGEs. This polypeptide is an inhibitor of phospholipase A_2 and thus quenches the production of PGEs leading to pain in the first place. This is expected to be a slower process than the analgesia produced by enkephalin. In addition, there are direct nervous connections between the hypothalamus and the adrenal medulla which lead to the release of epinephrine and of enkephalins in large amounts. The function of medulla enkephalin is presently unknown; however, it may have a positive action in counteracting pain and stress by peripheral actions, but its access to the central nervous system is unlikely in view of the blood–brain barrier.

H. Antihypertensive Renal Effects

In response to some stimulus (e.g., fright), catecholamines are secreted, causing renin to be released from the kidney juxtaglomerular apparatus. Renin stimulates production of angiotensin II (Fig. 15-8) and blood pressure elevation ensues from enhanced aldosterone production, Na^+ reabsorption, and constrictive effects on the vasculature. In response to the increased pressure, there is increased blood flow in the renal medulla resulting in the release of PGA_2 or PGE_2 (see Chapter 15).

I. The Platelet System

PGI_2 and TXA_2 generally produce opposite reactions in the platelet. TXA_2 produced in the platelet stimulates platelet aggregation while PGI_2

produced in the blood vessel wall inhibits platelet aggregation. It is not absolutely certain that TXA_2 is the active principle within the platelet, but there is good evidence supporting this conclusion. PGI_2 also relaxes coronary arteries whereas TXA_2 constricts them; PGI_2 lowers blood pressure and TXA_2 raises blood pressure.

The role of TXs and PGI_2 in platelet aggregation is suggested by Fig. 16-18. Wounding and exposure of collagen in the vascular wall is sufficient to cause platelet aggregation. Arachidonate is released from the platelet membrane and TXA_2 is produced. TXA_2 causes the release of

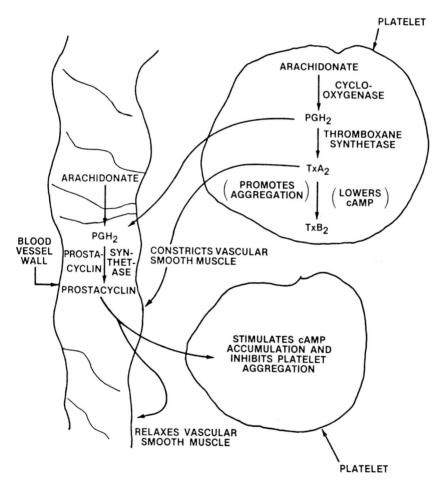

Figure 16-18. Model of human platelet homeostasis. Reproduced from R. R. Gorman, Modulation of human platelet function by prostacyclin and thromboxane A_2. *Fed. Proc. Fed. Am. Soc. Exp. Biol.* **38,** 83 (1979).

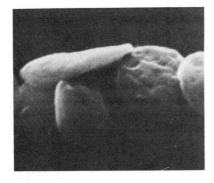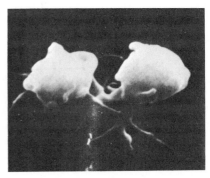

Figure 16-19. Platelets change shape when exposed to ADP which is liberated from platelet dense granules. Platelets are smooth flat disks shown in the electron micrograph at the left. Treatment with ADP causes long processes to protrude from the platelet, which swells to become an irregular "spiny sphere." The processes then adhere to a surface or to other platelets, shown on the right. Reproduced from M. B. Zucker, *Sci. Am.* **242**, 86–103 (1980).

Ca^{2+} from intracellular storage sites and the elevated Ca^{2+} inhibits adenylate cyclase, which is normally stimulated by circulating PGI_2 synthesized in the blood vessel walls. The elevated Ca^{2+} also stimulates the release of dense granules from the platelet which are rich in ADP and serotonin. ADP combines with the platelet, causing its surface to become sticky and the platelets to aggregate. The effect of ADP on platelets can be seen in Fig. 16-19.

A hemostatic plug of platelets is formed which aids in the repair process. The sequence of these events is diagrammed in Fig. 16-20. Under normal conditions when there is no stimulus to set off the production of TXA_2 in the platelet, the circulating PGI_2 continuously stimu-

Figure 16-20. Complex interactions of platelets, their constituents, and other substances involved in the formation of the hemostatic plug and of thrombi are still not understood. Some are diagrammed here. Contact of a platelet with collagen (1) in the presence of von Willebrand factor (a) initiates a pathway (b) that stimulates the secretion of ADP from the dense granules (c). The adhering platelet changes shape, spreads out along the collagen, and degranulates (2). Meanwhile, a number of steps involving tissue factor, calcium ions, and other clotting factors convert prothrombin in the plasma into thrombin (d), which is also formed on the platelet surface. Thrombin also stimulates secretion and converts fibrinogen (from the plasma and platelets) into fibrin. Platelets aggregate under the influence of collagen, ADP, and thrombin (3). Strands of fibrin reinforce the plug. The process may stop at this stage or may go on to form a larger thrombus with trapped red blood cells (4). Reproduced from M. B. Zucker, *Sci. Am.* **242**, 86–103 (1980).

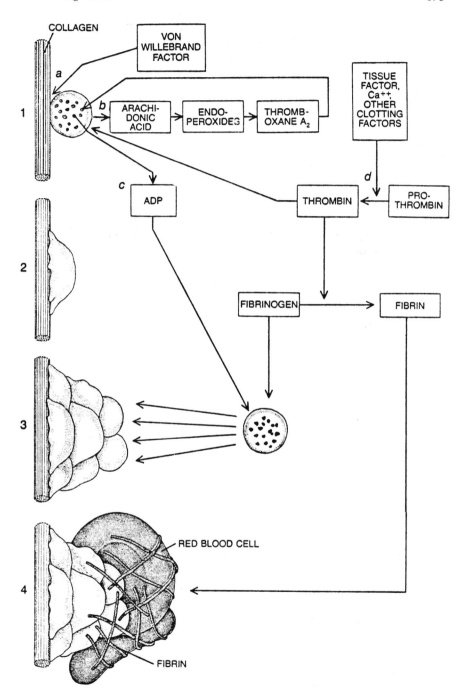

lates an elevated level of cyclic AMP in the platelet which inhibits mobilization of internal stores of Ca^{2+} and inhibits the activity of phospholipase A_2 and cyclooxygenase, although these latter conclusions remain to be elaborated. The overall activities in the platelet are shown in Fig. 16-21.

V. LEUKOTRIENES

A. Background

Although only recently discovered, these substances hold great promise for progress in diseases such as asthma. The LTs were identified as the principles of the slow-reacting substance of anaphylaxis (SRS or SRS-A). The LTs are closely related to immediate hypersensitivity reactions.

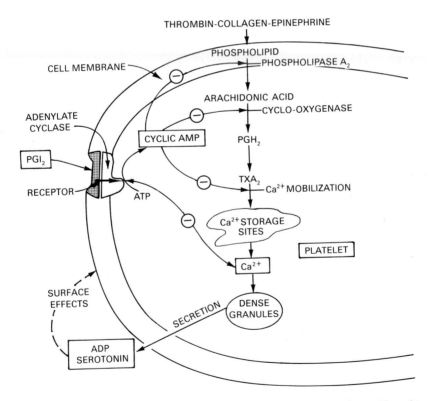

Figure 16-21. Interrelationships between platelet cell membrane stimulators (thrombin, collagen, epinephrine), TX (TXA$_2$), Ca^{2+}, PGI$_2$, and adenylate cyclase.

SRS causes slow contractile response of smooth muscle *in vitro* and has been isolated from the lung of pig and man. SRS-A from an asthmatic causes long-lasting bronchoconstriction and is extremely potent. SRS-A has been shown to be formed by incorporation of radiolabeled arachidonate and ^{35}S. SRS compounds have been characterized as LTs (see Fig. 16-12). LTA, LTB, and LTC were isolated from a murine mastocytoma cell line and from rabbit polymorphonuclear leukocytes. LTs are derivatives of arachidonic acid or of eicosapentenoic acid and many contain glutathione or cysteine.

B. LT and Asthma

Asthma is a complex disease resulting in part from narrowing of the airways. Mediators having various roles in this syndrome are derived from mast cells in the bronchus. These mediators either act directly on airway tissues or by indirect mechanisms which include recruitment of inflammatory cells. Some mediators are preformed within the mast cell whereas others are generated from the plasma membrane. The latter category includes the LTs, which may play a substantial role in asthma. The two classes of mediators are summarized in Fig. 16-22. One of the major secretions of the mast cell is histamine which, experimentally, causes a rapid and transient increase in airway resistance resulting from the action of histamine on bronchial smooth muscle. Other secretions include ECF-A (eosinophil chemotactic factor of anaphylaxis), NCF (neutrophil chemotactic factor of anaphylaxis), and those listed in Fig. 16-22. Precise roles of the enzymes secreted have not been clarified.

The membrane-derived factors are produced from arachidonic acid which is liberated by the action of phospholipase A_2 on phosphatidylcholine and other phospholipids. When an allergen interacts with IgE in the cell membrane (Fig. 16-23), cell membrane methyltransferases are activated and catalyze the conversion of phosphatidylethanolamine to phosphatidylcholine. This produces changes in the membrane and in the orientation of phospholipids and results in opening of the calcium ion gate, or constitution of the gate as the case may be, so that calcium is taken up from the extracellular space. This series of events is similar to other receptor systems (see Chapter 1). The increased level of calcium-activated membrane phospholipase A_2 (it is not clear whether calmodulin is required as in the GnRH-stimulated system, as shown in Fig. 3-14) results in the release of arachidonic acid from membrane phospholipid precursors. The cyclooxygenase-mediated metabolism of arachidonic acid would give rise to PGs, PGI_2, or TX, whereas lipoxygenase-mediated events would form LT and monohydroxy fatty acids.

676

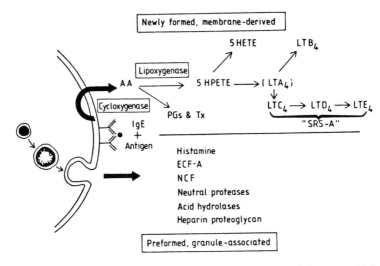

Figure 16-22. Mast cell-derived pharmacological mediators of hypersensitivity. Reproduced from A. B. Kay, *Eur. J. Respir. Dis.* **63,** Suppl. 122, 9–16 (1982). © 1982 Munksgaard International Publishers Ltd., Copenhagen, Denmark.

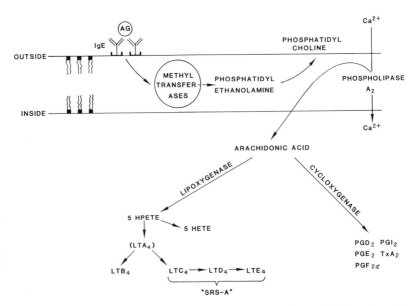

Figure 16-23. Membrane events and the release of free arachidonic acid. Reproduced from A. B. Kay, *Eur. J. Respir. Dis.* **63,** Suppl. 122, 9–16 (1982). © 1982 Munksgaard International Publishers Ltd., Copenhagen, Denmark.

The LTs are of special interest because they possess the activities of the "slow reacting substance of anaphylaxis." The precursor to the LTs is hydroperoxyeicosatetraenoic acid (5-HPETE) (Fig. 16-12). The LTs contain a 5-hydroxy group, three conjugated double bonds, and other polar substituents such as glutathione (GSH) (as in LTC_4), as shown in Fig. 16-12. The most potent LTs have one cis and two trans double bonds in the triene portion of the molecule (C-7). In most *in vitro* systems involving potency of smooth muscle contraction, the order of active substances is $LTD_4 > LTC_4 > LTE_4$. The polar LTs, LTB_4 especially (Fig. 16-12), are potent chemotactic factors.

The other PGs and TXA_2 also have effects on smooth muscle. PGD_2, $PGF_{2\alpha}$, and TXA_2 constrict, but PGE_2 has a slight dilatory effect. PGD_2, PGE_2, and PGI_2 add to the effects on permeability of histamine and bradykinin. Thus, while histamine gives a transient contraction of human lung smooth muscle *in vitro*, LTC_4 and LTD_4 cause prolonged responses and may be critical agents in asthma.

Thus, bronchial obstruction can be divided arbitrarily into three phases: a rapid spasmogenic phase, a late sustained phase, and a subacute inflammatory phase. These phases might occur in sequence following the initial release of agents from the mast cell resulting from the interaction of allergen and IgE or other nonimmunological stimuli, such as infection, exercise, or complement activation. These phases are represented in Fig. 16-24. The rapid phase is probably histamine mediated. A

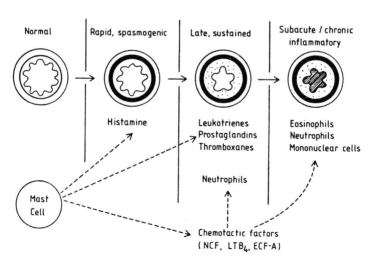

Figure 16-24. Mast cell mediators and airway obstruction in bronchial asthma. Reproduced from A. B. Kay, *Eur. J. Respir. Dis.* **63**, Suppl. 122, 9–16 (1982). © 1982 Munksgaard International Publishers Ltd., Copenhagen, Denmark.

more severe stage of the reaction is undoubtedly related to the LTs. The late reaction may be associated with reactivation of mast cells. LTs probably play a role in the late reaction as well since there is prolonged contraction of bronchial smooth muscle. Late reactions are inhibited by glucocorticoids which act to prevent the release of arachidonic acid by inducing the synthesis of a peptide (lipocortin) inhibitor of phospholipase A_2. This is the same reaction as discussed in connection with prostaglandin induced pain (Fig. 16-17). Corticosteroid-resistant asthma is a very serious problem in which LTs may play an influential part.

VI. CLINICAL ASPECTS

A. Abortion

There is good evidence that PGs participate in various aspects of the ovarian cycle. In particular, $PGF_{2\alpha}$ has been implicated as one of the factors effective in causing terminal contractions on the uterine myometrium. The levels of $PGF_{2\alpha}$ in amniotic fluid align with the progress of labor during the birth process. Administered PG inhibitors such as aspirin or indomethacin are known to delay the onset of labor. Administration of PG, often in the form of $PGF_{2\alpha}$, can produce side effects and should not be given to patients with a history of asthma. PGs are generally useful as abortifacients after the eighth week of pregnancy. In the second trimester, PGE_2 and $PGF_{2\alpha}$ can be given by the intrauterine route and other PGs given intramuscularly or vaginally to promote termination of pregnancy.

B. Myocardial Infarction

PGs play important roles in a number of organ systems, including the central nervous system, blood platelets (as described in this chapter), smooth muscles of the respiratory tract (also described here in connection with asthma), the peripheral nervous system, the gastrointestinal tract, and the cardiovascular system. In the kidney, PGs, possibly mainly PGAs, produce vasodilation and accelerate the removal of sodium ion into the urine. PGs can apparently act in the opposite direction by stimulating the renin–angiotensin–aldosterone system. In this case, as in many others, opposing actions of PGs occur as a homeostatic mechanism. Nonsteroidal antiinflammatory drugs, if administered chronically, can compromise the hypotensive activity of PGs in the kidney.

There is some reason to believe that activated platelet activity may play a role in plaque formation if the reaction is overresponsive and can contribute to some instances of myocardial infarction. Thus, TX production by platelets would be balanced by PGI$_2$ production. "Sticky" platelets could have a negative effect on development of myocardial infarction over the long term, and some claims have been made that chronic aspirin users could have a lower incidence of myocardial infarction, the explanation being that TX synthesis might be decreased in platelets and there would be a decreased contribution of sticky platelets to the formation of infarcts.

References

A. Books

Bergström, S., and Samuelson, B., eds. (1966). "Prostaglandins." Wiley (Interscience), New York.

Berti, F., and Velo, G. P., eds. (1979). "The Prostaglandin System." Plenum, New York.

Lefer, A. M., and Gee, M. H., eds. (1985). "Leukotrienes in Cardiovascular and Pulmonary Function." Alan R. Liss, New York.

Ramwell, P. W., ed. (1977). "The Prostaglandins," Vol. 3. Plenum, New York.

B. Review Articles

Bailey, J. M. (1979). Prostacyclins, thromboxanes, and cardiovascular disease. *Trends Biochem. Sci.* **4**, 68–71.

Bonta, I. L., and Parnham, M. J. (1978). Prostaglandins and chronic inflammation. *Biochem. Pharmacol.* **27**, 1611–1623.

Brody, M. J., and Kadowitz, P. J. (1974). Prostaglandins as modulators of the autonomic nervous system. *Fed. Proc., Fed. Am. Soc. Exp. Biol.* **33**, 48–60.

Dollery, C. T., and Hensby, C. N. (1978). Is prostacyclin a circulating anticoagulant? *Nature (London)* **273**, 706.

Gorman, R. R. (1979). Modulation of human platelet function by prostacyclin and thromboxane A$_2$. *Fed. Proc., Fed. Am. Soc. Exp. Biol.* **38**, 83–88.

Hammarström, S. (1984). The leukotrienes. *In* "Biochemical Actions of Hormones" (G. Litwack, ed.), Vol. 11, pp. 1–23. Academic Press, New York.

Horton, E. W. (1979). Prostaglandins and smooth muscle. *Br. Med. Bull.* **35**, 295–300.

Kay, A. B. (1982). Basic mechanisms in allergic asthma. *Eur. J. Respir. Dis.* **63**, Suppl. 122, 9–26.

McGiff, J. C., Crowshaw, K., and Itskovitz, H. D. (1974). Prostaglandins and renal function. *Fed. Proc., Fed. Am. Soc. Exp. Biol.* **33**, 39–47.

McGiff, J. C., Itskovitz, H. D., Terragno, A., and Wong, Y.-K. (1976). Modulation and mediation of the action of the renal kallikrein–kinin system by prostaglandins. *Fed. Proc., Fed. Am. Soc. Exp. Biol.* **35**, 175–180.

Mashiter, K., and Field, J. B. (1974). Prostaglandins and the thyroid gland. *Fed. Proc., Fed. Am. Soc. Exp. Biol.* **33**, 78–80.

Moncada, S., and Vane, J. R. (1978). Unstable metabolites of arachidonic acid and their role in hemostasis and thrombosis. *Br. Med. Bull.* **34**, 129–135.

Moncada, S., Korbut, R., Bunting, S., and Vane, J. R. (1978). Prostacyclin is a circulating hormone. *Nature (London)* **273**, 767–768.

Nasjletti, A., and Colina-Chourio, J. (1976). Interaction of mineralocorticoids, renal prostaglandins and the renal kallikrein–kinin system. *Fed. Proc., Fed. Am. Soc. Exp. Biol.* **35**, 189–193.

680

Nelson, N. A., Kelly, R. C., and Johnson, R. A. (1982). Prostaglandins and the arachidonic acid cascade. *Chem. Eng. News* Aug. 16, pp. 30–44.

Samuelsson, B., Goldyne, M., Granström, E., Hamberg, M., Hammarström, S., and Malmsten, C. (1978). Prostaglandins and thromboxanes. *Annu. Rev. Biochem.* **47**, 997–1029.

Tashjian, A. H., Jr., Voelkel, E. F., Goldhaber, P., and Levine, L. (1974). Prostaglandins, calcium metabolism and cancer. *Fed. Proc., Fed. Am. Soc. Exp. Biol.* **33**, 81–86.

Zucker, M. B. (1980). The functioning of blood platelets. *Sci. Am.* **242**, 86–103.

C. Research Papers

Brunton, L. L., Wikhund, R. A., van Arsdale, P. M., and Gilman, A. G. (1976). Binding of [^{3}H]prostaglandin E_1 to putative receptors linked to adenylate cyclase of cultured cell clones. *J. Biol. Chem.* **251**, 3037–3044.

Chassaing, G., Convert, O., and Lavielle, S. (1986). Preferential conformation of substance P in solution. *Eur. J. Biochem.* **154**, 77–850.

Dawson, W. (1980). SRS-A and the leukotrienes. *Nature (London)* **285**, 68.

Gorman, R. R., Hamilton, R. D., and Hopkins, N. K. (1979). Stimulation of human foreskin fibroblast adenosine 3′ :5′-cyclic monophosphate levels by prostacyclin. *J. Biol. Chem.* **254**, 1671–1676.

Langs, D. A., Erman, M., and DeTita, G. T. (1977). Conformations of prostaglandin $PGF_{2\alpha}$ and recognition of prostaglandins by their receptors. *Science* **197**, 1003–1005.

Langs, D. A., Fortier, S., Erman, M. G., and DeTita, G. T. (1979). Thromboxane molecules do not adopt the prostaglandin hairpin conformation. *Nature (London)* **281**, 237–238.

Lee, J. B. (1973). Hypertension, natriuresis and the renomedullary prostaglandins. *Prostaglandins* **3**, 551–579.

Miyamoto, T., Yamamoto, S., and Hayaishi, O. (1974). Prostaglandin synthetase system—resolution into oxygenase and isomerase components. *Proc. Natl. Acad. Sci. U.S.A.* **71**, 3645–3648.

Needleman, P. (1978). Experimental criteria for evaluating prostaglandin biosynthesis and intrinsic function. *Biochem. Pharmacol.* **27**, 1515–1518.

Orning, L., and Hammarström, S. (1980). Inhibition of leukotriene C and leukotriene D biosynthesis. *J. Biol. Chem.* **255**, 8023–8026.

Orning, L., Norin, E., Gustafsson, B., and Hammarström, S. (1986). *In vivo* metabolism of leukotriene C_4 in germ-free and conventional rats. Fecal excretion of *N*-acetyl-leukotriene E_4. *J. Biol. Chem.* **261**, 766–771.

Pek, S., Tai, T.-Y., Elster, A., and Fajans, S. S. (1975). Stimulation by prostaglandin E_2 of glucagon and insulin release from isolated rat pancreas. *Prostaglandins* **10**, 493–502.

Perry, G., Siegal, B., and Held, B. (1977). Second trimester abortion, Single dose intraamniotic injection of prostaglandin $PGF_{2\alpha}$ with intravenous oxytocin augmentation. *Prostaglandins* **13**, 987–994.

Saeed, S. A., McDonald-Gibson, W. J., Cuthbert, J., Copas, J. L., Schneider, C., Gardiner, P. J., Butt, N. M., and Collier, H. O. J. (1977). Endogenous inhibitor of prostaglandin synthetase. *Nature (London)* **270**, 32–36.

Van der Oudraa, F. J., Buytenhek, M., Nugteren, D. H., and van Dorp, D. A. (1980). Acetylation of prostaglandin endoperoxide synthetase with acetylsalicylic acid. *Eur. J. Biochem.* **109**, 1–8.

Weiss, J. W., Drazen, J. M., Coles, N., McFadden, Jr., E. R., Weller, P. F., Corey, E. J., Lewis, R. A., and Austen, K. F. (1982). Bronchoconstrictor effects of leukotriene C in humans. *Science* **216**, 196–198.

Wlodawer, P., and Hammarström, S. (1979). Some properties of prostacyclin synthase from pig aorta. *FEBS Lett* **97**, 32–36.

Thymus Hormones

I. INTRODUCTION

A. Background

It has become evident that the thymus gland and various polypeptides produced by thymus cells play a hormonal role in the functions of the immune system. A bewildering number of factors elaborated by thymus-derived cells appear to operate at one level or another in the growth of and immunoglobulin production by antibody-producing cells. The discussion here will be brief owing to the lack of biological characterization of many of these factors. Although there appears to be a multiplicity of thymic peptides, some will undoubtedly prove to be degradation products of others and the biology of these peptides is far from complete.

In addition to the central role of the thymus in the immune mechanism, there are hints emerging that the gland may produce components which regulate the secretion of hormones by other glands, for example, the release of prolactin from lactotrophs of the anterior pituitary. However, if the thymus produces hormones that regulate secretion of anterior pituitary hormones, then it is possible that feedback regulation

HORMONES

could exist, which in the case of prolactin might lead to the explanation of its pronounced increase in stress (see Chapter 10). Moreover, it would be of interest to know if regulatory functions of thymic peptides on other hormone-producing cells reside in the same substances which are operative in the immune system.

B. Immune System

There are approximately 10^6–10^8 antibody specificities referring to different antigenic structures (epitopes), and a specific antigenic molecule will interact with and activate only a small proportion ($<0.1\%$) of the antibody-producing cells. B cells are precursors of antibody-producing plasma cells and T cells are thymus-derived cells which produce a number of stimulatory agents for B cells. The ability of a B cell-derived immune (memory) cell to produce antibodies depends on a number of stimulatory factors as well as transpositions of variable genetic elements of the immunoglobulin structure, a subject of intense concentration in molecular genetics. Stimulatory activities are derived from thymus-derived cells (T cells), usually considered to be helper T cells (Fig. 17-1A).

Figure 17-1. (A) Summary of the T lymphocyte regulatory influences in the immune system. On the left in this diagram is the helper T cell. These cells can positively regulate B cells (upper) and stimulate their differentiation into mature antibody-secreting plasma cells. Helper T cells can also positively regulate precursors of T cells destined to become cytotoxic T cells (lower). A second category is suppressor T cells (right). These cells can negatively regulate differentiation of B lymphocytes or precursors of cytotoxic T lymphocytes directly or by interfering with the activity of helper T cells that would normally facilitate their development. Suppressor T cells directly inhibit the secretory function of matured plasma cells (upper right). Adapted with permission from D. H. Katz, The immune system: An overview. *In* "Basic and Clinical Immunology" (D. P. Stites, J. D. Stobo, H. H. Fudenberg, and J. V. Wells, eds.), 5th ed., pp. 13–20. Lange Medical Publications, Los Altos, California, 1984.
(B) The immunoglobulin antibody-producing system. This scheme illustrates interactions of regulatory cells participating in the development of a normal antibody response (although the figure specifies the involvement of the mechanism IgE, it is also applicable to other Ig classes). Carrier determinants of the allergen (antigen) are recognized by T cells and the haptenic determinants by B cells. Macrophages (MΦ) present the antigen in a favorable manner for induction of helper T cells which have specific receptors that interact with macrophage-associated cell interaction molecules. Soluble factors from the macrophage may be involved in induction of helper T cells. B cells interact with haptenic determinants with surface Ig receptors and then helper T cells interact with hapten-specific B cells. B cells differentiate into mature antibody-secreting plasma cells or memory cells. Soluble T cell factors may be involved in these interactions. In the absence of the macrophage participation, suppressor T cells can be induced by direct antigen binding and may interfere with these cell–cell interactions (broken arrows) by preventing activation of helper T cells, inhibiting helper T cell interactions with B lymphocytes, and by direct inhibition of B cell differentiation. Reproduced from D. P. Katz, J. D. Stobo, H. H. Fudenberg, and J. V. Wells, eds., "Basic and Clinical Immunology," 5th ed. Lange Medical Publications, Los Altos, California, 1984.

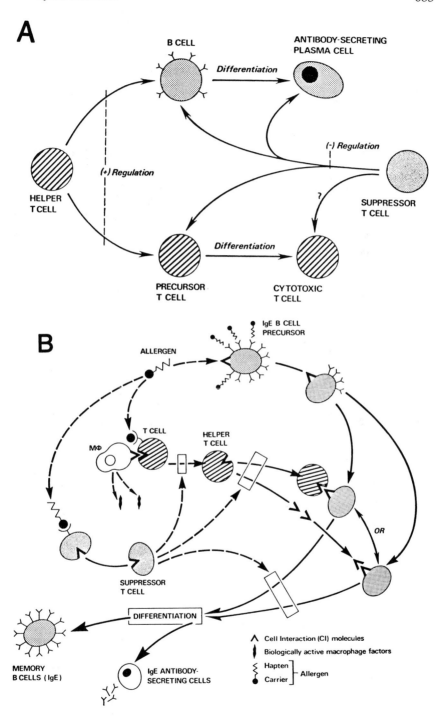

The thymus contains T cell lymphocytes which in turn produce factors to regulate expression of immunoglobulins by B cell lymphocytes. T cells enter the circulation from the thymus, as do B cells from bone marrow. Phagocytic cells are involved also in the immune process, as shown in Fig. 17-1B.

When an antigen (a foreign substance) enters the organism, B cells produce immunoglobulins with helper T cell action. Antibodies on the surface of T cells with the same specificity as those produced by the activated B cells bind the antigen, and the complex may then be transferred to a macrophage cell which may ingest and destroy the antigen. Although speculative, this scheme (Fig. 17-1) also depicts the factors contributed by helper T cells which may stimulate antibody production. This chapter concentrates on a family of peptide hormones which may regulate proliferation and maturation of precursor lymphocytes into immunologically competent cells.

II. ANATOMICAL AND MORPHOLOGICAL RELATIONSHIPS

The anatomy and histology of the thymus gland are pictured in Fig. 17-2. The gland lies above the heart, as shown in Fig. 17-2A, and is very much larger in the newborn than in the adult. Shrinkage of the gland with age to adult status is thought to be the result of increasing function of the adrenal cortex with higher circulating levels of glucocorticoid hormones. Thymocytes are sensitive to the action of glucocorticoids mediated by the glucocorticoid receptor and, as a result, the cells involute under hormonal action. The histology of the thymus is shown in Fig. 17-2B. Besides a capsule, there are two main layers of cells, the cortex and the medulla. The thymocyte idealized from electron microscopic examination is shown in Fig. 17-3. Thymocytes are similar to the lymphocytes of other lymphoid organs and to those in the circulation.

Figure 17-2. Anatomy and histology of the thymus gland. (A) Locations and comparative sizes at different stages of growth. Reproduced from W. Kahle, H. Leonhardt, and W. Platzer, "Color Atlas and Textbook of Human Anatomy," Vol. 2, p. 93. Year Book Medical Publishers, Chicago, Illinois, 1978. (B, p. 686) Histological organization of the thymus. The thymus is encapsulated and divided into lobules by septa. Densely packed dividing lymphocytes form a network of epithelioid cells in the cortex to the medulla. There are fewer lymphocytes in the medulla which contain more bone marrow-derived interdigitating cells. There is a close association of the developing lymphocytes with epithelial and interdigitating cells. Functions of the corpuscle structures are unknown. Reproduced from I. M. Roitt, J. Brostoff, and D. K. Male, "Immunology," p. 14.3. Gower Medical Pub. Ltd., 1985.

A

Lymphatic Organs: Thymus

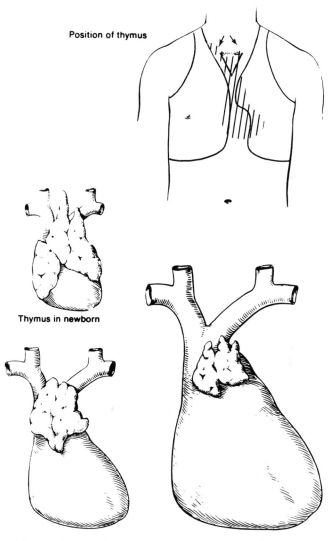

Position of thymus

Thymus in newborn

Thymus in 2-year-old child

Thymus in adult

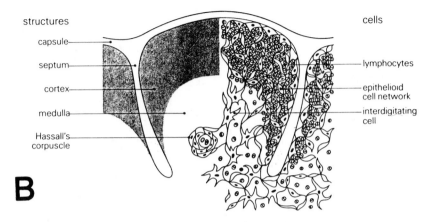

structures — cells

capsule
septum — lymphocytes
cortex — epithelioid cell network
medulla — interdigitating cell
Hassall's corpuscle

B

Figure 17-2B. See legend on p. 684.

The thymus arises from an epithelial outgrowth of the third and fourth branchial pouches to form the thymus gland. The human fetal thymus is predominantly lymphoid, a pattern which is preserved throughout childhood. Later the lymphoid component decreases, presumably under the influence of endogenous adrenal glucocorticoids (see Chapter 10). The lymphoid cells either divide and die in the thymus gland or populate the peripheral lymphatic organs. Lobules constitute the histological cores of the thymus gland. The lobular structure is not evident until the third intrauterine month (Fig. 17-4). Up to that time the thymus appears as an epithelial organ. The periphery of the lobes is bounded by a capsule which originates the connective tissue septa. Each lobule is composed of an outer darkly staining cortex and an inner paler staining medulla as visualized with hematoxylin and eosin (Fig. 17-4). The thymus gland proportionately to body weight is greatest at birth, but its absolute mass is greatest at puberty. Subsequently, there is involution and the thymic parenchyma is replaced by fat. This organ is the primary source of T lymphocytes.

III. CELL BIOLOGY

The immune system as a whole may be visualized as consisting of two major components: cellular and humoral immunity. Both respond to foreign proteins or other antigens. The gamma globulin fraction of plasma antibodies constitutes the humoral mechanism, whereas cellular immunity refers to lymphocyte products (lymphokines, e.g., the in-

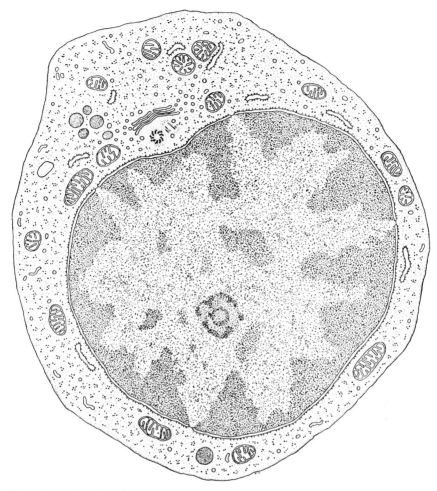

Figure 17-3. Drawing of an idealized thymocyte from electron microscopic observations. Reproduced from T. L. Lentz, "Cell Fine Structure," p. 53. Saunders, Philadelphia, Pennsylvania, 1971.

terleukins). The humoral mechanism protects against bacterial infection, whereas cellular immunity generates delayed allergic reactions and rejections of foreign tissue transplants or tumor cells. It neutralizes infections by viruses, fungi, and some bacteria. The development of these systems is outlined in Fig. 17-5. Precursor cells destined to become lymphocytes originate in the yolk sac and find their way into the developing fetus. Those populating the thymus mature under the stimulation of

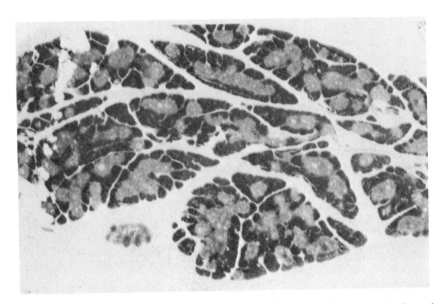

Figure 17-4. A normal child's thymus showing lobular structure. The thymus is derived from the entoderm of the third and fourth branchial arches with a probable contribution from the cervical sinus. Essentially the thymus is an epithelial organ and may be viewed as a foregut derivative. The characteristic lobular structure shown here appears in the third intrauterine month. Before then the rudimentary thymus is an epithelial organ. A capsule binds the periphery of the lobule from which are derived the connective tissue septa. Each lobule is composed of an outer darkly stained cortex and an inner paler staining medulla which is continuous throughout each half of the gland. Reproduced from W. F. Ganong, "Review of Medical Physiology," 12th ed., p. 425. Lange Medical Publications, Los Altos, California, 1985.

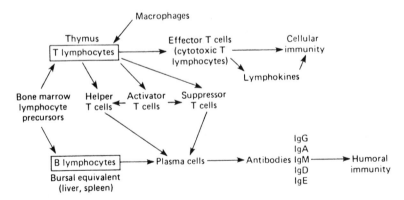

Figure 17-5. Basic aspects of the development of the immune system. Reproduced from W. F. Ganong, "Review of Medical Physiology," 12th ed., p. 425. Lange Medical Publications, Los Altos, California, 1985.

thymic hormones into T cell lymphocytes responsible for cellular immunity.

IV. CHEMISTRY AND BIOCHEMISTRY

A. Introduction

There are at the very least six peptides of the thymus called thymosins. These are described in Table 17-1 and appear to be acidic peptides in the molecular weight range 800–15,000. These "hormones" are produced in the thymus gland and control the development of the thymic-dependent lymphoid system as the thymus participates in the process of immune regulation. Among peptides isolated from the thymus, thymosin α_1, thymosin β_4, and polypeptide β_1 have been characterized fully and sequenced. The primary sequences of thymosin α_1, thymosin β_4, thymopoietin II, and facteur thymique serique (FTS) are shown in Fig. 17-6A and of prothymosin α in Fig. 17-6B. The thymosins modulate immunological responses *in vitro* and *in vivo* as well as regulating the differentiation of thymic-dependent lymphocytes. Polypeptide β_1 is homologous with ubiquitin (see later) and the N-terminal 74 amino acids of a nonhistone chromosomal protein which resembles a histone.

The primary sequence of ubiquitin is shown in Fig. 17-7. Although ubiquitin was discovered as a thymus polypeptide, it was soon learned

Table 17–1. Physical and Chemical Properties of Thymic Factors[a]

Compound	MW	Chemical properties	Origin
Thymosin fraction 5	1000–15,000	Family of heat-stable, acidic polypeptides	Bovine thymus
Thymosin α_1	3108	28 amino acid residues, pI 4.2	Bovine thymus + synthetic
Thymopoietin	5562	49 amino acid residues, heat stable, pI 5.2	Bovine thymus + synthetic
Thymopoietin pentapeptide		Amino acid residues, 32–36 in thymopoietin	Synthetic
Thymic humoral factor	3200	31 amino acid residues, heat labile, pI 5.7–5.9	Bovine thymus
Serum thymic factor	857	9 amino acid residues, heat labile, pI 7.3	Mouse, pig serum

[a] This is Table 3 from D. W. Wara, Thymic hormones and the immune system. *Adv. Pediatr.* **28**, 236 (1981).

A

THYMOSIN ALPHA₁

Ac–Ser Asp Ala Ala Val Asp Thr Ser Ser Glu Ile Thr Thr Lys Asp Leu Lys Glu Lys Lys Glu Val Val Glu Glu Ala Glu Asn

THYMOSIN BETA₄

Ac–Ser Asp Lys Pro Asp Met Ala Glu Ile Glu Lys Phe Asp Lys Ser Lys Leu Lys Lys Thr Glu Thr Gln Glu Lys Asn Pro Leu Pro Ser Lys Gly Thr Ile Glu Gln Glu Lys Gln Ala Gly Glu Ser

THYMOPOIETIN II

Ser Gln Phe Leu Glu Asp Pro Ser Val Leu Thr Lys Glu Lys Leu Lys Ser Glu Leu Val Ala Asn Asn Val Thr Leu Pro Ala Gly Glu Gln Arg Lys Asp Val Tyr Val Gln Leu Tyr Leu Gln Thr Leu Thr Ala Val Lys Arg

FTS

Glx Ala Lys Ser Glx Gly Gly Ser Asn

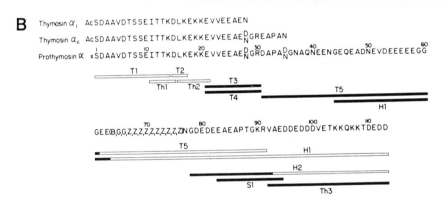

Figure 17-6. (A) Sequence of early-characterized thymic hormones: Thymosin α₁, thymosin β₄, thymopoietin II, and facteur thymique serique (FTS). From A. L. Goldstein, T. K. Low, G. B. Thurman, M. M. Zatz, N. Hall, J. Chen, S.-K. Hu, P. B. Naylor, and J. E. McClure, Current state of thymosin and other hormones of the thymus gland. *Recent Prog. Horm. Res.* **37**, 369–415 (1981). (B) The amino acid sequences of thymosins α₁ and α₁₁ isolated from calf thymus fraction 5 and of prothymosin isolated from rat thymus. The peptides used to establish the primary structure of prothymosin α are shown by the bars and letter, designated according to the cleavage methods used as follows: H, cleavage by hydroxylamine; S, *Staphylococcus aureus* V8 protease; T, trypsin; and Th, thermolysin. Sequences established by automated Edman degradation. The amino terminus is acetylated for all three peptides. The composition of the segment, including residues 64–76, is

1   10   20

NH_2–Met Gln Ile Phe Val Lys Thr Leu Thr Gly Lys Thr Ile Thr Leu Glu Val Glu Pro Ser

30   40

Asp Thr Ile Glu Asn Val Lys Ala Lys Ile Gln Asp Lys Glu Gly Ile Pro Pro Asp Gln

50   60

Gln Arg Leu Ile Phe Ala Gly Lys Gln Leu Glu Asp Gly Arg Thr Leu Ser Asp Tyr Asn

70

Ile Gln Lys Glu Ser Thr Leu His Leu Val Leu Arg Leu Arg–COOH

Figure 17-7. Amino acid sequence of ubiquitin. The sequence through 61 residues was obtained from automated sequence analysis of intact ubiquitin. From D. H. Schlesinger, G. Goldstein, and H. D. Niall, *Biochemistry* **14**, 2214–2218 (1975). Copyright 1975 American Chemical Society.

that it was present in a wide variety of tissues, consequently the name, ubiquitin. Although this protein occurs in chromatin often conjugated with histone, its function there is not very well understood. It has been characterized in another context, being identical to the heat-stable polypeptide of a proteolytic system in which it plays an important role in cellular protein breakdown. As a consequence of these findings, ubiquitin is not considered to be a thymic hormone.

B. Thymosin α_1

Thymosin α_1 was the initial polypeptide to be isolated among the fractions obtained from bovine thymus. It is very active in the process of T cell immunity and modulates the expression of terminal deoxynucleotidyltransferase. The N-terminal amino acid residue is blocked by an acetyl group. Inspection of Fig. 17-6A indicates no homology with the

---

shown in parentheses. The sequence of the first 20 residues is based on the composition of the peptides I1, T2, and Th1, and Th2 and the published sequences of thymosin α_1 and thymosin α_{II}. The COOH-terminal sequence Glu–Asp–AspOH was confirmed by the order of release of aspartic and glutamic acids by carboxypeptidase Y. The recommended one-letter notation for amino acids is used: A, Ala; R, Arg; N, Asn; D, Asp; B, Asp or Asn; C, Cys; Q, Gln; E, Glu; Z, Glu or Gln; G, Gly; H, His; I, Ile; L, Leu; K, Lys; M, Met; F, Phe; P, Pro; S, Ser; T, Thr; W, Trp; Y, Tyr; V, Val; X, unknown. Reproduced from A. A. Haritos, R. Bacher, S. Stein, J. Caldarella, and B. L. Horecker, Primary structure of rat prothymosin α. *Proc. Natl. Acad. Sci. U.S.A.* **82**, 343–346 (1985).

other well-characterized hormones and factors. According to A. Goldstein, who has conducted computer analysis with known sequences of other proteins, there are no known homologies with any of the primary sequences of thymosin α_1. More recent work designates prothymosin α as the true thymic hormone, inferring that thymosin α_1 may be a proteolyzed fragment (Fig. 17-6B).

As shown in Fig. 17-6A, the four thymic peptides fully characterized appear to be unrelated with regard to sequence homology. The multiplicity of peptides produced by the same tissue with different chemical structures suggests the possibility that although they share some common activities, they may also elicit highly individual functions in regulating the immune system. This would suggest either that homologous proteins have not yet been characterized or that the gene encoding this protein does not code for others with homologous sequences. Interestingly, limited homologies do show up with rabbit skeletal muscle tropomyosin α chain, 50 S ribosomal protein L7 from *Escherichia coli*, troponin I from rabbit skeletal muscle, and with bovine prothrombin. The sequences involved are shown in Fig. 17-8. Thymosin α_1 has been chemically synthesized and the product is equally active to the biological material. Thymosin α_1 mRNA has been translated in a wheat germ system using antiserum to this protein. These results suggest that a larger peptide of 16,000 molecular weight is a primary translation product which is degraded subsequently to the native hormone (3108 molecular weight). The oligodeoxynucleotide encoding thymosin α_1 has been synthesized, inserted into a plasmid, and cloned in *E. coli*, as shown in Fig. 17-9.

C. Thymosin β_4

Thymosin β_4 has a molecular weight of 4982 and also has its N-terminal amino acid residue blocked by an acetyl group (Fig. 17-6A). This protein induces expression of terminal deoxynucleotidyl transferase in transferase-negative mouse bone marrow cells *in vitro* and *in vivo* and increases the activity of this enzyme in hydrocortisone-immune suppressed mice *in vivo*. Thymosin β_4 therefore acts on lymphoid stem cells and in the early maturation process of thymus-dependent lymphocytes.

The primary sequence of thymosin β_4, like that of thymosin α_1, does not show homologies with sequences of other known proteins. However, there is an internal sequence duplication, as shown in Fig. 17-10. Although it would be attractive to consider thymosin β_4 as a discrete hormone of the thymus, it appears in many tissues. No pro- or prepro

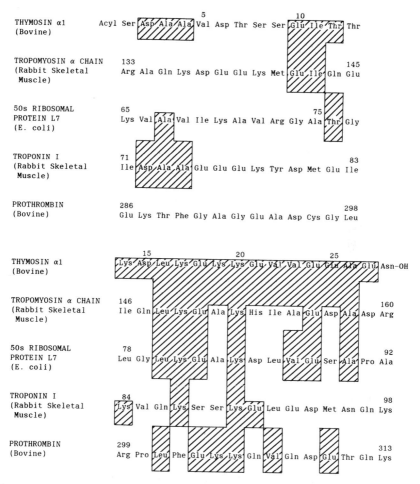

Figure 17-8. Sequence homology of thymosin α_1 to other proteins resulting from a computer search. From T. L. K. Low and A. L. Goldstein, *J. Biol. Chem.* **254,** 787–795 (1979).

peptide is formed as its precursor, and in mammalian tissues it is usually accompanied by a related peptide, thymosin β_{10} (B. Horecker laboratory). Horecker concludes that thymosin β_4 and β_{10} are not secretory peptide hormones.

Thymosin β_3 is another peptide completely related to thymosin β_4, but differs at the C-terminal end and has a molecular weight of 5500. It may also be a proteolytic fragment of thymosin β_4.

A

```
  1   2   3   4   5   6   7   8   9  10  11  12  13  14  15  16  17  18  19  20

Met Ser Asp Ala Ala Val Asp Thr Ser Ser Glu Ile Thr Thr Lys Asp Leu Lys Glu Lys Lys

   21  22  23  24  25  26  27  28

   Glu Val Val Glu Glu Ala Glu Asn-COOH
```

```
<------T1---------> <-----------T2--------------> <------T3------------> <------T4--
A A T T C A T G T C T G A T G C T G C T G T T G A T A C T T C T T C T G A G A T T A C

------------> <-----T9--------------> <-------T10-----------> <---------T11--------->
T A C T A A A G A T C T T A A G G A G A A G A A G G A A G T T G T C G A A G A G G C T

<-------T12-----------> <-----------T5-------------> <-----------T6-------> <------
G A G A A C T A A T A G G T A C A G A C T A C G A C G A C A A C T A T G A A G A A G A

---T7---------> <-----------T8-----------> <---------T13---------> <---------T14------->
C T C T A A T G A T G A T T T C T A G A A T T C C T C T T C T T C C T T C A A C A G C

---> <---------T15----------> <-----T16--------->
T T C T C C G A C T C T T G A T T A T C C T A G
```

B

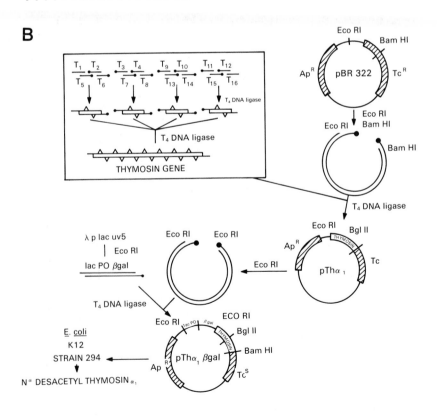

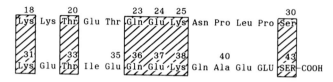

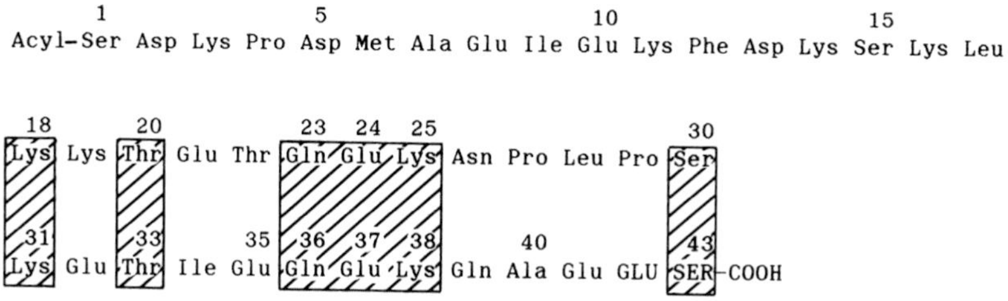

1 5 10 15
Acyl-Ser Asp Lys Pro Asp Met Ala Glu Ile Glu Lys Phe Asp Lys Ser Lys Leu
18 20 23 24 25 30
Lys Lys Thr Glu Thr Gln Glu Lys Asn Pro Leu Pro Ser
31 33 35 36 37 38 40 43
Lys Glu Thr Ile Glu Gln Glu Lys Gln Ala Glu GLU SER-COOH

Figure 17-10. Regions of internal sequence duplication of thymosin β_4. From A. L. Goldstein, T. L. K. Low, G. B. Thurman, M. M. Zatz, N. Hall, J. Chen, S.-K. Hu, P. B. Naylor, and J. E. McClure, *Recent Prog. Horm. Res.* **37,** 369–415 (1981).

V. BIOLOGICAL AND MOLECULAR ACTIONS

While thymosin peptides appear to act before and during the prothymocyte state, thymosin α_1 or prothymosin α acts at early as well as late stages of thymocyte maturation. It seems likely that thymosin β_3 is a proteolytic fragment of thymosin β_4.

By immunofluorescent microscopic methods, thymosin α_1 has been located in thymic epithelial cells of the medulla and in cells covering the cortical surface, whereas by the same methodology β_3 and β_4 were detected in cells covering the cortical surface. This finding aligns well with the known ability of β_3 in inducing terminal deoxynucleotide transferase expression and with the knowledge that cells containing this enzyme predominate in the thymic cortex. The thymic medulla, on the other hand, is terminal deoxynucleotide transferase negative and the action of thymosin α_1 is to suppress the expression of this enzyme.

Recent work implicates the autonomic and neuroendocrine systems in modulating the immune system. The thymus appears to play an integral role in the central nervous system regulation of the immune system. Figure 17-11 summarizes the interactions between the central nervous system and the neuroendocrine thymus. Apparently cholinergic recep-

---

Figure 17-9. Design of a synthetic oligonucleotide coding for the amino acid sequence in thymosin α_1 (A) and construction of the plasmid (B). The primary sequence of the DNA was developed from the amino acid sequence and preferred prokaryotic codons were used, eliminating codons with multiple specificity and minimizing AT or GC regions. The constructed gene was ligated into plasmids and expressed as part of a β-galactosidase chimeric protein by incorporation into the *lac* operon. From A. L. Goldstein, T. L. K. Low, G. B. Thurman, M. M. Zatz, N. Hall, J. Chen, S.-K. Hu, P. B. Naylor, and J. E. McClure, *Recent Prog. Horm. Res.* **37,** 369–415 (1981).

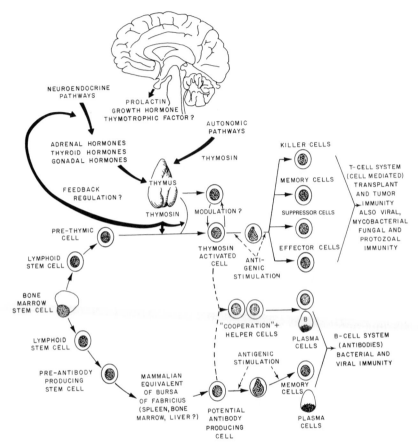

Figure 17-11. Hypothetical model illustrating the major interactions between the central nervous system and the neuroendocrine thymus. From A. L. Goldstein, T. L. K. Low, G. B. Thurman, M. M. Zatz, N. Hall, J. Chen, S.-K. Hu, P. B. Naylor, and J. E. McClure, *Recent Prog. Horm. Res.* **37,** 369–415 (1981).

tors occur on the surface of thymosin-producing epithelial cells. Cholinergic and β-adrenergic receptors occur on the surface of T lymphocytes. Detectable levels of gamma aminobutyric acid, a known neurotransmitter, have been observed in the thymus. In addition to neural regulation, various hormones are now believed to regulate thymosin production. Growth hormone increases levels of thymosin α_1. TSH may also have an influence. The role of glucocorticoids on the thymus (Chapter 10) is well known and there may be specific interactions between glucocorticoids and thymosin production.

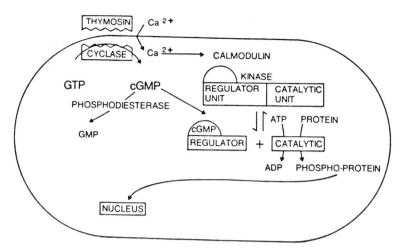

Figure 17-12. Mechanism of action of thymosin. From A. L. Goldstein, T. L. K. Low, G. B. Thurman, M. M. Zatz, N. Hall, J. Chen, S.-K. Hu, P. B. Naylor, and J. E. McClure, *Recent Prog. Horm. Res.* **37**, 369–415 (1981).

Thymosin appears to stimulate thymocyte cGMP levels (Fig. 17-12) as well as an influx of calcium. The increase in cGMP is calcium dependent. Thymosin apparently does not stimulate levels of cAMP. It is not known how calcium acts in this system or whether calmodulin calcium binding protein is actually involved. It is possible that cAMP may be increased by thymosin in earlier steps in thymocyte development and that cGMP and calcium are involved in later stages of differentiation.

VI. CLINICAL ASPECTS

Clearly the involvement of thymosin in the immune system makes it a potentially crucial agent in diseases of immunodeficiency and in several types of cancers. Clinical studies recently demonstrate prolonged survival of patients with immunodeficient diseases who have been treated with thymosin.

References

A. Books

Barness, L. A., ed. (1981). "Advances in Pediatrics," p. 229. Year Book Medical Publishers, Chicago, Illinois.

Friedman, H., ed. (1979). "Subcellular Factors in Immunity," Vol. 32. N. Y. Acad. Sci, New York.

Fudenberg, H. H., Stites, D. P., Caldwell, J. L., and Wells, J. V., eds. (1976). "Basic and Clinical Immunology," p. 92. Lange Medical Publications, Los Altos, California.

Ganong, W. F. (1975). "Review of Medical Physiology," p. 380. Lange Medical Publications, Los Altos, California.

Henry, K., and Farrer-Brown, G. (1982). "Thymus and Lymph Node Histopathology." Year Book Medical Publishers, Chicago, Illinois.

B. Review Articles

Goldstein, A. L., and White, A. (1970). The thymus as an endocrine gland: Hormones and their actions. In "Biochemical Actions of Hormones" (G. Litwack, ed.), Vol. 1, p. 465. Academic Press, New York.

Goldstein, A. L., Low, T. L. K., Thurman, G. B., Zatz, M. M., Hall, N., Chen, J., Hu, S.-K., Naylor, P. B., and McClure, J. E. (1981). Current status of thymosin and other hormones of the thymus gland. Recent Prog. Horm. Res. 37, 369.

Potash, M. J. (1981). B lymphocyte stimulation. Cell 23, 7–8.

Wara, D. W. (1981). Thymic hormones and the immune system. Adv. Pediat. 28, 236.

White, A. (1980). Chemistry and biological actions of products with thymic hormone-like activity. In "Biochemical Actions of Hormones" (G. Litwack, ed.), Vol. 7, p. 1. Academic Press, New York.

C. Research Papers

Audhya, T., Schlesinger, D. H., and Goldstein, G. (1981). Complete amino acid sequences of bovine thymopoietins I, II, and III: Closely homologous polypeptides. Biochemistry 20, 6195–6200.

Hannappel, E., Xu, G.-J., Morgan, J., Hempstead, J., and Horecker, B. (1982). Thymosin β_4: A ubiquitous peptide in rat and mouse tissues. Proc. Natl. Acad. Sci. U.S.A. 79, 2172–2175.

Haritos, A. A., Blacher, R., Stein, S., Caldarella, J., and Horecker, B. L. (1985). Primary structure of rat thymus prothymosin α. Proc. Natl. Acad. Sci. U.S.A. 82, 343–246.

Leonard, W. J., Depper, J. M., Kanehisa, M., Kronke, M., Peffer, N. J., Svetlik, P. B., Sullivan, M., and Greene, W. C. (1985). Structure of the human interleukin-2 receptor gene. Science 230, 633–639.

Low, T. L. K., and Goldstein, A. L. (1979). The chemistry and biology of thymosin. II. Amino acid sequence analysis of thymosin α_1 and polypeptide β_1. J. Biol. Chem. 254, 787–795.

Low, T. L. K., Thurman, G. B., McAdoo, M., McClure, J., Rossio, J. L., Naylor, P. H., and Goldstein, A. L. (1979). The chemistry and biology of thymosin. I. Isolation, characterization and biological activities of thymosin α_1 and polypeptide β_1 from calf thymus. J. Biol. Chem. 254, 981–981.

Low, T. L. K., Hu, S.-K., and Goldstein, A. L. (1981). Complete amino acid sequence of bovine thymosin β_4: A thymic hormone that induces terminal deoxynucleotidyl transferase activity in thymocyte populations. Proc. Natl. Acad. Sci. U.S.A. 78, 1162–1166.

Reichhart, R., Zeppezauer, M., and Jornvall, H. (1985). Preparations of homeostatic thymus hormones consist predominantly of histones 2A and 2B and suggest additional histone functions. Proc. Natl. Acad. Sci. U.S.A. 82, 4871–4875.

Pineal Hormones

I. INTRODUCTION

A. General Comments

The pineal gland is rather unique in respect to the magnitude of change characterizing its evolutionary development. In amphibians it is primarily a photoreceptive organ, but in higher forms it has evolved from this state to a gland producing hormones which receives light information by way of the lateral eyes and sympathetic nerves. Pineal products include melatonin, other methoxyindoles, serotonin, and acetylserotonin (see Fig. 18-1). Although vasotocin has been reported to be a pineal product, it is not clear whether significant amounts of vasotocin are actually synthesized in the pineal gland. Production of the methoxyindoles is dependent on light or darkness, and these hormones have been shown to regulate seasonal reproductive activities. There is some difference of opinion concerning the primacy of the hormones with

HORMONES

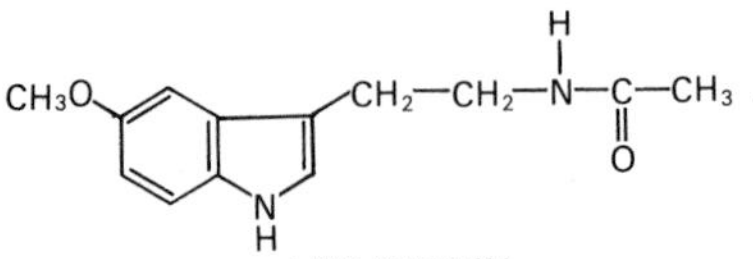

MELATONIN
(N-acetyl-5-methoxytryptamine)
Primary secreted product

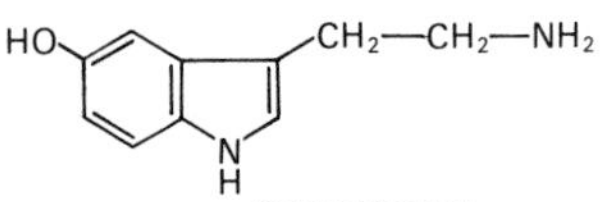

SEROTONIN
(5-hydroxytryptamine)
(may not be secreted)

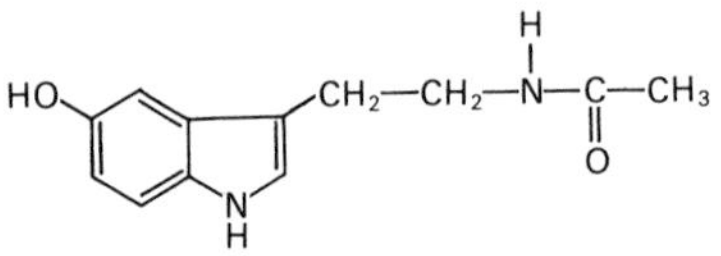

N-ACETYL-5-HYDROXYTRYPTAMINE
(N-acetylserotonin)
(may not be secreted)

Figure 18-1. Structure of pineal substance.

regard to physiological action. Melatonin is currently thought to be the principal active substance produced by the pineal. Secretion of melatonin from the pineal is generated by norepinephrine, which is released from neighboring neurons.

Of necessity the phenomenon of rhythmicity arises in connection with the pineal relating to its sensitivity to light and darkness. This translates directly to the development and seasonal cyclicity of the gonads and also may have effects on the pulsatile release of anterior pituitary hormones (see Chapter 5).

B. Evolutionary Aspects

The profundity of evolutionary alterations in the structure of this organ deserves some comment. In lower forms, the pineal organ functions as a light receptor and in this definition is often referred to as the "third vertebrate eye." In 1959, it was recognized that the ultrastructure of the receptor cells in the parietal eye of the lizard resembles that of retinal cones, and the most highly differentiated sensory elements of this type occur in the pineal vesicle of the lamprey, the frontal organ of the frog, and the parietal eye of the lizard. The similarities between the neuronal organization of the frog's pineal complex (epiphysis) and retina are evident in Fig. 18-2. In the frog, there appears to be a photolabile substance absorbing maximally at 560–580 nm, or around 500 nm in other species. Presumably light energy is converted to electrical energy and hormonal output.

The evolution of this organ consists first of photoreceptor cells which become gradually replaced by secretory rudimentary photoreceptor cells

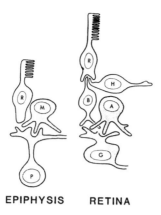

EPIPHYSIS   RETINA

Figure 18-2. Neuronal organization of the pineal complex of the frog in comparison to the neuronal circuitry in the retina. Epiphysis: R, photoreceptor cell; M, multipolar nerve cell (interneuron); P, neuron contributing to the pineal tract. Retina: R, receptor cell; B, bipolar cell; H, horizontal cell; A, amacrine cell; G, ganglion cell of the optic nerve. A, G, M, and P are acetylcholinesterase-positive elements. Reproduced from A. Oksche, The pineal organ—a component of photoneuroendocrine systems: Evolution, structure, function. *In* "Hormones, Adaptation and Evolution" (S. Ishii, T. Hirano, and M. Wada, eds.), p. 129. Jpn. Sci. Soc. Press, Tokyo, 1980.

and pinealocytes (Fig. 18-3). Sympathetic noradrenergic innervation becomes more pronounced so that light information coming in through the lateral eyes and sympathetic efferents replace the direct response to light characteristic of pinealocytes.

Ultimately the effects of pineal messages involve color change, endocrine control of reproduction, phototactic and locomotor reactions, detection of polarized light, and rhythmic phenomena. Clearly, the pineal gland is an important component of the photoneuroendocrine system.

R. Wurtman and J. Axelrod describe the pineal as a "neuroendocrine transducer which secretes a hormone, melatonin, in response to norepinephrine release from its sympathetic nerves, especially nocturnally, when the nerves are firing most frequently, and whose hormone provides the brain and possibly other organs with a time signal that cues other time-dependent physiological processes such as gonadal maturation, gonadal cyclicity, and perhaps sensitivity to environmental stimuli."

II. ANATOMY AND CELL BIOLOGY

In man the pineal gland is located in the brain grossly between the thalamus and the mesencephalon, as shown in Fig. 18-4. In the adult,

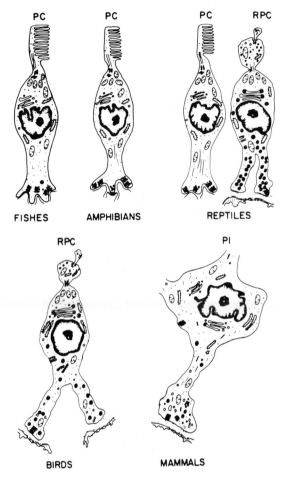

Figure 18-3. Vertebrate pineal cells showing evolution from a photoreceptor cell to a pinealocyte. Diagram of typical vertebrate pineal cells. PC, Photoreceptor cell; RPC, rudimentary photoreceptor cell; PI, pinealocyte. Reproduced from J. T. Hansen and M. Karasek, Neuron or endocrine cell? The pinealocyte as a paraneuron. *In* "The Pineal and Its Hormones" (R. J. Reiter, ed.), pp. 1–9. Alan R. Liss, Inc., New York, 1982.

the pineal is a flat, cone-shaped structure with dimensions about 5–8 mm long and 3–5 mm wide, weighing around 120 mg. It is located at the posterior border of the third ventricle above the roof of the diencephalon, being connected to it by a short stalk. The pineal is covered by a layer called the pia mater. From the pia mater connective tissue septa with blood vessels and unmyelinated nerve fibers enter the pineal to

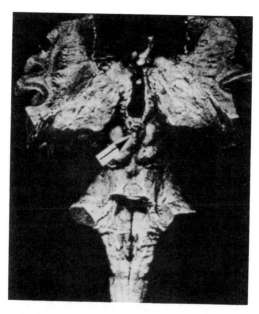

Figure 18-4. Photograph of a human brain stem showing the pineal gland (arrow) located at the posterior border of the third ventricle, between the superior colliculi (prominences) of the mesencephalon. This dissection and photography was carried out by Dr. S. Heil, Department of Anatomy, Johannes Gutenberg University, Mainz, Federal Republic of Germany. Reproduced with permission from L. Vollrath, Functional anatomy of the human pineal gland. *In* "The Pineal Gland" (R. J. Reiter, ed.), pp. 285–322. Raven, New York, 1984.

surround the cords of cells and follicles (alveoli) to form irregular lobules. Its location with respect to light stimuli is more clearly visualized in Fig. 18-5. The chain of events with regard to the photo effect is shown by light entering one of the eyes and the signal is carried to the suprachiasmic nuclei of the hypothalamus, the interomediolateral cell column of the spinal cord, then the superior cervical ganglia, and finally via the postganglionic sympathetic neurons, signaling the pineal, probably, via norepinephrine release.

In infants, the pineal is large and many cells are arranged in alveoli. Before puberty deposits of calcium, magnesium phosphate, and carbonate appear which usually render the pineal opaque to X rays.

There are several cell types in the adult pineal organ, but the major ones are pinealocytes and interstitial cells. The pineal is developed maximally at about 7 years of age. As mentioned, salts invest the capsule and septa. The organ is supplied with many blood vessels and both

704

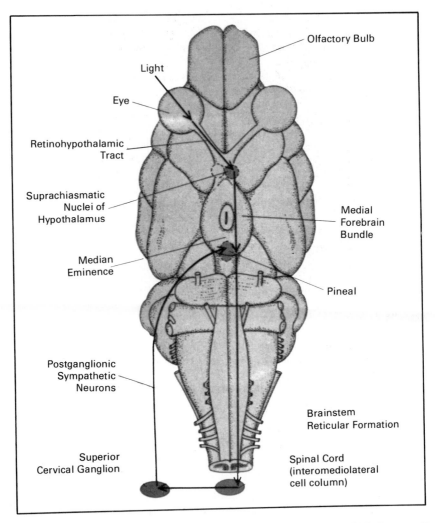

Figure 18-5. Anatomy of the pineal organ with respect to light stimulus. Light is transmitted from the retina along several brain pathways which merge at the superior cervical ganglia of the sympathetic nervous system, as do all neural impulses of central nervous system origin which travel to the pineal. These impulses affect the synthesis of melatonin through mediation of norepinephrine release and its stimulation of β-adrenergic receptors on the pineal cell membranes. This conversion of neural input identified the pineal as a neuroendocrine transducer. Reproduced from R. J. Wurtman, *In* "Neuroendocrinology" (D. T. Krieger and J. C. Hughes, eds.), p. 103. Sinauer Associates, Sunderland, Massachusetts, 1980. Courtesy Nancy Lou (Gahan) Makris.

myelineated and unmyelineated nerve fibers. Within the organ the capillaries are thin and fenestrated, but this may not apply to all species. The nerve fibers derive from the sympathetic autonomic nervous system. Nerve terminals may end directly on pineal cells. In Fig. 18-6 the human organ is shown to illustrate the cellular organization. The adrenergic nerve endings which regulate the pineal cells through release of norepinephrine are visualized. The neurosecretory granules housed in the nerve endings can be seen plainly. The nerve fibers, penetrating the pineal, lose the myelin sheath and the nerve endings shown in Fig. 18-6A end on pinealocytes. The neurosecretory granules containing norepinephrine are 40 nm in diameter. Serotonin is also present in the nerve endings as well as within the pinealocytes.

The pinealocytes have cytoplasmic processes that end in swellings (Fig. 18-7A). The other major cell type in the pineal organ is the interstitial cell, which is irregular in shape (Fig. 18-7B) and scattered among the pinealocytes. These cells resemble astrocytes and some consider them to be neuroglia.

III. CHEMISTRY

A major hormone secreted by the pinealocyte is melatonin, shown in Fig. 18-1. Serotonin and *N*-acetylserotonin also are important in the pineal, but they may not be secreted. Both melatonin and serotonin are derived from tryptophan, the characteristic feature of all of these compounds being the indole ring (Fig. 18-1). Other hydroxy- and methoxyindoles are present in the pinealocyte, as will be evident from the discussion of the biochemistry.

The pinealocyte may secrete a peptide, vasotocin (Fig. 18-1), which may have important activities in reproductive functions and which is related in structure to oxytocin and vasopressin (Fig. 4-4).

Recently, two neurophysins have been found in the pineal gland. Neurophysins are proteins derived from the same gene product as either vasopressin or oxytocin in the hypothalamus.

IV. BIOCHEMISTRY

Tryptophan is the precursor of melatonin. After uptake from the extracellular blood vascular system, this amino acid is converted in the pinealocyte to 5-hydroxytryptophan catalyzed by tryptophan hydrox-

706

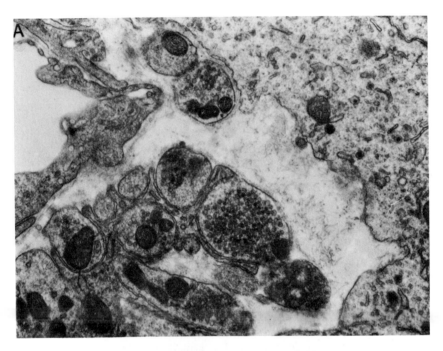

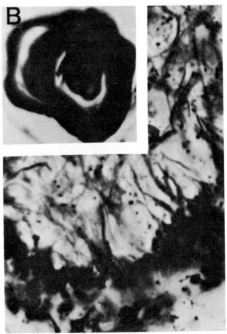

ylase. Serotonin is the product of the next step in the pathway achieved by the action of aromatic L-amino acid decarboxylase on 5-hydroxytryptophan.

Serotonin is the trivial name for 5-hydroxytryptamine. Serotonin concentration remains high in the pineal during the daylight hours as a result of the signaling mechanism reviewed in Fig. 18-8, but falls in darkness when serotonin either is converted to melatonin or falls in concentration for some other reason. Two enzymes achieve this conversion, serotonin, *N*-acetyltransferase, which converts serotonin to *N*-acetylserotonin, and hydroxyindole-*O*-methyltransferase (HIOMT), which catalyzes the transfer of a methyl group from *S*-adenosylmethionine (SAM) to the 5-hydroxyl of *N*-acetylserotonin. The product of this last reaction is melatonin (5-methoxy-*N*-acetyltryptamine). During darkness, there is an increased release of norepinephrine from the sympathetic neurons terminating on the pinealocytes (Fig. 18-8).

Melatonin circulates in the blood and is metabolized by the liver. Apparently, some or all of the melatonin is secreted either into the blood directly or into the cerebrospinal fluid before entering the bloodstream. It is unclear exactly how the metabolism of melatonin is partitioned between the liver and central nervous system, if the latter plays a role in this activity at all. Various effects of melatonin have been ascribed to occur in the central nervous system and perhaps elsewhere.

The biosynthesis of melatonin is shown in Fig. 18-9. In darkness, norepinephrine is secreted from adrenergic neurons ending on pinealocytes. The norepinephrine binds to the β-adrenergic receptor (see Chapter 11) on the pinealocyte membrane (may be a synapse) and results in the stimulation of intracellular cyclic AMP levels. The elevation of cyclic AMP probably operates as described elsewhere (Fig. 1-15) and stimulates protein kinase activity which in turn causes phosphorylation of specific proteins and results in the stimulation of the synthesis of *N*-acetyltransferase.

In cultured rat pineal glands during induction of serotonin *N*-acetyltransferase by catecholamine, a nuclear protein is phosphorylated in the early stages of enzyme induction. This protein is also phosphorylated

---

Figure 18-6. (A) Electron micrograph of adrenergic nerve endings in the pineal body. ×32,000. Reproduced from L. C. Junqueira, J. Carneiro, and A. N. Contopoulos, "Basic Histology," 2nd ed., p. 404. Lange Medical Publications, Los Altos, California, 1977. (B) Human pineal body in which the epithelioid cells are visualized with silver. Long branching processes of the cells terminate in bulbous endings. ×625. Inset: Acervulus ("brain sand"). ×250. Reproduced from T. S. Leeson and C. R. Leeson, "Histology," 4th ed., p. 481. Saunders, Philadelphia, Pennsylvania, 1981.

A

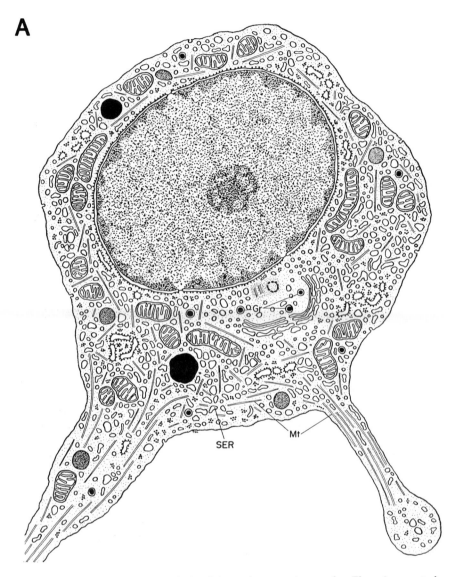

Figure 18-7. (A) A pinealocyte idealized from electron micrographs. There is a central nucleus with nucleolus. Large microtubules (Mt) are present in the cytoplasm extending in all directions within the cell body, but parallel to the long axis in the processes. There is an abundant smooth endoplasmic reticulum (SER). A large Golgi apparatus lies near the nucleus, with a pair of centrioles nearby. There are small dense membrane granules (Gr) throughout the cell and large numbers of mitochondria, some liposomes, and lipid droplets. The dense granules may contain hormones. Reproduced from T. L. Lentz, "Cell Fine

B

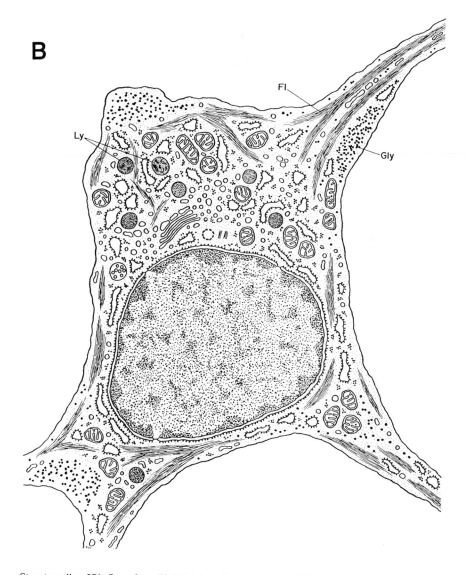

Structure," p. 351. Saunders, Philadelphia, Pennsylvania, 1971. (B) A pineal interstitial cell drawn from electron microscopic observations. There is a rounded nucleus and processes extending from the cell body. Filaments (Fl) occur in the cytoplasm in bundles and extend into the processes. There is rough endoplasmic reticulum studded with ribosomes and also free ribosomes. There are glycogen granules (Gly) and lysosomes (Ly). Mitochondria are small and well distributed. Reproduced from T. L. Lentz, "Cell Fine Structure," p. 353. Saunders, Philadelphia, Pennsylvania, 1971.

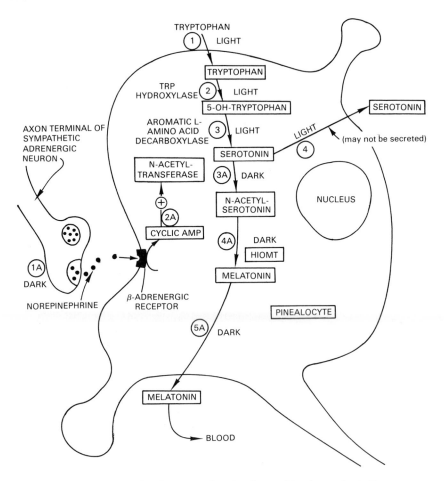

TRYPTOPHAN

LIGHT

TRYPTOPHAN

TRP HYDROXYLASE

LIGHT

5-OH-TRYPTOPHAN

AROMATIC L-AMINO ACID DECARBOXYLASE

LIGHT

SEROTONIN

LIGHT

SEROTONIN

(may not be secreted)

AXON TERMINAL OF SYMPATHETIC ADRENERGIC NEURON

N-ACETYL-TRANSFERASE

DARK

N-ACETYL-SEROTONIN

NUCLEUS

CYCLIC AMP

DARK

HIOMT

DARK

MELATONIN

NOREPINEPHRINE

β-ADRENERGIC RECEPTOR

PINEALOCYTE

DARK

DARK

MELATONIN

BLOOD

Figure 18-8. Biosynthesis of melatonin in the pinealocyte. Numbers refer to the sequence of events in the light. Numbers with (A) refer to dark-induced sequences of events.

when the glands are treated directly with dibutyryl cyclic AMP, over-stepping catecholamine ligand and its receptor. Increased levels of this enzyme lead to the conversion of serotonin to melatonin and its secretion from the cell probably into the bloodstream. Environmental light, perceived via the retinas, diminishes the flow of impulses along the pineal's sympathetic nerves, thus decreasing the release of norepinephrine onto pinealocytes. This decreases the activities of serotonin-N-acetyltransferase and HIOMT, suppressing the synthesis and secretion of melatonin. This pineal mechanism may mediate the stimulation of ovarian growth that occurs when young rats are placed under constant light.

The metabolic reactions involved in the conversion of tryptophan to melatonin are shown in Fig. 18-9. As shown in Fig. 18-10, the regulation of *N*-acetyltransferase is more elaborate than described up to this point. As mentioned before, the increased elaboration of norepinephrine, stimulated by the absence of light, results in enhanced synthesis of *N*-acetyl-

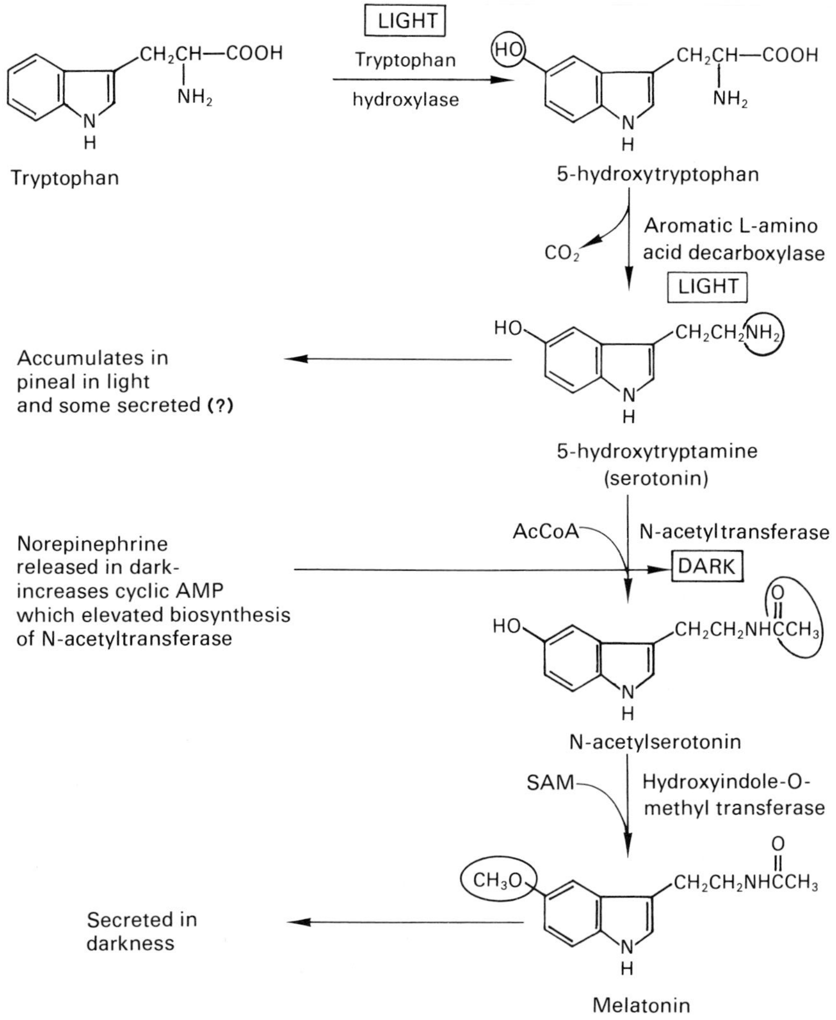

Figure 18-9. Reactions converting tryptophan to melatonin in pinealocytes.

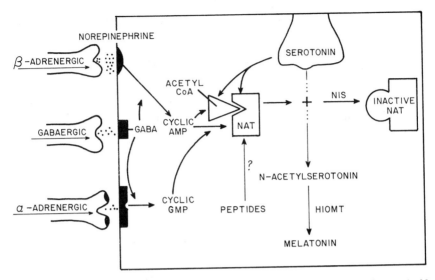

Figure 18-10. Regulation of *N*-acetyltransferase by pineal substances. NAT, Serotonin *N*-acetyltransferase; NIS, *N*-acetyltransferase inactivating substance. Reproduced from M. Ebadi, A. Chan, H. Hammad, P. Govitrapong, and S. Swanson, *in* "The Pineal and Its Hormones" (R. J. Reiter, ed.), pp. 21–33. Alan R. Liss, Inc., New York, 1982.

transferase and coenzyme A. There may be present an *N*-acetyltransfer-ase-inactivating substance (NIS). The NIS presumably would act when the concentration of acetyl CoA falls (light) to further reduce the production of melatonin. Other neurons are indicated in Fig. 18-10. Thus, γ-aminobutyric acid (GABA) could have a modulating effect on nor-epinephrine increases in *N*-acetyltransferase protein. Cyclic GMP may have some effect in this system, although the dominant effect of nor-epinephrine operates through cyclic AMP.

Although lighting is the synchronizer of this process, experiments have been done with animals housed in continuous darkness. Under these conditions, melatonin synthesis and secretion continue to exhibit circadian rhythms which require sympathetic nerves innervating the pineal. Obviously another cycling signal exists, perhaps originating in the suprachiasmic nuclei of the brain. Estrogens may exert some influ-ence on the system, modulating the production of melatonin, although the evidence is not strong. Melatonin clearly acts on the brain, but it may also act on the pituitary and other organs. In all species examined, melatonin has been found to reach peak concentrations in darkness in CSF, blood, and urine.

Melatonin is cleared in the urine for the most part by way of the liver, which contains a microsomal enzyme catalyzing 6-hydroxylation. Following hydroxylation, some of the product becomes esterified with sulfate and is excreted in that form (Fig. 18-11).

V. BIOLOGICAL AND MOLECULAR ACTIONS

A. General Comments

It is becoming clear that melatonin operates on the brain. For example, melatonin is known to produce drowsiness in humans.

The mechanism of melatonin secretion by pinealocytes is not understood. It is possible that this very lipid-soluble hormone leaves the cell by free diffusion, as pointed out by R. Wurtman, in relation to its ac-

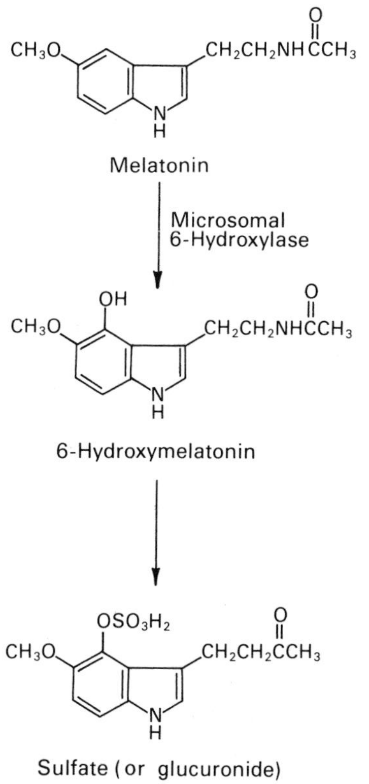

Figure 18-11. Metabolism of melatonin.

cumulation by the cell. In other words, the pinealocyte probably does not behave like a neuronal cell utilizing the process of exocytosis of neurosecretions.

B. Melatonin Receptor

To date, there is no firm evidence documenting a melatonin receptor; however, in 1978 a binding protein in cytosols of ovaries from hamster, rat, and human was reported which had many of the characteristics of a melatonin receptor (see Cohen et al., 1978). It was reasoned that because melatonin was a negative regulator of gonadal function under some circumstances, the activity of the hormone should be mediated by a receptor. This putative receptor has a dissociation constant, K_D, with respect to melatonin of 6 nM. A second class of sites produced a K_D of 550 nM, clearly the result of a low-affinity site. A similar binding site was found, in addition to ovarian tissue, in testis, uterus, skin, liver, and eye. These results may be indicative of a broader activity of melatonin than previously appreciated.

C. Actions of Melatonin on Anterior Pituitary

1. LH and FSH

Melatonin inhibits secretion of LH and FSH induced by GnRH. In particular, this has been demonstrated with anterior pituitary cells obtained from 1- to 20-day-old rats. The inhibition by melatonin was effective in the range of 0.1–1.0 nM when the cells were obtained from animals which were 5, 10, or 15 days of age. Suppression of anterior pituitary hormone release ranged to 50% of the full response to GnRH, as shown in Fig. 18-12. Melatonin interferes either with the GnRH stimulation of anterior pituitary hormone release or with the secretion process, probably through an indirect mechanism. Interestingly, pinealectomy results in an increase of ornithine decarboxylase activity in rat anterior pituitary, and this enhanced activity persists for several weeks, at least. Other reports that pinealectomy results in increased mitotic activity in the rat adenohypophysis align with the effect on ornithine decarboxylase activity which usually reflects mitotic activity. Whether this is related to release of LH and FSH in response to GnRH is unclear. Cells from 20- to 30-day-old animals no longer showed the response to melatonin, presumably contributing to the regulation of development of the reproductive system. In the rat, puberty occurs 2–3 weeks after melatonin's ability to inhibit the pituitary gland disappears. In humans,

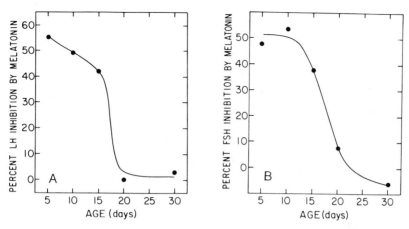

Figure 18-12. (A) Relationship between animal age and percentage of maximal inhibition by melatonin of pituitary LH response to LHRH (GnRH). The difference in LH values between groups treated with LHRH alone and groups treated with LHRH and 10 nM melatonin is expressed for each age as a percentage of stimulation over controls by LHRH alone. (B) Relationship between animal age and percentage of maximal inhibition by melatonin of pituitary FSH response to LHRH. The difference in FSH values between groups treated with LHRH alone and groups treated with 10 nM melatonin is expressed for each age as a percentage of stimulation over controls by LHRH alone. Reproduced from J. E. Martin and C. Sattler, *Endocrinology (Baltimore)* **105**, 1007–1012 (1979). © by The Endocrine Society (1979).

peak nocturnal plasma melatonin levels fall by about 75% between ages 7 and 12, when concurrently measured plasma LH is rising (Waldhauser *et al.*, 1984). This suggests that melatonin may have a role in timing human puberty.

2. Regulation of Growth Hormone Release

It has been suggested for some time that melatonin could inhibit release of growth hormone from the anterior pituitary. Recent work suggests that melatonin accomplishes this by stimulating the release of somatostatin which has been observed using explants of rat medial basal hypothalamus. The action of somatostatin on inhibiting growth hormone release is described in Fig. 5-23. Interestingly, melatonin concentrations effective in stimulating somatostatin release were in the range of 10–100 nM for explants of hypothalamus.

Relatively little is known about the specific actions of Arg-vasotocin and little or no information is available concerning an Arg-vasotocin receptor. In fact, some believe that vasotocin may not be present in the pineal at all.

VI. CLINICAL ASPECTS

Most inferences to pineal hormones and diseases have come from studies with experimental animals. Thus, pinealectomy at an early time in development in some species can lead to premature ovarian function, and treatment with melatonin can suppress ovarian function. As described above, the amounts of melatonin secreted nocturnally decline just prior to and during pubescence. Moreover, an acute oral dose (1–3 mg/kg) given to young adults causes prolactin to be secreted. A number of different kinds of tumors can affect the function of the pineal gland, usually resulting in central nervous system disturbances and either premature or delayed gonadal functioning, especially when these occur in the young.

There may be a point of interaction above the pituitary between melatonin and ACTH–corticosteroid secretion. An acute lowering of cortisol secretion in man (by metyrapone, for instance) stimulates melatonin secretion.

References

A. Books

Krieger, D. T., and Hughes, J. C., eds. (1980). "Neuroendocrinology." Sinauer Associates, Sunderland, Massachusetts.

Mess, B., Ruzsas, C., Tima, L., and Pevet, P., eds. (1985). "The Pineal Gland. Current State of Pineal Research." Elsevier, Amsterdam.

Reiter, R. J., ed. (1982). "The Pineal and Its Hormones." Alan R. Liss, New York.

B. Review Articles

Cardinali, D. P., Vacas, M. I., and Boyer, E. E. (1979). Specific binding of melatonin in bovine brain. *Endocrinology (Baltimore)* **105**, 437–441.

Cohen, M., Roselle, D., Chabner, B., Schmidt, T. J., and Lippman, M. (1978). Evidence for a cytoplasmic melatonin receptor. *Nature (London)* **274**, 894–895.

Martin, J. E., and Sattler, C. (1979). Developmental loss of the acute inhibitory effect of melatonin on the *in vitro* pituitary luteinizing hormone and follicle-stimulating hormone responses to luteinizing hormone-releasing hormone. *Endocrinology (Baltimore)* **105**, 1007–1012.

Richardson, S. B., Hollander, C. S., Prasad, J. A., and Hirooka, Y. (1981). Somatostatin release from rat hypothalamus *in vitro*: Effects of melatonin and serotonin. *Endocrinology (Baltimore)* **109**, 602–606.

Rivest, R. W., Lang, U., Aubert, M. L., and Sizonenko, P. C. (1985). Daily administration of melatonin delays rat vaginal opening and disrupts the first estrus cycles: Evidence that these effects are synchronized by the onset of light. *Endocrinology (Baltimore)* **116**, 779–787.

Scalabrino, G., Ferioli, M. E., Modena, D., and Fraschini, F. (1982). Enhancement of ornithine decarboxylase activity in rat adenohypophysis after pinealectomy. *Endocrinology (Baltimore)* **111,** 2132–2134.

Walhauser, F., and Wurtman, R. J. (1983). The secretion and action of melatonin. "Biochemical Action of Hormones," pp. 187–225. Academic Press, New York.

Walhauser, F., Frisch, H., Walhauser, M., Weiszenbacher, G., Zeitlhuber, U., and Wurtman, R. J. (1984). Fall in nocturnal serum melatonin during prepuberty and pubescence. *The Lancet,* Feb. 18, 362–365.

Winters, K. E., Morrissey, J. J., Loos, P. J., and Lovenberg, W. (1977). Pineal protein phosphorylation during serotonin N-acetyltransferase induction. *Proc. Natl. Acad. Sci. (Washington)* **74,** 1928–1931.

Wurtman, R. J. (1980). The pineal as a neuroendocrine transducer. *In* "Neuroendocrinology" (D. T. Kreiger and J. C. Hughes, eds.), pp. 102–108. Sinauer Associates, Sunderland, Massachusetts.

Wurtman, R. J., and Moskowitz, M. A. (1977). The pineal organ. *New Engl. J. Med.* **296,** 1329–1333; 1383–1386.

Chapter 19

Cell Growth Factors

I. INTRODUCTION

A. Background

Some of the polypeptide hormones already discussed in this book have growth factor activities. By that we mean that they can, among other actions, stimulate cells to divide or enter DNA synthesis at a greater rate. Serum-free defined media was an important development, principally by the laboratory of G. Sato, to identify cell types that respond to a specific growth factor. These actions begin with the interaction of the polypeptide growth factor or mitogen (a substance, usually a polypeptide, which stimulates cells to initiate mitosis) with a specific receptor on the cell membrane. Although the subsequent events leading directly to increased DNA synthesis and division, or mitosis, are not well understood, current ideas as to how this happens involve either (1) generation of a second messenger substance from the membrane interaction which has further effects leading to enhanced DNA synthetic rates, or (2) internalization of the hormone–receptor complex from the membrane, fusion with intracellular particles, such as lysosomes, and generation, perhaps by proteolytic degradation of the receptor (or its ligand), of a second messenger which acts subsequently to promote the DNA synthetic rate.

Hormones that have been discussed previously and fall within the category of cell growth factors are insulin (Chapter 7), somatomedins and growth hormone (Chapter 5), prolactin (Chapters 5 and 14), and erythropoietin (Chapter 15). In addition to these better known polypeptide hormones, an increasing list of polypeptides with cell growth-stimulating activities is being generated.

A partial list of growth factors and their properties is presented in Table 19-1. Virtually all of these are polypeptides and there are only minor exceptions to this which remain to be documented clearly. In general, growth factors have occurred in very low concentrations in tissues and their isolation, characterization, chemical synthesis, and genetic engineering, where possible, is a continuing effort.

B. Types of Hormonal Communication

As described in Chapter 1, hormones can be divided roughly into three types: endocrine, paracrine, and autocrine. The first concerns classical hormones which are secreted by cells located in one part of the body and travel over large distances to interact with target cells (which contain receptors for the endocrine hormone). Paracrine hormones operate over shorter distances to affect neighboring cells (and are not transformed systemically) and autocrine hormones affect the cells that produce them.

Growth factor hormones may be a mixture of all three types. Insulin-like growth factors (IGFs) are known to be secreted by the liver, for example, and to circulate in the blood complexed with a binding protein. These factors undoubtedly influence growth of hepatocytes, but also

Table 19-1. Summary of Some Known Growth Factors

Growth factor	Chemistry	Molecular weight	Origins	Targets	Receptors and actions
Insulin	Peptide, 2 chains	6,000 (monomer) 12,000 (dimer)	β cell (pancreas), brain	Hepatocyte, adipocyte, muscle cells, many others	$α_2$ (125,000), $β_2$ (90,000); resembles IgG structure; is a protein kinase; phosphorylates receptor
Insulin-like growth factors (IGF-I and somatomedins, cell multiplication factors)	Polypeptide homology with insulin; diverged from common ancester	7500	Hepatocyte, kidney cells, intestinal cells(?), stimulated by GH	Same as sources + bone (sulfation factor)	Cell membranes; IGF-I receptor similar in structure to insulin receptor (350 kDa); IGF-II receptor single peptide chain (250 kDa)
Nerve growth factor (NGF)	3 chain peptide, α subunit (26,000), β subunit (13,250), γ subunit (~28,000); has Arg esteropeptidase activity	130,000 as $α_2$: $β_2$: $γ_2$	Submaxillary gland	Stimulates DNA synthesis of ganglia as neuroblast division nears conclusion	Receptor = 135,000 from rabbit superior cervical ganglia; 2 types in intact sensory neurons: K_d 2×10^{-11} M and 1.4×10^{-9} M; internalization of membrane receptor
Epidermal growth factor (EGF)	Peptide	6000	Submaxillary gland; urogastrone in urine	Many cells	Protein kinase; phosphorylates tyrosine; cell membrane receptors internalized; actions resemble *src* gene product (protein

(continued)

Table 19-1. (*Continued*)

Growth factor	Chemistry	Molecular weight	Origins	Targets	Receptors and actions
					kinase); EGF receptor, 160 kDa single chain
Growth hormone (GH)	Peptide	21,500 (human)	Anterior pituitary	Hepatocyte	Cell membrane, hormone stimulates release of somatomedins; other direct effects at membrane
Platelet-derived growth factor (PDGF)	Peptide, 2 chains, 14,000 and 17,000	30,000–35,000	Platelet α granules and blood from this source	Fibroblasts, arterial smooth muscle cells	Cell membrane receptor stimulates DNA synthesis, cell migration, amino acid transport, protein synthesis, cholesterol ester synthesis, phospholipid turnover, PGI$_2$ synthesis, modulates binding of EGF, LH, low-density lipoprotein, somatomedin C to their receptors;

Name	Type	Molecular weight	Source	Target cells	Comments
Transforming growth factor (TGFs)	Peptides	6,000–25,000	In neoplastic normal cells which synthesize them; "autocrine" hormones; β TGF from human platelets (also human placenta and bovine kidney)	May interact in some way with EGF receptor and these factors may be related to *src* gene product	PDGF receptor, 170 kDa single chain; Cell membrane binding; TGF α induces phosphorylation of Tyr in EGF receptor; TGF α competes with EGF for membrane binding; TGF β does not compete with EGF binding; TGF β fully potentiates colony-forming response with EGF; TGF γ does not compete with EGF binding and is not required in anchorage-dependent growth of NRK cells; TGF β accelerates wound healing in rats
Glial growth factor (GGF)	Peptide	31,000	Anterior and posterior pituitary and other parts of brain	Schwann cells (astrocytes, rat muscle fibroblasts)	Stimulates cells to divide

growth of other tissue cells as well. Many of the growth factors to be described here have been uncovered and studied extensively in tissue culture. Growth factors often act like paracrine and autocrine hormones affecting other cells in their neighborhood as well as the cell of origin.

C. Comparison of Gross Structures of Insulin-Related Growth Factors

The trophic hormones, insulin, relaxin, and IGF all act to promote cellular growth and have certain similarities in their general structures. Nerve growth factor (NGF) promotes neurite outgrowth. These are shown in Fig. 19-1. In addition to similarities in gross structure, there also exist homologies in primary amino acid sequences, to be pointed out later. Similarities of general structures between this particular group of IGFs suggest a common origin. Relatedness in the structures of receptors for these hormones is evident in the case of insulin and IGF-I receptors. More information will be forthcoming on the receptors for NGF

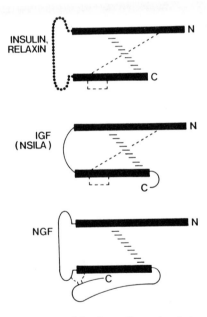

Figure 19-1. Schematic comparison of the three-dimensional structure of the four insulin-related growth factors. Heavy segments represent the B and A chain regions. The conserved disulfide is emphasized. The C region of prorelaxin is inferred. Reproduced from R. Bradshaw and H. D. Niall, *Trends Biochem. Sci.* **3,** 274–278 (1978).

and for relaxin. Identification of similarities between these and other growth factors (Table 19-1) remains for the future.

Since many of the newer growth factors are studied in the context of cell culture systems, it cannot be stated with any assurance what their relative roles are qualitatively or quantitatively in the whole animal.

In the case of insulin and epidermal growth factor (EGF), insulin-like growth factor 1 (IGF-1), and platelet-derived growth factor (PDGF), their receptors have been shown to have protein kinase activity which is specific for tyrosine residues. This activity resembles the *src* gene product and other phenotypes of oncogenes. Oncogenes occur in viruses and in cells. When they become active in a cell, they express phenotypes, sometimes growth factors, receptors, or part of growth factor receptors whose action is to release the cell's regulation so as to allow unrestricted division. There is conjecture on the possibility that normal cells and cancer cells may differ at some point in the numbers of receptors per cell which are specific for growth factors, and the quantitative differences in such receptors may explain the tremendous growth potential of tumor cells. Thus, the "problem" of growth factor hormones may be close to the heart of the cancer problem.

In this chapter, some of the currently known growth factors are reviewed in terms of structures and modes of action.

II. ANATOMICAL ASPECTS

Fibroblasts

Fibroblasts are involved in the formation of connective tissue fibers and amorphous ground substance. They are spindle-shaped cells, in general, and they usually produce collagen. Many experiments leading to conclusions about the existence of cellular growth factors have been carried out with fibroblastic cells in tissue culture, notably mouse 3T3 cells and other similar lines. An example of fibroblasts growing in culture is shown in Fig. 19-2. Untransformed fibroblasts of this general type can be maintained in culture for over 200 generations when cell-to-cell contact is limited. When they are grown under conditions of extensive cell-to-cell contact, the fibroblasts become transformed or tumorigenic within 30 generations.

An advantage of these fibroblast cells is that many hormone receptors are retained in their cell membranes, and it is possible to determine

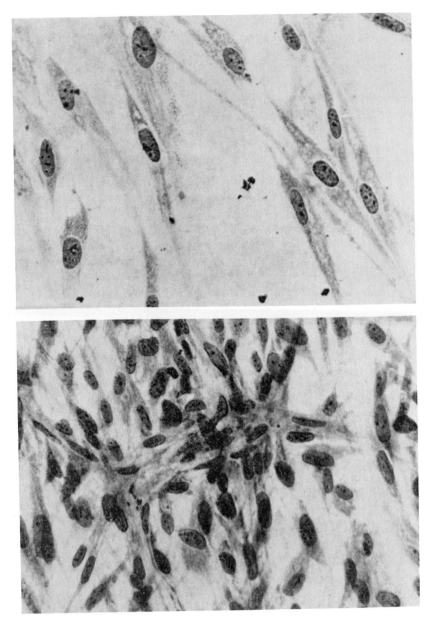

Figure 19-2. Fibroblastic-type cells in tissue culture. Reproduced from J. Paul, "Cell and Tissue Culture," 5th ed., p. 20. Churchill-Livingstone, Edinburgh and London, 1975.

effects of hormones and growth factors on the cells as well as regulation of receptor functions. However, growth factors discovered from cell culture experiments will ultimately have to be assessed in the whole organism.

III. CHEMISTRY

The chemistry and primary amino acid sequences of insulin (Figs. 7-6, 7-7, and 7-8) and growth hormone (Figs. 5-4 and 5-5) have been presented previously in Chapters 5 and 7.

A. Epidermal Growth Factor (EGF)

This hormone consists of a single polypeptide chain of 6045 Da. The 53 amino acid primary structure of mouse EGF is shown in Fig. 19-3. It is a heat-stable protein stabilized by three disulfide linkages. It is devoid of alanine, phenylalanine, and lysine residues as well as of free sulfhydryl groups and sugar substituents. The isoelectric point is about pH 4.6. Intact disulfide bonds are required for activity. There is little α-helical structure, about 25% β helix, and 75% random coil. Human urogastrone is similar to mouse EGF and is apparently the excreted form of the same hormone. A comparison of the amino acid sequences of these two proteins is shown in Fig. 19-4. Of the sequences of the two proteins, 70%

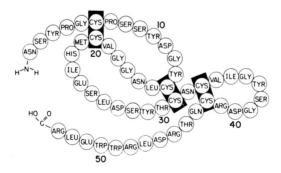

Figure 19-3. Amino acid sequence and location of disulfide linkages of mouse-derived EGF. Reproduced from G. Carpenter and J. G. Zendegui, Epidermal growth factor, its receptor, and related proteins. *Exp. Cell Res.* **162,** 1–10.

are homologous, the differences being attributed to species variation. Urogastrone has the biological activity of EGF and is now recognized as the same protein.

There is a high-molecular-weight form of mouse EGF which represents its storage form (74,000 Da). It is composed of two molecules of active EGF (each 6045 Da) and two molecules of a protein to which EGF is bound (Fig. 19-5), each of which is 29,300 Da. The binding protein is similar to the γ subunit of NGF (see later) in that it expresses arginine esteropeptidase activity (Table 19-1). It is also similar in molecular weight, antigenic cross-reactivity, and amino acid composition. The NGF γ subunit and the EGF binding protein are similar but not identical proteins based on amino acid sequence; EGF binding protein does not substitute for NGF γ subunit in the formation of 7 S (high molecular weight) NGF.

B. Nerve Growth Factor (NGF)

NGF is composed of three kinds of subunits, α, β, and γ. The β subunit is the biologically active component with a molecular weight of 13,250. It exists as a dimer and is active in this form in the absence of α and γ subunits. The γ subunit has a molecular weight of 26,000 and is an

									10		
Asn	Ser	Tyr	Pro	Gly	Cys	Pro	Ser	Ser	Tyr	Asp	Gly
Asn	Ser	Asp	Ser	Glu	Cys	Pro	Leu	Ser	His	Asp	Gly
							20				
Tyr	Cys	Leu	Asn	Gly	Gly	Val	Cys	Met	His	Ile	Glu
Tyr	Cys	Leu	His	Asp	Gly	Val	Cys	Met	Tyr	Ile	Glu
					30						
Ser	Leu	Asp	Ser	Tyr	Thr	Cys	Asn	Cys	Val	Ile	Gly
Ala	Leu	Asp	Lys	Tyr	Ala	Cys	Asn	Cys	Val	Val	Gly
			40								
Tyr	Ser	Gly	Asp	Arg	Cys	Gln	Thr	Arg	Asp	Leu	Arg
Tyr	Ile	Gly	Glu	Arg	Cys	Gln	Tyr	Arg	Asp	Leu	Lys
	50										
Trp	Trp	Glu	Leu	Arg	——	EGF (mouse)					
Trp	Trp	Glu	Leu	Arg	——	UROGASTRONE					

Figure 19-4. Amino acid sequences of mouse EGF and human urogastrone. Reproduced from H. Gregory, *Nature (London)* **257,** 325 (1975). © 1975 Macmillan Journals Limited.

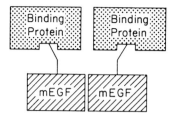

Figure 19-5. High-molecular-weight mouse EGF (mEGF). Reproduced from L. E. Underwood and J. J. van Wyk, *in* "Textbook of Endocrinology" (R. H. Williams, ed.), 7th ed., p. 172. Saunders, Philadelphia, Pennsylvania, 1985.

arginine esteropeptidase. The precise function of the α subunit is not clear; its molecular weight is 26,500. The α and γ subunits show about 80% sequence identity, but the α subunit has no catalytic activity. A high-molecular-weight form of NGF exists as a 7 S aggregate and consists of dimers of α, β, and γ subunits, as diagrammed in Fig. 19-6, with a molecular weight of 130,000. The gene for human NGF has been cloned.

C. Platelet-Derived Growth Factor (PDGF)

The platelet-derived growth factor (PDGF) is involved in wound healing *in vivo* and is stable to high temperatures and to acid. PDGF may also be involved in atherosclerosis. It has an isoelectric point around 10 and a molecular weight of 30,000–35,000. Reduction of the polypeptide results in two inactive chains of 14,000 and 17,000 Da. In the native polypeptide these two chains are probably linked together by disulfide bonds. Re-

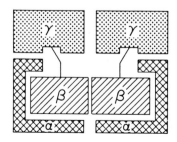

Figure 19-6. Mouse 7 S nerve growth factor (NGF). Reproduced from L. E. Underwood and J. J. van Wyk, *in* "Textbook of Endocrinology" (R. H. Williams, ed.), 7th ed., p. 172. Saunders, Philadelphia, Pennsylvania, 1985.

cent reports suggest that active PDGF may be heterogeneous and separation of two forms has been accomplished by gel filtration. The second form could derive from the first by enzymatic cleavage, since the difference in the molecular weight of one of the constituent chains is about 2000 Da. Amino acid analysis shows a predominance of basic amino acids. A landmark development has shown that PDGF is related to the oncogene v-*sis*. Relationships between oncogenes and growth factors are mentioned later.

D. Insulin-Like Growth Factors (IGF-I and IGF-II)

IGFs probably are comprised of a family of polypeptides in the range of 7500 Da. Other related factors are the somatomedins (see Fig. 5-24) and cell multiplication factors. They all appear to derive from the same family and some may be identical. C. H. Li's laboratory has shown that IGF-I is identical to somatomedin C; it has been synthesized chemically and is being produced by genetic engineering. There are two well-known IGFs, IGF-I and IGF-II. These polypeptides, which have homologies with the insulin molecule, bind to discrete receptors. As indicated in Chapter 5, some of the growth effects of growth hormone on somatic cells are mediated by these factors.

These polypeptides contain three disulfide bridges, and 45% of the amino acids composing IGF-I, IGF-II, and insulin are identical. This suggests that IGF and insulin were derived from a common ancestral gene. The primary amino acid sequence of IGF-I is shown in Fig. 19-7. As seen, there is striking homology with the insulin–proinsulin sequence.

Recently, J. Van Wyk's laboratory has shown that human IGF-I is identical to somatomedin C. Figure 19-8 stresses the general structural

Ala Ser Lys Ala Pro Lys Leu Pro Ala Cys Tyr Met Glu Leu Arg Arg

Leu Asp Cys Ser Arg Phe Cys Cys Glu Asp Val Ile Gly Thr Gln Pro

Ala Arg Arg Ser Ser Ser Gly Tyr Gly Thr Pro Lys Asn Phe Tyr Phe

Gly Arg Asp Gly Cys Val Phe Gln Leu Ala Asp Val Leu Glu Ala Gly

Cys Leu Thr Glu Pro Gly

Figure 19-7. Structure of IGF-I. The amino acids that are underlined denote those in identical positions as in the A and B chain of human insulin. Reproduced from E. R. Froesch, J. Zapf, E. Rinderknecht, B. Morell, E. Schoenle, and R. E. Humbel, *Cold Spring Harbor Conf. Cell Proliferation* **6**, 62 (1979).

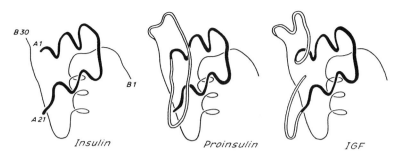

Figure 19-8. Schematic representation of the three-dimensional structure of insulin based on X ray of rhombohedral porcine 2-Zn insulin crystals and proposed confirmation based on model building for proinsulin and IGF-I showing the close structural homology. Reproduced from E. R. Froesch, J. Zapf, E. Rinderknecht, B. Morell, E. Schoenle, and R. E. Humbel, *Cold Spring Harbor Conf. Cell Proliferation* **6**, 62 (1979).

similarities between insulin, proinsulin, and IGF. Further homologies may be extended to NGF and relaxin, as shown in Fig. 19-9.

Somatomedin A has been purified, but its amino acid sequence has not been described. In its amino acid composition it resembles IGF-I, although not as extensively as does somatomedin C. Consequently, unlike somatomedin B, it is a true member of the IGF family.

A comparison of the sequences of IGF-I and IGF-II is shown in Fig. 19-10.

E. Transforming Growth Factor (TGF)

TGFs were named on the basis of their activity in causing anchorage-independent growth of NRK cells in soft agar. This apparent "transformation" is not a permanent change in the cell phenotype or genotype and is reversible. TGFs are represented by a heterogeneous family of polypeptides with a range of molecular weights between 6000 and 25,000. They are acidic, heat stable, and stabilized structurally by disulfide bridges. Disulfides are required for biological activity, since disulfide reducing agents cause inactivation. These factors have been classified into two types, α and β, depending on whether they interact with the EGF receptor and their requirement for EGF for transforming activity. TGFs are widely distributed and conveniently extracted by classical peptide extraction using acid-ethanol. TGFs are found in both normal and neoplastic tissues. Other factors, such as "sarcoma growth factor" (SGF), fit into the TGF category. Some of the TGFs have structural ho-

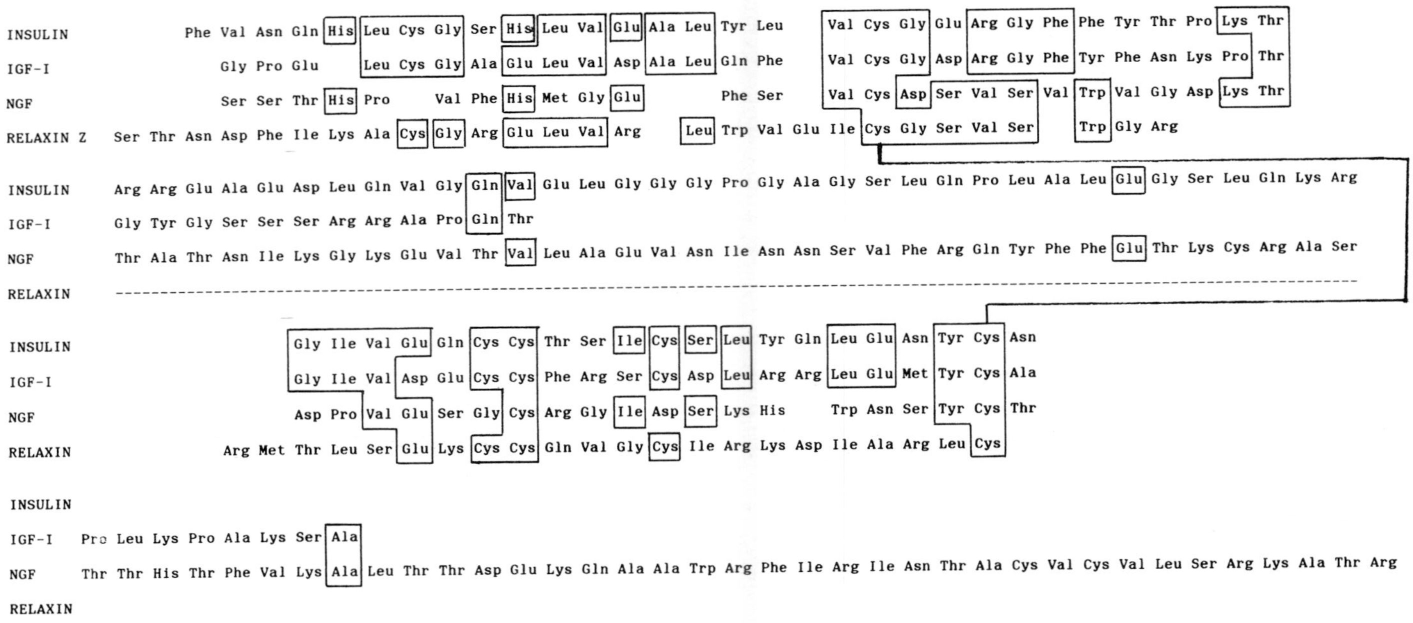

Figure 19-9. Comparison of amino acid sequences of human proinsulin, IGF-I, NGF, and relaxin. Solid boxes indicate residues identical in at least two of the polypeptides. Deletions were inserted arbitrarily to increase identities. The connecting line between the half cystinyl (C) residues of the A and B segments represents the one disulfide bond conserved in all four hormones. Reproduced from R. A. Bradshaw and H. D. Niall, *Trends Biochem. Sci.* **3**, 277 (1978).

INSULIN   Phe Val Asn Gln His Leu Val Glu Ala Leu Tyr Leu   Val Cys Gly Glu Arg Gly Phe Phe Tyr Thr Pro Lys Thr
IGF-I   Gly Pro Glu   Leu Cys Gly Ala Glu Leu Val Asp Ala Leu Gln Phe   Val Cys Gly Asp Arg Gly Phe Tyr Phe Asn Lys Pro Thr
NGF   Ser Ser Thr His Pro   Val Phe His Met Gly Glu   Phe Ser   Val Cys Asp Ser Val Ser Val Trp Val Gly Asp Lys Thr
RELAXIN Z   Ser Thr Asn Asp Phe Ile Lys Ala Cys Gly Arg Glu Leu Val Arg Leu Trp Val Glu Ile Cys Gly Ser Val Ser   Trp Gly Arg

INSULIN   Arg Arg Glu Ala Glu Asp Leu Gln Val Gly Gln Val Glu Leu Gly Gly Gly Pro Gly Ala Gly Ser Leu Gln Pro Leu Ala Leu Glu Gly Ser Leu Gln Lys Arg
IGF-I   Gly Tyr Gly Ser Ser Ser Arg Arg Ala Pro Gln Thr
NGF   Thr Ala Thr Asn Ile Lys Gly Lys Glu Val Thr Val Leu Ala Glu Val Asn Ile Asn Asn Ser Val Phe Arg Gln Tyr Phe Phe Glu Thr Lys Cys Arg Ala Ser
RELAXIN

INSULIN   Gly Ile Val Glu Gln Cys Cys Thr Ser Ile Cys Ser Leu Tyr Gln Leu Glu Asn Tyr Cys Asn
IGF-I   Gly Ile Val Asp Glu Cys Cys Phe Arg Ser Cys Asp Leu Arg Arg Leu Glu Met Tyr Cys Ala
NGF   Asp Pro Val Glu Ser Gly Cys Arg Gly Ile Asp Ser Lys His Trp Asn Ser Tyr Cys Thr
RELAXIN   Arg Met Thr Leu Ser Glu Lys Cys Cys Gln Val Gly Cys Ile Arg Lys Asp Ile Ala Arg Leu Cys

INSULIN

IGF-I   Pro Leu Lys Pro Ala Lys Ser Ala
NGF   Thr Thr His Thr Phe Val Lys Ala Leu Thr Thr Asp Glu Lys Gln Ala Ala Trp Arg Phe Ile Arg Ile Asp Thr Ala Cys Val Cys Val Leu Ser Arg Lys Ala Thr Arg
RELAXIN

732

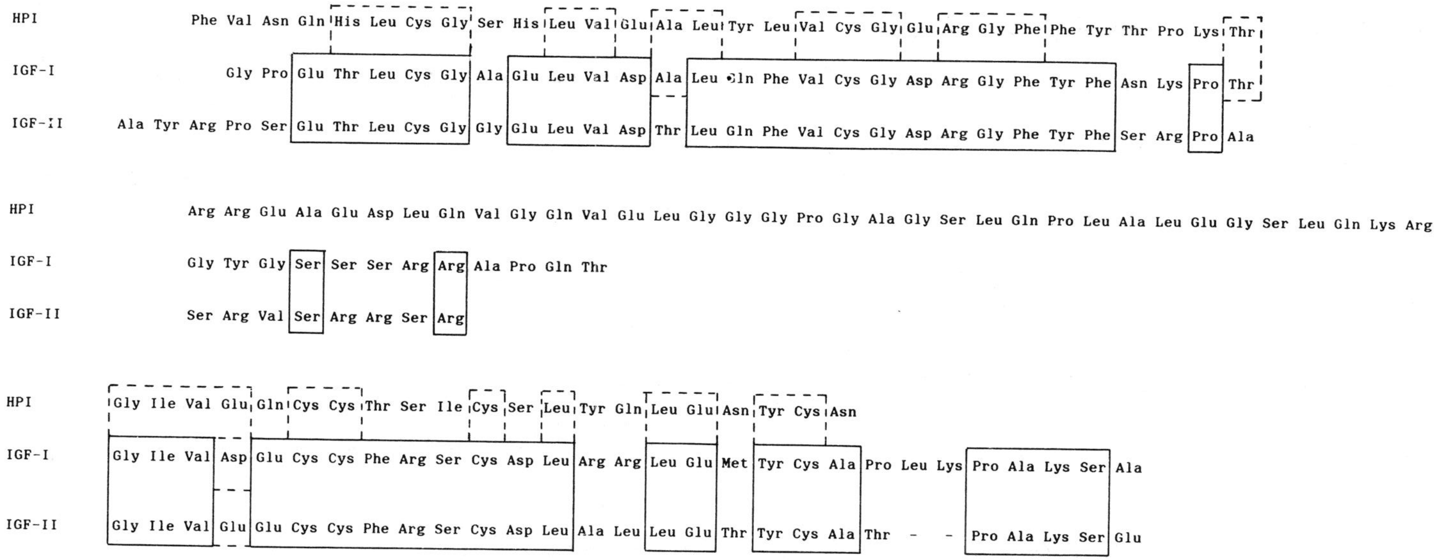

Figure 19-10. Primary structure of human proinsulin (HPI), IGF-I, and IGF-II. Alignment was chosen for maximal homology. Boxes with solid lines, residues identical in IGF-I and IGF-II; dashed lined boxes, residues identical in HPI and in IGF-I and/or IGF-II. Reproduced from E. R. Froesch, J. Zapf, E. Rinderknecht, B. Morell, E. Schoenle, and R. E. Humbel, *Cold Spring Harbor Conf. Cell Proliferation* **6**, 63 (1979).

mology to EGF in spite of being antigenically non-cross-reactive with anti-EGF. The general occurrence of TGFs is summarized in Table 19-2.

F. Fibroblast Growth Factor (FGF)

FGF was first characterized by D. Gospodarowicz. It has been purified by R. Bradshaw and collaborators to near homogeneity, and good sources are brain and pituitary, although the latter has been claimed to yield a product of higher purity. This factor stimulates incorporation of radioactive thymidine in 3T3 cells, frequently used to assess the activity of FGF. It has a molecular weight in the range of 15,000; it is acid- and heat-labile, has a basic pI, and is insensitive to reducing agents. Receptors for this growth factor have not been identified.

G. Glial Growth Factor (GGF)

A polypeptide growth factor present in brain and pituitary extracts, termed glial growth factor (GGF), stimulates the rate of division of purified rat Schwann cells in tissue culture. The molecular weight of this substance is 31,000. It stimulates the division of astrocytes (star-shaped cells with extending cytoplasmic processes often terminating on the surfaces of blood vessels; protoplasmic astrocytes occur in gray matter; fibrous astrocytes occur in white matter) and of fibroblasts from newborn rat muscle cultures. This factor has not yet been purified to homogeneity. It has some properties reminiscent of PDGF. It is basic in charge

Table 19–2. Occurrence of Transforming Growth Factors (TGFs)[a]

TGF group	Source
Extracellular (conditioned medium)	Virally transformed cells (mouse, rat); chemically transformed cells (mouse, rat); nonneoplastic cells (mouse); tumor cell lines (human)
Intracellular (tissues or cells)	Embryonic tissue (mouse); tumor tissue (mouse, rat); virally transformed cells (mouse); nonneoplastic adult tissue and cells (human, bovine, mouse); tumor cell lines (human); blood platelets (human, bovine)

[a] Reproduced from A. B. Roberts, C. A. Frolik, M. A. Anzano, and M. B. Sporn, Transforming growth factors from neoplastic and nonneoplastic tissues. *Fed. Proc., Fed. Am. Soc. Exp. Biol.* **42**, 2621–2626 (1983).

and heat resistant. This factor and PDGF may derive from the same family of polypeptides. Future examination of primary sequences will be of interest.

H. Other Growth Factors

1. Erythropoietin

Erythropoietin is a polypeptide produced by the kidney in cases of anemia or hypoxia which is essential for the normal production of red blood cells (Chapter 15). It can be considered to be a growth factor. Its deficiency is thought to be a major factor in anemia characteristic of renal failure. This hormone can stimulate many cycles of proliferations of primitive stem cells prior to stimulating terminal mitosis of pro-erythrocytes to generate hemoglobin-synthesizing cells. It is a glycoprotein of 39,000 Da, but the human urinary form has a molecular weight of about 25,000, possibly because it has been desialated or it represents a different form of the hormone. The regulation of the synthesis of this growth factor is shown in Fig. 19-11.

2. Estromedins

The estromedins are polypeptides produced in uterus, kidney, or liver under the influence of estrogens. These growth factors stimulate the growth of estrogen-responsive tumor cells. The molecular weight range of estromedins (uterus) is about 60,000–70,000 and that from hamster liver >65,000, but also 5,000–10,000.

3. Mammary Growth Factor

This factor apparently has been purified to homogeneity, and it has been characterized as phosphoethanolamine and ethanolamine. It is found in the pituitary in amounts equivalent to other pituitary hormones and it functions as a growth factor for a hormone-dependent mammary tumor cell line. Its exact function is unclear.

IV. BIOCHEMISTRY

Aside from examples of similarities in the structures of some groups of these hormones, such as the insulin-related growth factors, these growth factors share several biochemical activities, to be described here together with some information about the nature of their receptors.

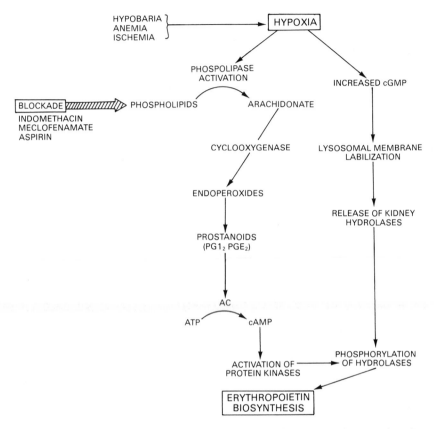

Figure 19-11. Schematic model for hypoxic stimulation of kidney production of erythropoietin. AC, Adenylate cyclase. Reproduced from J. W. Fisher, *Proc. Soc. Exp. Biol. Med.* **173,** 289–305 (1983).

A. Structures of Receptors of Growth Factors

The use of protein cross-linking agents has permitted the characterization of polypeptide hormone–receptor complexes. Using this methodology, it has been learned that the insulin receptor and the IGF-I receptor have four subunits ($\alpha_2\beta_2$) in the same general configuration as the immunoglobulins. Receptors for other growth factors so far studied, such as IGF-II, NGF, EGF, TGF, and PDGF, appear to have less complex structures and may consist of single polypeptide chains. Gross structures of these receptors are shown in Fig. 19-12. As reviewed in Fig. 7-24, the insulin receptor has been found to be a glycoprotein. The receptor for IGF-I has high affinity for IGF-I and low affinity for insulin, but it appears to be quite similar in structure to the insulin receptor. The

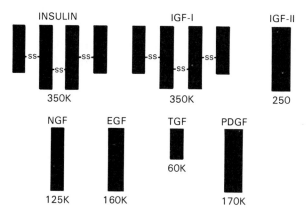

Figure 19-12. Minimum subunit structures for several growth factor receptors derived from affinity labeling data. Subunits other than indicated could be present which were not affinity labeled under conditions of experiments. Homobifunctional hydroxysuccinimide cross-linker, disuccinimidyl suberate, has been used to affinity label receptors for insulin, IGF-I, IGF-II, EGF, TGF, and PDGF. TGF receptor is more complex in structure than shown here. It may have two subunits and the 60K form shown here may be a cleavage fragment of a larger form (possibly a 560K receptor; communicated by M. Czech). This reagent was ineffective in affinity labeling the NGF receptor, but the heterobifunctional photoactive reagent hydroxysuccinimide azidobenzoate was used successfully. Reproduced from M. P. Czech, C. L. Oppenheimer, and J. Massague, *Fed. Proc., Fed. Am. Soc. Exp. Biol.* **42,** 2598–2601 (1983).

IGF-II receptor has high affinity for IGF-II and lower affinity for IGF-I, with little or no affinity for insulin. The IGF-II receptor does not appear to be linked to additional subunits through disulfide bonds. This is also the case for the receptors of the polypeptides: EGF, NGF, TGF, and PDGF, as shown in Fig. 19-12. It is not clear whether any structural homology exists between these receptors. However, some evidence indicates that there may be a form of communication between receptors. An example of this possibility is that one effect of the insulin receptor interaction in different cells isolated or in culture (adipocytes and H-35 hepatoma cells) is a marked stimulation in the affinity of IGF-II receptor for IGF-II. This may explain the growth-promoting effects of insulin, in whole or in part, in addition to the cellular metabolic effects generated directly by the insulin–receptor interaction.

B. Ligand–Receptor Interactions and Biochemical Effects

Some of the insulin-related growth factors as well as insulin itself, after complexing with receptor, generate two or three reactions: autophosphorylation and phosphorylation of unique proteins, both usually involving tyrosine residues; the formation of intracellular peptides (in the case of insulin), which may give rise to metabolic effects by regulating activities of phosphoprotein phosphatases, and internalization which can result in intracellular release of hormone (intact or degraded) and degraded receptor fragments. Generation of a second messenger of insulin action from the cell membrane is still controversial, and some view the second messenger as a cytoplasmic protein(s) which has become phosphorylated through the insulin action on its receptor.

Thus, the early events after growth factor binding to receptor may involve change in conformation of the receptor, autophosphorylation of tyrosine residues in the receptor, and tyrosine residue phosphorylation of other proteins which may appear in the cytoplasm. These activities are known variously for insulin and EGF as well as one or two others. It is likely that autophosphorylation of the receptor's protein kinase may lead to further phosphorylation of a specific polypeptide. Perhaps this factor would then play a more proximate role in events leading to mitosis (DNA replication).

1. Second Messengers of Insulin–Receptor Complex as a Possible Model for Actions of Some Growth Factors

After insulin binds to its cell membrane receptor, a protease in the membrane, either discrete or related to the receptor, may cleave out a fragment, perhaps from the cell membrane, which constitutes the second message of insulin action. This fragment would stimulate the activity of phosphoprotein phosphatase whose actions would result in the stimulation of cell membrane ion-transporting ATPase and inhibition of cell membrane adenylate cyclase and cyclic AMP phosphodiesterase of the smooth endoplasmic reticulum, while elevating activities of glycogen synthetase and of mitochondrial pyruvate dehydrogenase. These actions come about by removing phosphate groups from enzymes that are active in the dephosphorylated state and decreasing activities of enzymes that are inactive in the dephosphorylated state. The overall hypothetical mechanism restricted to glycogen synthetase and pyruvate dehydrogenase is shown in Fig. 19-13. This mechanism may serve as a model for testing other insulin-related growth factor polypeptides and the consequences of interactions with their respective receptors. It should be mentioned that this hypothesis of insulin control of metabolism does not have unanimous acceptance.

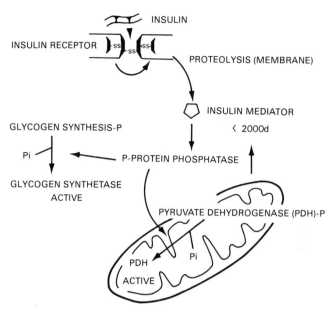

Figure 19-13. A speculative scheme to demonstrate the action of insulin through its membrane receptor in generating a cytoplasmic second messenger. Reproduced from G. Litwack, *in* "Altered Endocrine Status During Aging" (V. Cristofalo, G. T. Baker, III, R. C. Adelman, and J. Roberts, eds.), p. 5. Alan R. Liss, Inc., New York, 1984.

2. Internalization of Hormone–Receptor Complexes

Complexes of receptors for EGF, NGF, and insulin have been shown to concentrate at the membrane and undergo an internalization process involving invagination and pinching off in the cytoplasm forming a vesicle. The vesicle may fuse with lysosomes and, subsequent to enzymatic action, may lead to degradative actions, including breakdown of the hormone and receptor. There is some conjecture that the intact or partially proteolysed hormone may have further activities mediated by receptors on the perinuclear membrane. Some evidence for this concept is available in the case of insulin (see later). The internalized vesicle may also fuse with the Golgi apparatus and the fate of this fusion may be the recycling of receptors to the outer cell membrane. This renewal process is called "up regulation," while the loss of receptors from the cell surface as a result of the internalization reaction is termed "down regulation." The internalization process in the case of NGF is pictured in Fig. 19-14

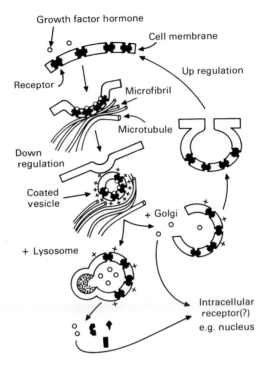

Figure 19-14. Diagrammatic scheme for the internalization of NGF. Reproduced from G. Litwack, *in* "Altered Endocrine Status During Aging" (V. Cristofalo, G. T. Baker, III, R. C. Adelman, and J. Roberts, eds.), p. 6. Alan R. Liss, Inc., New York, 1984. This drawing is based on one in G. L. Nicholson, *in* "Biological Regulation and Development" (R. F. Goldberger and K. R. Yamamoto, eds.), Vol. 3A, p. 243. Plenum, New York, 1982.

and the early postulated steps in the internalization process are summarized in Fig. 19-15.

3. Possible Role of Nuclear Receptors

A major problem is to understand the nature of the second messenger of mitogenic hormone–receptor interaction. As pointed out before, this internal signal could be generated at the cell membrane by a mechanism similar to that shown in Fig. 19-13, although this theory remains controversial. Presumably the signal generated in this way would act (via the nucleus?) to promote DNA synthesis and cell division. An alternative is that the intact internalized receptor or a receptor product is released in the cytoplasm and is able to somehow carry a message to the nucleus. Alternatively, it is possible that insulin itself could survive the inter-

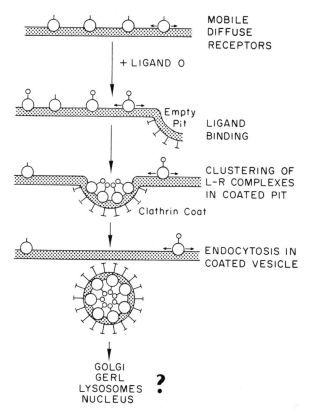

MOBILE
DIFFUSE
RECEPTORS

+ LIGAND O

Empty
Pit

LIGAND
BINDING

CLUSTERING OF
L–R COMPLEXES
IN COATED PIT

Clathrin Coat

ENDOCYTOSIS IN
COATED VESICLE

GOLGI
GERL
LYSOSOMES **?**
NUCLEUS

Figure 19-15. Model for receptor-mediated endocytosis. Reproduced from F. R. Maxfield, M. C. Willingham, J. Schlessinger, P. J. A. Davies, and I. Pastan, *Cold Spring Harbor Conf. Cell Proliferation* **6,** 165 (1979).

nalization process, enter the lumen of the endoplasmic reticulum, and gain access to the nuclear envelope. There it could bind to specific receptors on the perinuclear membrane. There is some evidence for this idea with respect to the mitogenic activity of insulin. A recent suggestion is that the perinuclear insulin–receptor complex leads to an enhanced rate of mRNA efflux from the nucleus to the cytoplasm by the hormonal stimulation of a phosphatase whose action would stimulate an NTPase coupled to the outward transport of mRNA (Fig. 19-16). This activity would be expected to stimulate the rate of translation of mRNAs and some of the translation products could be involved directly in the process of mitogenesis.

742

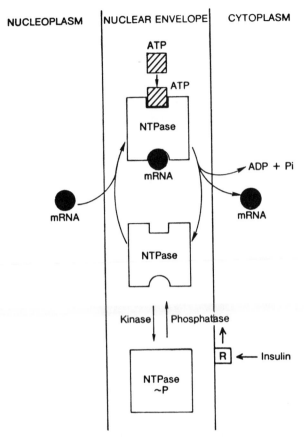

NUCLEOPLASM | NUCLEAR ENVELOPE | CYTOPLASM

Figure 19-16. Speculative proposal of insulin regulation of mRNA efflux from the nucleus mediated by nuclear insulin receptors. Reproduced from F. Purrello, D. B. Burnham, and I. D. Goldfine, *Proc. Natl. Acad. Sci. U.S.A.* **80**, 1189–1193 (1983).

4. Protein Kinase Activity of Membrane Receptors

Many growth receptors have been found to have protein kinase activity. In the case of the insulin receptor, for example, the β subunit is a tyrosine kinase which autophosphorylates the β subunit in an insulin-dependent fashion. In some cases receptor autophosphorylation results in enhanced receptor kinase activity. A hypothetical model of a sequence of phosphorylation reactions dependent on hormone binding is shown, for the insulin receptor, in Fig. 19-17. The end result is an activated kinase which could achieve a biological action through localized phosphorylations of specific membrane or cytoplasmic proteins.

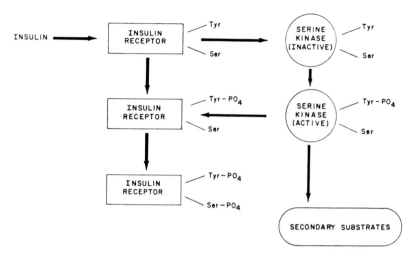

Figure 19-17. Proposed cascade of insulin receptor phosphorylation. Reproduced from C. R. Kahn, J. A. Hedo, and M. Kasuga, *in* "Biochemical Actions of Hormones" (G. Litwack, ed.), Vol. 11, p. 128. Academic Press, Orlando, Florida, 1984.

C. Growth Factors and Oncogenes

Oncogenes are genes that cause cancer and important breakthroughs in the cancer problem developed when oncogene products were shown to be major portions of growth factors or growth factor receptors. These "aberrant" phenotypes are produced and function in the transformed cell like their normal counterparts except that they may be "turned on" permanently, thus escaping normal regulation. For example, if the oncogene product is a receptor, it may lack the ligand binding site and, after deposition in the cell or cell membrane, may function continuously as an activated receptor without a requirement for availability of the growth factor hormone and its binding to the receptor's binding site. Normally, this interaction would render a conformation of the receptor complex in the active form, allowing the receptor to perform a function (e.g., phosphorylation); however, the oncogene product could be permanently in this form, thus escaping normal regulation, and the cell will have lost the normal growth control.

Known oncogenes and their products and functions are summarized in Table 19-3. The actions of oncogenes through their cellular products are summarized in Fig. 19-18.

Table 19-3. Known Oncogenes, Their Products and Functions[a]

Name of oncogene	Retrovirus	Tumor	Cellular location	Oncogenic protein		
				Function	Class	
src	Chicken sarcoma	—	Plasma membrane			
yes	Chicken sarcoma	—	Plasma membrane (?)			
fgr	Cat sarcoma	—	(?)	Tyrosine-specific pro-tein kinase	Class 1 (cytoplasmic tyrosine protein kinases)	
abl	Mouse leukemia	Human leukemia	Plasma membrane			
fps	Chicken sarcoma	—	Cytoplasm (plasma membrane?)			
fes	Cat sarcoma	—	Cytoplasm (cytoskeleton?) (?)			
ros	Chicken sarcoma	—				
erb-B	Chicken leukemia	—	Plasma and cytoplasmic membranes	EGF receptor's cytoplasmic tyrosine-specific protein-kinase do-main		
fms	Cat sarcoma	—	Plasma and cytoplasmic membranes	Cytoplasmic domain of a growth-factor receptor (?)	Class 1-related (poten-tial protein kinases)	
mil	Chicken carcinoma	—	Cytoplasm	(?)		
raf	Mouse sarcoma	—	Cytoplasm	(?)		
mos	Mouse sarcoma	Mouse leukemia	Cytoplasm	(?)		

744

	Source (viral oncogene)	Human and animal tumors	Secreted	PDGF-like growth factor	Class 2 (growth factors)
sis	Monkey sarcoma	—	Secreted	PDGF-like growth factor	Class 2 (growth factors)
Ha-ras	Rat sarcoma	Human carcinoma, rat carcinoma	Plasma membrane	GTP binding	Class 3 (cytoplasmic, GTP binding)
Ki-ras	Rat sarcoma	Human carcinoma, leukemia and sarcoma	Plasma membrane		
N-ras	—	Human leukemia and carcinoma	Plasma membrane		
fos	Mouse sarcoma	—	Nucleus	(?)	Class 4 (nuclear)
myc	Chicken leukemia	Human lymphoma	Nucleus	DNA binding	
myb	Chicken leukemia	Human leukemia	Nucleus	(?)	
B-lym		Chicken lymphoma, human lymphoma	Nucleus (?)	(?)	
ski	Chicken sarcoma	—	Nucleus (?)	(?)	Unclassified
rel	Turkey leukemia	—		(?)	
erb-A	Chicken leukemia	—		(?)	
ets	Chicken leukemia	—		(?)	

a The second column gives the source from which each viral oncogene was first isolated and the cancer induced by the oncogene. Some names, such as *fps* and *fes*, may be equivalent genes in birds and mammals. The third column lists human and animal tumors caused by agents other than viruses in which the *ras* oncogene or an inappropriately expressed protooncogene has been identified. Reproduced from T. Hunter, The proteins of oncogenes. *Sci. Am.* **251**, 70–79 (1984).

746

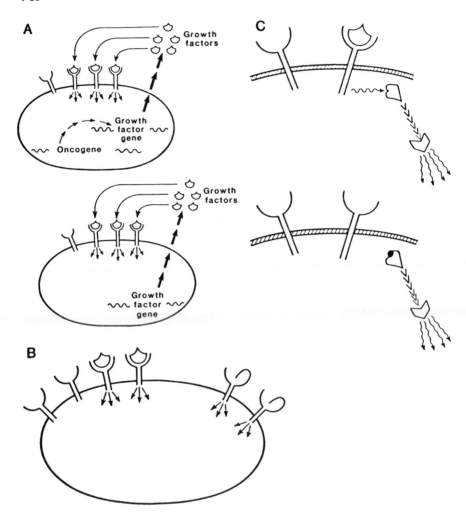

Figure 19-18. Three mechanisms by which oncogenes can allow a cell to escape dependence on exogenous growth factors: (A) By autocrine mechanism where the oncogene product is a growth factor active ligand and overstimulates its receptor; (B) by receptor alteration so that receptor is "permanently turned on" without a requirement for growth factor binding; and (C) by transducer alteration where the intermediate between the receptor and its resultant activity, i.e., the GTP stimulatory protein, is permanently turned on uncoupling the normal requirement of ligand-receptor binding. Reproduced from R. A. Weinberg, The action of oncogenes in the cytoplasm and nucleus. *Science* **230**, 770–776 (1985). Copyright 1985 by the AAAS.

V. CLINICAL ASPECTS

In most cases the functions of growth factors in the complex organism remain to be tested, but it is possible that various disease states will be linked to the underproduction of some of these substances.

References

A. Books

Pollack, R. (1975). "Readings in Mammalian Cell Culture," Rev. Ed. Cold Spring Harbor Lab., Cold Spring Harbor, New York.

Sato, G. H., and Ross, R. (1979). "Hormones and Cell Culture." Cold Spring Harbor Lab., Cold Spring Harbor, New York.

B. Review Articles

Antoniades, H. N., and Williams, L. T. (1983). Human platelet-derived growth factor: Structure and function. *Fed. Proc., Fed. Am. Soc. Exp. Biol.* **42**, 2630–2634.

Bradshaw, R. A. (1983). What cloned genes can tell us about nerve growth factor. *Nature (London)* **303**, 751.

Bradshaw, R. A. (1983). Nerve growth factor and related hormones. *In* "Biochemical Action of Hormones" (G. Litwack, ed.), Vol. 10, pp. 91–114. Academic Press, New York.

Bradshaw, R. A., and Niall, H. D. (1978). Insulin-related growth factors. *Trends Biochem. Sci.* **3**, 274–278.

Czech, M. P., Oppenheimer, C. L., and Massague, J. (1983). Interrelationships among receptor structures for insulin and peptide growth factors. *Fed. Proc., Fed. Am. Soc. Exp. Biol.* **42**, 2598–2601.

Fisher, J. W. (1983). Control of erythropoietin production. *Proc. Soc. Exp. Biol. Med.* **173**, 289–305.

Fox, C. F., Vale, R., Peterson, S. W., and Das. M. (1979). The EGF receptor: Identification and functional modulation. Hormones and cell culture. *Cold Spring Harbor Conf. Cell Proliferation* **6**, 143–157.

Froesch, E. R., Zapf, J., Rinderknecht, E., Morell, B., Schoenle, E., and Humbel, R. E. (1979). Insulin-like growth factor (IGF-NSILA), structure, function, and physiology. *Cold Spring Harbor Conf. Cell Proliferation* **6**, 61–77.

Goldfine, I. D. (1981). Effects of insulin on intracellular functions. *In* "Biochemical Actions of Hormones" (G. Litwack, ed.), Vol. 8, pp. 274–307. Academic Press, New York.

Hunter, T. (1984). The proteins of oncogenes. *Sci. Am.* **251**, 70–79.

James, R., and Bradshaw, R. A. (1984). Polypeptide growth factors. *Ann. Rev. Biochem.* **53**, 259–292.

Kahn, C. R., Hedo, J. A., and Kasuga, M. (1984). Antibodies to the insulin receptor: Studies of receptor structure and function. *In* "Biochemical Actions of Hormones" (G. Litwack, ed.), Vol. 11, pp. 128–162. Academic Press, Orlando, Florida.

Kano-Sueoka, T., Errick, J. E., and Cohen, D. W. (1979). Effects of hormones and a novel mammary growth factor on a rat mammary carcinoma in culture. *Cold Spring Harbor Conf. Cell Proliferation* **6**, 499–512.

Kingston, R. E., Baldwin, A. S., and Sharp, P. A. (1985). Transcription control by oncogenes. *Cell* **41**, 3–5.

Lemke, G. E., and Brockes, J. P. (1983). Glial growth factor: A mitogenic polypeptide of the brain and pituitary. *Fed. Proc., Fed. Am. Soc. Exp. Biol.* **42**, 2627–2629.

Marx, J. L. (1983). *onc* gene related to growth factor gene. *Science* **221**, 248.

Roberts, A. B., Frolik, C. A., Anzano, M. A., and Sporn, M. B. (1983). Transforming growth factors from neoplastic and nonneoplastic tissues. *Fed. Proc., Fed. Am. Soc. Exp. Biol.* **42**, 2621–2626.

Sirbasku, D. A., and Benson, R. H. (1979). Estrogen-inducible growth factors that may act as mediators (estromedins) of estrogen-promoted tumor cell growth. *Cold Spring Harbor Conf. Cell Proliferation* **6**, 477–498.

Underwood, L. E., and Van Wyk, J. J. (1981). Hormones in normal and aberrant growth. *In* "Textbook of Endocrinology" (R. H. Williams, ed.), 6th ed., pp. 1149–1191. Saunders, Philadelphia, Pennsylvania.

Weinberg, R. A. (1985). The action of oncogenes in the cytoplasm and nucleus. *Science* **230**, 770–776.

C. Research Papers

Aaronson, S. A., and Todaro, G. J. (1968). Basis for the acquisition of malignant potential by mouse cells cultivated *in vitro*. *Science* **162**, 245–247.

Blundell, T. L., Bedarkar, S., Rinderknecht, E., and Humbel, R. E. (1978). Insulin-like growth factor: A model for tertiary structure accounting for immunoreactivity and receptor binding. *Proc. Natl. Acad. Sci. U.S.A.* **75**, 180–184.

Cohen, S., Carpenter, G., and King, L., Jr. (1980). Epidermal growth factor–receptor–protein kinase interactions. *J. Biol. Chem.* **255**, 4834–4842.

Haigler, H., Ash, J. F., Singer, S. J., and Cohen, S. (1978). Visualization by fluorescence of the binding and internalization of epidermal growth factor in human carcinoma cells A-431. *Proc. Natl. Acad. Sci. U.S.A.* **75**, 3317–3321.

Klapper, D. G., Svoboda, M. E., and van Wyk, J. J. (1983). Sequence analysis of somatomedin C: Confirmation of identity with insulin-like growth factor I. *Endocrinology (Baltimore)* **112**, 2215–2217.

Lemmon, S. K., and Bradshaw, R. A. (1983). Purification and partial characterization of bovine pituitary fibroblast growth factor. *J. Cell. Biochem.* **21**, 195–208.

Maxfield, F. R., Davies, P. J. A., Klempner, L., Willingham, M. C., and Pastan, I. (1979). Epidermal growth factor stimulation of DNA synthesis is potentiated by compounds that inhibit its clustering in coated pits. *Proc. Natl. Acad. Sci. U.S.A.* **76**, 5731–5735.

Appendix A. Compilation of Known Hormones in Higher Mammals and Humans[a]

Trivial name and class abbreviation	Source	Action
Amino acid-derived hormones		
Adrenals		
Epinephrine (EP) (adren-aline)	Adrenal medulla (CNS)	Glycogenolysis in liver; increases blood pressure
Intestine		
Histamine	Gut, CNS, mast cells, many tissues	Gastric secretion; may affect CNS
Bursa of Fabricius (chickens)		
Bursin	Bursa of Fabricius	A tripeptide inducing differentiation of avian and mammalian B-precursor cells
Nervous system		
(Acetylcholine)	Neurons	Variety of activities in nervous system; innervates adrenal medulla
Dopamine (also believed to be PIF)	CNS	Inhibits PRL release (and other actions)
γ-Aminobutyric acid (GABA)	CNS	Neurotransmitter; inhibits release of CRF and PRL
Norepinephrine (NEP) (noradrenaline)	CNS neurons	Neurotransmitter; increases blood pressure
Serotonin	CNS neurons, gut	Affects smooth muscles + nerves; stimulates release of GH, TSH, ACTH (CRF), and inhibits LH release
Pineal gland		
Acetylserotonin		Affects GH release from anterior pituitary
Melatonin		Inhibits GH release from anterior pituitary; affects reproductive functions
Octopamine		Inhibition of monoamine oxidase
Thyroid/parathyroid gland		
Thyroxine (T_4) and tri-iodothyrone (T_3)	Thyroid gland	Increases oxidation rates in tissues
Autoimmune antibodies acting like unregulated hormones		
Autoimmune antiinsulin	Human	Produces diabetes-like syndrome
Long-acting thyroid stimulator (LATS)	Human	Stimulates thyroid-like TSH, but is not regulated by thyroid hormone

(continued)

Appendix A. (*Continued*)

Trivial name and class abbreviation	Source	Action
Fatty acid (arachidonic acid) -derived hormones		
Blood		
Prostacyclin (PGI$_2$)	Vascular endothelium, blood	Prevents aggregation of platelets
Thromboxane B$_2$ (TXB$_2$)	Platelets	Metabolite of TXA$_2$
Lung		
Leukotrienes (LT)		Long-acting bronchoconstrictor
Leukotriene A$_5$ (LTA$_5$)		Long-acting bronchoconstrictor
Leukotriene C (LTC)		Long-acting bronchoconstrictor
Leukotriene A$_4$ (LTC$_4$)		Long-acting bronchoconstrictor
Leukotriene C$_5$ (LTC$_5$)		Long-acting bronchoconstrictor
Leukotriene B (LTB)		Long-acting bronchoconstrictor
Thromboxane A$_2$ (TXA$_2$)	Platelets, lung, etc.	Causes platelet aggregation
Prostaglandins		
Prostaglandin E$_1$ + E$_2$ (PGE$_1$ or PGE$_2$)	Wide variety of cells	Stimulates cyclic AMP
Prostaglandin F$_{1\alpha}$ + F$_{2\alpha}$ (PGF$_{1\alpha}$ or PGF$_{2\alpha}$)	Wide variety of cells	Active in dissolution of corpus luteum; ovulation + parturition contractions
Prostaglandin A$_2$ (PGA$_2$)	Kidney	Hypotensive effect
Polypeptides		
Adrenals		
Met-enkephalin + Leu-enkephalin	Adrenal medulla and CNS cells	Analgesic actions in CNS; other unknown effects
Blood		
Angiotensin II	Blood, lungs, brain, many tissues	*Zona glomerulosa* cells of adrenal cortex to stimulate synthesis + release of aldosterone
Bradykinin	Plasma, gut, other tissues	Vasodilator; lowers blood pressure
Osteoclast-activating factor (OAF)	Human leukocytes	Stimulates bone resorption *in vitro*
Platelet growth factor	Platelets	Similar to FGF
Heart		
Atrial natriuretic factor (ANF; also known as	Atria	Blood pressure lowering; stimulates renal sodium

(*continued*)

Appendix A. (*Continued*)

Trivial name and class abbreviation	Source	Action
atriopeptin)		excretion; increases GFR and urine volume
Hypothalamus hormones		
Arg-vasotocin	Hypothalamus and pineal gland	Regulates reproductive glands
Corticotropic-releasing factor (CRF)	Hypothalamus	Releases ACTH + β-endorphin in anterior pituitary
Gonadotropic-releasing hormone (GRH)	Hypothalamus, distributed in CNS; milk; gonadal cells containing GRH receptors	Releases FSH and LH in anterior pituitary
Growth hormone release inhibiting hormone (somatostatin)	Hypothalamus, extrahypothalamic brain, spinal cord, pancreas, stomach, and intestine	Inhibits release of GH and TSH in anterior pituitary; regulates pancreatic hormones
Growth hormone releasing factor (GRF)		Releases GH in anterior pituitary
Melanotropin release inhibiting factor (MIF)		Prevents release of MSH in anterior pituitary; probably not in man
Melanotropin releasing factor (MRF)		Releases MSH in anterior pituitary; probably not in man
Neurotensin	Hypothalamus, intestine (mucosa)	May have neurotransmitter actions; in pharmacological amounts, has several effects on gut
Prolactin releasing factor (PRH or TRH)		Releases PRL in anterior pituitary
Substance P (SP)	Hypothalamus and CNS, intestine	Transmits pain and other functions; increases smooth muscle contractions of GI tract
Thyrotropic releasing hormone (TRH)	Hypothalamus, extrahypothalamic brain, spinal cord, and brain stem	Releases TSH and PRL in anterior pituitary
Intestine		
Bombesin	Nerves + endocrine cells of gut	Hypothermic hormone; increases gastrin + gastric

(*continued*)

Appendix A. (*Continued*)

Trivial name and class abbreviation	Source	Action
		acid secretion; many other actions
Cholecystokinin (CCK) (pancreozymin)		Stimulates gallbladder contraction + bile flow; enhances secretion of pancreatic enzymes
Enteroglucagon (different from pancreatic glucagon) (GLI, glucagon-like immunoreactivity)	Gut, L cells of ileum and colon, brain	May have some role in glucose homeostasis
Gastric inhibitory polypeptide (GIP)	Duodenum	Inhibits gastric acid secretion; stimulates insulin secretion when blood glucose level >25 mg/dl above fasting level
Glicentin		Glucagon-like activity
Gastrin	G cells in midpyloric glands, in stomach antrum	Increases secretion of gastric acid + pepsin + many other effects
Secretin	Duodenum when pH of its contents is less than 4.5	Stimulates pancreatic acinar cells to release bicarbonate + water which are transported to duodenum to elevate pH
Vasointestinal peptide (VIP)	GI tract, hypothalamus, + elsewhere	Neurotransmitters in peripheral autonomic nervous system; relaxes smooth muscles of circulation; increases secretion of water and electrolytes from pancreas and gut
Kidney Erythropoietin		Acts on bone marrow to induce terminal differentiation + initiation of hemoglobin synthesis
Liver Somatomedins (IGF and IGF_2 = insulin-like growth factors)	Liver, muscle, kidney, + other tissue	Cartilage sulfation; somatic cell growth, insulin-like effect
Lung Eosinophil chemotactic	Lung mast cells	After release, selective chemo-

(*continued*)

Appendix A. (*Continued*)

Trivial name and class abbreviation	Source	Action
factor of anaphylaxis		attractants for eosinophils
Other		
Colony-stimulating factor; macrophage growth factor	Kidney, lung, spleen, peritoneal exudates	Stimulates conversion of white blood cell precursors to granulocytes and mononuclear phagocytes
HLA antigen: somatomedin(s) (IGF and IGF$_2$ = insulin-like growth factors)	Liver, muscle, kidney, + other tissues	Cartilage sulfation; somatic cell growth; insulin-like effects
Ovaries		
Relaxin	Corpus luteum	Increases during gestation (may inhibit myometrial contractions)
Pancreas		
Glucagon	A cells	Glycogenolysis in liver; increases cyclic AMP
Insulin	B cells	Glucose utilization in liver; promotes synthesis of glycogen
Pancreatic polypeptide (PP)	Pancreatic islets (peripheral cells of)	Has a number of effects on gut in pharmacological amounts
Proinsulin	B cells	Precursor to insulin
Pituitary		
Adrenocorticotrophic hormone (ACTH)	Adenohypophysis	Stimulates synthesis and release of cortisol and dehydroepiandrosterone from adrenal cortex
Arg-vasopressin (AVP or ADH)	Posterior pituitary	Increases water reabsorption in kidney
β-Endorphin	*Pars intermedia* and CNS cells	Analgesic actions in CNS
Fibroblast growth factor (FGF)		Stimulates proliferation of cells derived from endoderm and mesoderm in presence of serum
Follicle-stimulating hormone (FSH)	Adenohypophysis	Stimulates development of ovarian follicle and secretion of estrogen; stimulates seminal tubules and spermatogenesis
Growth hormone	Adenohypophysis	Somatic cell growth medi-

(*continued*)

Appendix A. (*Continued*)

Trivial name and class abbreviation	Source	Action
(somatomammotropin or somatotropin) (GH)		ated by somatomedins, hyperglycemia, liver steroid metabolism, bone sulfation reactions
Lipotropin (LPH)	Adenohypophysis	Fat mobilization; source of opioid peptides
Luteinizing hormone (formerly "interstitial cell regulating hormone" in reference to male) (LH)	Adenohypophysis	Stimulates Leydig (interstitial) cell development in male + production of testosterone; stimulates corpus luteum and its production of progesterone in female
Melanocyte-stimulating hormone (MSH)	Adenohypophysis pars intermedia	CNS functions (e.g., in memory retention) and skin-darkening reaction
Motilin	Duodenum (jejunum), pineal, pituitary	Acts on GI tract to alter motility; stimulates contraction of fundus + antrum + decreases gastric emptying
Ovarian growth factor		Prolongs ovarian cell survival
Oxytocin	Posterior pituitary, hypothalamus	Lactating mammary gland, milk letdown; uterine contraction at parturition
Prolactin (PRL)	Adenohypophysis	Synthesis of milk constituents in mammary gland; stimulates testosterone production; secondary growth hormone effects in liver (e.g., as hyperglycemic agent); mammary gland secretory cell differentiation
Thyroid-stimulating hormone (TSH)	Adenohypophysis	Stimulates thyroid gland follicles to secrete thyroid hormone
Placenta		
Human chorionic gonadotropin (hCG)		LH-like functions, maintains progesterone productivity during pregnancy
Human placental lactogen (hPL)		Acts like PRL and like GH because of large amount of hPL produced

(*continued*)

Appendix A. (*Continued*)

Trivial name and class abbreviation	Source	Action
Salivary gland		
Epidermal growth factor (EGF), formerly urogastrone		Stimulates proliferation of cells of ectodermal and mesodermal origin with serum; inhibits gastric secretion
Skin		
Alytesian	Amphibian skin	Stimulates gastric acid secretion
Cerulein	Frog skin	Similar to CCK + gastrins
Litorin	Amphibian skin	Stimulates gastric secretion
Ranatensin	Amphibian skin	Stimulates gastric secretion
Submaxillary gland		
Nerve growth factor (NGF)		Differentiation and growth of embryonic dorsal root ganglia
Testes		
Antimullerian hormone	Fetal Sertoli cells of the testes	Mediates involution of the mullerian ducts
Inhibin	Seminiferous tubule (and ovary)	Negative feedback inhibitors of FSH secretion from anterior pituitary
Thymus		
Thymic humoral factor (THF)		Activates adenylate cyclase in thymus + spleen cells
Thymopoietin I and II, α-thymosin		Stimulates phagocytes; stimulates differentiation of precursors into immune competent T cells
Thyroid/parathyroid		
Calcitonin (CT)	Parafollicular C cells of thyroid gland	Lowers serum calcium
Parathyroid hormone (PTH)	Parathyroid glands	Stimulates bone resorption; stimulates phosphate excretion by the kidney
Steroid hormones		
Adrenals		
Aldosterone and 11-deoxycorticosterone (DOC)	*Zona glomerulosa* of adrenal cortex	Salt retention in kidney
Cortisol (hydrocortisone)	*Zona fasciculata* and *zona reticularis* of adrenal cortex	Antistress hormone; carbohydrate metabolism; circulating glucose increased; liver glycogen increased;

(*continued*)

Appendix A. (*Continued*)

Trivial name and class abbreviation	Source	Action
		depresses immune system; antiinflammatory agent
Dehydroepiandrosterone (DHEA)	*Zona reticularis* of adrenal cortex	Weak androgen; major secretion of fetal adrenal cortex; can be converted to estrogen; may have other unknown actions
Brain		
Catecholestrogens		Stimulates catecholamine receptors in CNS
Kidney		
1,25-Dihydroxyvitamin D_3 (1,25-dihydroxycholecalciferol)		Stimulates a Ca^{2+} binding protein in variety of tissues, especially in intestine, and causes stimulation of Ca^{2+} transport
24R,25-Dihydroxyvitamin D_3 (24R,25-dihydroxycholecalciferol)		Has receptor in chondrocytes (also parathyroid gland)
Ovaries		
17β-Estradiol and estriol	Ovarian follicle (corpus luteum)	Uterine endometrium development, female tissues
Progesterone	Corpus luteum, placenta (ovarian follicle)	Breast development; uterine endometrium development
Testes		
Dihydrotestosterone	Seminiferous tubule + other male tissues (e.g., prostate)	Conversion product of testosterone which binds to androgen receptor
Testosterone	Leydig cells (interstitial cells of testis) (adrenal)	Spermatogenesis/male characteristics
Second messenger substances		
Arachidonic acid	All cell membranes	Precursor of prostaglandins
Ca^{2+} (and calmodulin)	All cells	Required for secretory activity; enzyme regulator
Cyclic AMP	Many cells	Protein phosphorylation
Cyclic GMP	Many cells	
Diadenosinetetraphosphate	Many cells	Ligand of binder associated with DNA polymerase α
Insect hormones		
Ecdysone (steroid)		Stimulates molting
Juvenile hormone (JH) (hydrocarbon terpenoid)		Controls molting

(*continued*)

Appendix A. (*Continued*)

Trivial name and class abbreviation	Source	Action
Plant hormones		
Auxins (indoleacetic acid)	All higher plants and some lower plants	Stimulates extension growth and cell division in cambrium and foot
Giberellins (diterpenoid cells)	Widespread plant regulators	Stimulates extension growth
Kinins (N-substituted)		Promotes cell division

a This table tabulates all the known hormones of higher animals and man. At the first level it tabulates hormones by structure (amino acid-derived hormones, autoimmune antibodies acting like unregulated hormones, fatty acid-derived hormones, polypeptide hormones, steroid hormones, second messenger substances, insect hormones, and plant hormones). Each of these categories is then subdivided, where appropriate, by organ; finally, the individual hormones in a category are entered alphabetically.

Appendix B. Human Blood Concentrations of Major Hormones[a]

Hormone	Blood concentration
cAMP	15 ± 3 nM
cGMP	5.1 ± 7 nM
PGE	385 ± 30 pg/ml
PGF	141 ± 15 pg/ml
15-Keto-PGF$_{2\alpha}$	0.5 ng/ml
15-Keto-PGE$_2$	<50 pg/ml
TRH	7–30 pg/ml (rat)
GnRH	1–80 pg/ml
Somatostatin	
Melatonin (human)	14 ± 0.5 pg/ml (day)
	66 ± 5.3 pg/ml (night)
Neurotensin	40–60 fmol/ml rat
	20–40 fmol/ml rabbit sheep
Gonadotropins (human FSH)	
Children	5 mIU/ml
Men	10–15 mIU/ml
Women (midcycle)	20–30 mIU/ml
Rest of cycle	10–20 mIU/ml
Human LH	
Children	2–4 mIU/ml
Men	10–12 mIU/ml
Women (midcycle)	80 mIU/ml
Rest of cycle	10–30 mIU/ml
Prolactin	Up to 25 ng/ml serum
Growth hormone	Less than 5 mg/ml
ACTH	6 a.m.; <120 pg/ml; mean: 55 pg/ml; 6 p.m.: <75 pg/ml; mean: 35 pg/ml
α-MSH	Not detectable
TSH	<0.5–10 μU/ml
Oxytocin	
Men	2 pg/ml
Women (nonlactating)	2 pg/ml
Pregnant women	40 ± 8 (33–40 weeks)
Vasopressin	
Hydrated	0.45 pg/ml
Dehydrated	3.7 pg/ml
Calcitonin	<100 pg/ml
T3 and T4	
T3 (mean)	138 ng/100 ml
T4 (mean)	7.4 μg/100 ml
rT3	450 ± 200 pg/ml
PTH	200–400 pg/ml
Erythropoietin	4.9 ± 0.2 mU/ml (male)
	4.3 ± 0.2 mU/ml (female)

(*continued*)

Appendix B. (*Continued*)

Hormone	Blood concentration
Vitamin D metabolites	
25-OHD	4–55 ng/ml
1,25(OH)$_2$D	33 ± 6 pg/ml
24,25(OH)$_2$D	1–5 ng/ml
Gastrin	<120 pg/ml; mean, 70 pg/mml
Secretin	37 ± 8 pg/ml
CCK-PZ	60.4 pg/ml; 25% <5 pg/ml
Serotonin	168 ± 13 ng/ml whole blood, 341 ng/10^9 platelets
GIP	<125–400 pg/ml
VIP	4.5 ± 2 pmol/liter
Insulin	Fasting: 1–25 μU/ml; mean, 8.44 ± 0.35 μU/ml
Proinsulin	Fasting: 0.05–0.5 ng/ml; mean, 0.156 ± 0.014 ng/ml
C peptide	Fasting: 0.5–2.0 ng/ml
Glucagon	50–150 pg/ml; mean, 75 ± 4 pg/ml
Pancreatic polypeptide	50–200 pg/ml (human)
	100–200 pg/ml (dog)
Estrogens	
Estradiol	
Menstrual cycle (days)	
1–10	50 pg/ml
10–12	100–150 pg/ml
12–14	350–600 pg/ml
14–28	200–400 pg/ml
Estriol	
Weeks of pregnancy	
22–30	3–5 ng/ml
32–37	6–11 ng/ml
38–41	25–17 ng/ml
Estrone	
Weeks of pregnancy	
22–30	3–5 ng/ml
32–37	5–6 ng/ml
38–41	7–10 ng/ml
Progesterone	
Menstrual	
Follicular	0.4–0.6 ng/ml
Midluteal	7.7–12.1 ng/ml
Pregnancy (weeks)	
16–18	48.4 ± 18 ng/ml
28–30	98 ± 28 ng/ml
38–40	178.5 ± 48 ng/ml
Androgens	
Testosterone	
Males	4.0–12.0 ng/ml
Females	0.3–1.0 ng/ml

(*continued*)

Appendix B. (*Continued*)

Hormone	Blood concentration
Dihydrotestosterone (DHT)	
Males	3.0–8.0 ng/ml
Females	0.1–1.0 ng/ml
Mineralocorticoids	
Aldosterone	60 ng/100 ml
Deoxycorticosterone (DOC)	5 ng/100 ml, *ad lib* diet
18-OHDOC	5 ng/100 ml, *ad lib* diet; 90 ng/100 ml, 10 meq Na diet
Glucocorticoids	
Cortisol	5–20 μg/100
Corticosterone	0.4–2 μg/100 ml
Compound S	0.1–0.3 μg/100 ml
HCG	Human pregnancy
	Primary peak (first trimester), 163,000 mIU/ml
	Nadir (second trimester), 12,000 mIU/ml
	Secondary peak (third trimester), 63,000 mIU/ml
Prolactin (PL)	4.9 μg/ml (human), 10.15 μg/ml (monkey), 0.5–1.6 μg/ml (ovine)
Relaxin	Before day 100 gestation (pig), <2 ng/ml
	Day 100 until 2 days preceding parturition, 5–40 ng/ml
	Day preceding parturition, 100–200 ng/ml
	Day following parturition, <2 ng/ml
Bradykinin	70 pg/ml
Renin (angiotensin II)	11.2 ± 3.4 pg/ml
EGF	Up to 10 pg/ml (mouse)
NGF	6–10 ng NGF immunoreactivity/ml
NSILA-s	350 ± 66 mU/liter
Somatomedin A	1.00 ± 0.23 U/ml
Somatomedin C	1.49 ± 0.25 U/ml

[a] Abstracted principally from B. M. Jaffe and H. R. Behrman, eds., "Methods of Hormone Radioimmunoassay," 2nd ed. Academic Press, New York, 1979.

Appendix C. Clinically Relevant Endocrine Disorders[a]

Disease	Description
Acromegaly	Inappropriate and continued secretion of growth hormone by a tumor of pituitary cells which leads usually in the third or fourth decade to soft tissue swelling and hypertrophy of the skeletal extremities
Addison's disease	Adrenocorticol insufficiency resulting from a deficient production of glucocorticoids and/or mineralocorticoids due to a destruction of the adrenal cortex
Bartter's syndrome	Characterized by increased angiotensin II, renin, aldosterone, secretion, hypokalemia, and alkalosis, and hyperplasia of the renal juxtaglomerular cells, but with normal blood pressure; the disease, which is possibly an autosomal-dominant disorder, usually appears in late infancy or early childhood; the primary defect may be a lesion in chloride reabsorption in the kidney loop of Henle
Celiac disease	An intestinal malabsorption disorder occurring in some individuals who may lack an enzyme necessary for the hydrolysis of N-glutamyl peptides in the small intestine; as a consequence, the affected individual is intolerant of some proteins—usually those derived from wheat, oats, barley, or rye; the disease is also referred to as gluten-sensitive enteropathy
Chiari–Frommel syndrome	The occurrence of galactorrhea (non-nursing-related lactation) and amenorrhea (absence of expected menstrual periods) during the postpartum period; the disease may be due to the presence of a prolactin-secreting tumor
Cretinism	Characterized by a permanent neurological and skeletal retardation and results from an inadequate output of thyroid hormone during uterine and neonatal life; may be caused by iodine deficiency, thyroid hypoplasia, genetic enzyme defects, or excessive maternal intake of goitrogens
Cushing's disease	Hypercortisolism resulting from the presence of small pituitary tumors which secrete ACTH leading to excess production of cortisol by the adrenals
Cushing's syndrome	The circumstance of glucocorticoid excess without specification of the specific etiology; it may result from endogenous causes but is more commonly iatrogenic

(*continued*)

Appendix C. (*Continued*)

Disease	Description
Diabetes insipidus	A deficient secretion of vasopressin which is manifested clinically as diabetes insipidus; it is a disorder characterized by the excretion of an increased volume of dilute urine
Diabetes mellitus	A disease characterized by a chronic disorder of intermediary metabolism due to a relative lack of insulin which is characterized by hyperglycemia in both the postprandial and fasting state (see also Types I and II diabetes mellitus)
Diabetes mellitus (insulin dependent or Type I diabetes)	The form of diabetes which appears in the second and third decade of life and is characterized by a destruction of the pancreas B cells; this form of the disease is normally treated with daily administration of insulin
Diabetes mellitus (insulin independent or Type II diabetes)	The form of diabetes arising after the fourth decade, usually in obese individuals; this form of the disease does not normally require treatment with insulin
Empty sella syndrome	Empty sella is a term that describes sellae that fill with air during pneumoencephalography; it is frequently associated with the flattening of the pituitary gland; the etiology of the disease is unknown; the pituitary function is usually normal
Fanconi syndrome	A renal tubular defect in the absorption of a variety of substances including H_2O, phosphate, sodium, bicarbonate, and amino acids; frequently an osteomalacic bone disease and a distal tubular acidosis may accompany the disease
Feminization	Feminization of males, usually as manifested by enlargement of the breasts (gynecomastia) which can be attributed to an increase in estrogen levels relative to the prevailing androgen levels
Froehlich's syndrome	A condition usually caused by craniopharyngioma (a tumor of the hypothalamus) which results in a combination of obesity and hypogonadism; sometimes termed adiposogenital dystrophy
Galactorrhea	The persistent discharge from the breast of a fluid that resembles milk and that occurs in the absence of parturition or else persists postpartum (4–6 months) after the cessation of nursing
Gigantism	This condition appears in the first year of life and is characterized by a rapid weight and height gain; affected children usually have a large head and mental retardation; to date no specific endocrine

(*continued*)

Appendix C. (*Continued*)

Disease	Description
	abnormalities have been detected
Goiter	Goiter may be defined as a thyroid gland that is twice its normal size; endemic goiter is the major thyroid disease throughout the world; goiter is frequently associated with a dietary iodine deficiency; in instances of sporadic goiter it may occur as a consequence of a congenital defect in thyroid hormone synthesis
Gynecomastia	Abnormal breast enlargement which may occur in males during puberty
Hartnup's disease	An intestinal transport disorder; the condition may be diagnosed by the massive urinary excretion of monoamino-monocarboxylic amino acids; frequently there are pellagra-like rashes after exposure to sunlight as well as attacks of cerebellar ataxia
Hermaphroditism	True hermaphroditism is defined as the presence of both testicullar and ovarian tissue in the same individual; pseudohermaphroditism is a discrepancy between gonadal and somatic sex
Hirsutism	An increase in facial hair in women which is beyond that cosmetically acceptable; this condition may be associated with a number of masculinizing disorders including Cushing's syndrome, congenital adrenal hyperplasia, and polycystic ovary syndrome
Hyperaldosteronism	An inappropriate secretion of aldosterone; it can occur as a primary adrenal problem (e.g., adrenal tumor) or can be secondary to other metabolic derangements that stimulate its release; it is often characterized by inappropriately high levels of plasma renin
Hyperparathyroidism	Inappropriately high secretion of PTH leading to hypercalcemia; frequently associated with the hyperparathyroidism is a metabolic bone disease characterized by excessive bone calcium reabsorption; frequently attributable to an adenoma of the parathyroid gland
Hypoparathyroidism	Inappropriately low secretion of PTH leading to hypocalcemia; the disease is either idiopathic or iatrogenically induced
Hypophosphatasia	An autosomal recessive trait characterized by elevated serum and urine inorganic pyrophosphate, a low serum alkaline phosphatase, and frequently

(*continued*)

Appendix C. (*Continued*)

Disease	Description
	hypercalcemia; may be related to a dysfunction of the osteoblasts
Klinefelter's syndrome	Typically characterized by male hypogonadism; the presence of extra X chromosomes is likely the fundamental underlying etiological factor; it is characterized by varying degrees of decreased Leydig cell function and seminiferous tubule failure
Milk–alkali syndrome	Affected subjects have hypercalcemia, nephrocalcinosis, soft tissue calcification, renal impairment, alkalosis, and hyperphosphatemia; the syndrome can result as a consequence of an excessive dietary intake of milk and other absorbable alkali (e.g., Na_2CO_3 or $NaHCO_3$); it is uncommon today
Myxedema	Hypothyroidism clinically manifested by the presence of a mucinous edema; the disease may appear at any time throughout life and is attributable to disorders of the thyroid gland or to pituitary insufficiency
Nelson's syndrome	A pituitary adenoma occurring in 10% of patients with Cushing's disease; afflicted subjects have a severe skin pigmentation
Osteomalacia	A bone disease in adults characterized by a failure of the skeletal osteoid to calcify; it is usually caused by an absence of adequate access to vitamin D
Pseudohypoparathyroidism	A familial disorder characterized by hypocalcemia, increased circulating levels of PTH, and a peripheral unresponsiveness to the hormone; afflicted individuals frequently are of short stature, with mental retardation and short metacarpals and/or metatarsals
Rickets	A failure in the child of the skeletal osteoid to calcify; it is usually caused by an absence of adequate amounts of vitamin D; it is characterized by a bowing of the femur, tibia, and fibias
Turner's syndrome	A condition present in females with a 45, XO chromosome pattern (i.e., complete absence of the X chromosome); the XO individual is typically short with a thick neck and trunk and no obvious secondary sex characteristics
Waterhouse–Friedericksen syndrome	Acute adrenal insufficiency resulting from severe systemic infection by meningococcus characterized by a high fever, meningeal irritation, and vascular collapse

(*continued*)

Appendix C. (*Continued*)

Disease	Description
Werner's syndrome	Multiple endocrine neoplasia, type I, caused by an autosomal recessive inheritance; it is often characterized by a severe testicular atrophy and a mild insulin-resistant diabetes
Zollinger–Ellison syndrome	Tumors of the pancreas which result in excessive secretion of gastrin; the afflicted subject has recurrent duodenal ulcers and diarrhea caused by hypersecretion of gastric acid

[a] This list was abstracted from the United States National Library of Medicine—Medical Subject Headings—Tree Structures—1983. Nat. Tech. Inf. Serv., pp. 115–120. U.S. Department of Commerce, Washington, D.C., 1982. The diseases were included in the National Library of Medicine table on the basis of frequency of publication of papers about the given disease topics.

Appendix D. Incidences of Principal Disease Diagnoses (Number and Percentage Distribution by Principal Medical Diagnosis of Visits to Physician's Office in the United States)[a]

Principal diagnosis (for 1977)	Number of office visits (in thousands)	Percentage distribution
Infective and parasitic diseases	22,668	4.0
Neoplasms	14,286	2.5
Endocrine, nutritional, and metabolic diseases	24,287	4.3
Mental disorders	24,522	4.3
Diseases of the nervous system and sense organs	48,291	8.5
Diseases of the circulatory system	54,702	9.6
Diseases of the respiratory system	82,466	14.5
Diseases of the digestive system	18,451	3.2
Diseases of the genitourinary system	36,473	6.4
Diseases of the skin and subcutaneous tissue	31,910	5.6
Diseases of the musculoskeletal system	32,983	5.8
Symptoms and ill-defined conditions	25,695	4.5
Accidents, poisonings, and violence	43,761	7.7
Special conditions and examinations without sickness	96,009	16.8
All other diagnoses	13,550	2.4
All diagnoses:	570,052	100.0

[a] Abstracted from Table 5 of "Standard Medical Almanac," 2nd ed., p. 422. Marquis Academic Media, Chicago, Illinois, 1979.

Appendix E. Summary of Nobel Prizes in Endocrinology and Related Fields[a]

Year	Field[b]	Awardee(s)	Achievement
1909	P/M	Emil Kocher	Physiology, pathology, and surgery of thyroid gland
1923	P/M	Sir F. G. Banting, J. J. R. Macleod	Discovery of insulin
1927	Chemistry	Heinrich Wieland	Research into the constitution of bile acids
1928	Chemistry	Adolf Windaus	Constitution of sterols and their connection with vitamins
1929	P/M	Christiaan Eijkman	Discovery of antineuritic vitamin
1929	P/M	Sir F. Hopkins	Discovery of growth-stimulating vitamins
1939	Chemistry	Adolf Butenandt	Work on sexual hormones
1943	P/M	Henrik Dam	Discovery of vitamin K
1943	P/M	Edward A. Doisy	Discovery of chemical nature of vitamin K
1947	P/M	Carl F. Cori, Gerty T. Cori	Discovery of how glycogen is catalytically converted
1947	P/M	Bernardo Houssay	Pituitary hormone function in sugar metabolism
1950	P/M	Philip S. Hench, Edward C. Kendall, Tadeusz Reichstein	Research on adrenal cortex hormones, their structure and biological effects
1955	Chemistry	Vincent Du Vigneaud	First synthesis of a polypeptide hormone
1958	Chemistry	Frederick Sanger	Determination of the structure of the insulin molecule
1958	P/M	George W. Beadle, Edward L. Tatum	Genetic regulation of chemical processes
1958	P/M	Joshua Lederberg	Genetic recombination
1962	P/M	Francis H. C. Crick, James D. Watson, Maurice Wilkins	Discoveries concerning the molecular structure of deoxyribonucleic acid
1964	P/M	Dorothy Crowfoot-Hodgkin	Determination of three-dimensional structure of insulin
1965	Chemistry	Robert B. Woodward	Synthesis of sterols, chlorophyll, and other complex natural products
1966	P/M	Charles B. Huggins, Frances P. Rous	Research on causes and treatment of cancer
1968	P/M	Robert W. Holley, H.	Deciphering of the genetic

(*continued*)

Appendix E. (*Continued*)

Year	Field[b]	Awardee(s)	Achievement
		Gobind Khorana, Marshall W. Nirenberg	code
1971	P/M	Earl W. Sutherland, Jr.	Action of hormones
1975	Chemistry	J. W. Cornforth, Vladimir Prelog	Work in stereochemistry related to steroids
1977	P/M	Rosalyn S. Yalow, Roger Guillemin, Andrew Schally	Development of radioimmunoassay; research on pituitary hormones
1980	Chemistry	Paul Berg, Walter Gilbert, Frederick Sanger	Sequencing of nucleic acids
1984	Chemistry	R. Bruce Merrifield	Solid-phase synthesis of peptides/proteins
1984	P/M	Cesar Milstein, Georges Kohler, Niels Jerne	Development of hybridoma techniques for production of monoclonal antibodies
1985	P/M	Michael S. Brown, Joseph L. Goldstein	Description of cell surface receptor-mediated endocytosis for low-density lipoprotein (LDL)
1986	P/M	Rita Levi-Montecini, Stanley Cohen	Nerve growth factor (NGF) and epidermal growth factor (EGF)

[a] Abstracted from "Encyclopaedia Britannica," Micropaedia VII, pp. 369–372. (1980). Encyclopaedic Britannica, Inc., Chicago, Illinois.

[b] P/M, Physiology or medicine.

Appendix F. The Genetic Code*a*

First position (5' end)	Second position				Third position (3' end)
	U	C	A	G	
U	Phe	Ser	Tyr	Cys	U
	Phe	Ser	Tyr	Cys	C
	Leu	Ser	C.T.	C.T.	A
	Leu	Ser	C.T.	Trp	G
C	Leu	Pro	His	Arg	U
	Leu	Pro	His	Arg	C
	Leu	Pro	Gln	Arg	A
	Leu	Pro	Gln	Arg	G
A	Ile	Thr	Asn	Ser	U
	Ile	Thr	Asn	Ser	C
	Ile	Thr	Lys	Arg	A
	Met	Thr	Lys	Arg	G
G	Val	Ala	Asp	Gly	U
	Val	Ala	Asp	Gly	C
	Val	Ala	Glu	Gly	A
	Val	Ala	Glu	Gly	G

a The code is expressed in terms of triplet sequences as they would appear in a natural messenger RNA molecule. The sequence of each codon is read from left to right, starting with the 5' end and going toward the 3' end. The codons UAA, UAG, and UGA result in chain termination (CT) and are used to indicate the end of a polypeptide chain. No separate code is required to start the polypeptide chain, since the first amino acid is always methionine (Met).

Appendix G. Amino Acid Abbreviations

Amino acid	Three letter	Single letter
Alanine	Ala	A
Arginine	Arg	R
Asparagine	Asn	N
Aspartic acid	Asp	D
Cysteine	Cys	C
Glutamic acid	Glu	E
Glutamine	Gln	Q
Glycine	Gly	G
Histidine	His	H
Isoleucine	Ile	I
Leucine	Leu	L
Lysine	Lys	K
Methionine	Met	M
Phenylalanine	Phe	F
Proline	Pro	P
Serine	Ser	S
Threonine	Thr	T
Tryptophan	Trp	W
Tyrosine	Tyr	Y
Valine	Val	V

Appendix H. Units of Measurement in Biological Systems

The Systemé International d'Unités (SI units), which is now generally accepted as the universal scientific system of measure, is based on the meter and kilogram (m kgs) rather than the centimeter and gram of the older cgs system. It has seven basic units of measurements:

Quantity	SI unit	Symbol
Amount of substance	mole	mol
Mass	kilogram	kg
Time	second	s
Length	meter	m
Electric current	ampere	A
Thermodynamic temperature	kelvin	K
Light intensity	candela	cd

Several important units employed in biological systems which are derived from SI units include the following:

Quantity to be measured	Definition in terms of basic units	SI unit	Symbol
Volume	10^{-3} m^3	liter	L
Frequency	s^{-1}	hertz	Hz
Pressure	kg m^{-1} s^{-2}	pascal	Pa
Energy[a]	kg m^2 s^{-1}	joule	J

[a] One calorie is the energy required to heat 1 cm^3 of water from 14.5 to 15.5°C. One Calorie, which is equivalent to 1000 calories or 1.0 kilocalorie, is the standard unit employed nutritionally. To convert calories into joules, multiply by the conversion factor of 4.185.

For a complete description of SI units see the IUPAC Manual of Symbols and Terminology for Physicochemical Quantities and Units (1970). *Pure Appl. Chem.* **21,** 3–44.

Other units employed in biological systems include the following:

Unit	Abbreviation	Comment
Mole	mol	
Becquerel	Bq	Units of radioactivity[a]
Curie	Ci	
Calorie	cal	
Kilocalorie	kcal or Cal	
Svedburg	S	(1 S = 10^{-13} sec)

[a] 1 becquerel = 1 dps or 60 dpm, while 1 Ci = 3.7 × 10^{10} Bq.

(*continued*)

Appendix H. (*Continued*)

The following prefixes and symbols are used to indicate multiples or decimal fractions of the SI units.

Prefix	Factor	Symbol
exa	10^{18}	E
peta	10^{15}	P
tera	10^{12}	T
giga	10^{9}	G
mega	10^{6}	M
kilo	10^{3}	k
hecto	10^{2}	h
deca	10^{1}	da
deci	10^{-1}	d
centi	10^{-2}	c
milli	10^{-3}	m
micro	10^{-6}	μ
nano	10^{-9}	n
pico	10^{-12}	p
femto	10^{-15}	f
atto	10^{-18}	a

Index